The GALE ENCYCLOPEDIA of SURGERY AND MEDICAL TESTS

SECOND EDITION

The GALE
ENCYCLOPEDIA *of*
SURGERY AND
MEDICAL TESTS

SECOND EDITION

VOLUME

1

A–C

BRIGHAM NARINS, EDITOR

GALE
CENGAGE Learning·

Detroit • New York • San Francisco • New Haven, Conn • Waterville, Maine • London

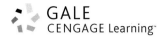
GALE
CENGAGE Learning

Gale Encyclopedia of Surgery and Medical Tests, Second Edition

Project Editor: Brigham Narins

Editorial: Donna Batten, Amy Kwolek, Jeffrey Wilson

Product Manager: Kate Hanley

Editorial Support Services: Andrea Lopeman

Indexing Services: Katherine Jensen, Indexes, etc.

Rights Acquisition and Management: Margaret Chamberlain-Gaston, Kelly A. Quin, and Robyn V. Young

Composition: Evi Abou-El-Seoud

Manufacturing: Wendy Blurton

Imaging: Lezlie Light

Product Design: Pam Galbreath

For product information and technology assistance, contact us at
Gale Customer Support, 1-800-877-4253.
For permission to use material from this text or product,
submit all requests online at **www.cengage.com/permissions.**
Further permissions questions can be emailed to
permissionrequest@cengage.com

While every effort has been made to ensure the reliability of the information presented in this publication, Gale, a part of Cengage Learning, does not guarantee the accuracy of the data contained herein. Gale accepts no payment for listing; and inclusion in the publication of any organization, agency, institution, publication, service, or individual does not imply endorsement of the editors or publisher. Errors brought to the attention of the publisher and verified to the satisfaction of the publisher will be corrected in future editions.

Library of Congress Cataloging-in-Publication Data

The Gale encyclopedia of surgery and medical tests : a guide for patients and caregivers / Brigham Narins, editor. -- 2nd ed.
    p. cm.
    Includes bibliographical references and index.
    ISBN-13: 978-1-4144-4884-8 (set : alk. paper)
    ISBN-13: 978-1-4144-4885-5 (vol. 1 : alk. paper)
    ISBN-13: 978-1-4144-4886-2 (vol. 2 : alk. paper)
    ISBN-13: 978-1-4144-4887-9 (vol. 3 : alk. paper)
    [etc.]
    1. Surgery--Encyclopedias. 2. Diagnosis--Encyclopedias. I. Narins, Brigham, 1962-.

RD17.G342 2008
617.003--dc22   2008020207

Gale
27500 Drake Rd.
Farmington Hills, MI, 48331-3535

ISBN-13: 978-1-4144-4884-8 (set)   ISBN-10: 1-4144-4884-8 (set)
ISBN-13: 978-1-4144-4885-5 (vol. 1)   ISBN-10: 1-4144-4885-6 (vol. 1)
ISBN-13: 978-1-4144-4886-2 (vol. 2   ISBN-10: 1-4144-4886-4 (vol. 2)
ISBN-13: 978-1-4144-4887-9 (vol. 3)   ISBN-10: 1-4144-4887-2 (vol. 3)
ISBN-13: 978-1-4144-4888-6 (vol. 4)   ISBN-10: 1-4144-4888-0 (vol. 4)

This title is also available as an e-book.
ISBN-13: 978-1-4144-4889-3 ISBN-10: 1-4144-4889-9
Contact your Gale, Cengage Learning sales representative for ordering information.

Printed in China
1 2 3 4 5 6 7 12 11 10 09 08

CONTENTS

LIST OF ENTRIES

H

Hair transplantation
Hammer, claw, and mallet toe surgery
Hand surgery
Health care proxy
Health history
Health Maintenance Organization (HMO)
Heart surgery for congenital defects
Heart transplantation
Heart-lung machines
Heart-lung transplantation
Heller myotomy
Hemangioma excision
Hematocrit
Hemispherectomy
Hemoglobin test
Hemoperfusion
Hemorrhoidectomy
Hepatectomy
Hiatal hernia
HIDA Scan
Hip osteotomy
Hip replacement
Hip revision surgery
Home care
Hospice
Hospital services
Hospital-acquired infections
Human leukocyte antigen test
Hydrocelectomy
Hypophysectomy
Hypospadias repair
Hysterectomy
Hysteroscopy

I

Ileal conduit surgery
Ileoanal anastomosis
Ileoanal reservoir surgery
Ileostomy
Immunoassay tests

Immunologic therapies
Immunosuppressant drugs
Implantable cardioverter-defibrillator
In vitro fertilization
Incision care
Incisional hernia repair
Informed consent
Inguinal hernia repair
Intensive care unit
Intensive care unit equipment
Intestinal obstruction repair
Intra-Operative Parathyroid Hormone Measurement
Intravenous rehydration
Intussusception reduction
Iridectomy
Islet cell transplantation

K

Kidney dialysis
Kidney function tests
Kidney transplantation
Knee arthroscopic surgery
Knee osteotomy
Knee replacement
Knee revision surgery
Kneecap removal

L

Laceration repair
Laminectomy
Laparoscopy
Laparoscopy for endometriosis
Laparotomy, exploratory
Laryngectomy
Laser in-situ keratomileusis (LASIK)
Laser iridotomy
Laser posterior capsulotomy
Laser skin resurfacing
Laser surgery
Laxatives

LDL cholesterol test
Leg lengthening or shortening
Length of hospital stay
Limb salvage
Lipid profile
Lipid tests
Liposuction
Lithotripsy
Liver biopsy
Liver function tests
Liver transplantation
Living will
Lobectomy, pulmonary
Long-term care insurance
Lumpectomy
Lung biopsy
Lung transplantation
Lymphadenectomy

M

Magnetic resonance angiogram
Magnetic resonance imaging
Magnetic resonance venogram
Mammography
Managed care plans
Mantoux test
Mastectomy
Mastoidectomy
Maze procedure for atrial fibrillation
Mechanical circulation support
Mechanical ventilation
Meckel's diverticulectomy
Mediastinoscopy
Medicaid
Medical charts
Medical co-morbidities
Medical errors
Medicare
Medication Monitoring
Meningocele repair
Mental health assessment
Mentoplasty
Microsurgery

LIST OF ENTRIES BY BODY SYSTEM

Cardiovascular

Angiography
Angioplasty
Aortic aneurysm repair
Aortic valve replacement
Arteriovenous fistula
Balloon valvuloplasty
Cardiac catheterization
Cardiac event monitor
Cardiac marker tests
Cardiac monitor
Cardiopulmonary resuscitation
Cardioversion
Carotid endarterectomy
Coronary artery bypass graft
  surgery
Coronary stenting
Defibrillation
Echocardiography
Electrocardiogram
Electrocardiography
Electrophysiology study of the
  heart
Endovascular stent surgery
Femoral hernia repair
Heart surgery for congenital
  defects
Heart transplantation
Heart-lung machines
Heart-lung transplantation
Hemangioma excision
Implantable cardioverter-
  defibrillator
Magnetic resonance angiogram

Magnetic resonance venogram
Maze procedure for atrial
  fibrillation
Mechanical circulation support
Minimally invasive heart surgery
Mitral valve repair
Mitral valve replacement
Multiple-gated acquisition
  (MUGA) scan
Myocardial resection
Pacemakers
Pericardiocentesis
Peripheral endarterectomy
Peripheral vascular bypass
  surgery
Portal vein bypass
Sclerotherapy for varicose veins
Stress test
Vascular surgery
Vein ligation and stripping
Venous thrombosis prevention
Ventricular assist device
Ventricular shunt

Endocrine

Adenoidectomy
Adrenalectomy
Endoscopic retrograde
  cholangiopancreatography
Hypophysectomy
Intra-Operative Parathyroid
  Hormone Measurement
Islet cell transplantation
Oral glucose tolerance test

Pancreas transplantation
Pancreatectomy
Parathyroidectomy
Sestamibi scan
Thyroidectomy
Whipple procedure

Gastrointestinal

Antrectomy
Appendectomy
Artificial sphincter insertion
Barium enema
Biliary stenting
Bowel preparation
Bowel resection
Bowel resection, small intestine
Cholecystectomy
Colonic stent
Colonoscopy
Colorectal surgery
Colostomy
Defecography
Diverticulitis
Endoscopic ultrasound
Esophageal atresia repair
Esophageal function tests
Esophageal resection
Esophagogastrectomy
Esophagogastroduodenoscopy
Gastrectomy
Gastric acid inhibitors
Gastric bypass
Gastroduodenostomy

Gastroenterologic surgery

Gastroesophageal reflux scan

Gastroesophageal reflux surgery

Gastrostomy

Glossectomy

Heller myotomy

Hemorrhoidectomy

Hepatectomy

HIDA Scan

Ileoanal anastomosis

Ileoanal reservoir surgery

Ileostomy

Intestinal obstruction repair

Intussusception reduction

Liver biopsy

Liver transplantation

Laxatives

Parotidectomy

Pyloroplasty

Rectal prolapse repair

Rectal resection

Sclerotherapy for esophageal varices

Sigmoidoscopy

Tube enterostomy

Upper GI exam

Vagotomy

Vertical banded gastroplasty

Hematological

ABO blood typing

Alanine aminotransferase test

Albumin Test, Blood

Anticoagulant and antiplatelet drugs

Arterial blood gases (ABG)

Aspartate aminotransferase test

Autologous blood donation

Blood Ca (calcium) level

Blood carbon dioxide level

Blood culture

Blood donation and registry

Bloodless surgery

Blood phosphate level

Blood potassium level

Blood pressure measurement

Blood salvage

Blood sodium level

Blood type test

Blood urea nitrogen test

Bone marrow aspiration and biopsy

Bone marrow transplantation

BUN-creatinine ratio

Chemistry screen

Cholesterol and triglyceride tests

Complete blood count

Creatine phosphokinase (CPK)

Electrolyte tests

Enhanced external counterpulsation

Hematocrit

Hemoglobin test

Hemoperfusion

Human leukocyte antigen test

LDL cholesterol test

Lipid profile

Lipid tests

Liver function tests

Meckel's diverticulectomy

Partial thromboplastin time

Phlebography

Phlebotomy

Photocoagulation therapy

Prothrombin time

Pulse oximeter

Red blood cell indices

Rh blood typing

Rheumatoid factor testing

Sedimentation rate

Serum chloride level

Serum creatinine level

Serum glucose level

Sphygmomanometer

Thrombolytic therapy

Transfusion

Type and screen

White blood cell count and differential

Integumentary

Bedsores

Blepharoplasty

Cleft lip repair

Debridement

Dermabrasion

Face lift

Fasciotomy

Forehead lift

Laceration repair

Laser skin resurfacing

Mohs surgery

Skin grafting

Webbed finger or toe repair

Musculoskeletal

Abdominal wall defect repair

Abdominoplasty

Amputation

Arthrography

Arthroplasty

Arthroscopic surgery

Bankart procedure

Bone grafting

Bone x rays

Bunionectomy

Club foot repair

Craniofacial reconstruction

Disk removal

Eye muscle surgery

Finger reattachment

Fracture repair

Ganglion cyst removal

Hammer, claw, and mallet toe surgery

Hand surgery

Hiatal hernia

Hip osteotomy

Hip replacement

Hip revision surgery

Incisional hernia repair
Inguinal hernia repair
Knee arthroscopic surgery
Knee osteotomy
Knee replacement
Knee revision surgery
Kneecap removal
Laminectomy
Leg lengthening or shortening
Limb salvage
Mastoidectomy
Mentoplasty
Orthopedic surgery
Pectus excavatum repair
Rotator cuff repair
Shoulder joint replacement
Shoulder resection arthroplasty
Skull x rays
Spinal fusion
Spinal instrumentation
Tendon repair
Tenotomy
Traction
Umbilical hernia repair
Wrist replacement

Neurological

Anterior temporal lobectomy
Bispectral index
Carpal tunnel release
Cerebral aneurysm repair
Cerebrospinal fluid (CSF)
  analysis
Corpus callosotomy
Craniotomy
Deep brain stimulation
Electroencephalography
Hemispherectomy
Meningocele repair
Myelography
Neurosurgery
Pallidotomy
Rhizotomy
Stereotactic radiosurgery
Sympathectomy
Vagal nerve stimulation

Reproductive, Female

Abortion, induced
Amniocentesis
Breast biopsy
Breast implants
Breast reconstruction
Breast reduction
Cervical cerclage
Cervical cryotherapy
Cesarean section
Colporrhaphy
Colposcopy
Colpotomy
Cone biopsy
Dilatation and curettage
Episiotomy
Fallopian tube implants
Fetal surgery
Fetoscopy
Hysterectomy
Hysteroscopy
In vitro fertilization
Laparoscopy for endometriosis
Lumpectomy
Mammography
Mastectomy
Modified radical mastectomy
Myomectomy
Obstetric and gynecologic surgery
Oophorectomy
Quadrantectomy
Salpingo-oophorectomy
Salpingostomy
Simple mastectomy
Tubal ligation
Uterine stimulants

Reproductive, Male

Circumcision
Hydrocelectomy
Hypospadias repair

Open prostatectomy
Orchiectomy
Orchiopexy
Penile prostheses
Transurethral resection of the
  prostate
Vasectomy
Vasovasostomy

Respiratory

Bronchoscopy
Chest tube insertion
Cricothyroidotomy
Endoscopic sinus surgery
Endotracheal intubation
Laryngectomy
Lobectomy, pulmonary
Lung biopsy
Lung transplantation
Mantoux test
Mechanical ventilation
Mediastinoscopy
Pharyngectomy
Pneumonectomy
Septoplasty
Snoring surgery
Spirometry tests
Tracheotomy

Sensory

Cochlear implants
Corneal transplantation
Cryotherapy for cataracts
Cyclocryotherapy
Endolymphatic shunt
Enucleation, eye
Extracapsular cataract extraction
Goniotomy
Iridectomy
Laser in-situ keratomileusis
  (LASIK)
Laser iridotomy
Laser posterior capsulotomy
Myringotomy and ear tubes

Ophthalmologic surgery
Ophthalmoscopy
Otoplasty
Phacoemulsification for cataracts
Photorefractive keratectomy (PRK)
Retinal cryopexy
Scleral buckling
Sclerostomy
Stapedectomy
Tarsorrhaphy
Trabeculectomy
Tube-shunt surgery
Tympanoplasty

Urinary

Bladder augmentation
Catheterization, female
Catheterization, male
Collagen periurethral injection
Cystectomy
Cystocele repair
Cystoscopy
Gallstone removal
Ileal conduit surgery
Kidney dialysis
Kidney function tests
Kidney transplantation
Lithotripsy
Needle bladder neck suspension
Nephrectomy
Nephrolithotomy, percutaneous
Nephrostomy
Patent urachus repair
Retropubic suspension
Sacral nerve stimulation
Sling procedure
Transurethral bladder resection
Ureteral stenting
Ureterosigmoidoscopy
Ureterostomy, cutaneous
Urinalysis
Urinary anti-infectives

Urine culture
Urologic surgery

Other Surgeries

Abscess incision and drainage
Axillary dissection
Curettage and electrosurgery
Ear, nose, and throat surgery
Elective surgery
Emergency surgery
Essential surgery
Exenteration
General surgery
Gingivectomy
Laparoscopy
Laparotomy, exploratory
Laser surgery
Lymphadenectomy
Microsurgery
Necessary surgery
Omphalocele repair
Outpatient surgery
Pediatric surgery
Plastic, reconstructive, and cosmetic surgery
Radical neck dissection
Rhinoplasty
Robot-assisted surgery
Root canal treatment
Scar revision surgery
Second-look surgery
Segmentectomy
Sex reassignment surgery
Splenectomy
Telesurgery
Thoracic surgery
Thoracotomy
Tonsillectomy
Tooth extraction
Tooth replantation
Trabeculectomy
Transplant surgery
Tumor removal

Other Tests & Procedures

Abdominal ultrasound
Anaerobic bacteria culture
Antibody tests, immunoglobulins
Biofeedback
Chest x ray
Cryotherapy
CT scans
Dental implants
Epidural therapy
Glucose tests
Hair transplantation
Immunoassay tests
Immunologic therapies
Intravenous rehydration
Liposuction
Magnetic resonance imaging
Medication Monitoring
Mental health assessment
Oxygen therapy
Paracentesis
Parentage testing
Pelvic ultrasound
Peritoneovenous shunt
pH monitoring
Physical examination
Positron emission tomography (PET)
Sentinel lymph node biopsy
Temperature measurement
Tumor marker tests
Ultrasound
Weight management

Drugs

Acetaminophen
Adrenergic drugs
Analgesics
Analgesics, opioid
Anesthesia evaluation
Anesthesia, general
Anesthesia, local

Antianxiety drugs
Antibiotics
Antibiotics, topical
Antihypertensive drugs
Antinausea drugs
Antiseptics
Aspirin
Barbiturates
Cephalosporins
Corticosteroids
Diuretics
Erythromycins
Fluoroquinolones
Immunosuppressant drugs
Muscle relaxants
Nonsteroidal anti-inflammatory
  drugs
Prophylaxis, antibiotic
Proton pump inhibitors
Scopolamine patch
Sedation, conscious
Sulfonamides
Tetracyclines

Related Issues & Topics

Admission to the hospital
Adult day care
Ambulatory surgery centers
Anesthesiologist's role
Aseptic technique
Bandages and dressings
Body temperature

Closures: stitches, staples, and
  glue
Death and dying
Discharge from the hospital
Do not resuscitate (DNR) order
Drug-resistant organisms
Exercise
Fibrin sealants
Finding a surgeon
Health care proxy
Health history
Health Maintenance
  Organization (HMO)Home care
Hospice
Hospital services
Hospital-acquired infections
Incision care
Informed consent
Intensive care unit
Intensive care unit equipment
Length of hospital stay
Living will
Long-term care insurance
Managed care plans
Medicaid
Medical charts
Medical co-morbidities
Medical errors
Medicare
Medication Monitoring
Mental health assessment
Negative pressure rooms
Nursing homes
Operating room

Pain management
Patient confidentiality
Patient rights
Patient-controlled analgesia
Pediatric concerns
Planning a hospital stay
Postoperative care
Post-surgical infections
Post-surgical pain
Power of attorney
Preoperative care
Preparing for surgery
Presurgical testing
Private insurance plans
Recovery at home
Recovery room
Reoperation
Second opinion
Smoking cessation
Stethoscope
Surgical instruments
Surgical mesh
Surgical oncology
Surgical risk
Surgical team
Surgical training
Surgical triage
Syringe and needle
Talking to the doctor
Thermometer
Trocars
Vital signs
Wound care
Wound culture

PLEASE READ—IMPORTANT INFORMATION

The *Gale Encyclopedia of Surgery and Medical Tests, 2nd Edition* is a health reference product designed to inform and educate readers about a wide variety of surgeries, tests, diseases and conditions, treatments and drugs, equipment, and other issues associated with surgical and medical practice. Cengage Learning believes the product to be comprehensive, but not necessarily definitive. It is intended to supplement, not replace, consultation with physicians or other healthcare practitioners. While Cengage Learning has made substantial efforts to provide information that is accurate, comprehensive, and up-to-date, Cengage Learning makes no representations or warranties of any kind, including without limitation, warranties of merchantability or fitness for a particular purpose, nor does it guarantee the accuracy, comprehensiveness, or timeliness of the information contained in this product. Readers should be aware that the universe of medical knowledge is constantly growing and changing, and that differences of opinion exist among authorities. Readers are also advised to seek professional diagnosis and treatment for any medical condition, and to discuss information obtained from this book with their healthcare provider.

INTRODUCTION

The *Gale Encyclopedia of Surgery and Medical Tests, 2ⁿᵈ Edition* is a unique and invaluable source of information. This collection of 535 entries provides in-depth coverage of various issues related to surgery, medical tests, diseases and conditions, hospitalization, and general health care. These entries generally follow a standard format, including a definition, purpose, demographics, description, diagnosis/preparation, aftercare, precautions, risks, side effects, interactions, morbidity and mortality rates, alternatives, normal results, questions to ask your doctor, and information about who performs the procedures and where they are performed. Topics of a more general nature related to surgical hospitalization and medical testing round out the set. Examples of this coverage include entries on Adult day care, Ambulatory surgery centers, Death and dying, Discharge from the hospital, Do not resuscitate (DNR) order, Exercise, Finding a surgeon, Hospice, Hospital services, Informed consent, Living will, Long-term care insurance, Managed care plans, Medicaid, Medicare, Patient rights, Planning a hospital stay, Power of attorney, Private insurance plans, Second opinion, Talking to the doctor, and others.

Scope

The *Gale Encyclopedia of Surgery and Medical Tests, 2ⁿᵈ Edition* covers a wide variety of topics relevant to the user. Entries follow a standardized format that provides information at a glance. Rubrics include the following (not every entry will make use of all of them):

- Definition
- Description
- Purpose
- Demographics
- Diagnosis/preparation
- Aftercare
- Precautions
- Risks
- Side effects
- Interactions
- Morbidity and mortality rates
- Alternatives
- Normal results
- "Questions to ask the doctor"
- "Who performs the procedure and where is it performed?"
- Resources
- Key Terms

Inclusion criteria

A preliminary list of topics was compiled from a wide variety of sources, including health reference books, general medical encyclopedias, and consumer health guides. The advisory board evaluated the topics and made suggestions for inclusion. Final selection of topics to include was made by the advisory board in conjunction with the editor.

About the contributors

The essays were compiled by experienced medical writers, including medical doctors, pharmacists, and registered nurses. The advisers reviewed the completed essays to ensure that they are appropriate, up-to-date, and accurate.

How to use this book

The *Gale Encyclopedia of Surgery and Medical Tests, 2ⁿᵈ Edition* has been designed with ready reference in mind.

- Straight **alphabetical arrangement** of topics allows users to locate information quickly.
- **Bold-faced terms** within entries direct the reader to related articles.
- **Cross-references** placed throughout the encyclopedia direct readers from alternate names and related topics to entries.
- A list of **Key terms** is provided where appropriate to define terms or concepts that may be unfamiliar to the user. A **glossary** of key terms in the back of the fourth volume contains a concise list of terms arranged alphabetically.
- The **Resources** section directs readers to additional sources of information on a topic.
- Valuable **contact information** for health organizations is included with most entries. An Appendix of **organizations** in the back of the fourth volume contains an extensive list of organizations arranged alphabetically.
- A comprehensive **general index** guides readers to significant topics mentioned in the text.

Graphics

The *Gale Encyclopedia of Surgery and Medical Tests, 2nd Edition* is also enhanced by color photographs, illustrations, and tables.

Acknowledgements

The editor wishes to thank all of the people who contributed to this encyclopedia. There are too many names to list here, so the reader is urged to review the Advisory board and Contributors pages for the list of writers, physicians, and health-care experts to whom he is indebted. Special thanks must go to Rosalyn Carson-DeWitt for all the writing, updating, and advising she did; the project could not have been completed without her. L. Fleming Fallon provided invaluable assistance at every step of the way; his writing, advice, and good humor made this project a pleasure. Laurie Cataldo's expertise in so many areas helped make this book as good as it is. And Maria Basile provided not only many beautifully written entries, but she performed some last-minute review work for which the editor is most grateful. To all of you, my deepest thanks.

ADVISORS

A number of experts in the medical community provided invaluable assistance in the formulation of this encyclopedia. Our advisory board performed a myriad of duties, from defining the scope of coverage to reviewing individual entries for accuracy and accessibility. The editor would like to express his appreciation to them.

Rosalyn Carson-DeWitt, MD
Medical Writer
Durham, NC

Laura Jean Cataldo, RN, EdD
Nurse, Medical Consultant,
*   Educator*
Germantown, MD

L. Fleming Fallon, Jr, MD, DrPH
Professor of Public Health

Bowling Green State University
Bowling Green, OH

Chitra Venkatasubramanian, MD
Clinical Assistant Professor,
*   Neurology and Neurological*
*   Sciences*
Stanford University School of
    Medicine
Palo Alto, CA

CONTRIBUTORS

Laurie Barclay, MD
Neurological Consulting
  Services
Tampa, FL

Jeanine Barone
Nutritionist, Exercise Physiologist
New York, NY

Julia Barrett
Science Writer
Madison, WI

Donald G. Barstow, RN
Clinical Nurse Specialist
Oklahoma City, OK

Maria Basile, PhD
Neuropharmacologist
Roselle, NJ

Mary Bekker
Medical Writer
Willow Grove, PA

**Mark A. Best, MD, MPH,
  MBA**
Associate Professor of Pathology
St. Matthew's University
Grand Cayman, BWI

Randall J. Blazic, MD, DDS
Oral and Maxillofacial Surgeon
Goodyear, AZ

Robert Bockstiegel
Medical Writer
Portland, OR

Maggie Boleyn, RN, BSN
Medical Writer
Oak Park, MN

Susan Joanne Cadwallader
Medical Writer
Cedarburg, WI

Diane M. Calabrese
*Medical Sciences and Technology
  Writer*
Silver Spring, MD

Richard H. Camer
Editor
International Medical News Group
Silver Spring, MD

Rosalyn Carson-DeWitt, MD
Medical Writer
Durham, NC

Laura Jean Cataldo, RN, EdD
*Nurse, Medical Consultant,
  Educator*
Germantown, MD

Lisa Christenson, Ph.D.
Science Writer
Hamden, CT

Rhonda Cloos, RN
Medical Writer
Austin, TX

Constance Clyde
Medical Writer
Dana Point, CA

Angela M. Costello
Medical writer
Cleveland, OH

L. Lee Culvert, PhD
Health writer
Alna, ME

Tish Davidson, AM
Medical Writer
Fremont, CA

Lori De Milto
Medical Writer
Sicklerville, NJ

Victoria E. DeMoranville
Medical Writer
Lakeville, MA

Altha Roberts Edgren
Medical Writer
Medical Ink
St. Paul, MN

Lorraine K. Ehresman
Medical Writer
Northfield, Quebec, Canada

Abraham F. Ettaher, MD

**L. Fleming Fallon, Jr, MD,
  DrPH**
Professor of Public Health
Bowling Green State
  University
Bowling Green, OH

Paula Ford-Martin
Medical Writer
Warwick, RI

Janie F. Franz
Journalist
Grand Forks, ND

Rebecca J. Frey, PhD
Medical Writer
New Haven, CT

Debra Gordon
Medical Writer
Nazareth, PA

Jill Granger, MS
Sr. Research Associate
Dept. of Pathology
University of Michigan Medical
  Center
Ann Arbor, MI

Peter Gregutt
Medical Writer
Asheville, NC

Laith Farid Gulli, MD, MS
Consultant Psychotherapist in Private Practice
Lathrup Village, MI

Stephen John Hage, AAAS, RT(R), FAHRA
Medical Writer
Chatsworth, CA

Maureen Haggerty
Medical Writer
Ambler, PA

Robert Harr
Associate Professor and Chair
Department of Public and Allied Health
Bowling Green State University
Bowling Green, OH

Dan Harvey
Medical Writer
Wilmington, DE

Katherine Hauswirth, APRN
Medical Writer
Deep River, CT

Caroline A. Helwick
Medical Writer
New Orleans, LA

Lisette Hilton
Medical Writer
Boca Raton, FL

Fran Hodgkins
Medical Writer
Sparks, MD

René A. Jackson, RN
Medical Writer
Port Charlotte, FL

Nadine M. Jacobson, RN
Medical Writer
Takoma Park, MD

Randi B. Jenkins, BA
Copy Chief
Fission Communications
New York, NY

Michelle L. Johnson, MS, JD
Patent Attorney
ZymoGenetics, Inc.
Seattle, WA

Paul Johnson
Medical Writer
San Diego, CA

Cindy L. A. Jones, PhD
Biomedical Writer
Sagescript Communications
Lakewood, CO

Linda D. Jones, BA, PBT (ASCP)
Medical Writer
Asheboro, NY

Crystal H. Kaczkowski, MSc
Health writer
Chicago, IL

Beth A. Kapes
Medical Writer
Bay Village, OH

Mary Jeanne Krob, MD, FACS
Physician, writer
Pittsburgh, PA

Monique Laberge, PhD
Sr. Res. Investigator
Dept. of Biochemistry & Biophysics, School of Medicine
University of Pennsylvania
Philadelphia, PA

Richard H. Lampert
Senior Medical Editor
W.B. Saunders Co.
Philadelphia, PA

Renee Laux, MS
Medical Writer
Manlius, NY

Victor Leipzig, PhD
Biological Consultant
Huntington Beach, CA

Lorraine Lica, PhD
Medical Writer
San Diego, CA

John T. Lohr, PhD
Assistant Director, Biotechnology Center
Utah State University
Logan, UT

Jennifer Lee Losey, RN
Medical Writer
Madison Heights, MI

Nicole Mallory, MS, PA-C
Medical Student, Wayne State University
Detroit, MI

Jacqueline N. Martin, MS
Medical Writer
Albrightsville, PA

Nancy McKenzie, PhD
Public Health Consultant
Brooklyn, NY

Mercedes McLaughlin
Medical Writer
Phoenixville, CA

Miguel A. Melgar, MD, PhD
Neurosurgeon
New Orleans, LA

Christine Miner Minderovic, BS, RT, RDMS
Medical Writer
Ann Arbor, MI

Mark Mitchell, MD, MPH, MBA
Medical Writer
Bothell, WA

Alfredo Mori, MD, FACEM, FFAEM
Emergency Physician
The Alfred Hospital
Victoria, Australia

Bilal Nasser, MD, MS
Senior Medical Student, Wayne State University
Detroit, MI

Erika J. Norris
Medical Writer
Oak Harbor, WA

Teresa Norris, RN
Medical Writer
Ute Park, NM

Debra Novograd, BS, RT(R)(M)
Medical Writer
Royal Oak, MI

Jane E. Phillips, PhD
Medical Writer
Chapel Hill, NC

J. Ricker Polsdorfer, MD
Medical Writer
Phoenix, AZ

Elaine R. Proseus, MBA/TM, BSRT, RT(R)
Medical Writer
Farmington Hills, MI

Robert Ramirez, BS
Medical Student
University of Medicine & Dentistry of New Jersey
Stratford, NJ

Esther Csapo Rastegari, RN, BSN, EdM
Medical Writer
Holbrook, MA

Martha Reilly, OD
Clinical Optometrist, Medical Writer
Madison, WI

Toni Rizzo
Medical Writer
Salt Lake City, UT

Richard Robinson
Medical Writer
Sherborn, MA

Nancy Ross-Flanigan
Science Writer
Belleville, MI

Belinda Rowland, PhD
Medical Writer
Voorheesville, NY

Laura Ruth, PhD
Medical, Science, & Technology Writer
Los Angeles, CA

Uchechukwu Sampson, MD, MPH, MBA

Kausalya Santhanam, PhD
Technical Writer
Branford, CT

Joan M. Schonbeck
Medical Writer
Nursing
Massachusetts Department of Mental Health
Marlborough, MA

Stephanie Dionne Sherk
Medical Writer
University of Michigan
Ann Arbor, MI

Lee A. Shratter, MD
Consulting Radiologist
Kentfield, CA

Jennifer E. Sisk, MA
Medical Writer
Havertown, PA

Allison Joan Spiwak, MSBME
Circulation Technologist
The Ohio State University
Columbus, OH

Kurt Richard Sternlof
Science Writer
New Rochelle, NY

Margaret A Stockley, RGN
Medical Writer
Boxborough, MA

Dorothy Elinor Stonely
Medical Writer
Los Gatos, CA

Bethany Thivierge
Biotechnical Writer and Editor
Technicality Resources
Rockland, ME

Carol A. Turkington
Medical Writer
Lancaster, PA

Samuel D. Uretsky, PharmD
Medical Writer
Wantagh, NY

Chitra Venkatasubramanian, MD
Clinical Assistant Professor, Neurology and Neurological Sciences
Stanford University School of Medicine
Palo Alto, CA

Ellen S. Weber, MSN
Medical Writer
Fort Wayne, IN

Barbara Wexler
Medical Writer
Chatsworth, CA

Abby Wojahn, RN, BSN, CCRN
Medical Writer
Milwaukee, WI

Kathleen D. Wright, RN
Medical Writer
Delmar, DE

Mary Zoll, PhD
Science Writer
Newton Center, MA

Michael Zuck, PhD
Medical Writer
Boulder, CO

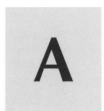

A

Abdominal ultrasound

Definition

Abdominal **ultrasound** uses high-frequency sound waves to produce two-dimensional images of the body's soft tissues, which are used for a variety of clinical applications, including diagnosis and guidance of treatment procedures. Ultrasound does not use ionizing radiation to produce images, and, in comparison to other diagnostic imaging modalities, it is inexpensive, safe, fast, and versatile.

Purpose

Abdominal ultrasound is used in the hospital radiology department and emergency department, as well as in physician offices, for a number of clinical applications. Ultrasound has a great advantage over x-ray imaging technologies in that it does not damage tissues with ionizing radiation. Ultrasound is also generally far better than plain x rays at distinguishing the subtle variations of soft tissue structures, and can be used in any of several modes, depending on the area of interest.

As an imaging tool, abdominal ultrasound is generally indicated for patients afflicted with chronic or acute abdominal pain; abdominal trauma; an obvious or suspected abdominal mass; symptoms of liver or biliary tract disease, pancreatic disease, gallstones, spleen disease, kidney disease, and urinary blockage; evaluation of ascites; or symptoms of an abdominal aortic aneurysm.

The specifics include:

- Abdominal pain. Whether acute or chronic, pain can signal a serious problem—from organ malfunction or injury to the presence of malignant growths. Ultrasound scanning can help doctors quickly sort through potential causes when presented with general or ambiguous symptoms. All of the major abdominal organs can

be studied for signs of disease that appear as changes in size, shape, or internal structure.

- Abdominal trauma. After a serious accident such as a car crash or a fall, internal bleeding from injured abdominal organs is often the most serious threat to survival. Neither the injuries nor the bleeding may be immediately apparent. Ultrasound is very useful as an initial scan when abdominal trauma is suspected, and it can be used to pinpoint the location, cause, and severity of hemorrhaging. In the case of puncture wounds, from a bullet for example, ultrasound can locate the foreign object and provide a preliminary survey of the damage. (Computed tomography [CT] scans are sometimes used in trauma settings.)

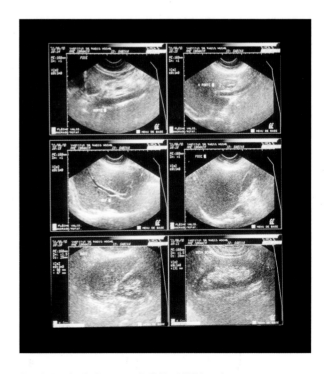

An abdominal ultrasound. *(Mike Hill/Alamy)*

KEY TERMS

Accessory organ—A lump of tissue adjacent to an organ that is similar to it, but which serves no important purpose (if it functions at all). While not necessarily harmful, such organs can cause problems if they are confused with a mass, or in rare cases, if they grow too large or become cancerous.

Ascites—Free fluid in the abdominal cavity.

Benign—In medical usage, benign is the opposite of malignant. It describes an abnormal growth that is stable, treatable, and generally not life-threatening.

Biopsy—The surgical removal and analysis of a tissue sample for diagnostic purposes. Usually the term refers to the collection and analysis of tissue from a suspected tumor to establish malignancy.

Calculus—Any type of hard concretion (stone) in the body, but usually found in the gallbladder, pancreas, and kidneys. Calculi (the plural form) are formed by the accumulation of excess mineral salts and other organic material, such as blood or mucous. They can cause problems by lodging in and obstructing the

proper flow of fluids, such as bile to the intestines or urine to the bladder.

Cirrhosis—A chronic liver disease characterized by the degeneration of proper functioning. Jaundice is often an accompanying symptom. Causes of cirrhosis include hepatitis, alcoholism, and metabolic diseases.

Common bile duct—The branching passage through which bile—a necessary digestive enzyme—travels from the liver and gallbladder into the small intestine. Digestive enzymes from the pancreas also enter the intestines through the common bile duct.

Computed tomography scan (CT scan)—A specialized type of x-ray imaging that uses highly focused and relatively low-energy radiation to produce detailed two-dimensional images of soft-tissue structures, such as the brain or abdomen. CT scans are the chief competitor to ultrasound and can yield higher-quality images not disrupted by bone or gas. They are, however, more cumbersome, time consuming, and expensive to perform, and they use ionizing radiation.

- Abdominal mass. Abnormal growths—tumors, cysts, abscesses, scar tissue, and accessory organs—can be located and tentatively identified with ultrasound. In particular, potentially malignant solid tumors can be distinguished from benign fluid-filled cysts. Masses and malformations in any organ or part of the abdomen can be found.

- Liver disease. The types and underlying causes of liver disease are numerous, though jaundice tends to be a general symptom. Sometimes, liver disease manifests as abnormal laboratory results, such as abnormal liver function tests. Ultrasound can differentiate between many of the types and causes of liver malfunction, and it is particularly good at identifying obstruction of the bile ducts and cirrhosis, which is characterized by abnormal fibrous growths and altered blood flow.

- Pancreatic disease. Inflammation of the pancreas—caused by, for example, abnormal fluid collections surrounding the organ (pseudocysts)—can be identified by ultrasound. Pancreatic stones (calculi), which can disrupt proper functioning, can also be detected.

- Gallstones. These are an extremely common cause of hospital admissions. In the non-emergency or non-acute setting, gallstones can present as abdominal pain, or fatty-food intolerance. These calculi can cause painful

inflammation of the gallbladder and obstruct the bile ducts that carry digestive enzymes from the gallbladder and liver to the intestines. Gallstones are readily identifiable with ultrasound.

- Spleen disease. The spleen is particularly prone to injury during abdominal trauma. It may also become painfully inflamed when infected or cancerous. The spleen can become enlarged with some forms of liver disease.

- Kidney disease. The kidneys are also prone to traumatic injury and are the organs most likely to form calculi, which can block the flow of urine and cause further systemic problems. A variety of diseases causing distinct changes in kidney morphology can also lead to complete kidney failure. Ultrasound imaging has proved extremely useful in diagnosing kidney disorders, including blockage and obstruction.

- Abdominal aortic aneurysm. This aneurysm is a bulging weak spot in the abdominal aorta, which supplies blood directly from the heart to the entire lower body. A ruptured aortic aneurysm is imminently life-threatening. However, it can readily be identified and monitored with ultrasound before acute complications result.

- Appendicitis. Ultrasound is useful in diagnosing appendicitis, which causes abdominal pain.

Doppler—The Doppler effect refers to the apparent change in frequency of sound-wave echoes returning to a stationary source from a moving target. If the object is moving toward the source, the frequency increases; if the object is moving away, the frequency decreases. The size of this frequency shift can be used to compute the object's speed—be it a car on the road or blood in an artery.

Frequency—Sound, whether traveling through air or the human body, produces vibrations—molecules bouncing into each other—as the shock wave travels along. The frequency of a sound is the number of vibrations per second. Within the audible range, frequency means pitch: the higher the frequency, the higher a sound's pitch.

Ionizing radiation—A type of radiation that can damage living tissue by disrupting and destroying individual cells at the molecular level. All types of nuclear radiation, including x rays, gamma rays, and beta rays, are potentially ionizing. Sound waves physically vibrate the material through which they pass, but do not ionize it.

Jaundice—A condition that results in a yellow tint to the skin, eyes, and body fluids. Bile retention in the liver, gallbladder, and pancreas is the immediate cause, but the underlying cause could be as simple as obstruction of the common bile duct by a gallstone or as serious as pancreatic cancer. Ultrasound can distinguish between these conditions.

Malignant—The term literally means growing worse and resisting treatment. It is used as a synonym for cancerous and connotes a harmful condition that generally is life threatening.

Morphology—Literally, the study of form. In medicine, morphology refers to the size, shape, and structure rather than the function of a given organ. As a diagnostic imaging technique, ultrasound facilitates the recognition of abnormal morphologies as symptoms of underlying conditions.

Ultrasound technology can also be used for treatment purposes, most frequently as a visual aid during surgical procedures, such as guiding needle placement to drain fluid from a cyst, or to guide biopsies.

Description

Ultrasound includes all sound waves above the frequency of human hearing—about 20 thousand hertz (Hz), or cycles per second. Medical ultrasound generally uses frequencies between 1 and 10 megahertz (1–10 MHz). Higher-frequency ultrasound waves produce more detailed images, but they are also more readily absorbed and so cannot penetrate as deeply into the body. Abdominal ultrasound imaging is generally performed at frequencies between 2–5 MHz.

An ultrasound scanner consists of two parts, the transducer and the data processing unit. The transducer both produces the sound waves that penetrate the body and receives the reflected echoes. Transducers are built around piezoelectric ceramic chips. (Piezoelectric refers to electricity that is produced when pressure is put on certain crystals, such as quartz.) These ceramic chips react to electric pulses by producing sound waves (transmitting) and react to sound waves by producing electric pulses (receiving). Bursts of high-frequency electric pulses supplied to the transducer cause it to produce the scanning sound waves. The transducer then receives the returning echoes, translates them back into electric pulses, and sends them to the data processing unit, a computer that organizes the data into an image on a television screen.

Because sound waves travel through all the body's tissues at nearly the same speed—about 3,400 miles per hour—the microseconds it takes for each echo to be received can be plotted on the screen as a distance into the body. (The longer it takes to receive the echo, the farther away the reflective surface must be.) The relative strength of each echo, a function of the specific tissue or organ boundary that produced it, can be plotted as a point of varying brightness. In this way, the echoes are translated into an image.

Four different modes of ultrasound are used in medical imaging:

- A-mode. This is the simplest type of ultrasound in which a single transducer scans a line through the body with the echoes plotted on screen as a function of depth. This method is used to measure distances within the body and the size of internal organs.
- B-mode. In B-mode ultrasound, which is the most common use, a linear array of transducers simultaneously scans a plane through the body that can be viewed as a two-dimensional image on screen.

- M-Mode. The M stands for motion. A rapid sequence of B-mode scans whose images follow each other in sequence on screen enables doctors to see and measure range of motion, as the organ boundaries that produce reflections move relative to the probe. M-mode ultrasound has been put to particular use in studying heart motion.

- Doppler mode. Doppler ultrasonography includes the capability of accurately measuring velocities of moving material, such as blood in arteries and veins. The principle is the same as that used in radar guns that measure the speed of a car on the highway. Doppler capability is most often combined with B-mode scanning to produce images of blood vessels from which blood flow can be directly measured. This technique is used extensively to investigate valve defects, arteriosclerosis, and hypertension, particularly in the heart, but also in the abdominal aorta and the portal vein of the liver.

The actual procedure for a patient undergoing an abdominal ultrasound is relatively simple, regardless of the type of scan or its purpose. Fasting for at least eight hours prior to the procedure ensures that the patient's stomach is empty and as small as possible, and that the intestines and bowels are relatively inactive. This also helps the gallbladder become more visible. Prior to scanning, an acoustic gel is applied to the skin of the patient's abdomen to allow the ultrasound probe to glide easily across the skin and to better transmit and receive ultrasonic pulses. The probe is moved around the abdomen's surface to obtain different views of the target areas. The patient will likely be asked to change positions from side to side and to hold the breath as necessary to obtain the desired views. Usually, a scan will take from 20 to 45 minutes, depending on the patient's condition and the anatomical area being scanned.

Ultrasound scanners are available in different configurations, with different scanning features. Portable units, which weigh only a few pounds and can be carried by hand, are available for bedside use, office use, or use outside the hospital, such as at sporting events and in ambulances. Portable scanners range in cost from $10,000 to $50,000. Mobile ultrasound scanners, which can be pushed to the patient's bedside and between hospital departments, are the most common configuration and range in cost from $100,000 to more than $250,000, depending on the scanning features purchased.

Preparation

A patient undergoing abdominal ultrasound will be advised by his or her physician about what to expect and how to prepare. As mentioned above, preparations generally include fasting.

Aftercare

In general, no aftercare related to the abdominal ultrasound procedure itself is required. Discomfort during the procedure is minimal.

Risks

Properly performed, ultrasound imaging is virtually without risk or side effects.

Results

As a diagnostic imaging technique, a normal abdominal ultrasound is one that indicates the absence of the suspected condition that prompted the scan. For example, symptoms such as abdominal pain radiating to the back suggest the possibility of, among other things, an abdominal aortic aneurysm. An ultrasound scan that indicates the absence of an aneurysm would rule out this life-threatening condition and point to other, less serious causes.

Because abdominal ultrasound imaging is generally undertaken to confirm a suspected condition, the results of a scan often will confirm the diagnosis, be it kidney stones, cirrhosis of the liver, or an aortic aneurysm. At that point, appropriate medical treatment as prescribed by a patient's physician is in order.

Ultrasound scanning should be performed by a registered and trained ultrasonographer, either a technologist or a physician (radiologist, obstetrician/gynecologist). Ultrasound scanning in the emergency department may be performed by an emergency medicine physician, who should have appropriate training and experience in ultrasonography.

Resources

BOOKS

Grainger, RG, et al. *Grainger & Allison's Diagnostic Radiology: A Textbook of Medical Imaging*. 4th ed. Philadelphia: Saunders, 2001.

Mettler, FA. *Essentials of Radiology*. 2nd ed. Philadelphia: Saunders, 2005.

Townsend, CM et al. *Sabiston Textbook of Surgery*. 17th ed. Philadelphia: Saunders, 2004.

PERIODICALS

Kuhn, M., R. L. L. Bonnin, M. J. Davey, J. L. Rowland, and S. Langlois. "Emergency Department Ultrasound Scanning for Abdominal Aortic Aneurysm: Accessible, Accurate, Advantageous." *Annals of Emergency Medicine* 36, No. 3 (September 2000): 219–223.

Sisk, Jennifer. "Ultrasound in the Emergency Department: Toward a Standard of Care." *Radiology Today* 2, No. 1 (June 4, 2001): 8–10.

ORGANIZATIONS

American College of Radiology. 1891 Preston White Drive, Reston, VA 20191-4397. (800) 227-5463. http://www.acr.org (accessed March 6, 2008).

American Institute of Ultrasound in Medicine. 14750 Sweitzer Lane, Suite 100, Laurel, MD 20707-5906. (301) 498-4100. http://www.aium.org (accessed March 6, 2008).

American Registry of Diagnostic Medical Sonographers. 600 Jefferson Plaza, Suite 360, Rockville, MD 20852-1150. (800) 541-9754. http://www.ardms.org (accessed March 6, 2008).

American Society of Radiologic Technologists (ASRT). 15000 Central Avenue SE, Albuquerque, NM 87123-2778. (800) 444-2778. http://www.asrt.org (accessed March 6, 2008).

Radiological Society of North America. 820 Jorie Boulevard, Oak Brook, IL 60523-2251. (630) 571-2670. http://www.rsna.org (accessed March 6, 2008).

Society of Diagnostic Medical Sonography. 12770 Coit Road, Suite 708, Dallas, TX 75251-1319. (972) 239-7367. http://www.sdms.org (accessed March 6, 2008).

Jennifer E. Sisk, MA
Lee A. Shratter, MD
Rosalyn Carson-DeWitt, MD

Abdominal wall defect repair

Definition

Abdominal wall defect repair is a surgery performed to correct one of two birth defects of the abdominal wall: gastroschisis or omphalocele. Depending on the defect treated, the procedure is also known as omphalocele repair/closure or gastroschisis repair/closure.

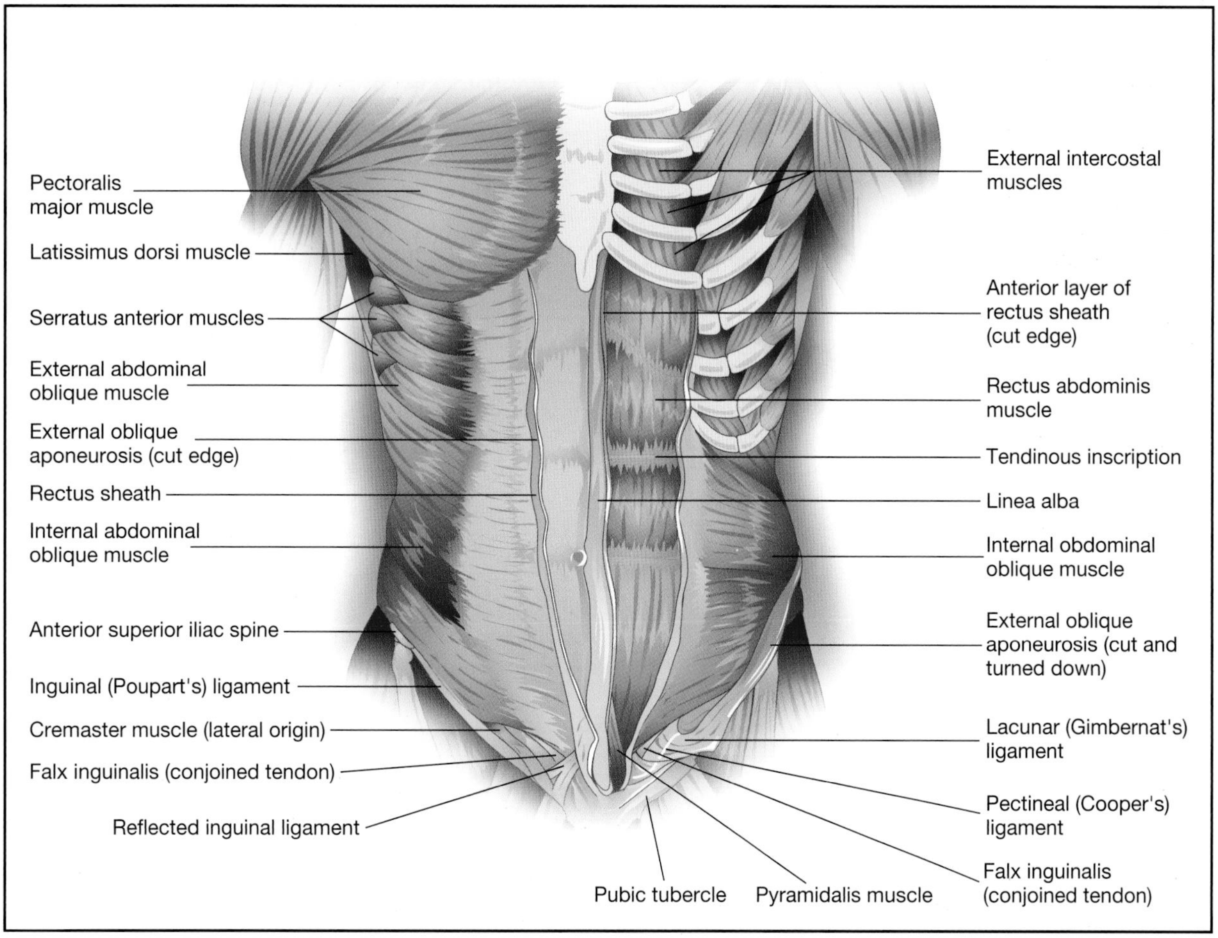
Pectoralis major muscle
Latissimus dorsi muscle
Serratus anterior muscles
External abdominal oblique muscle
External oblique aponeurosis (cut edge)
Rectus sheath
Internal abdominal oblique muscle
Anterior superior iliac spine
Inguinal (Poupart's) ligament
Cremaster muscle (lateral origin)
Falx inguinalis (conjoined tendon)
Reflected inguinal ligament
Pubic tubercle
Pyramidalis muscle
External intercostal muscles
Anterior layer of rectus sheath (cut edge)
Rectus abdominis muscle
Tendinous inscription
Linea alba
Internal obdominal oblique muscle
External oblique aponeurosis (cut and turned down)
Lacunar (Gimbernat's) ligament
Pectineal (Cooper's) ligament
Falx inguinalis (conjoined tendon)

Muscles of the abdomen. *(Illustration by Electronic Illustrators Group.)*

Purpose

In some cases, for some unknown reason, while in utero, the abdominal wall muscles do not form correctly. And, when the abdominal wall is incompletely formed at birth, the internal organs of the infant can either protrude into the umbilical cord (omphalocele) or to the side of the navel (gastroschisis). The size of an omphalocele varies: some are very small, about the size of a ping pong ball, while others may be as big as a grapefruit. **Omphalocele repair** is performed to repair the omphalocele defect in which all or part of the bowel and other internal organs lie on the outside of the abdomen in a hernia (sac). Gastroschisis repair is performed to repair the other abdominal wall defect through which the bowel protrudes with no protective sac present. Gastroschisis is a life-threatening condition that requires immediate medical intervention. Surgery for abdominal wall defects aims to return the abdominal organs back to the abdominal cavity, and to repair the defect if possible. It can also be performed to create a pouch to protect the intestines until they are inserted back into the abdomen.

Demographics

Abdominal wall defects occurs in the United States at a rate of one case per 2,000 births, which means that some 2,360 cases are diagnosed per year. Mothers below the age of 20 are four times as likely as mothers in their late twenties to give birth to affected babies.

Description

Abdominal wall defect surgery is performed soon after birth. The protruding organs are covered with **dressings**, and a tube is inserted into the stomach to prevent the baby from choking or from breathing in the contents of the stomach into the lungs. The surgery is performed under **general anesthesia**. First, the pediatric surgeon enlarges the hole in the abdominal wall in order to examine the bowel for damage or other birth defects. Damaged portions of the bowel are removed and the healthy bowel is reconnected with **stitches**. The exposed organs are replaced within the abdominal cavity, and the opening is closed. Sometimes closure of the opening is not possible, for example when the abdominal cavity is too small or when the organs are too large or swollen to close the skin. In such cases, the surgeon will place a plastic covering pouch, commonly called a silo because of its shape, over the abdominal organs on the outside of the infant to protect the organs. Gradually, the organs are squeezed through the pouch into the opening and returned to the body. This procedure can take up to

a week, and final closure may be performed a few weeks later. More surgery may be required to repair the abdominal muscles at a later time.

Diagnosis/Preparation

Prenatal screening can detect approximately 85% of abdominal wall defects. Gastroschisis and omphalocele are usually diagnosed by **ultrasound** examinations before birth. These tests can determine the size of the abdominal wall defect and identify the affected organs. The surgery is performed immediately after delivery, as soon as the newborn is stable.

KEY TERMS

Abdomen—The portion of the body that lies between the thorax and the pelvis. It contains a cavity with many organs.

Amniotic membrane—A thin membrane that contains the fetus and the protective amniotic fluid surrounding the fetus.

Anesthesia—A combination of drugs administered by a variety of techniques by trained professionals that provide sedation, amnesia, analgesia, and immobility adequate for the accomplishment of the surgical procedure with minimal discomfort, and without injury, to the patient.

Gastroschisis—A defect of the abdominal wall caused by rupture of the amniotic membrane or by the delayed closure of the umbilical ring. It is usually accompanied by protrusion of internal organs in the abdomen.

Hernia—The protrusion or thrusting forward of an organ or tissue through an abnormal opening into the abdominal sac.

Omphalocele—A hernia that occurs at the navel.

Peritonitis—Inflammation of the membrane lining the abdominal cavity. It causes abdominal pain and tenderness, constipation, vomiting, and fever.

Short bowel syndrome—A condition in which digestion and absorption in the small intestine are impaired.

Ultrasound—An imaging technology that allows various organs in the body to be examined.

Umbilical ring—An opening through which the umbilical vessels pass to the fetus; it is closed after birth and its site is indicated by the navel.

WHO PERFORMS THE PROCEDURE AND WHERE IS IT PERFORMED?

Abdominal wall defect surgery is performed by a pediatric surgeon. A pediatric surgeon is specialized in the surgical care of children. He or she must have graduated from medical school, and completed five years of postgraduate general surgery training in an accredited training program. A pediatric surgeon must complete an additional accredited two-year fellowship program in pediatric surgery and be board-eligible or board-certified in general surgery. (Board certification is granted when a fully trained surgeon has taken and passed first a written, then an oral examination.) Once the general surgery boards are passed, a fellowship-trained pediatric surgeon becomes eligible to take the pediatric surgery examination. Other credentials may include membership in the American College of Surgeons, the American Pediatric Surgical Association, and/or the American Academy of Pediatrics. Each of these organizations require that fellows meet well-established standards of training, clinical knowledge, and professional conduct.

If prenatal screening indicates that abdominal wall defects are present in the fetus, delivery should occur at a hospital with an neonatal intensive care unit (NICU) and a pediatric surgeon on staff.

Aftercare

After surgery, the infant is transferred to an **intensive care unit** (ICU) and placed in an incubator to keep warm and to prevent infection. Oxygen is provided. When organs are placed back into the abdominal cavity, this may increase pressure on the abdomen and make breathing difficult. In such cases, the infant is provided with a breathing tube and ventilator until the swelling of the abdominal organs has decreased. Intravenous fluids, **antibiotics**, and pain medication are also administered. A tube is also placed in the stomach to empty gastric secretions. Feedings are started very slowly, using a nasal tube as soon as bowel function starts. Babies born with omphaloceles can stay in the hospital from one week to one month after surgery, depending on the size of the defect. Babies are discharged from the hospital when they are taking all their feedings by mouth and gaining weight.

Risks

The risks of abdominal wall repair surgery include peritonitis and temporary paralysis of the small bowel. If a large segment of the small intestine is damaged, the baby may develop short bowel syndrome and have digestive problems.

Normal results

In most cases, the defect can be corrected with surgery. The outcome depends on the amount of damage to the bowel.

Morbidity and mortality rates

The size of the abdominal wall defect, the extent to which organs protrude out of the abdomen, and the presence of other birth defects influence the outcome of the surgery. The occurrence of other birth defects is uncommon in infants with gastroschisis, and 85% survive. Approximately half of the babies diagnosed with omphalocele have heart defects or other birth defects, and approximately 60% survive to age one.

Alternatives

Gastroschisis is a life-threatening condition requiring immediate surgical intervention. There is no alternative to surgery for either gastroschisis or omphalocele.

Resources

BOOKS

Feldman, M, et al. *Sleisenger & Fordtran's Gastrointestinal and Liver Disease.* 8th ed. St. Louis: Mosby, 2005.

Khatri, VP and JA Asensio. *Operative Surgery Manual.* 1st ed. Philadelphia: Saunders, 2003.

Townsend, CM et al. *Sabiston Textbook of Surgery.* 17th ed. Philadelphia: Saunders, 2004.

PERIODICALS

Lenke, R. "Benefits of term delivery in infants with antenatally diagnosed gastroschisis." *Obstetrics and Gynecology* 101 (February 2003): 418–419.

Sydorak, R. M., A. Nijagal, L. Sbragia, et al. "Gastroschisis: small hole, big cost." *Journal of Pediatric Surgery* 37 (December 2002): 1669–1672.

ORGANIZATIONS

American Academy of Pediatrics. 141 Northwest Point Boulevard, Elk Grove Village, IL 60007-1098. (847) 434-4000. http://www.aap.org (accessed March 6, 2008).

OTHER

National Birth Defects Prevention Network. January 27, 2003. http://www.nbdpn.org (accessed March 6, 2008).

Monique Laberge, PhD
Rosalyn Carson-DeWitt, MD

Abdominoplasty

Definition

Also known as a tummy tuck, abdominoplasty is a surgical procedure in which excess skin and fat in the abdominal area is removed and the abdominal muscles are tightened.

Purpose

Abdominoplasty is a cosmetic procedure that treats loose or sagging abdominal skin, resulting in a protruding abdomen that typically occurs after significant weight loss. Good candidates for abdominoplasty are individuals in good health who have one or more of the above conditions and who have tried to address these issues with diet and **exercise** with little or no results.

Women who have had multiple pregnancies often seek abdominoplasty as a means of ridding themselves of loose abdominal skin. While in many cases diet and exercise are sufficient in reducing abdominal fat and loose skin after pregnancy, in some women these conditions may persist. Abdominoplasty is not recommended for women who wish to have further pregnancies, as the beneficial effects of the surgery may be undone.

Another common reason for abdominoplasty is to remove excess skin from a person who has lost a large amount of weight or is obese. A large area of overhanging skin is called a pannus. Older patients are at

> **KEY TERMS**
>
> **Abdominal hernia**—A defect in the abdominal wall through which the abdominal organs protrude.
>
> **Morbidly obese**—A term defining individuals who are more than 100 lb (45 kg) over their ideal body weight.

an increased risk of developing a pannus because skin loses elasticity as one ages. Problems with hygiene or wound formation can result in a patient who has multiple hanging folds of abdominal skin and fat. If a large area of excess tissue is removed, the procedure is called a panniculectomy.

In some instances, abdominoplasty is performed simultaneously or directly following gynecologic surgery such as **hysterectomy** (removal of the uterus). One study found that the removal of a large amount of excess abdominal skin and fat from morbidly obese patients during gynecologic surgery results in better exposure to the operating field and improved wound healing.

Contraindications

Certain patients should not undergo abdominoplasty. Poor candidates for the surgery include:

- Women who wish to have subsequent pregnancies.
- Individuals who wish to lose a large amount of weight following surgery.
- Patients with unrealistic expectations (those who think the surgery will give them a "perfect" figure).
- Those who are unable to deal with the post-surgical scars.
- Patients who have had previous abdominal surgery.
- Heavy smokers.

Demographics

According to the American Academy of Plastic Surgeons, in 2005 there were approximately 169,314 abdominoplasties performed in the United States, relating to 4% of all **plastic surgery** patients and less than 0.5% of all plastic surgery procedures. Female patients accounted for 97% of all abdominoplasties. Most patients undergoing cosmetic plastic surgery were between the ages of 35 and 50 (47%), with patients between 19 and 35 years of age accounting for 24%, and patients between the ages of 51 and 64 accounting for 24%. Eighty percent of all plastic surgery patients during 2001 were white, 9% were Hispanic, 6% were African American, and 6% were Asian American.

Description

The patient is usually placed under **general anesthesia** for the duration of surgery. The advantages to general anesthesia are that the patient remains unconscious during the procedure, which may take from two to five hours to complete; no pain will be experienced nor will the patient have any memory of the procedure; and the patient's muscles remain completely relaxed, lending to safer surgery.

Once an adequate level of anesthesia has been reached, an incision is made across the lower abdomen. For a complete abdominoplasty, the incision will stretch from hipbone to hipbone. The skin will be lifted off the abdominal muscles from the incision up to the ribs, with a separate incision being made to free the umbilicus (belly button). The vertical abdominal muscles may be tightened by stitching them closer together. The skin is then stretched back over the abdomen and excess skin and fat are cut away. Another incision will be made across the stretched skin through which the umbilicus will be located and stitched into position. A temporary drain may be placed to remove excess fluid from beneath the incision. All incisions are then stitched closed and covered with **dressings**.

Individuals who have excess skin and fat limited to the lower abdomen (i.e., below the navel) may be candidates for partial abdominoplasty. During this procedure, the muscle wall is not tightened. Rather, the skin is stretched over a smaller incision made just above the pubic hairline, and excess skin is cut away. The incision is then closed with **stitches**. The umbilicus is not repositioned during a partial abdominoplasty; its shape, therefore, may change as the skin is stretched downward.

Additional procedures

In some cases, additional procedures may be performed during or directly following abdominoplasty. **Liposuction**, also called suction lipectomy or lipoplasty, is a technique that removes fat that cannot be removed by diet or exercise. During the procedure, which is generally performed in an outpatient surgical facility, the patient is anesthetized and a hollow tube called a cannula is inserted under the skin into a fat deposit. By physical manipulation, the fat deposit is loosened and sucked out of the body. Liposuction may be used during abdominoplasty to remove fat deposits from the torso, hips, or other areas. This may create a more desired body contour.

Some patients may choose to undergo breast augmentation, reduction, or lift during abdominoplasty. Breast augmentation involves the insertion of a silicone- or saline-filled implant into the breast, most often behind the breast tissue or chest muscle wall. A **breast reduction** may be performed on patients who have large breasts that cause an array of symptoms such as back and neck pain. Breast reduction removes excess breast skin and fat and moves the nipple and area around the nipple (called the areola) to a higher position. A breast lift, also called a mastopexy, is performed on women who have low, sagging breasts, often due to pregnancy, nursing, or aging. The surgical procedure is similar to a breast reduction, but only excess skin is removed; **breast implants** may also be inserted.

Breast reconstruction

A modified version of abdominoplasty may be used to reconstruct a breast in a patient who has undergone **mastectomy** (surgical removal of the breast, usually as a treatment for cancer). Transverse rectus abdominis myocutaneous (TRAM) flap reconstruction may be performed at the time of mastectomy or as a later, separate procedure. Good candidates for the surgery include women who have had or will have a large portion of breast tissue removed and also have excess skin and fat in the lower abdominal region. Women who are not in good health, are obese, have had a previous abdominoplasty, or wish to have additional children are not considered good candidates for TRAM flap reconstruction.

The procedure is usually performed in three separate steps. The first step is the TRAM flap surgery. In a procedure similar to traditional abdominoplasty, excess skin and fat is removed from the lower abdomen, and then stitched into place to create a breast. The construction of a nipple takes place several months later to enable to the tissue to heal adequately. Finally, once the new breast has healed and softened, tattooing may be performed to add color to the constructed nipple.

Costs

Because abdominoplasty is considered to be an elective cosmetic procedure, most insurance policies will not cover the procedure, unless it is being performed for medical reasons (for example, if an abdominal hernia is the cause of the protruding abdomen).

A number of fees must be taken into consideration when calculating the total cost of the procedure. Typically, fees include those paid to the surgeon, the anesthesiologist, and the facility where the surgery is performed. If liposuction or breast surgery is to be performed, additional costs may be incurred. The average cost of abdominoplasty is $6,500, but may range between $5,000–$9,000, depending on the surgeon and the complexity of the procedure.

Diagnosis/Preparation

There are a number of steps that the patient and plastic surgeon must take before an abdominoplasty may be performed. The surgeon will generally schedule an initial consultation, during which a **physical examination** will be performed. The surgeon will assess a number of factors that may impact the success of the surgery. These include:

- the patient's general health
- the size and shape of the abdomen and torso
- the location of abdominal fat deposits
- the patient's skin elasticity
- what medications the patient may be taking

It is important that the patient come prepared to ask questions of the surgeon during the initial consultation. The surgeon will describe the procedure, where it will be performed, associated risks, the method of anesthesia and pain relief, any additional procedures that may be performed, and post-surgical care. The patient may also meet with a staff member to discuss how much the procedure will cost and what options for payment are available.

The patient will also receive instructions on how to prepare for abdominoplasty. Certain medications should be avoided for several weeks before and after the surgery; for example, medications containing **aspirin** may interfere with the blood's ability to clot. Because tobacco can interfere with blood circulation and wound healing, smokers are recommended to quit for several weeks before and after the procedure. A medicated antibacterial soap may be prescribed prior to surgery to decrease levels of bacteria on the skin around the incision site.

Aftercare

The patient may remain in the hospital or surgical facility overnight, or return home the day of surgery after spending several hours recovering from the procedure and anesthesia. Before leaving the facility, the patient will receive the following instructions on post-surgical care:

- For the first several days after surgery, it is recommended that the patient remain flexed at the hips (i.e., avoid straightening the torso) to prevent unnecessary tension on the surgical site.
- Walking as soon as possible after the procedure is recommended to improve recovery time and prevent blood clots in the legs.
- Mild exercise that does not cause pain to the surgical site is recommended to improve muscle tone and decrease swelling.

- The patient should not shower until any drains are removed from the surgical site; sponge baths are permitted.
- Work may be resumed in two to four weeks, depending on the level of physical activity required.

Surgical drains will be removed within one week after abdominoplasty, and stitches from one to two weeks after surgery. Swelling, bruising, and pain in the abdominal area are to be expected and may last from two to six weeks. Recovery will be faster, however, in the patient who is in good health with relatively strong abdominal muscles. The incisions will remain a noticeable red or pink for several months, but will begin to fade by nine months to a year after the procedure. Because of their location, scars should be easily hidden under clothing, including bathing suits.

Risks

There are a number of complications that may arise during or after abdominoplasty. Complications are more often seen among patients who smoke, are overweight, are unfit, have diabetes or other health problems, or have scarring from previous abdominal surgery. Risks inherent to the use of general anesthesia include nausea, vomiting, sore throat, fatigue, headache, and muscle soreness; more rarely, blood pressure problems, allergic reaction, heart attack, or stroke may occur.

Risks associated with the procedure include:

- bleeding
- wound infection
- delayed wound healing
- skin or fat necrosis (death)
- hematoma (collection of blood in a tissue)
- seroma (collection of serum in a tissue)
- blood clots
- pulmonary embolism (a blood clot that travels to the lungs)
- numbness to the abdominal region or thighs (due to damage to nerves during surgery)

Normal results

In most cases, abdominoplasty is successful in providing a trimmer abdominal contour in patients with excess skin and fat and weak abdominal muscles. A number of factors will influence how long the optimal results of abdominoplasty will last, including age, skin elasticity, and physical fitness. Generally, however, good results will be long lasting if the patient remains in good health, maintains a stable weight,

WHO PERFORMS THE PROCEDURE AND WHERE IS IT PERFORMED?

Abdominoplasty is usually performed by a plastic surgeon, a medical doctor who has completed specialized training in the repair or reconstruction of physical defects or the cosmetic enhancement of the human body. In order for a plastic surgeon to be considered board certified by the American Board of Plastic Surgery, he or she must meet a set of strict criteria (including a minimum of five years of training in general surgery and plastic surgery) and pass a series of examinations. The procedure may be performed in a hospital operating room or a specialized outpatient surgical facility.

QUESTIONS TO ASK THE DOCTOR

- How long have you been practicing plastic surgery?
- Are you certified by the American Board of Plastic Surgeons?
- How many abdominoplasties have you performed, and how often?
- What is your rate of complications?
- How extensive will the post-surgical scars be?
- What method of anesthesia will be used?
- What are the costs associated with this procedure?
- Will my insurance pay for part or all of the surgery?
- Do you provide revision surgery (i.e., if I experience suboptimal results)?

and exercises regularly. One study surveying patient satisfaction following abdominoplasty indicated that 95% felt their symptoms (excess skin and fat) were improved, 86% were satisfied with the results of the surgery, and 86% would recommend the procedure to a friend.

Morbidity and mortality rates

The overall rate of complications associated with abdominoplasty is approximately 32%. This percentage, however, is higher among patients who are overweight; one study placed the complication rate among obese patients at 80%. Rates are also higher among patients who smoke or are diabetic. The rate of major complications requiring hospitalization has been reported at 1.4%.

Alternatives

Before seeking abdominoplasty, an individual will want to be sure that loose and excess abdominal skin and fat cannot be decreased through a regimen of diet and exercise. Abdominoplasty should not be viewed as an alternative to weight loss. In fact, some doctors would suggest that a patient be no more than 15% over his or her ideal body weight in order to undergo the procedure.

Liposuction is a surgical alternative to abdominoplasty. There are several advantages to liposuction. It is less expensive (an average of $2,000 per body area treated compared to $6,500 for abdominoplasty). It also is associated with a faster recovery, use of less anesthesia, a smaller rate of complications, and significantly smaller incisions. What liposuction cannot do is remove excess skin. Liposuction is a good choice for patients with localized deposits of fat, while abdominoplasty is a better choice for patients with excess abdominal skin and fat.

Resources

BOOKS

Khatri, VP and JA Asensio. *Operative Surgery Manual.* 1st ed. Philadelphia: Saunders, 2003.

Townsend, CM et al. *Sabiston Textbook of Surgery.* 17th ed. Philadelphia: Saunders, 2004.

ORGANIZATIONS

American Academy of Cosmetic Surgery. 737 N. Michigan Ave., Suite 820, Chicago, IL 60611. (312) 981-6760. http://www.cosmeticsurgery.org (accessed March 6, 2008).

American Board of Plastic Surgery, Inc. 7 Penn Center, Suite 400, 1635 Market St., Philadelphia, PA 19103-2204. (215) 587-9322. http://www.abplsurg.org (accessed March 6, 2008).

American Society of Plastic Surgeons. 444 E. Algonquin Rd., Arlington Heights, IL 60005. (888) 4-PLASTIC. http://www.plasticsurgery.org (accessed March 6, 2008).

OTHER

"2001 Statistics." American Society of Plastic Surgeons, 2003. http://www.plasticsurgery.org/media/statistics/2001statistics.cfm (accessed March 6, 2008).

"Abdominoplasty." *American Society of Plastic Surgeons,* 2003. http://www.plasticsurgery.org/public_education/procedures/Abdominoplasty.cfm (accessed March 6, 2008).

Gallagher, Susan. "Panniculectomy: Implications for Care." *Perspectives in Nursing,* 2003. http://www.

perspectivesinnursing.org/v3n3/panniculectomy.html (accessed March 6, 2008).

"Training Requirements." *American Board of Plastic Surgery,* July 2002. http://www.abplsurg.org/training_require ments.html (accessed March 6, 2008).

"Tummy Tuck." *The American Society for Aesthetic Plastic Surgery,* 2000. http://www.surgery.org/q1 (accessed March 6, 2008).

Zenn, Michael R. "Breast Reconstruction: TRAM, Unipe-dicled." *eMedicine,* December 13, 2001. http://www. emedicine.com/plastic/topic141.htm (accessed March 6, 2008).

Stephanie Dionne Sherk
Rosalyn Carson-DeWitt, MD

WHO PERFORMS THE PROCEDURE AND WHERE IS IT PERFORMED?

ABO blood typing involves personnel from several allied health disciplines. A phlebotomist usually obtains an initial blood sample. A medical technologist typically runs the tests to determine specific blood types. A physician or surgeon commonly prescribes blood or blood products. A nurse typically administers the blood or blood products to a recipient.

ABO blood typing

Definition

Of the many different bases for typing blood, the most commonly used and the most important are the ABO groups. Specific combinations of antigens and antibodies defines the blood type of all humans and many primates.

Purpose

The purpose of the ABO typing system is to allow successful sharing of blood and blood products by avoiding rejections after transfusions.

Description

The ABO blood groups were discovered by Karl Landsteiner in 1900 and 1901 at the University of Vienna. All humans and most other primates can be

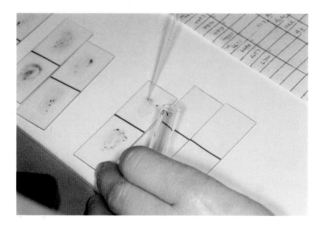

Testing blood type. *(Image Source Black / Alamy)*

typed using the ABO blood group system. Four principal blood types have been defined on the basis of antigens and antibodies.

- Type A blood is positive for antigen A and anti-B antibody and is negative for Antigen B and anti-A antibody.

- Type B blood is positive for antigen B and anti-A antibody and is negative for Antigen A and anti-B antibody.

- Type O blood is negative for both antigen A and antigen B and is positive for both anti-A antibody and anti-B antibody.

- Type AB blood is positive for both antigen A and antigen B and is negative for both anti-A antibody and anti-B antibody.

The presence or absence of antigens and antibodies determines the type of blood that a person can give (donate) or receive. People will not destroy blood of their own type but will destroy other types of blood. For example, the absence of anti-A antibodies allows people with type A blood to receive type A blood. However, the anti-B antibodies in type A blood will destroy type B blood. This immune system mechanism protects people from alien organisms.

Individuals with type O blood do not produce any ABO antigens. As a consequence, their blood usually will not be rejected when it is given to others with different ABO types. People with type O blood are called universal donors for transfusions. However, they can only receive type O blood. Persons having type AB blood do not have any ABO antibodies. They are universal receivers for transfusions, but their blood will be rejected when given to people with every other type because they produce both kinds of antigens.

KEY TERMS

Agglutination—An immunochemical reaction. It is termed positive when two chemicals that are mixed cause clumps to form.

Hematoma—An accumulation of blood outside of the circulatory system

Phlebotomist—a person trained to obtain a blood sample.

Rhesus factor—A secondary component of ABO typing that was first observed in rhesus monkeys.

To determine an individual's ABO type, serum containing anti-A antibodies is mixed with a few drops pf their blood. Another serum containing anti-B antibodies is mixed with a different few drops of blood. The results determine the ABO type by a process of elimination.

ABO blood types are inherited through genes on chromosome 9, and they do not change as a result of environmental influences during life.

The Rhesus factor is a associates with ABO blood typing. This further describes the reactivity of each type. The Rhesus factors are positive (+) and negative (-). The Rhesus factor is abbreviated as Rh. The Rh factors of a donor and recipient must match to avoid sensitization or rejection. Thus, for example, type O blood includes O+ and O-. Including the Rh factor, the ABO system includes 8 different blood types: A +, A-, B +. B-, AB +, AB-, O + and O-.

Precautions

ABO typing is not routinely used to determine genetic inheritance patterns from their parents. In fact, paternity in the U.S. and many other nations can no longer be legally established based on conventional blood typing. HLA types or DNA sequencing are more precise than ABO typing. DNA is the most costly test to use.

Risks

The risks associated with obtaining a blood sample are minimal. They include fainting, feeling light-headed, pain from the needle used to obtain a blood sample (venipuncture), bleeding at the site of venipuncture, blood accumulating at the venipuncture site (hematoma), and infection.

Side effects

The most common physical side effect of ABO typing is a bruise at the site of venipuncture used to obtain a blood sample. A lab error has the potential to sensitize or kill a recipient if blood of the wrong type is given.

Interactions

ABO blood typing does not interact with pharmaceutical products.

Resources

BOOKS

Fischbach, F. T. and M. B. Dunning. *A Manual of Laboratory and Diagnostic Tests*. 8th ed. Philadelphia: Lippincott Williams & Wilkins, 2008.

McGhee, M. *A Guide to Laboratory Investigations*. 5th ed. Oxford, UK: Radcliffe Publishing Ltd, 2008.

Price, C. P. *Evidence-Based Laboratory Medicine: Principles, Practice, and Outcomes*. 2nd ed. Washington, DC: AACC Press, 2007.

Scott, M.G., A. M. Gronowski, and C. S. Eby. *Tietz's Applied Laboratory Medicine*. 2nd ed. New York: Wiley-Liss, 2007.

Springhouse, A. M.. *Diagnostic Tests Made Incredibly Easy!*. 2nd ed. Philadelphia: Lippincott Williams & Wilkins, 2008.

PERIODICALS

Cho, D., J. S. Lee, M. H. Yazar, et al. "Chimerism and mosaicism are important causes of ABO phenotype and genotype discrepancies." *Immunohematology* 22, no. 4 (2006): 183–187.

Deng, Z. H., J. Q. Zeng, Q. Yu, et al. "Genotyping of samples lacking expected antibodies in ABO blood group." *Journal of Clinical Laboratory Analysis* 21, no. 6 (2007): 363–366.

Fung, M. K., K. A. Downws, and I. A. Shulman. "Transfusion of platelets containing ABO-incompatible plasma: a survey of 3156 North American laboratories." *Archives of Pathology and Laboratory Medicine* 131, no. 6 (2007): 909–916.

Grim, S. A., T. Pham, J. Thielke, et al. "Infectious complications associated with the use of rituximab for ABO-incompatible and positive cross-match renal transplant recipients." *Clinical Transplantation* 21, no. 5 (2007): 628–632.

Yazer, M. H., and D. J. Triulzi. "Immune hemolysis following ABO-mismatched stem cell or solid organ transplantation." *Current Opinions in Hematology* 14, no. 6 (2007): 664–670.

ORGANIZATIONS

American Association for Clinical Chemistry. http://www.aacc.org/AACC/.

American Society for Clinical Laboratory Science. http://www.ascls.org/.

American Society of Clinical Pathologists. http://www.ascp.org/.

College of American Pathologists. http://www.cap.org/apps/cap.portal.

OTHER

American Clinical Laboratory Association. "Information about clinical chemistry." 2008 [cited February 24, 2008]. http://www.clinical-labs.org/.

Clinical Laboratory Management Association. "Information about clinical chemistry." 2008 [cited February 22, 2008]. http://www.clma.org/.

Lab Tests On Line. "Information about lab tests." 2008 [cited February 24, 2008]. http://www.labtestsonline.org/.

National Accreditation Agency for Clinical Laboratory Sciences. "Information about laboratory tests." 2008 [cited February 25, 2008]. http://www.naacls.org/.

L. Fleming Fallon, Jr, MD, DrPH

Abortion, induced

Definition

Induced abortion is the intentional termination of a pregnancy before the fetus can live independently. An abortion may be elective, based on a woman's personal choice; or therapeutic, to preserve the health or save the life of a pregnant woman.

Purpose

An abortion may be performed whenever there is some compelling reason to end a pregnancy. An abortion is termed "induced" to differentiate it from a spontaneous abortion in which the products of conception are lost naturally. A spontaneous abortion is also called a miscarriage.

An abortion is considered to be elective if a woman chooses to end her pregnancy, and it is not for maternal or fetal health reasons. Some reasons a woman might choose to have an elective abortion are:

- continuation of the pregnancy may cause emotional or financial hardship;
- the woman is not ready to become a parent;
- the pregnancy was unintended;
- the woman is pressured into aborting by her partner, parents, or others; and
- the pregnancy was the result of rape or incest.

A therapeutic abortion is performed in order to preserve the health or save the life of a pregnant woman. A health care provider might recommend a therapeutic abortion if the fetus is diagnosed with significant abnormalities or not expected to live, or if it has died *in utero*. Therapeutic abortion may also be used to reduce the number of fetuses if a woman is pregnant with multiples; this procedure is called multifetal pregnancy reduction (MFPR).

A therapeutic abortion may be indicated if a woman has a pregnancy-related health condition that endangers her life. Some examples of such conditions include:

- severe hypertension (high blood pressure);
- cardiac disease;
- severe depression or other psychiatric conditions;
- serious kidney or liver disease;
- certain types of infection;
- malignancy (cancer); and
- multifetal pregnancy.

Demographics

Abortion has been a legal procedure in the United States since 1973. Since then, more than 39 million abortions have taken place. It is estimated that approximately 1.3–1.4 million abortions occur in the United States annually. Induced abortions terminate approximately half of the estimated three million unplanned pregnancies each year and approximately one-fifth of all pregnancies.

The total number of abortions performed has declined from 1.31 million in 2000, to 1.21 million performed in 2005. From 1973 through 2005, more than 45 million legal abortions took place. The estimated number of abortions during 2004–2006 were 1,287,000. In 2000 an estimated 21 out of 1,000 women aged 15–44 had an abortion. Out of every 100 pregnancies that year that ended in live birth or abortion, approximately 24 were elective terminations. The highest abortion rates in 2000 occurred in New Jersey, New York, California, Delaware, Florida, and Nevada (greater than 30 per 1,000 women of reproductive age). Kentucky, South Dakota, Wyoming, Idaho, Mississippi, Utah, and West Virginia had the lowest rates (less than seven per 1,000 women).

In 2000 and 2001, the highest percentage of abortions were performed on women between the ages of 20 and 30, with women ages 20–24 having the highest rate (47 per 1,000 women). Adolescents ages 15–19 accounted for 19% of elective abortions, while 25% were performed on women older than 30. Approximately 73% of women having an abortion had previously been pregnant; 48% of those had a previous abortion.

Abortion, induced

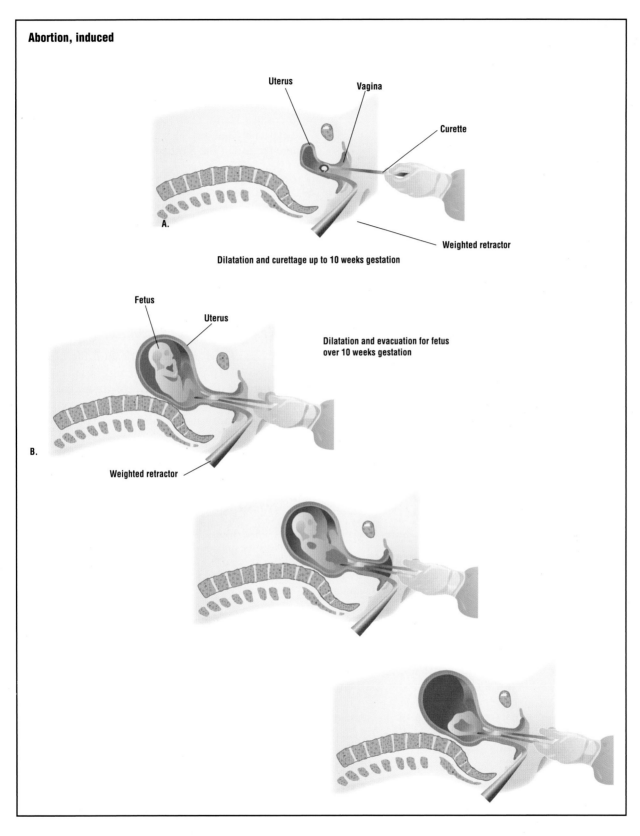

Uterus

Vagina

Curette

A.

Weighted retractor

Dilatation and curettage up to 10 weeks gestation

Fetus

Uterus

Dilatation and evacuation for fetus
over 10 weeks gestation

B.

Weighted retractor

A dilatation and curettage is used to perform an abortion up to 10 weeks gestation (A). Over 10 weeks, the physician may use dilatation and evacuation to achieve the abortion (B). *(Illustration by GGS Information Services. Cengage Learning, Gale.)*

KEY TERMS

Curette—A spoon-shaped instrument used to remove tissue from the inner lining of the uterus.

Endocarditis—An infection of the inner membrane lining of the heart.

Fibroid tumors—Non-cancerous (benign) growths in the uterus; they occur in 30–40% of women over age 40 and do not need to be removed unless they are causing symptoms that interfere with a woman's normal activities.

Lupus erythematosus—A chronic inflammatory disease in which inappropriate immune system reactions cause abnormalities in the blood vessels and connective tissue.

Prostaglandin—Responsible for various hormonal reactions such as muscle contraction.

Rh negative—Lacking the Rh factor, which are genetically determined antigens in red blood cells that produce immune responses. If an Rh-negative woman is pregnant with an Rh-positive fetus, her body will produce antibodies against the fetus's blood, causing a disease known as Rh disease. Sensitization to the disease occurs when the women's blood is exposed to the fetus's blood. Rh immune globulin (RhoGAM) is a vaccine that must be given to a woman after an abortion, miscarriage, or prenatal tests in order to prevent sensitization to Rh disease.

Non-Hispanic, white women reported the highest percentage of abortions in 2000 and 2001 (41%). African American women accounted for 32%, Hispanic women for 20%, Asian and Pacific Islander women for 6%, and Native American women for 1%. The highest abortion rates occurred among African American women (49 per 1,000 women), with Hispanic and Asian women also reporting higher-than-average rates (33 and 31 per 1,000 women, respectively). The rate was the lowest among white women (13 per 1,000 women). As of 2005, 50% of women in the United States who obtained abortions were younger than age 25, 33% of those having abortions were between the ages of 20–25, and 17% were teenagers. About 60% of women having abortions were women who already had one or more children.

Description

Abortions are safest when performed within the first six to 10 weeks after the last menstrual period (LMP). This calculation is used by health care providers to determine the stage of pregnancy. About 90% of women who have abortions do so in the first trimester of pregnancy (before 13 weeks) and experience few complications. Abortions performed between 13 and 24 weeks (during the second trimester) have a higher rate of complications. Abortions after 24 weeks are extremely rare and are usually limited to situations where the life of the mother is in danger.

Although it is safer to have an abortion during the first trimester, some second trimester abortions may be inevitable. The results of genetic testing are often not available until 16 weeks gestation. In addition, women, especially teens, may not have recognized the pregnancy or come to terms with it emotionally soon enough to have a first trimester abortion. Teens make up the largest group having second trimester abortions.

Very early abortions cost between $200 and $400. Later abortions cost more. The cost increases about $100 per week between the thirteenth and sixteenth week. Second trimester abortions are much more costly because they often involve more risk, more services, anesthesia, and sometimes a hospital stay. Private insurance carriers may or may not cover the procedure. Federal law prohibits federal funds (including **Medicaid**) from being used to pay for an elective abortion.

Medical abortions

Medical abortions are brought about by taking medications that end the pregnancy. The advantages of a first trimester medical abortion are:

- the procedure is non-invasive, so no surgical instruments are used;
- anesthesia is not required;
- drugs are administered either orally or by injection; and
- the outcome resembles a natural miscarriage.

Disadvantages of a medical abortion are:

- the effectiveness decreases after the seventh week;
- the procedure may require multiple visits to the doctor;
- bleeding after the abortion lasts longer than after a surgical abortion; and
- the woman may see the contents of her womb as it is expelled.

As of 2003, two drugs were available in the United States to induce abortion: methotrexate and mifepristone.

METHOTREXATE. Methotrexate (Rheumatrex) targets rapidly dividing fetal cells, thus preventing the fetus from further developing. It is used in conjunction with misoprostol (Cytotec), a prostaglandin that stimulates contractions of the uterus. Methotrexate may be taken up to 49 days after the first day of the last menstrual period.

On the first visit to the doctor, the woman receives an injection of methotrexate. On the second visit, about a week later, she is given misoprostol tablets vaginally to stimulate contractions of the uterus. Within two weeks, the woman will expel the contents of her uterus, ending the pregnancy. A follow-up visit to the doctor is necessary to assure that the abortion is complete.

With this procedure, a woman will feel cramping and may feel nauseated from the misoprostol. This combination of drugs is approximately 92–96% effective in ending pregnancy. Approximately 50% of women will experience the abortion soon after taking the misoprostol; 35–40% will have the abortion up to seven days later.

Methotrexate is not recommended for women with liver or kidney disease, inflammatory bowel disease, clotting disorders, documented immunodeficiency, or certain blood disorders.

MIFEPRISTONE. Mifepristone (RU-486), which goes by the brand name Mifeprex, works by blocking the action of progesterone, a hormone needed for pregnancy to continue. It was approved by the Food and Drug Administration (FDA) in September 2000 as an alternative to surgical abortion. Mifepristone can be taken up to 49 days after the first day of a woman's last period.

On the first visit to the doctor, a woman takes a mifepristone pill. Two days later she returns and, if the miscarriage has not occurred, takes two misoprostol pills, which causes the uterus to contract. Approximately 10% will experience the abortion before receiving the dose of misoprostol.

Within four days, 90% of women have expelled the contents of their uterus and completed the abortion. Within 14 days, 95–97% of women have completed the abortion. A third follow-up visit to the doctor is necessary to confirm through observation or **ultrasound** that the procedure is complete. In the event that it is not, a surgical abortion is performed. Studies show that 4.5–8% of women need surgery or a blood **transfusion** after taking mifepristone, and the pregnancy persists in about 1%. Surgical abortion is then recommended because the fetus may be damaged. Side effects include nausea, vaginal bleeding, and heavy cramping. The bleeding is typically heavier than a normal period and may last up to 16 days.

Mifepristone is not recommended for women with ectopic pregnancy or an intrauterine device (IUD), or those who have been taking long-term steroidal therapy, have bleeding abnormalities, or on blood-thinners such as Coumadin.

In 2005, 57% of abortion providers performed one or more medication induced abortions (a 70% increase from medication induced abortions during the first half of 2001). In 2005, 13% of all abortions were attributable to medication induced abortions and the incidence of medication induced abortions performed outside a traditional hospital setting was estimated to total about 161,100.

Surgical abortions

MANUAL VACUUM ASPIRATION. Up to 10 weeks gestation, a pregnancy can be ended by a procedure called manual vacuum aspiration (MVA). This procedure is also called menstrual extraction, mini-suction, or early abortion. The contents of the uterus are suctioned out through a thin plastic tube that is inserted through the cervix; suction is applied by a syringe. The procedure generally lasts about 15 minutes.

A 1998 study of women undergoing MVA indicated that the procedure was 99.5% effective in terminating pregnancy and was associated with a very low risk of complications (less than 1%). Menstrual extractions are safe, but because the amount of fetal material is so small at this stage of development, it is easy to miss. This results in an incomplete abortion that means the pregnancy continues.

DILATATION AND SUCTION CURETTAGE. Dilation and suction curettage may also be called D & C, suction dilation, vacuum curettage, or suction curettage. The procedure involves gentle stretching of the cervix with a series of dilators or specific medications. The contents of the uterus are then removed with a tube attached to a suction machine, and walls of the uterus are cleaned using a narrow loop called a curette.

Advantages of an abortion of this type are:

- it is usually done as a one-day outpatient procedure;
- the procedure takes only 10–15 minutes;
- bleeding after the abortion lasts five days or less; and
- the woman does not see the contents of her womb being removed.

Disadvantages include:

- the procedure is invasive, so surgical instruments are used; and
- infection may occur.

The procedure is 97–99% effective. The amount of discomfort a woman feels varies considerably. **Local anesthesia** is often given to numb the cervix, but it does not mask uterine cramping. After a few hours of rest, the woman may return home.

DILATATION AND EVACUATION. Some second trimester abortions are performed as a dilatation and evacuation (D & E). The procedures are similar to those used in a D & C, but a larger suction tube must be used because more material must be removed. This increases the amount of cervical dilation necessary and increases the risk and discomfort of the procedure. A combination of suction and manual extraction using medical instruments is used to remove the contents of the uterus.

OTHER SURGICAL OPTIONS. Other surgical procedures are available for performing second trimester abortions, although are rarely used. These include:

- Dilatation and extraction (D & X)—the cervix is prepared by means similar to those used in a dilatation and evacuation; however, the fetus is removed mostly intact although the head must be collapsed to fit through the cervix. This procedure is sometimes called a partial-birth abortion. D & X accounted for only 0.17% of all abortions in 2000.

- Induction—in this procedure, an abortion occurs by means of inducing labor. Prior to induction, the patient may have rods inserted into her cervix to help dilate it or receive medications to soften the cervix and speed up labor. On the day of the abortion, drugs (usually prostaglandin or a salt solution) are injected into the uterus to induce contractions. The fetus is delivered within eight to 72 hours. Side effects of this procedure include nausea, vomiting, and diarrhea from the prostaglandin, and pain from uterine contractions. Anesthesia of the sort used in childbirth can be given to reduce pain. Many women are able to go home a few hours after the procedure.

- Hysterotomy—a surgical incision is made into the uterus and the contents of the uterus removed through the incision. This procedure is generally used if induction methods fail to deliver the fetus.

Diagnosis/Preparation

The doctor must know accurately the stage of a woman's pregnancy before an abortion is performed. The doctor will ask the woman questions about her menstrual cycle and also do a **physical examination** to confirm the stage of pregnancy. This may be done at an office visit before the abortion or on the day of the abortion.

Pre-abortion counseling is important in helping a woman resolve any questions she may have about having the procedure. Some states require a waiting period (most often of 24 hours) following counseling before the abortion may be obtained. Most states require parental consent or notification if the patient is under the age of 18.

Aftercare

Regardless of the method used to perform the abortion, a woman will be observed for a period of time to make sure her blood pressure is stable and that bleeding is controlled. The doctor may prescribe **antibiotics** to reduce the chance of infection. Women who are Rh negative (lacking genetically determined antigens in their red blood cells that produce immune responses) should be given an injection of human Rh immune globulin (RhoGAM) after the procedure unless the father of the fetus is also Rh negative. This prevents blood incompatibility complications in future pregnancies.

Bleeding will continue for about five days in a surgical abortion and longer in a medical abortion. To decrease the risk of infection, a woman should avoid intercourse, tampons, and douches for two weeks after the abortion.

A follow-up visit is a necessary part of the woman's aftercare. Contraception will be offered to women who wish to avoid future pregnancies, because menstrual periods normally resume within a few weeks.

Risks

Complications from abortions can include:

- uncontrolled bleeding;
- infection;
- blood clots accumulating in the uterus;
- a tear in the cervix or uterus;
- missed abortion (the pregnancy is not terminated); and
- incomplete abortion where some material from the pregnancy remains in the uterus.

Women who experience any of the following symptoms of post-abortion complications should call the clinic or doctor who performed the abortion immediately:

- severe pain;
- fever over 100.4°F (38.2°C);
- heavy bleeding that soaks through more than one sanitary pad per hour;
- foul-smelling discharge from the vagina; and
- continuing symptoms of pregnancy.

WHO PERFORMS THE PROCEDURE AND WHERE IS IT PERFORMED?

An induced abortion must be done under the supervision of a physician. Under normal circumstances, the abortion is performed by a licensed obstetrician or gynecologist. In some states, advanced clinicians such as nurse practitioners, certified nurse midwives, or physician assistants can perform an abortion under the direct supervision of a physician.

Most women are able to have abortions at clinics or outpatient facilities if the procedure is performed early in pregnancy and the woman is in relatively good health. Women with heart disease, previous endocarditis, asthma, lupus erythematosus, uterine fibroid tumors, blood clotting disorders, poorly controlled epilepsy, or some psychological disorders usually need to be hospitalized in order to receive special monitoring and medications during the procedure. In 2000, over 93% of abortions were performed in a clinic setting; clinics accounted for nearly half (46%) of all abortion providers. Hospitals were the site of 5% of abortions (accounting for 33% of abortion providers), while only 3% of abortions were performed at physician offices (21% of abortion providers).

Normal results

Usually the pregnancy is ended without complication and without altering future fertility.

Morbidity and mortality rates

Serious complications resulting from abortions performed before 13 weeks are rare. Of the 90% of women who have abortions in this time period, 2.5% have minor complications that can be handled without hospitalization. Less than 0.5% have complications that require a hospital stay. The rate of complications increases as the pregnancy progresses.

Only one maternal **death** occurs per 530,000 abortions performed at eight weeks gestation or less; this increases to one death per 17,000 abortions performed from 16 to 20 weeks, and one death per 6,000 abortions performed over 20 weeks.

Alternatives

Adoption is an option for pregnant women who do not want to raise a child but are unwilling or unable

QUESTIONS TO ASK THE DOCTOR

- What abortion options are available to me based on my stage of pregnancy?
- What are the short- and long-term complications of the procedure?
- What type of pain relief/anesthesia is available to me?
- Who can be in the procedure room with me?
- What will the abortion cost? What do the fees include?
- Is pre-abortion counseling offered?
- How is follow-up or emergency care provided?
- Does the doctor who will perform the abortion have admitting privileges at a hospital in case of a problem?

to have an abortion. Adoption agencies, crisis pregnancy centers, family service agencies, family planning clinics, or state social service agencies are available for women to contact for more information about the adoption process.

Resources

PERIODICALS

Elam-Evans, Laurie D., Lilo T. Strauss, Joy Herndon, Wilda Y. Parker, Sara Whitehead, and Cynthia J. Berg. "Abortion Surveillance—United States, 1999." *Morbidity and Mortality Weekly Report* 51 (November 29, 2002): 1–9.

Finer, L. B. and S. K. Henshaw. "Abortion Incidence and Services in the United States in 2000." *Perspectives on Sexual and Reproductive Health* 35, no. 1 (January/February 2003): 6–15.

Jones, R. K., J. E. Darroch, and S. K. Henshaw. "Patterns in the Socioeconomic Characteristics of Women Obtaining Abortions in 2000–2001." *Perspectives on Sexual and Reproductive Health* 34, no. 5 (September/October 2002): 226–235.

OTHER

"Abortion After the First Trimester in the United States." *Planned Parenthood Federation of America* May 2007. http://www.plannedparenthood.org/issues-action/abortion/trimester-abortion-6140.htm.

"Choosing Abortion: Questions and Answers." *Planned Parenthood Federation of America* February 2003. http://www.plannedparenthood.org/health-topics/abortion/choosing-abortion.htm (February 26, 2003).

"Facts on Induced Abortion in the United States." *Gutt-macher Institute*. January 2008. http://www.guttmacher.org/pubs/fb_induced_abortion.html.

James, Denise and Natalie E. Roche. "Therapeutic Abortion." *eMedicine* May 22, 2002. http://www.emedicine.com/med/topic3311.htm (February 26, 2003).

"Manual Vacuum Aspiration." *Reproductive Health Technologies Project* 2002 http://www.rhtp.org/abortion/mva/default.asp (February 26, 2003).

Trupin, Suzanne R. "Abortion." *eMedicine* December 2, 2002. http://www.emedicine.com/med/topic5.htm (February 26, 2003).

ORGANIZATIONS

Alan Guttmacher Institute, 1301 Connecticut Ave., NW, Suite 700, Washington, DC, 20036, (202) 296-4012, http://www.guttmacher.org.

Centers for Disease Control and Prevention, Division of Reproductive Health, 4770 Buford Highway, NE, Mail Stop K-20, Atlanta, GA, 30341-3717, (770) 488-5200, http://www.cdc.gov/reproductivehealth/.

National Abortion Federation, 1660 L Street, NW, Suite 450, Washington, DC, 20036, (202) 667-5881, http://www.prochoice.org.

Planned Parenthood Federation of America, 434 West 33rd St., New York, NY, 10001, (212) 541-7800, http://www.plannedparenthood.org.

Debra Gordon
Stephanie Dionne Sherk
Laura Jean Cataldo, R.N., Ed.D.

Abscess incision and drainage

Definition

An abscess is an infected skin nodule containing pus. It may need to be drained via an incision (cut) if the pus does not resolve with treatment by **antibiotics**. This allows the pus to escape, the infection to be treated, and the abscess to heal.

Purpose

An abscess is a pus-filled sore, usually caused by a bacterial infection. The pus is comprised of both living and dead organisms. It also contains destroyed tissue due to the action of white blood cells that were carried to the area to fight the infection. Abscesses are often found in the soft tissue under the skin such as the armpit or the groin. However, they may develop in any organ, and are commonly found in the breast and gums. Abscesses are far more serious and call for more specific treatment if they are located in deep organs such as the lung, liver, or brain.

White blood cells—Cells that protect the body against infection.

Because the lining of an abscess cavity tends to interfere with the amount of drug that can penetrate the source of infection from the blood, the cavity itself may require draining. Once an abscess has fully formed, it often does not respond to antibiotics. Even if the antibiotic does penetrate into the abscess, it does not function as well in that environment.

Demographics

Abcess drainage is a minor and common surgical procedure that is often performed in a professional medical office. Accurate records concerning the number of procedures are kept in private medical office rather than hospital records. For these reasons, it is impossible to accurately tally the number of abscess incision and drainage procedures performed in a year. The procedure increases in frequency with increasing age.

Description

A doctor will cut into the lining of an abscess, allowing the pus to escape either through a drainage tube or by leaving the cavity open to the skin. The size of the incision depends on the volume of the abscess and how quickly the pus is encountered.

Cells normally formed for the surface of the skin often migrate into an abscess. They line the abscess cavity. This process is called epithelialization. This lining prevents drugs from reaching an abscess. It also promotes recurrence of the abscess. The lining must be removed when an abscess is drained to prevent recurrence.

Once an abscess is opened, the pus drained, and the epithelial lining removed, the doctor will clean and irrigate the wound thoroughly with saline. If it is not too large or deep, the doctor may simply pack the abscess wound with gauze for 24–48 hours to absorb the pus and discharge.

If it is a deeper abscess, the doctor or surgeon may insert a drainage tube after cleaning out the wound. Once the tube is in place, the surgeon closes the incision with simple **stitches** and applies a sterile dressing. Drainage is maintained for several days to

Abscesses are most commonly incised and drained by general surgeons. Occasionally, a family physician or dermatologist may drain a superficial abscess. These procedures may be performed in a professional office or in an outpatient facility. The skin and surrounding area may be numbed by a topical anesthetic.

Brain abscesses are usually drained by neurosurgeons. Thoracic surgeons drain abscesses in the lung. Otolaryngologists drain abscesses in the neck. These procedures are performed in a hospital operating room. General anesthesia is used.

help prevent the abscess from reforming. The tube is removed, and the abscess allowed to finish closing and healing.

Diagnosis/Preparation

An abscess can usually be diagnosed visually, although an imaging technique such as a computed tomography (CT) scan or **ultrasound** may be used to confirm the extent of the abscess before drainage. Such procedures may also be needed to localize internal abscesses such as those in the abdominal cavity or brain.

Prior to incision, the skin over an abscess will be cleansed by swabbing gently with an antiseptic solution.

Aftercare

Much of the pain around an abscess will be gone after the surgery. Healing is usually very rapid. After the drainage tube is removed, antibiotics may be continued for several days. Applying heat and keeping the affected area elevated may help relieve inflammation.

Risks

Any scarring is likely to become much less noticeable as time goes on, and eventually become almost invisible. Occasionally, an abscess within a vital organ (such as the brain) damages enough surrounding tissue that there is some permanent loss of normal function.

Other risks include incomplete drainage and prolonged infection. Occasionally, an abscess may require

a second incision and drainage procedure. This is frequently due to retained epithelial cells that line the abscess cavity.

Normal results

Most abscesses heal after drainage alone. Others may require more prolonged drainage and antibiotic drug treatment.

Morbidity and mortality rates

Morbidity associated with an abscess incision and drainage is very uncommon. Post-surgical problems are usually associated with infection or an adverse reaction to antibiotic drugs prescribed. Mortality is virtually unknown.

Alternatives

There is no reliable alternative to surgical incision and drainage of an abscess. Heat alone may cause small superficial abscesses to resolve. The degree of epithelialization usually determines if the abscess reappears.

Resources

BOOKS

Bland, K. I., W. G. Cioffi, and M. G. Sarr. *Practice of General Surgery*. Philadelphia: Saunders, 2001.

Braunwald, E., Longo, D. L., and J. L. Jameson. *Harrison's Principles of Internal Medicine, 15th Edition*. New York: McGraw-Hill, 2001.

Goldman, L., and J. C. Bennett. *Cecil Textbook of Medicine, 21st Edition*. Philadelphia: Saunders, 1999.

Schwartz, S. I., J. E. Fischer, F. C. Spencer, G. T. Shires, and J. M. Daly. *Principles of Surgery, 7th Edition*. New York: McGraw Hill, 1998.

Townsend, C., K. L. Mattox, R. D. Beauchamp, B. M. Evers, and D. C. Sabiston. *Sabiston's Review of Surgery, 3rd Edition*. Philadelphia: Saunders, 2001.

PERIODICALS

Cmejrek, R. C., J. M. Coticchia, and J. E. Arnold. "Presentation, Diagnosis, and Management of Deep-neck Abscesses in Infants." *Archives of*

Otolaryngology Head and Neck Surgery, 128(12) 2002: 1361–1364.

Douglass, A. B., and J. M. Douglass. "Common Dental Emergencies." *American Family Physician,* 67(3) 2003: 511–516.

Usdan, L. S., and C. Massinople. "Multiple Pyogenic Liver Abscesses Associated with Occult Appendicitis and Possible Crohn's Disease." *Tennessee Medicine,* 95(11) 2002: 463–464.

Wang, L. F., W. R. Kuo, C. S. Lin, K. W. Lee, and K. J. Huang. "Space Infection of the Head and Neck." *Kaohsiung Journal of Medical Sciences,* 18(8) 2002: 386–392.

ORGANIZATIONS

American Academy of Otolaryngology-Head and Neck Surgery. One Prince St., Alexandria, VA 22314-3357. (703) 836-4444. http://www.entnet.org/index2. cfm.

American College of Surgeons. 633 North St. Clair Street, Chicago, IL 60611-32311. (312) 202-5000; Fax: (312) 202-5001. Web site: http://www.facs.org. E-mail: postmaster@facs.org.

American Medical Association. 515 N. State Street, Chicago, IL 60610. (312) 464-5000. http://www.ama-assn.org.

American Osteopathic College of Otolaryngology-Head and Neck Surgery. 405 W. Grand Avenue, Dayton, OH 45405. (937) 222-8820 or (800) 455-9404; Fax (937) 222-8840. Email: info@aocoohns.org.

American Society of Colon and Rectal Surgeons. 85 W. Algonquin Rd., Suite 550, Arlington Heights, IL 60005. (847) 290-9184; Fax: (847) 290-9203. http://www.fascrs. org. Email: ascrs@fascrs.org.

OTHER

American Society of Colon and Rectal Surgeons, (April 4, 2003). http://www.fascrs.org/brochures/anal-abscess.html.

Merck Manual, (April 5, 2003). http://www.merck.com/ pubs/mmanual/section6/chapter74/74a.htm.

National Library of Medicine, (April 4, 2003). http://www. nlm.nih.gov/medlineplus/ency/article/001353.htm.

Oregon Health and Science University, (April 4, 2003). http://www.ohsu.edu/cliniweb/C1/C1.539.830.25.html.

Vanderbilt University Medical Center, (April 4, 2003). http://www.mc.vanderbilt.edu/peds/pidl/neuro/ brainabs.htm.

L. Fleming Fallon, Jr, MD, DrPH

Acetaminophen

Definition

Acetaminophen is a medicine used to relieve pain and reduce fever.

Purpose

Acetaminophen is used to relieve many kinds of minor aches and pains, including headaches, muscle aches, backaches, toothaches, menstrual cramps, arthritis, and the aches and pains that often accompany colds. It is suitable for control of pain following minor surgery, or for **post-surgical pain** after the need for stronger pain relievers has been reduced. Acetaminophen is also used in combination with narcotic **analgesics** both to increase pain relief and reduce the risk that the narcotics will be abused.

Description

This drug is available without a prescription. Acetaminophen (APAP) is sold under various brand names, including Tylenol, Panadol, Aspirin-Free Anacin, and Bayer Select Maximum Strength Headache Pain Relief Formula. Many multi-symptom cold, flu, and sinus medicines also contain acetaminophen. Persons are advised to check the ingredients listed on the container to see if acetaminophen is included in the product.

Acetaminophen is also included in some prescription-only combinations. These usually contain a narcotic in addition to acetaminophen; it is combined with oxycodone in Percocet, and is included in Tylenol with Codeine.

Studies have shown that acetaminophen relieves pain and reduces fever about as well as **aspirin**. But differences between these two common drugs exist. Acetaminophen is less likely than aspirin to irritate the stomach. However, unlike aspirin, acetaminophen does not reduce the redness, stiffness, or swelling that accompany arthritis.

Recommended dosage

The usual dosage for adults and children age 12 and over is 325–650 mg every four to six hours as needed. No more than 4 g (4,000 mg) should be taken in 24 hours. Because the drug can potentially harm the liver, people who drink alcohol in large quantities should take considerably less acetaminophen and possibly should avoid the drug completely.

For children ages six to 11 years, the usual dose is 150–300 mg, three to four times a day. People are advised to check with a physician for dosages for children under six years of age.

Precautions

A person should never take more than the recommended dosage of acetaminophen unless told to do so by a physician or dentist.

KEY TERMS

Arthritis—Inflammation of the joints; the condition causes pain and swelling.

Fatigue—Physical or mental weariness.

Inflammation—A response to irritation, infection, or injury, resulting in pain, redness, and swelling.

Because acetaminophen is included in both prescription and non-prescription combinations, it is important to check the total amount of acetaminophen taken each day from all sources in order to avoid taking more than the recommended maximum dose.

Patients should not use acetaminophen for more than 10 days to relieve pain (five days for children) or for more than three days to reduce fever, unless directed to do so by a physician. If symptoms do not go away, or if they get worse, the patient should contact a physician. Anyone who drinks three or more alcoholic beverages a day should check with a physician before using this drug and should never take more than the recommended dosage. People who already have kidney or liver disease or liver infections should also consult with a physician before using the drug. Women who are pregnant or breastfeeding should also consult with a physician before using acetaminophen.

Smoking cigarettes may interfere with the effectiveness of acetaminophen. Smokers may need to take higher doses of the medicine, but should not take more than the recommended daily dosage unless told to do so by a physician.

Many drugs can interact with one another. People should consult a physician or pharmacist before combining acetaminophen with any other medicine, and they should not use two different acetaminophen-containing products at the same time, unless instructed by a physician or dentist.

Some products, such as Nyquil, contain acetaminophen in combination with alcohol. While these products are safe for people who do not drink alcoholic beverages, people who consume alcoholic drinks regularly, even in moderation, should use extra care before using acetaminophen-alcohol combinations.

Acetaminophen interferes with the results of some medical tests. Before having medical tests done, a person should check to see whether taking acetaminophen would affect the results. Avoiding the drug for a few days before the tests may be necessary.

Side effects

Acetaminophen causes few side effects. The most common one is lightheadedness. Some people may experience trembling and pain in the side or the lower back. Allergic reactions do occur in some people, but they are rare. Anyone who develops symptoms such as rash, swelling, or difficulty breathing after taking acetaminophen should stop taking the drug and get immediate medical attention. Other rare side effects include yellow skin or eyes, unusual bleeding or bruising, weakness, fatigue, bloody or black stools, bloody or cloudy urine, and a sudden decrease in the amount of urine.

Overdoses of acetaminophen may cause nausea, vomiting, sweating, and exhaustion. Very large overdoses can cause liver damage. In case of an overdose, a person is advised to get immediate medical attention.

Interactions

Acetaminophen may interact with a variety of other medicines. When this happens, the effects of one or both of the drugs may change or the risk of side effects may be greater. Among the drugs that may interact with acetaminophen are alcohol, **nonsteroidal anti-inflammatory drugs** (NSAIDs) such as Motrin, oral contraceptives, the anti-seizure drug phenytoin (Dilantin), the blood-thinning drug warfarin (Coumadin), the cholesterol-lowering drug cholestyramine (Questran), the antibiotic Isoniazid, and zidovudine (Retrovir, AZT). People should check with a physician or pharmacist before combining acetaminophen with any other prescription or nonprescription (over-the-counter) medicine.

Resources

BOOKS

Brody, T.M., J. Larner, K.P. Minneman, and H.C. Neu. *Human Pharmacology: Molecular to Clinical, 2nd ed.* St. Louis: Mosby Year-Book, 1998.

Griffith, H.W., and S. Moore. *2001 Complete Guide to Prescription and Nonprescription Drugs.* New York: Berkely Publishing Group, 2001.

OTHER

"Acetaminophen." Federal Drug Administration. Center for Drug Evaluation and Research. [cited May 2003] http://www.fda.gov/cder/foi/nda/2000/75077_ Acetaminophen.pdf.

"Acetaminophen." Medline Plus Drug Information. [cited May 2003] http://www.nlm.nih.gov/medlineplus/ druginfo/medmaster/a681004.html.

"Acetaminophen, Systemic." Medline Plus Drug Information. [cited May 2003] http://www.nlm.nih.gov/medlineplus/druginfo/uspdi/202001.html.

Nancy Ross-Flanigan
Sam Uretsky, PharmD

Acid reducers *see* **Gastric acid inhibitors**

Adenoidectomy

Definition

An adenoidectomy is the surgical removal of the adenoids—small lumps of tissue that lie in the back of the throat behind the nose.

Purpose

The adenoids are removed if they block breathing through the nose and if they cause chronic earaches or deafness. The adenoids consist of lymphoid tissue—white blood cells from the immune system. They are located near the tonsils, two other lumps of similar lymphoid tissue. In childhood, adenoids and tonsils are believed to play a role in fighting infections by producing antibodies that attack bacteria entering the body through the mouth and nose. In adulthood however, it is unlikely that the adenoids are involved in maintaining health, and they normally shrink and disappear. Between the ages of two and six, the adenoids can become chronically infected, swelling up and becoming inflamed. This can cause breathing difficulties, especially during sleep. The swelling can also block the eustachian tubes that connect the back

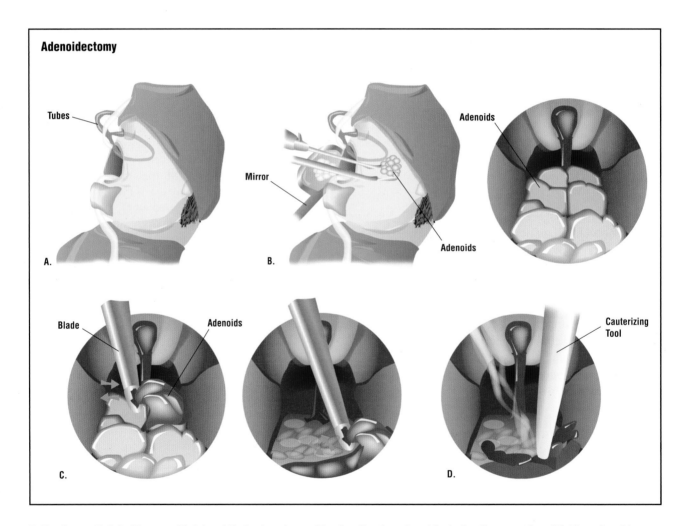

Adenoidectomy

Patient's mouth is held open with tubes (A). A mirror is used to visualize the adenoids during the procedure (B). The adenoids are removed with a side-to-side or front-to-back motion (C). Bleeding is controlled with a cauterizing tool (D). *(Illustration by GGS Information Services. Cengage Learning, Gale.)*

of the throat to the ears, leading to hearing problems until the blockage is relieved. The purpose of an adenoidectomy is thus to remove infected adenoids. Since they are often associated with infected tonsils, they are often removed as part of a combined operation that also removes the tonsils, called a T&A (**tonsillectomy** and adenoidectomy).

Demographics

Demographics information is difficult to provide because adenoidectomy is routinely performed in an outpatient setting, for which demographic data are not well recorded. Good information is available from the 1970s and 1980s when the surgery was performed in an inpatient setting. In the United States in 1971, more than one million combined T&As, tonsillectomies alone, or adenoidectomies alone were performed, with 50,000 of these procedures consisting of adenoidectomy alone. In 1987, 250,000 combined or single procedures were performed, with 15,000 consisting of adenoidectomy alone. Now, almost all adenoidectomies are performed on an outpatient basis unless other medical problems require hospital admission or an overnight stay. T&A is considered the most common major surgical procedure in the United States.

Description

An adenoidectomy is performed under **general anesthesia**. The surgeon removes the adenoids from behind the palate. **Stitches** are usually not required.

Excision through the mouth

The adenoids are most commonly removed through the mouth after placing an instrument to open the mouth and retract the palate. A mirror is used to see the adenoids behind the nasal cavity. Several instruments can then be used to remove the adenoids.

- Curette removal. The most common method of removal is using the adenoid curette, an instrument that has a sharp edge in a perpendicular position to its long handle. Various sizes of curettes are available.
- Adenoid punch instrument. An adenoid punch is a curved instrument with a chamber that is placed over the adenoids. The chamber has a knife blade sliding-door to section off the adenoids that are then housed in the chamber and removed with the instrument.

- Magill forceps. A Magill forceps is a curved instrument used to remove residual adenoid, usually located deeper in the posterior nasal cavity, after attempted removal with curettes or adenoid punches.
- Electrocautery with a suction Bovie. The adenoids can also be removed by electrocautery with a suction Bovie, an instrument with a hollow center to suction blood and a rim of metal to achieve coagulation.
- Laser. The Nd:YAG laser has also been used to remove the adenoids. However, this technique has caused scarring of tissue and is usually avoided.

Excision through the nose

Adenoids may also be removed through the nasal cavity with a surgical suction instrument called a microdebrider. With this procedure, bleeding is controlled either with packing or suction cautery.

Diagnosis/Preparation

The primary methods used to determine whether adenoids need removal are:

- medical history
- physical examination
- throat bacterial cultures
- x rays
- blood tests

When the patient arrives at the hospital or the day-surgery unit, a nurse or a doctor will ask questions concerning the patient's general health to make sure he or she is fit to undergo surgery. They will also check that the patient has not had anything to eat or drink and will record pulse and blood pressure. The doctor or nurse must be informed if the patient has had any allergic or unusual reactions to drugs in the past. The patient will be asked to put on a hospital gown and to remove any loose orthodontic braces, false teeth, and jewelry. In the past, an adenoidectomy usually called for an overnight stay in hospital. However, it is increasingly more common to have this operation on an outpatient basis, meaning that the patient goes home on the same day. The surgery is usually performed early in the morning to allow a sufficient observation period after the operation.

Aftercare

After surgery, the patient wakes up in the recovery area and is given medication to reduce swelling and pain. When the patient has recovered from surgery, he or she is sent home and usually given a week's course of **antibiotics** to be taken by mouth. The patient may also develop a sore throat, especially when swallowing or speaking, or moderate pain at the back of the nose and throat, for which pain medication is prescribed. Normally, the pain goes away after a week. A child who has undergone an adenoidectomy should rest at home for at least one week to avoid possible infections at school. Swimming should not be allowed for at least 10 days after the operation. If there is any sign of bleeding or infection (fever, increased pain), the treating physician should be immediately contacted.

Risks

Risks and complications include those generally associated with surgery and anesthesia. Very few complications are known to occur after this operation, except, very rarely, bleeding (which occurs in 0.4% of cases). Bleeding is more a concern with a very young child because he or she often will not notice. For this reason, a child is always kept in observation at the hospital or clinic for a few hours after the operation. If bleeding does occur, the surgeon may insert a pack of gauze into the nose to stop the blood flow for subsequent removal after a day or two. The other possible complications are those associated with any operation, including infection of the operated area, which may result in light bleeding, increased pain, and fever. Infection is usually treated with antibiotics and bed rest.

Normal results

Adenoidectomy is an operation that has very good outcomes, and patients are expected to make a full and quick recovery once the initial pain has subsided. Adenoid tissue rarely regrows, but some instances have been reported. The exact mechanism is unknown but may be related to incomplete removal.

Alternatives

There is no good evidence supporting any curative non-surgical therapy for chronic infection of the adenoid. Antibiotics have been used for as long as six weeks in lymphoid tissue infection, but with failure to eradicate the bacteria. With reported incidences of drug-resistant bacteria, use of long-term antibiotics is not a recommended alternative to surgical removal of infected adenoids.

Some studies indicate some benefit from using topical nasal steroids. Studies show that while using the medication, the adenoids may shrink up to 10% and help relieve nasal blockage. However, once the steroid medication is stopped, the adenoids can again enlarge and continue to cause symptoms. In a child with nasal obstructive symptoms, a trial of topical nasal steroid spray and saline spray may be attempted for controlling symptoms.

Resources

BOOKS

Bluestone, C. D. *Pediatric otolaryngology* Philadelphia: Saunders, 2003.

Lee, K. J. *Essential otolaryngology: head and neck surgery.* New York: McGraw-Hill Medical Pub. Division, 2003.

Markel, H. and F. A. Oski. *The Practical Pediatrician: The A to Z Guide to Your Child's Health, Behavior, and Safety.* New York: W. H. Freeman and Co., 1995.

PERIODICALS

Felder-Puig, R., A. Maksys, C. Noestlinger, et al. "Using a children's book to prepare children and parents for elective ENT surgery: results of a randomized clinical trial." *International Journal of Pediatrics and Otorhinolaryngology* 67 (January 2003): 35–41.

Homer, J. J., J. Swallow, and P. Semple. " Audit of pain management at home following tonsillectomy in children." *Journal of Laryngology and Otology* 115 (March 2001): 205–208.

Kokki, H. and R. Ahonen. "Pain and activity disturbance after paediatric day case adenoidectomy." *Paediatric Anaesthesiology* 7 (1997): 227–231.

Kvaerner, K. J., P. Nafstad, and J. J. Jaakkola. "Otolaryngological surgery and upper respiratory tract infections in children: an epidemiological study." *Annals of Otology, Rhinology and Laryngology* 111 (November 2002): 1034–1039.

McClay, J. E. "Resistant bacteria in the adenoids: a preliminary report." *Archives of Otolaryngology: Head and Neck Surgery* 123 (May 2000): 625–629.

ORGANIZATIONS

American Academy of Otolaryngology - Head and Neck Surgery. One Prince Street, Alexandria, VA 22314. (703) 806-4444. http://www.entnet.org.

American College of Surgeons. 633 N. Saint Claire St., Chicago, IL 60611. (312) 202-5000. http://www.faacs.org.

OTHER

American College of Surgeons. "Tonsillectomy and Adenoidectomy." February 21, 2003 [cited April 23, 2003]. http://www.facs.org/public_info/operation/aboutbroch.html.

BUPA. "Adenoidectomy." [cited April 23, 2003]. http://www.bupa.com.

Texas Pediatric Surgical Associates. "Adenoids and Adenoidectomy." [cited April 23, 2003]. http://www.pedisurg.com/PtEducENT/adenoids.htm.

Monique Laberge, Ph.D.

Admission to the hospital

Definition

Hospital admission involves staying at a hospital for at least one night or more.

Purpose

Staying in the hospital overnight is done because the individual is too sick to stay at home, requires 24-hour nursing care, and/or is receiving medications and undergoing tests and/or surgery that can be performed only in a hospital setting.

Description

An individual may be admitted to the hospital for a positive experience, such as having a baby, or because of undergoing an **elective surgery** or procedure, or because of being admitted through the emergency department. Being admitted through the emergency department is the most stressful of these circumstances because the event is unexpected and may be a major life crisis.

Before the person is taken to a patient room, admitting procedures are performed. The person's personal data is recorded and entered into the hospital's computer database. This data may include:

- name
- address
- home and work telephone numbers
- date of birth
- place of employment
- occupation
- emergency contact information, or the names and telephone numbers of those individuals the hospital should contact if the person being admitted needs emergency care or his or her condition worsens significantly
- insurance coverage

- reason for hospitalization
- allergies to medications or foods
- religious preference, including whether the patient wishes a visit from a clergy member

There may be several forms to fill out. One form may be a detailed medical and medication history. This history will include past hospitalizations and surgeries. Having this information readily available will help the admission process move faster and can allow a family member or friend who is accompanying the person to help fill out the forms more easily. The hospital may ask if there are any advance directives. This refers to forms that have been filled out indicating what medical decisions the patient wants others to make on his or her behalf. One form is called a **living will** and clearly tells which specific resuscitation efforts the person does or does not want to have performed in order to save or extend his or her life. Another form may be a durable **power of attorney**. This is a form stating whom the patient wishes to make medical decisions for him or her if the patient becomes unable to do so, such as if the patient falls into a coma. Some hospitals have blank forms that the individual can use to make these designations; others may just ask if the forms have been filled out, and, if so, to add copies of them into the person's medical record. These forms are considered legally binding, and an attorney can assist in filling them out. During the time spent in the admitting department, a plastic bracelet will be placed on the person's wrist that details name, age, date of birth, room number, and medical record number. A separate bracelet is added that lists allergies. Forms are completed and signed, so that the patient is giving full consent to have the hospital personnel take care of him or her while in the hospital during that particular hospital stay. Subsequent hospital stays require new consent forms.

Once all the admitting forms have been completed, the person is taken to a patient room. Most people stay in a semi-private room, which means that there are two people in the room. In some circumstances, a person's medical condition may require staying in a private room. If there are private rooms available, and the individual is willing to pay the extra cost (insurance companies generally only cover the cost of a semi-private room), it may be possible to have a private room. Once the patient is taken to a room, the nurse will go over the medical and medication history, and orient the patient to the room by explaining how to adjust bed height, how to use the nurse call button, where the bathroom is located, and

how to use the bedside telephone and television. The cost for the telephone and television are not usually covered by insurance. There may be limitations on using the bathroom, for example, if the patient's doctor feels that the patient should not get out of bed. These decisions are made with the patient's safety and medical condition in mind. Another safety practice is raising the side rails of the bed to prevent the patient from falling out of bed. The nurse will review the doctor's orders, such as what tests have been scheduled, whether the patient can get out of bed to use the bathroom or to walk around the unit, what medications the patient will be getting, and whether there are food restrictions. The hospital will supply towels, sheets, and blankets, but some people like to bring something personal with them from home. If a person does choose to bring in a personal item, the item should be washed with warm or hot water and soap upon returning home to ensure that germs are not brought home from the hospital.

Sometimes a person needs extremely close observation that can only be provided with specialized care in an **intensive care unit** (ICU). Because of the patient's medical condition, visiting hours are more restricted than in the regular rooms. It may be that only one or two people can visit at a time, and only for a few minutes at a time. Once the person's condition improves, he or she may then be transferred to a room with a less rigid visitation policy. If an individual has a surgical procedure performed, he or she will spend a few hours in a recovery area. This is to make sure that the person's condition is stable before returning to the regular room. Visiting is limited in the recovery area, and the person may spend most of the time sleeping, as the effects of the surgical anesthesia wear off.

If the person entering the hospital is a child, the parents or guardian will fill out the hospital forms.

Most hospitals allow parents and guardians to stay overnight in the hospital with the child, and to be with him or her 24 hours a day. Many hospitals have special areas for children to play in.

Preparation

If the hospitalization is prearranged, there are preparations that will make the process go more smoothly. For example, a list of all medications currently being taken, the dosages, how often they are taken, and why they are taken is helpful. The list should also include any allergies to food and medications, including a description of the reaction, and when the food or medication was last taken. The list should include over-the-counter (OTC) and prescription medications, vitamins, supplements, and herbal and home remedies.

If the hospital stay involves surgery in which there is the potential for significant blood loss, it may be possible to arrange to have blood drawn and stored so that, in the event of a **transfusion**, the individual receives his or her own blood.

If the hospital stay is an extended one, a list of family and friends, with their telephone numbers, can make it easier to stay in touch with people who can come and visit, or offer support by telephone. It is not a good idea to bring anything of value to the hospital as there are many times when the patient could be out of the room. However, it may be helpful to have some pocket change available to make some small purchases at the hospital gift shop, such as a newspaper.

A small bag can be brought into the hospital that contains:

- night clothes (the hospital supplies gowns, but some people like to wear familiar clothing)
- a robe
- slippers
- clothes for the return trip home
- reading material
- hobby materials, such as knitting or a book of crossword puzzles
- reading glasses
- personal care items such as comb, brush, and toothbrush (most hospitals supply these items, but many individuals prefer to have their own from home)

It is best not to bring in any medication from home unless it has been prearranged with the physician and hospital staff prior to hospitalization. This is to prevent an error from occurring by having the person taking one dose from his or her own medicine and then being given another dose from the hospital pharmacy.

Resources

BOOKS

Perry, Anne Griffin. *Clinical Nursing Skills and Techniques.* Mosby, 1998.

ORGANIZATIONS

American Hospital Association. One North Franklin, Chicago, IL 60606. (312) 422-3000. http://www.aha.org (accessed March 6, 2008).

Nemours Center for Children's Health Media. http://kidshealth.org (accessed March 6, 2008).

Esther Csapo Rastegari, RN, BSN, EdM
Fran Hodgkins

Adrenal gland removal *see* **Adrenalectomy**

Adrenalectomy

Definition

Adrenalectomy is the surgical removal of one or both adrenal glands. The adrenal glands are paired endocrine glands—one located above each kidney—that produce hormones such as epinephrine, norepinephrine, androgens, estrogens, aldosterone, and cortisol. Adrenalectomy is usually performed by conventional (open) surgery; however, in selected patients, surgeons may use **laparoscopy**. With laparoscopy, adrenalectomy can be accomplished through four very small incisions.

Purpose

Adrenalectomy is usually advised for patients with tumors of the adrenal glands. Adrenal gland tumors may be malignant or benign, but all typically excrete excessive amounts of one or more hormones. When malignant, they are usually neuroblastoma cancers. A successful procedure will aid in correcting hormone imbalances, and may also remove cancerous tumors before they invade other parts of the body. Occasionally, adrenalectomy may be recommended when hormones produced by the adrenal glands aggravate another condition such as breast cancer.

Demographics

Neuroblastoma is one of the few cancer types known to secrete hormones. It occurs most often in

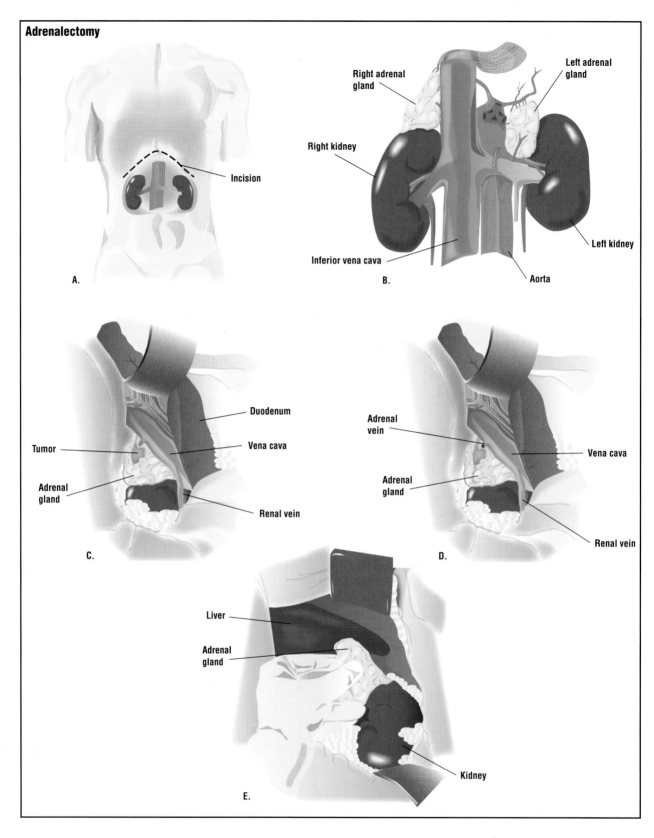

Adrenalectomy

A.

B.

Right adrenal gland

Left adrenal gland

Right kidney

Left kidney

Inferior vena cava

Aorta

C.

Tumor

Duodenum

Vena cava

Adrenal gland

Renal vein

D.

Adrenal vein

Vena cava

Adrenal gland

Renal vein

E.

Liver

Adrenal gland

Kidney

To remove the adrenal glands, an incision is made below the patient's ribcage (A). The adrenal gland, which sits on top of the kidney (B), is visualized (C). The vein emerging from the gland is tied off and cut (D), and the adrenal is removed (E). *(Illustration by GGS Information Services. Cengage Learning, Gale.)*

children, and it is the third most common cancer that occurs in children. In the united States, approximately 7.5% of the childhood cancers diagnosed in 2001 were neuroblastomas, affecting one in 80,000 to 100,000 children. Close to 50% of cases of neuroblastoma occur in children younger than two years old. The disease is sometimes present at birth, but is usually not noticed until later. Approximately one-third of neuroblastomas start in the adrenal glands. According to some reports, African-American children develop the disease at a slightly higher rate than Caucasian children (8.7 per million compared to 8.0 per million cases diagnosed).

Description

Open adrenalectomy

The surgeon may operate from any of four directions, depending on the exact problem and the patient's body type.

In the anterior approach, the surgeon cuts into the abdominal wall. Usually the incision will be horizontal, just under the rib cage. If the surgeon intends to operate on only one of the adrenal glands, the incision will run under just the right or the left side of the rib cage. Sometimes a vertical incision in the middle of the abdomen provides a better approach, especially if both adrenal glands are involved.

In the posterior approach, the surgeon cuts into the back, just beneath the rib cage. If both glands are to be removed, an incision is made on each side of the body. This approach is the most direct route to the adrenal glands, but it does not provide quite as clear a view of the surrounding structures as the anterior approach.

In the flank approach, the surgeon cuts into the patient's side. This is particularly useful in massively obese patients. If both glands need to be removed, the surgeon must remove one gland, repair the surgical wound, turn the patient onto the other side, and repeat the entire process.

The last approach involves an incision into the chest cavity, either with or without part of the incision into the abdominal cavity. It is used when the surgeon anticipates a very large tumor, or if the surgeon needs to examine or remove nearby structures as well.

Laparoscopic adrenalectomy

This technique does not require the surgeon to open the body cavity. Instead, four small incisions (about 0.5

in [1.27 cm] diameter each) are made into a patient's flank, just under the rib cage. A laparoscope enabling the surgeon to visualize the inside of the abdominal cavity on a television monitor is placed through one of the incisions. The other incisions are for tubes that carry miniaturized versions of surgical tools. These tools are designed to be operated by manipulations that the surgeon makes outside the body.

Diagnosis/Preparation

Most aspects of preparation are the same as in other major operations. In addition, hormone imbalances are often a major challenge. Whenever possible, physicians will try to correct hormone imbalances through medication in the days or weeks before surgery. Adrenal tumors may cause other problems such as hypertension or inadequate potassium in the blood, and these problems also should be resolved if possible before surgery is performed. Therefore, a patient may take specific medicines for days or weeks before surgery.

Most adrenal tumors can be imaged very well with a **CT scan** or MRI, and benign tumors tend to look different on these tests than do cancerous tumors. Surgeons may order a CT scan, MRI, or scintigraphy (viewing of the location of a tiny amount of radioactive agent) to help locate exactly where the tumor is located.

The day before surgery, patients will probably have an enema to clear the bowels. In patients with lung problems or clotting problems, physicians may advise special preparations.

Aftercare

Patients stay in the hospital for various lengths of time after adrenalectomy. The longest hospital stays are required for open surgery using an anterior approach; hospital stays of about three days are indicated for open surgery using the posterior approach or for laparoscopic adrenalectomy.

The special concern after adrenalectomy is the patient's hormone balance. There may be several sets of required lab tests to define hormone problems and monitor the results of drug treatment. In addition, blood pressure problems and infections are more common after removal of certain types of adrenal tumors.

As with most open surgery, surgeons are also concerned about blood clots forming in the legs and traveling to the lungs (venous thromboembolism), bowel problems, and postoperative pain. With laparoscopic adrenalectomy, these problems are somewhat less prevalent, but they are still present.

Risks

The risks of adrenalectomy include major hormone imbalances, caused by the underlying disease, the surgery, or both. These can include problems with healing, blood pressure fluctuations, and other metabolic problems.

Other risks are typical of many operations. These include:

- bleeding
- damage to adjacent organs (spleen, pancreas)
- loss of bowel function
- blood clots in the lungs
- lung problems
- surgical infections
- pain
- scarring

Normal results

The outcome of an adrenalectomy depends on the condition for which it was performed. For example, in the case of hyperaldosteronism, the surgical removal of the adrenal glands provides excellent results, with the majority of patients being cured. In the case of patients diagnosed with pheochromocytoma, long-term cures are rare in cases of malignant pheochromocytomas. In cases of metastatic disease, five-year survival rates as high as 36% have been reported.

Morbidity and mortality rates

There is wide agreement that laparoscopic approaches decrease operative morbidity. The laparoscopic approach is commonly used to treat smaller adrenal tumors. At many laparoscopic centers, the laparoscopic adrenalectomy has become the standard practice. Several centers recommend a particular approach or laparoscopic method, but regardless of which approach is preferred, the cure and morbidity rates are similar for laparoscopic and open adrenalectomy (in the case of small tumors). No method is suitable for all patients. In general, selecting the approach based on patient and tumor characteristics while considering the familiarity of the surgeon yields the best results.

Alternatives

Alternatives to adrenalectomy depend on the medical condition underlying the decision to perform the surgery. In some cases, drug therapy may be considered as an alternative when the condition being treated in benign.

Resources

BOOKS

Bradley, Edward L., III. *The Patient's Guide to Surgery.* Philadelphia: University of Pennsylvania Press, 1994.

Fauci, Anthony S., et al., ed. *Harrison's Principles of Internal Medicine.* New York: McGraw-Hill, 1997.

Little, M., and D. C. Garrell. *The Endocrine System: The Healthy Body.* New York: Chelsea House, 1990.

PERIODICALS

Del Pizzo, J. J. "Transabdominal laparoscopic adrenalectomy." *Current Urology Reports* 4 (February 2003): 81–86.

Desai, M. M., I. S. Gill, J. H. Kaouk, S. F. Matin, G. T. Sung, and E. L. Bravo. "Robotic-assisted laparoscopic adrenalectomy." *Urology* 60 (December 2002): 1104–1107.

Hawn, M. T., D. Cook, C. Deveney, and B. C. Sheppard. "Quality of life after laparoscopic bilateral adrenalectomy for Cushing's disease." *Surgery* 132 (December 2002): 1068–1069.

Ikeda, Y., H. Takami, G. Tajima, Y. Sasaki, J. Takayama, H. Kurihara, M. Niimi. "Laparoscopic partial adrenalectomy." *Biomedical Pharmacotherapy* 56 (2002) suppl.1: 126s–131s.

Martinez, D. G. "Adrenalectomy for primary aldosteronism." *Annals of Internal Medicine* 138 (January 2003): 157–159.

Munver, R., J. J. Del Pizzo, and R. E. Sosa. "Adrenal-preserving Minimally Invasive Surgery: The Role of Laparoscopic Partial Adrenalectomy, Cryosurgery, and Radiofrequency Ablation of the Adrenal Gland." *Current Urology Reports* 4 (February 2003): 87–92.

ORGANIZATIONS

American Association of Clinical Endoctrinologists. 1000 Riverside Ave., Suite 205, Jacksonville, FL 32204. (904) 353-7878. http://www.aace.com.

American College of Surgeons. 633 N. Saint Clar St., Chicago, IL 60611-3211. (312) 202-5000. http://www.facs.org.

OTHER

"Adrenalectomy." http://www.dundee.ac.uk/medicine/tayendoweb/images/adrenalectomy.htm.

"Laparoscopic Adrenalectomy: The preferred operation for benign adrenal tumors." http://www.endocrineweb.com/laparo.html.

"Laparoscopic Removal of the Adrenal Gland." 2001. http://mininvasive.med.nyu.edu/urology/adrenalectomy.html.

Richard H. Lampert
Monique Laberge, Ph.D.

Adrenergic drugs

Definition

Adrenergic amines are drugs that stimulate the sympathetic nervous system, also called the adrenergic nervous system. These compounds are known as sympathomimetic drugs. The sympathetic nervous system is the part of the autonomic nervous system that originates in the thoracic, or chest, and lumbar, or lower back regions of the spinal cord and regulates involuntary reactions to stress. It stimulates the heartbeat, sweating, breathing rate, and other stress-related body processes.

Purpose

Adrenergic drugs have many uses. They are used to increase the output of the heart, to raise blood pressure, and to increase urine flow as part of the treatment of shock. Adrenergics are also used as heart stimulants. They may be given to a patient to reverse the drop in blood pressure that is sometimes caused by **general anesthesia**. They may be used to stop bleeding by causing the blood vessels to constrict, and to keep local anesthetics in a small area of the body by closing off the nearby blood vessels that would otherwise spread the anesthetic to other parts of the body. This ability to make blood vessels constrict makes adrenergics useful in reducing nasal stuffiness associated with colds and allergies. They may also be given to open the bronchi, the tubes leading to the lungs, for treatment of asthma and chronic obstructive pulmonary disease (COPD).

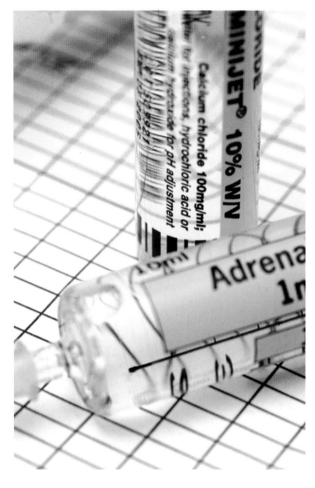

(Medical-on-Line / Alamy)

- Dobutamine (Dobutrex and generic forms)—used to stimulate the heart during surgery or after a heart attack or cardiac arrest;

- Dopamine (Intropin)—used to increase cardiac output, blood pressure, and urine flow in treating patients with shock;

- Epinephrine (Adrenalin)—used locally to control bleeding from arterioles and capillaries during surgery. It is used to treat shock, as a heart stimulant, and as a decongestant. Epinephrine may be added to local anesthetics to keep the anesthetic in the area where it is applied. Epinephrine may also be applied to the eye to reduce the symptoms of conjunctivitis (red eye);

- Isoproteranol—most widely used to ease breathing problems in asthma and COPD, but also used to control several types of irregular heartbeat until a pacemaker can be implanted;

- Metaraminol (Aramine)—used to raise the blood pressure and stimulate the heart in treating patients with shock;

- Norepinephrine (Levophed)—used to increase the output of the heart and raise blood pressure as part of the treatment of shock; and

- Phenylephrine (Neo-Synephrine)—used to treat shock and low blood pressure; also used in the form of nose drops or spray to relieve nasal congestion from colds and allergies.

Recommended dosage

The recommended dosage of an adrenergic drug depends on the specific compound, the purpose for which it is given, and the route of administration (oral or intravenous).

People who use adrenergic amines to treat breathing problems or conjunctivitis (red eye) should not use over-the-counter preparations of these drugs as an alternative to seeking professional care. These medications may temporarily relieve the symptoms of some disorders but will not cure the underlying problems, which may be serious.

Precautions

When adrenergic amines are given during surgery, they will be administered by an anesthesiologist or other health care professional skilled in their use. It is the anesthesiologist's responsibility to **exercise** appropriate care when these drugs are used during an operation.

Description

There are several types of adrenergic receptors in the human body. Although all types of adrenergic receptors, or nerve endings, respond to the same drugs, the effects depend on which specific receptors are stimulated. The alpha receptors make the heart beat faster, the pupils of the eyes dilate, and the muscles contract. The beta receptors have similar effects and also cause the bronchi in the lungs to open up. Both alpha and beta receptors are divided into subgroups—alpha-1, alpha-2, beta-1, and beta-2—each with its own specific effects. A hormone called norepinephrine that is secreted in the body affects all types of adrenergic receptors; the drugs used in medicine and surgery, however, have been developed to affect only specific types of receptors.

There are several adrenergic amines in common use:

- Albuterol (Alupent, Ventolin, others)—given by mouth or as a nasal spray to improve breathing;

KEY TERMS

Adrenergic—Characteristic of or releasing epinephrine or related substances. The term often refers to the nerve fibers in the sympathetic nervous system that release norepinephrine as a neurotransmitter.

Amine—A chemical compound that contains NH_3 (a nitrogen-hydrogen combination) as part of its structure.

Autonomic nervous system—The part of the nervous system that regulates the activity of heart muscle, smooth muscle, and glands.

Bronchi—The large air tubes leading from the trachea to the lungs that convey air to and from the lungs.

Conjunctivitis—Inflammation of the conjunctiva, the membrane on the inner part of the eyelids and the covering of the white of the eye.

Norepinephrine—A naturally occurring hormone that acts as a neurotransmitter and affects both alpha- and beta-adrenergic receptors. It is also known as noradrenaline.

Receptor—A sensory nerve ending that responds to chemical or other stimuli of various kinds.

Shock—A serious condition in which the body's blood circulation and metabolism is severely impaired by injury, pain, blood loss, or certain diseases. The symptoms of shock include a pale complexion, very low blood pressure, and a weak pulse.

Sympathetic nervous system—The part of the nervous system stimulated by adrenergic drugs. It regulates such involuntary reactions to stress as changes in the heartbeat and breathing rate, sweating, and changes in digestive secretions.

Sympathomimetic drugs—Another name for adrenergic drugs.

The following are some of the hazards associated with the use of adrenergic amines. Patients under anesthesia may not be aware of these side effects:

- nervousness;
- rapid heart beat;
- high blood pressure;
- irregular heart beat;
- rapid heartbeat;
- chest pain;
- dizziness;
- dry mouth;

- headache;
- flushing;
- nausea;
- vomiting; and
- weakness.

Before undergoing procedures that may involve the use of an adrenergic amine, people with any of these medical problems should make sure their physicians know about them:

- narrow-angle glaucoma;
- liver disease;
- enlarged heart;
- disorders affecting the arteries and veins; and
- diseases and disorders affecting the blood supply to the brain.

Side effects

The most common side effects of adrenergic amines are nervousness, agitation, and wakefulness. These side effects do not usually cause problems when the drugs are given during surgery or in combination with local anesthetics.

The following side effects sometimes occur when adrenergic amines are used to treat nasal congestion due to allergies or infections:

- rapid heartbeat;
- increased sweating;
- nervousness;
- hallucinations;
- sleep disturbances; and
- paleness.

Other rare side effects may occur. Anyone who has unusual symptoms after taking adrenergic amines should contact his or her physician right away.

Interactions

Adrenergic amines may interact with many different types of drugs. People should discuss the use of these drugs with their pharmacist or physician before using over-the-counter preparations that contain them for colds or allergies. Patients scheduled for surgery should be sure to give the surgeon and anesthesiologist a list of all the drugs they take, including nonprescription, herbal, and alternative preparations. Some drugs that interact with adrenergic amines should be discontinued several days before surgery, since they last for a long time after the last dose.

Drugs that may interact with adrenergic amines include:

- furazolidone (Furoxone);
- tricyclic antidepressants (Adapin, Asendin, Aventyl, Elavil, Endep, Norpramin, Pamelor, Sinequan, Surmontil, Tofranil, Vivactil);
- guanethidine (Ismelin); and
- methyldopa (Aldomet).

Herbs that have been reported to interact with adrenergic amines include ephedra (ma huang), often sold in over-the-counter weight loss formulas; St. John's wort, a popular remedy for anxiety or depression; alfalfa; hibiscus; ginseng; angelica (dong quai); and yohimbe.

The list above does not include every drug or herb that may interact with adrenergic amines. People should consult their physician or pharmacist before combining adrenergic amines with any other prescription or nonprescription (over-the-counter) medicine.

Resources

BOOKS

Beers, M. H., R. S. Porter, T. V. Jones, J. L. Kaplan, and M. Berkwits, eds. *The Merck Manual of Diagnosis and Therapy,* 18th ed. Whitehouse Station, NJ: Merck Research Laboratories, 2006.

Brody, T. M., J. Larner, and K. P. Minneman. *Human Pharmacology: Molecular to Clinical,* 3rd ed. St. Louis: Mosby, 1998.

Sweetman, Sean C., ed. *Martindale: The Complete Drug Reference,* 35th ed. London: The Pharmaceutical Press, 2007.

PERIODICALS

Brumley, C. "Herbs and the Perioperative Patient." *AORN Journal* 72, no. 5 (November 2000): 785–794, 796.

OTHER

"Adrenergic Drugs." Lutherans Online 2004. www. lutheransonline.com/servlet/lo_ProcServ/dbpage = page&GID = 011580013609860643656196186 PG = 012680013610164047208153 96.

"Adrenergic Bronchodilator Overdose." Medline Plus Drug Information. October 29, 2007. http://www.nlm.nih. gov/medlineplus/ency/article/002594.htm.

ORGANIZATIONS

American Herbal Products Association, 8484 Georgia Avenue, Suite 370, Silver Spring, MD, 20910, (301) 588-1171, http://www.ahpa.org.

American Society of Health-System Pharmacists, 7272 Wisconsin Avenue, Bethesda, MD, 20814, (301) 657-3000, http://www.ashp.org.

U.S. Food and Drug Administration, 5600 Fishers Lane, Rockville, MD, 20857-0001, (888) INFO-FDA, http:// www.fda.gov.

Samuel Uretsky, Pharm.D.
Laura Jean Cataldo, R.N., Ed.D.

Adult day care

Definition

Adult day care includes programs, services, and facilities designed to assist physically or mentally impaired adults remain in their homes and communities. These are persons who might otherwise require institutional or long-term care and rehabilitation.

Purpose

There are two general purposes for adult day-care. The first is to provide an alternative to placement in a residential institution. The second is to create a respite for care-givers, often the children of the persons for whom the care is being provided.

Description

There are two general types of adult day care programs. One is based on a medical model and the other on a social model. The medical model provides comprehensive medical, therapeutic, and rehabilitation treatment, usually during normal working hours. The social model offers supervised activities, peer support, companionship, and recreation. Both models assist older adults and those with chronic conditions to remain as independent as possible, for as long as possible.

Programs organized along medical model lines are often called adult day health care to distinguish them from social programs. Adult day health care programs offer health services such as physician visits, nursing care, and podiatry, as well as rehabilitation services such as physical, occupational, and speech therapy in a secure environment. This model of adult day care is offered to persons with a variety of chronic medical conditions including the following:

- adults with Alzheimer's disease, other forms of dementia, or depression;
- persons recovering from strokes or head or spinal cord injuries;
- people with chronic conditions such as diabetes or cardiovascular disease;
- adults with developmental disabilities such as Down syndrome;
- adults suffering from mental illnesses; and
- weak or frail older adults requiring nursing care or assistance with daily living activities.

The social model of adult day care emphasizes supervised group activities such as crafts, gardening, music, and **exercise**. Participants in this model may require some assistance with the activities of daily living (e.g., eating, bathing, dressing) but they generally do not require skilled nursing care. Like adult day health care facilities, these social programs generally provide transportation and a midday meal for participants, as well as caregiver support groups, information and referral services, and community outreach programs.

In 2008, an estimated 37 million Americans will be aged 65 or older. According to statistics from the U.S. Department of Labor, the fastest growing segment of older adults is the population aged 85 and older. Historically, approximately 80% of the frail elderly remain in their communities and are cared for by relatives, most commonly by adult daughters; however, as of the early twenty-first century, an increasing number of women aged 35–54 are in the workforce and unable to care for aging parents or disabled adult children living at home.

Although the participants of adult day care are adults who attend the programs daily or several times each week, adult day care also meets the needs of families and other caregivers. Before women entered the workforce, they were available to care for relatives at home. In the early 2000s, adult day care provides a secure, alternative source of care for women who work outside the home. It also offers respite, or much needed breaks, for caregivers. Older adults caring for spouses, or children caring for aging parents find that adult day care helps ease the burden of caring for ill, confused, or disabled family members.

The first adult day care centers opened in England during the 1940s and 1950s. Established by psychiatric hospitals, these centers were designed to reduce the frequency of hospital admissions. The first adult day care centers in the United States appeared during the early 1970s. Today, there are more than 4,500 services and centers. Most centers and programs operate during normal business hours, Monday through Friday, but some offer weekend and evening care.

As of 2007, 35 states offer licensure of adult day care, but only 26 require such licensure. Adult day care services or programs may be affiliated with hospitals,

nursing homes, home health agencies, or senior centers, but many are unaffiliated, independent programs. They may be located in storefronts, senior centers, community health and medical centers, and nursing homes.

Among centers responding to a 1997 National Adult Day Services Association (NADSA) survey, the average number of persons in an adult day care facility was approximately 40 and the average age of persons served was 76. About three out of four persons receiving adult day care services lived with family. Nearly 80% of adult day centers offered nursing services, and approximately 90% were not-for-profit. Fees ranged from $1 to $200 per day, with an average of $28 to $43 dollars per day. As of 2003, **Medicare** does not pay for any type of adult day care; however, in 35 states, **Medicaid** can be used to pay for adult day care services for individuals that meet financial criteria.

Though fees for adult day care vary widely, the service is generally considered to be cost effective when compared with the cost of institutional care, such as skilled nursing facilities or even home health care. More importantly, adult day care enables older adults, persons with physical disabilities, and those with cognitive impairments to maintain their independence. Research has demonstrated that adult day care also reduces the risks and frequency of hospitalization for older adults. Adult day care satisfies two requirements of care. It provides a secure, protected environment and is often the least restrictive setting in which care may be delivered.

Quality and standards of care vary from state to state and from one center or program to another. NADSA and the National Council on the Aging have developed standards and benchmarks for care, but adherence to these standards is voluntary. NADSA is developing a certification program for adult day center administrators and directors. A certification process for program assistants also exists. Since no uniform national standards exist, it is difficult for consumers to know whether a program or center is staffed by qualified personnel or provides appropriate services.

Generally, quality adult day care centers or programs conduct thorough assessments of each person and develop individualized plans of care and activities to meet the needs of impaired, disabled, or frail older adults. The plans for each individual describe objectives in terms of improvement or maintenance of health status, functional capabilities, and emotional well being. Centers must have sufficient staff to ensure safety, supervision, and close attention. Further, all personnel and volunteers should be qualified, trained, and sensitive to the special needs of older adults. For example, centers and services for persons with Alzheimer's disease or other dementias must take special precautions to ensure that people do not wander away from the facility.

Results

The aging population in the United States, the increasing incidence of Alzheimer's disease, and rising popularity of adult day care have created new and additional opportunities for health professionals and other care-giving and service personnel.

Resources

BOOKS

Buelow, J. R. *Listening to the Voices of Long-Term Care*. Lanham, MD: University Press of America, 2007.

Capezuti, E. A., E. L. Siegler, and M. D. Mezey. *Encyclopedia of Elder Care*, 2nd ed. New York: Springer Publishing, 2007.

Mace, N. L., and P. V. Rabins. *The 36-Hour Day: A Family Guide to Caring for People with Alzheimer Disease, Other Dementias, and Memory Loss in Later Life*, 4th ed. Baltimore: Johns Hopkins University Press, 2006.

Moore, K. D., L. D. Geboy, and G. D. Weisman. *Designing a Better Day: Guidelines for Adult and Dementia Day Services Centers*. Baltimore: Johns Hopkins University Press, 2006.

PERIODICALS

Cohen-Mansfield, J., and B. Jensen. "Changes in habits related to self-care in dementia: the nursing home versus adult day care." *American Journal of Alzheimer's Disease and Other Dementias* 23, no. 3 (2007): 184–189.

Gerdner, L. A., T. Tripp-Reimer, and H. C. Simpson. "Hard lives, God's help, and struggling through: caregiving in Arkansas Delta." *Journal of Cross-Cultural Gerontology* 22, no. 4 (December 2007): 355–374.

Walker, R. J., and H. A. Kiyak. "The impact of providing dental services to frail older adults: perceptions of elders in adult day health centers." *Special Care in Dentistry* 27, no. 4 (July 2007): 139–143.

Yan, E., T. Kwok, C. Tang, and F. Ho. "Factors associated with life satisfaction of personal care workers delivering dementia care in day care centers." *Social Work in Health Care* 46, no. 1 (2007): 37–45.

OTHER

"Adult Day Care: One Form of Respite for Older Adults." *ARCH National Respite Network* Fact Sheet 54, April 2002. http://www.archrespite.org/archfs54.htm (March 20, 2008).

"Adult Day Care Fact Sheet." *Eldercare, U.S. Department of Health and Human Services* July 6, 2005. http://www.eldercare.gov/eldercare/Public/resources/fact_sheets/adult_day.asp (December 24, 2007).

"Nursing Homes." *Medicare, U.S. Department of Health and Human Services* April 10, 2007. http://www.medicare.gov/Nursing/Alternatives/Pace.asp (December 24, 2007).

"Adult Day Services: The Facts." *National Adult Day Services Association*. http://www.nadsa.org/adsfacts/default.asp (March 20, 2008).

ORGANIZATIONS

Alzheimer's Association, 225 N. Michigan Ave., Fl. 17, Chicago, IL, 60601-7633, (312) 335-8700, (800) 272-3900, (866) 699-1246, info@alz.org, http://www.alz.org.

California Association for Adult Day Services, 921 11th Street Suite 1101, Sacramento, CA, 95814, (916) 552-7400, (916) 552-7404, caads@caads.org, http://www.caads.org.

National Adult Day Services Association, 85 South Washington, Suite 316, Seattle, WA, 98104, (877) 745-1440, (206) 461-3218, info@nadsa.org, http://www.nadsa.org.

U.S. Administration on Aging, One Massachusetts Ave., Washington, DC, 20201, (202) 619-0724, AoAInfo@aoa.hhs.gov, http://www.aoa.gov.

L. Fleming Fallon, Jr., M.D., Dr.P.H.

AICD *see* **Implantable cardioverter-defibrillator**

Alanine aminotransferase test

Definition

The alanine aminotransferase test, also known as ALT, is one of a group of tests known as **liver function tests** (or LFTs) and is used to monitor damage to the liver.

Purpose

ALT levels are used to detect liver abnormalities. Since the alanine aminotransferase enzyme is also found in muscle, tests indicating elevated ALT levels may indicate muscle damage; however, other tests, such as the levels of the MB fraction of creatine kinase should indicate whether the abnormal test levels are because of muscle or liver damage.

Demographics

The number of ALT tests administered each year can only be estimated. Since statins are the most prescribed drugs in the United States and standards of care call for quarterly liver function tests, the number of ALTs can easily exceed 500 million per year.

Description

The alanine aminotransferase test (ALT) can reveal liver damage. It is probably the most specific test for liver damage; however, the severity of the liver damage is not necessarily shown by the ALT test since the amount of dead liver tissue does not correspond to higher ALT levels. Also, persons with normal, or declining, ALT levels may experience serious liver damage without an increase in ALT.

Nevertheless, ALT is widely used, and useful, because ALT levels are elevated in most patients with liver disease. Although ALT levels do not necessarily indicate the severity of the damage to the liver, they may indicate how much of the liver has been damaged. ALT levels, when compared to the levels of a similar enzyme, aspartate aminotransferase (AST), may provide important clues to the nature of the liver disease. For example, within a certain range of values, a ratio of 2:1 or greater for AST:ALT might indicate that a person suffers from alcoholic liver disease. Other diagnostic data may be gleaned from ALT tests to indicate abnormal results.

Preparation

No special preparations are necessary for this test.

Aftercare

This test involves blood being drawn, usually from a vein in the person's elbow. The person being tested should keep the wound from the needle puncture covered with a bandage until the bleeding stops. Individuals should report any unusual symptoms to their physician.

Risks

The greatest risk associated with an ALT test is bleeding. The odds of experiencing uncontrolled bleeding are fewer than one in a million.

Normal results

Normal values vary from laboratory to laboratory, and should be available to physicians at the time of the test. An informal survey of some laboratories indicates many laboratories find values from approximately 7 to 50 IU/L (international units per liter) to be normal.

Abnormal results

Mildly elevated levels of ALT (generally below 300 IU/L) may indicate any kind of liver disease. Levels above 1,000 IU/L generally indicate extensive liver damage from toxins or drugs, viral hepatitis, or a lack of oxygen (usually resulting from very low blood pressure or a heart attack). A briefly elevated ALT above 1,000 IU/L that resolves in 24–48 hours may indicate a blockage of the bile duct. More moderate levels of ALT (300–1,000 IU/L) may support a diagnosis of acute or chronic hepatitis.

It is important to note that persons with normal livers may have slightly elevated levels of ALT. This is a normal finding.

Morbidity and mortality rates

Morbidity rates are excessively miniscule. The most common problems are minor bleeding and bruising. Since neither are reportable events, morbidity can only be estimated. Mortality is essentially zero.

Alternatives Resources

There are no alternatives to an alanine amino transferase test.

Precautions

The only precaution needed is to clean the venipuncture site with alcohol.

Side effects

The most common side effects of an alanine amino transferase test are minor bleeding and bruising.

Interactions

There are no known interactions with an alanine amino transferase test.

Resources

BOOKS

Fischbach, F. T. and M. B. Dunning. *A Manual of Laboratory and Diagnostic Tests,* 8th ed. Philadelphia: Lippincott Williams & Wilkins, 2008.

McGhee, M. *A Guide to Laboratory Investigations,* 5th ed. Oxford, UK: Radcliffe Publishing Ltd., 2008.

Price, C. P. *Evidence-Based Laboratory Medicine: Principles, Practice, and Outcomes,* 2nd ed. Washington, DC: AACC Press, 2007.

Scott, M. G., A. M. Gronowski, and C. S. Eby. *Tietz's Applied Laboratory Medicine,* 2nd ed. New York: Wiley-Liss, 2007.

Springhouse Corp. *Diagnostic Tests Made Incredibly Easy!,* 2nd ed. Philadelphia: Lippincott Williams & Wilkins, 2008.

PERIODICALS

Inoue, K., M. Matsumoto, Y. Miyoshi, and Y. Kobayashi. "Elevated liver enzymes in women with a family history of diabetes." *Diabetes Research in Clinical Practice* 79, no. 3 (February 2008): e4–e7.

Kansu, A. "Treatment of chronic hepatitis B in children." *Recent Patents on Anti-Infectious Drug Discoveries* 3, no. 1 (January 2008): 64–69.

Lampe, E., C. F. Yoshida, R. V. De Oliveira, G. M. Lauer, and L. L. Lewis-Ximenez. "Molecular analysis and patterns of ALT and hepatitis C virus seroconversion in haemodialysis patients with acute hepatitis." *Nephrology (Carlton)* 13, no. 3 (June 2008): 186–192.

Lazo, M., E. Selvin, and J. M. Clark. "Brief communication: clinical implications of short-term variability in liver function test results." *Annals of Internal Medicine* 148, no. 5 (March 2008): 348–352.

OTHER

American Clinical Laboratory Association. Information about clinical chemistry. http://www.clinical-labs.org/ (February 24, 2008).

Clinical Laboratory Management Association. Information about clinical chemistry. http://www.clma.org/ (February 22, 2008).

Lab Tests Online. Information about lab tests. http://www.labtestsonline.org/ (February 24, 2008).

National Accreditation Agency for Clinical Laboratory Sciences. Information about laboratory tests. http://www.naacls.org/ (February 25, 2008).

ORGANIZATIONS

American Association for Clinical Chemistry, 1850 K Street, NW, Suite 625, Washington, DC, 20006, (800) 892-1400, http://www.aacc.org/AACC/.

American Society for Clinical Laboratory Science, 6701 Democracy Blvd., Suite 300, Bethesda, MD, 20817, (301) 657-2768, http://www.ascls.org/.

American Society for Clinical Pathology, 1225 New York Ave., NW, Suite 250, Washington, DC, 20005, (202) 347-4450, http://www.ascp.org/.

College of American Pathologists, 325 Waukegan Rd., Northfield, IL, 60093-2750, (800) 323-4040, http://www.cap.org/apps/cap.portal.

L. Fleming Fallon, Jr., M.D., Dr.P.H.

Albumin test *see* **Liver function tests**

Albumin Test, Blood

Definition

Albumin is a type of protein found in the plasma (liquid) portion of the blood. Of all the types of protein in plasma, albumin is found in the highest concentrations, constituting about two-thirds of total plasma protein.

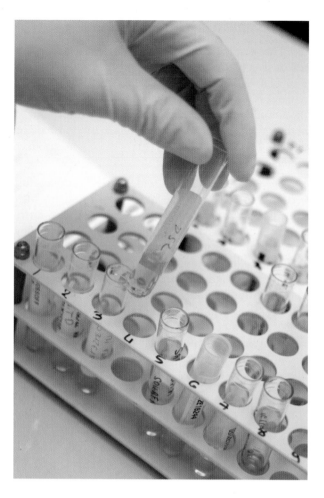

Vials of blood serum. *(AJP / Hop Americain / Photo Researchers, Inc.)*

Albumin serves a number of important purposes. It transports a variety of other important chemicals in the blood, allowing them to be delivered to various organs and tissues. Chemicals that bind to albumin include thyroxine, bilirubin, penicillin, cortisol, estrogen, free fatty acids, warfarin, calcium, magnesium, and heme. Appropriate levels of albumin are also necessary in order to maintain sufficient quantities of fluid within the blood vessels. When the correct concentration of albumin is present in the blood's serum, fluid remains in the blood vessels in order to reach a chemical equilibrium of protein concentrations in and outside of the blood vessels. When there is an insufficient amount of albumin in the serum, fluid will leak out of the blood vessels in response to the considerably higher concentration of protein in the surrounding tissues. This can result in visible swelling of the lower legs (referred to as edema), or in ascites (an abnormal collection of fluid in the abdomen).

Purpose

Albumin levels are tested in order to monitor liver and kidney functioning, and in order to ascertain an individual's nutritional status. Albumin levels may be checked if there is new edema or ascites. Albumin is manufactured in the liver, therefore, low albumin levels may indicate liver damage. Under normal circumstances, no albumin leaves the body in urine; however, when the kidneys are damaged, they may become leaky, allowing albumin to be excreted in the urine. This happens, for example, in nephrotic syndrome, and in pregnant women with pre-eclampsia and eclampsia. Individuals who have poor diets, with an extremely low dietary intake of protein, may also have low serum albumin.

An increased concentration of albumin may suggest that an individual has become dehydrated. High albumin levels may also occur when an individual is using insulin, growth hormones, androgens, or anabolic steroids.

Precautions

Individuals who have been on intravenous fluids may not have an accurate serum albumin reading. Additionally, it's important to remember that women have lower-than-normal serum albumin levels during pregnancy. Individuals using certain medications, such as insulin, growth hormones, androgens, or anabolic steroids, may also have an abnormal serum albumin level.

Description

This test is usually performed as part of a panel of blood tests, in which a single sample of blood is tested for a variety of chemical elements. Serum albumin levels are often tested along with total protein levels. A blood test for serum albumin requires vein puncture with a needle, and is usually performed by a nurse of phlebotomist (an individual who has been trained to draw blood).

Preparation

There are no restrictions on diet or physical activity, either before or after the blood test.

Aftercare

As with any blood tests, discomfort, bruising, and/or a very small amount of bleeding is common at the puncture site. Immediately after the needle is withdrawn, it is helpful to put pressure on the puncture site until the bleeding has stopped. This decreases

---

> ## KEY TERMS
>
> **Ascites**—An abnormal collection of fluid within the abdomen, often suggests liver disease such as cirrhosis.
>
> **Cirrhosis**—Liver disease that results in damage and scarring to the liver.
>
> **Dehydration**—Low overall levels of body fluid. May occur due to increased loss of fluids through sweating, vomiting, or diarrhea.
>
> **Eclampsia**—A serious, life-threatening complication of pregnancy, in which high blood pressure results in a variety of problems, including seizures.
>
> **Nephrotic syndrome**—A kidney disorder which causes a cluster of symptoms, including low serum protein, loss of protein in the urine, and body swelling.
>
> **Plasma**—The fluid component of blood which contains such substances as proteins, vitamins, minerals, enzymes, and sugars.
>
> **Pre-eclampsia**—High blood pressure in pregnancy, which can result in protein in the urine; untreated, pre-eclampsia may lead to the life-threatening condition known as eclampsia, which is characterized by seizures.

the chance of significant bruising. Warm packs may relieve minor discomfort. Some individuals may feel briefly woozy after a blood test, and they should be encouraged to lie down and rest until they feel better.

Risks

Basic blood tests, such as serum albumin levels, do not carry any significant risks, other than slight bruising and the chance of brief dizziness.

Normal results

In general, the normal range of serum albumin is 3.4 to 5.4 g/dL (grams per deciliter). Different labs may have slightly different values listed for the normal range of serum albumin. If total serum proteins are also being tested, the fraction that is made up of albumin should be about 60%.

Abnormal results

Low albumin may indicate:

- liver disease, such as cirrhosis, hepatitis, or hepato-cellular necrosis (death of liver cells);

- kidney disease, such as nephritic syndrome or glomerulonephritis;
- severe malnutrition, as occurs in developing countries where protein deficiencies are common. This type of malnutrition is referred to as kwashiorkor, and results in the stereotypical "potbelly" often associated with malnourished children;
- malnourishment due to chronic diseases such as HIV or cancer, or due to the effects of an eating disorder such as anorexia nervosa;
- inability to absorb and digest protein, as occurs in Crohn's disease, Whipple's disease, or sprue;
- loss of protein from severe or chronic diarrhea;
- inflammation;
- severe burns; or
- shock.

High albumin levels can result from dehydration or the presence of certain medications.

Resources

BOOKS

Brenner, B. M., and F. C. Rector, eds. *Brenner & Rector's The Kidney,* 7th ed. Philadelphia: Saunders, 2004.

Feldman, M., L. S. Friedman, and L. J. Brandt. *Sleisenger & Fordtran's Gastrointestinal and Liver Disease,* 8th ed. St. Louis: Mosby, 2006.

McPherson R. A., and M. R. Pincus, eds. *Henry's Clinical Diagnosis and Management by Laboratory Methods,* 21st ed. Philadelphia: Saunders, 2006.

OTHER

Medical Encyclopedia. Medline Plus. U. S. National Library of Science and the National Institutes of Health. http://www.nlm.nih.gov/medlineplus/encyclopedia.html (February 10, 2008).

ORGANIZATIONS

American Association for Clinical Chemistry, 1850 K Street, NW, Suite 625, Washington, DC, 20006, (800) 892-1400, http://www.aacc.org.

Rosalyn Carson-DeWitt, M.D.

Allogenic transplant *see* **Bone marrow transplantation**

Ambulatory surgery centers

Definition

Ambulatory surgery centers (ASCs) are medical facilities that specialize in elective same-day or outpatient surgical procedures. They do not offer emergency care.

The word ambulatory comes from the Latin verb *ambulare,* which means "to walk." It means that the patients treated in these surgical centers do not require admission to a hospital and are well enough to go home after the procedure. Ambulatory surgical centers are also known as surgicenters.

Demographics

As of 2008, there were more than 5,300 ambulatory surgical centers in the United States, up from about 3,700 in 2003. In 1980, only 275 such centers existed. This rapid increase reflects a general trend toward surgeries performed on an outpatient basis. According to *American Medical News,* 70% of all surgical procedures performed in the United States in 2000 were done in outpatient facilities, compared to 15% in 1980. As of 2003, over seven million surgeries are performed annually in American ASCs. Between 1990 and 2000, the number of operations performed annually in these centers rose 191%, from 2.3 million procedures in 1990 to 6.7 million in 2000.

The types of surgical procedures performed in ASCs have also undergone significant changes in recent years. Many of the early ASCs were outpatient centers for **plastic surgery**. Advances in minimally invasive surgical techniques in other specialties, however, led to the establishment of ASCs for orthopedic, dental, and ophthalmologic procedures. According to the Federated Ambulatory Surgery Association (FASA), gastroenterology accounted for only 10% of all procedures performed in ASCs in 1995, while plastic surgery still represented 20%. These proportions changed rapidly. By 1998, only three years later, ophthalmology accounted for more procedures performed in ASCs than any other surgical specialty (26.8%), followed by gastroenterology (18.8%), **orthopedic surgery** (9.8%), gynecology (9.5%), plastic surgery (7.7%), and otolaryngology (6.9%). The remaining 20.6% included dental, urological, neurological, podiatric, and pain block procedures.

As of 2003, ASCs are not distributed evenly across the United States; they tend to be concentrated in urban areas, particularly those with a high ratio of physicians to the general population.

Description

Ambulatory surgical centers are sometimes classified as either hospital-associated or freestanding. The term freestanding is somewhat confusing because some hospital-associated ASCs are located in buildings that may be several blocks away from the main hospital. As a result, some states have defined an ASC for legal purposes as "a facility primarily organized or established for the purpose of performing surgery for outpatients and...a separate identifiable legal entity from any other health care facility." More recently, some ASCs have sought institutional relationships with academic medical centers, hoping to benefit from the prestige associated with teaching and research.

Ambulatory surgery centers should not be confused with office-based surgery practices or with other outpatient centers that provide diagnostic services or primary health care, such as urgent care centers, community health centers, mobile diagnostic units, or rural health clinics. ASCs are distinguished from these other health care facilities by their use of a referral system for accepting patients and their maintenance of a dedicated **operating room**. The first characteristic means that any patient who wants to be treated in an ambulatory surgery center must first consult their primary health care provider, or PCP, and choose to have their condition treated by surgery rather than an alternative approach. The second feature means that the surgical facility must have at least one room that is used only for operations.

Accreditation and ownership

The Joint Commission on Accreditation of Healthcare Organizations (JCAHO) lists nine types of ASCs that it presently accredits:

- cosmetic and facial surgery centers
- endoscopy centers
- ophthalmology practices
- laser eye surgery centers
- centers for oral and maxillofacial surgery
- orthopedic surgery centers
- plastic surgery centers
- podiatry clinics
- multi-specialty surgery centers

Medicare inspection and certification of ambulatory surgery centers is a separate process from professional accreditation. An ASC does not have to be certified by Medicare in order to be accredited by JCAHO. Office-based surgical practices are accredited by JCAHO under a specialized Office-Based Surgery Accreditation program.

ASCs are sometimes categorized on the basis of ownership. Some are owned by hospitals and others are owned by the physicians who treat patients in them; about half, however, are operated by investor-owned businesses. The rapid growth of ASCs is in part a reflection of the general commercialization of health care in the United States over the past two decades.

Patient care

A patient in an ambulatory surgical center is asked to observe some of the same precautions and preparations that hospital patients undergo, including routine blood tests and a thorough medical history to make certain that they will not have an adverse reaction to anesthesia. In most cases the patient will be told to avoid eating and drinking before the procedure. Patients are asked to have a friend or family member drive them home after surgery; some ASCs request that the friend or relative come with the patient in the morning and stay at the center in a waiting area until the patient feels well enough to leave.

On average, patients leave the ASC within two hours after their surgery. If the patient needs overnight care or has a serious complication, he or she is transferred to an acute care hospital. Most ASCs that are not hospital-owned have arrangements with nearby hospitals to cover emergency situations.

Historical background

The first ambulatory surgical center was opened in 1970 by a group of anesthesiologists in Phoenix, Arizona. Relatively few ASCs were built, however, until the mid-1980s. Two factors that encouraged the rapid spread of ASCs after that point were the development of accreditation programs and standards on the one hand and government approval on the other. In 1980 the American Society of Plastic and Reconstructive Surgeons (ASPRS) established the American

Association for Accreditation of Ambulatory Plastic Surgery Facilities, or AAAAPSF, in order to guarantee the quality of outpatient surgical facilities. The AAAAPSF then formed the American Association for Accreditation of Ambulatory Surgical Facilities, or AAAASF, to establish standards for single-specialty and multi-specialty ASCs owned or operated by surgeons who are board-certified in other types of surgery. In 1982 procedures performed at ASCs were made eligible for Medicare payments on the grounds that they were low-risk surgeries provided in less expensive settings. As of 2003, 85% of the ASCs in the United States are certified by Medicare.

Other factors involved in the expansion of ASCs include:

- Advances in medical technology. The development of instruments that made minimally invasive procedures possible made certain types of surgery less complicated to perform and less painful for the patient. The most important single development that made outpatient surgery increasingly safe, however, is the discovery of new anesthetic agents combined with better techniques for administering anesthesia. The number of anesthesia-related deaths has dropped sharply since the 1980s, from 1:10,000 operations in 1982 to 1:400,000 in 2002.

- Demographic changes. Instead of a shortage, by the late 1990s there was an oversupply of physicians as well as hospital beds in the United States. This situation has led to increasing competition for patients among both doctors and hospital managers.

- The increasing commercialization of health care. The rise of investor-owned hospitals and ambulatory surgery centers encouraged many doctors to invest money in these facilities, particularly the ASCs. Since ambulatory surgery centers accept patients only on a referral basis, questions have been raised about the legitimacy of doctors referring patients to facilities in which they have a financial interest. The former editor of the *New England Journal of Medicine* cites a Florida study revealing that almost 40% of the doctors practicing in that state had money invested in the ASCs to which they sent their patients.

Advantages of ASCs

Surgeons as well as patients tend to prefer ambulatory surgery centers for outpatient procedures for several reasons:

- Cost. In many cases, an outpatient procedure done in an ASC costs between one-half and one-third as much as the same procedure done in a hospital. It is important, however, for patients to compare costs carefully, because some ASC procedures may cost as much as or even more than hospital-based procedures. For example, the Medicare Payment Advisory Commission found that whereas a cataract operation cost only $942 at an ambulatory surgery center in 2001 as opposed to $1334 at a hospital, after-cataract laser surgery cost $429 at the ASC versus $246 at a hospital. Figures for an endoscopy and biopsy of the upper digestive tract were $429 and $359 respectively; for a diagnostic colonoscopy, $429 and $401; and for epidural anesthesia, $320 and $183.

- Convenience. There is much less administrative paperwork and "red tape" at an ambulatory surgical center compared to the admissions process at most hospitals. Patients also like the fact that they can leave an ASC relatively quickly after their surgery, which translates into less time lost from work.

- Presence of family and friends. Whereas most hospitals keep patients recovering from a surgical procedure in separate rooms, in an ASC the patient can usually spend the recovery period after surgery with their loved ones.

- Greater efficiency. This advantage is particularly important to surgeons. It takes much less time to prepare an operating room in a specialized ASC for the next patient than in a standard hospital. Improved efficiency allows the surgeon to treat more patients in the same amount of time than he or she would be able to do in a hospital; some surgeons maintain that they can do three times the number of procedures in an ASC as they could in a hospital setting.

- Greater control over procedures and standards. Many doctors prefer working in an ASC because they can set the standards for staffing, safety precautions, postoperative care, etc., rather than having these things decided for them by a hospital manager.

ASCs within the American health care system

As of 2003, there are several areas of tension in the health care system related to ambulatory surgical centers. One is opposition from hospitals. Most hospitals have relied on income from surgical procedures to make up for losses incurred by treating other patients who cannot afford to pay. The movement toward freestanding ambulatory surgery centers means a considerable loss of income for many hospitals.

On the other hand, there is also increasing competition between ASCs and office-based surgical practices. The same improvements in anesthesia and surgical equipment that made **outpatient surgery** in an ASC safe to perform have also made it safe to do a growing number of fairly complex procedures in a doctor's office. Such procedures as hernia repair, arthroscopic joint repair, and **liposuction** are now being performed in office-based facilities. It is estimated that by 2005, 10 million surgical procedures will be performed annually in American doctors' offices, or twice as many as were done in 1995. The American Society of Anesthesiologists predicts that office-based surgical procedures will account for a steadily growing proportion of outpatient surgeries. The ASA has stated that "... the trend toward office-based surgery is growing at least as fast [as of 2003] as the trend toward ambulatory surgery grew a few years ago."

Legal and regulatory issues

The growing number of for-profit ASCs as well as government involvement with outpatient facilities through the Medicare program has led to a number of legal and regulatory questions. One issue concerns the level of Medicare reimbursement for procedures performed in ASCs. The present Medicare fee schedule is based on data from 1986, when the operating costs of many ambulatory surgical centers were higher than they are in 2003, due to advances in technology. As a result, some observers think that ASCs are being overpaid for services to Medicare patients. Another issue is a proposal to add more procedures to the list approved by Medicare for ASC patients. The present list has not been updated since 1995. The proposed additions would increase ASC services available to Medicare patients by 20%.

The major legal question facing surgeons who own or have investments in ambulatory surgical centers is whether they are breaking the law by referring patients to ASCs in which they have invested or in which they perform surgery. The existing laws are not entirely clear on this point, but experts in health law do not expect the confusion to be resolved in the near future.

Resources

PERIODICALS

Aker, J. "Safety of Ambulatory Surgery." *Journal of Perianesthesia Nursing* 16 (December 2001): 353–358.

Baker, J. J. "Medicare Payment System for Ambulatory Surgical Centers." *Journal of Health Care Finance* 28 (Spring 2002): 76–87.

Becker, S. and M. Biala. "Ambulatory Surgery Centers—Current Business and Legal Issues." *Journal of Health Care Finance* 27 (Winter 2000): 1–7.

Becker, S. and N. Harned. "The Fraud and Abuse Statute and Investor-Owned Ambulatory Surgery Centers." *Health Care Law Monthly* (April 2002): 13–23.

Hawryluk, Markian. "Ambulatory Surgery Centers' Medicare Pay Rate Questioned." *American Medical News* November 25, 2002 [cited March 12, 2003]. http://www.ama-assn.org/sci-pubs/amnews/pick_02/gvsa1125.htm.

Jackson, Cheryl. "Cutting Into the Market: Rise of Ambulatory Surgical Centers." *American Medical News*, April 15, 2002. [cited March 12, 2003]. http://www.ama-assn.org/sci-pubs/amnews/pick_02/bisa0415.htm.

Lynk, W. J. and C. S. Longley. "The Effect of Physician-Owned Surgicenters on Hospital Outpatient Surgery." *Health Affairs (Millwood)* 21 (July-August 2002): 215–221.

Mamel, J. J. and H. J. Nord. "Endoscopic Ambulatory Surgery Centers in the Academic Medical Center. We Can Do It Too!" *Gastrointestinal Endoscopy Clinics of North America* 12 (April 2002): 275–284.

O'Brien, D. "Acute Postoperative Delirium: Definitions, Incidence, Recognition, and Interventions." *Journal of Perianesthesia Nursing* 17 (December 2002): 384–392.

Relman, Arnold S., MD. "Canada's Romance with Market Medicine." *American Prospect* 13 (October 21, 2002) [cited March 12, 2003]. http://www.prospect.org/print_friendly/print/V13/19/relman-a.html.

Relman, Arnold S., MD. "What Market Values Are Doing to Medicine." *Atlantic Monthly* 269 (March 1992): 99–106.

ORGANIZATIONS

Accreditation Association for Ambulatory Health Care (AAAHC). 3201 Old Glenview Road, Suite 300, Wilmette, IL 60091-2992. (847) 853-6060. http://www.aahc.org.

American Association for Accreditation of Ambulatory Surgery Facilities (AAAASF). 1202 Allanson Road, Mundelein, IL 60060. (888) 545-5222.

American Association of Ambulatory Surgical Centers (AAASC). P. O. Box 23220, San Diego, CA 92193. (800) 237-3768. http://www.aaasc.org.

American Health Lawyers Association. Suite 600, 1025 Connecticut Avenue NW, Washington, DC 20036-5405. (202) 833-1100. http://www.healthlawyers.org.

American Society of Anesthesiologists (ASA). 520 N. Northwest Highway, Park Ridge, IL 60068-2573. (847) 825-5586. http://www.asahq.org.

Federated Ambulatory Surgery Association (FASA). 700 North Fairfax Street, #306, Alexandria, VA 22314. (703) 836-8808. http://www.fasa.org.

Joint Commission on Accreditation of Healthcare Organizations (JCAHO). One Renaissance Boulevard, Oakbrook Terrace, IL 60181. (630) 792-5000. http://www.jcaho.org.

OTHER

American Society of Anesthesiologists. *Office-Based Anesthesia and Surgery.* [cited March 13, 2003]. http://www.asahq.org/patientEducation/officebased.htm.

Rebecca Frey, Ph.D.

Ammonia (blood) test *see* **Liver function tests**

Amniocentesis

Definition

Amniocentesis is a procedure used to diagnose fetal defects in the early second trimester of pregnancy. A sample of the amniotic fluid, which surrounds a fetus in the womb, is collected through a pregnant woman's abdomen using a needle and syringe. Tests performed on fetal cells found in the amniotic fluid can reveal the presence of many types of genetic disorders. Early diagnosis allows doctors and prospective parents to make important decisions about treatment and intervention prior to birth.

Purpose

Since the mid-1970s, amniocentesis has been used routinely to test for Down syndrome, by far the most common, nonhereditary, genetic birth defect, afflicting about one in every 1,000 babies. By 1997, approximately 800 different diagnostic tests were available, most of them for hereditary genetic disorders such as Tay-Sachs disease, sickle cell disease, hemophilia, muscular dystrophy, and cystic fibrosis.

Amniocentesis, often called amnio, is recommended for women who will be older than 35 on their due date. It is also recommended for women who have already borne children with birth defects, or when either of the parents has a family history of a birth defect for which a diagnostic test is available. Another reason for the procedure is to confirm indications of Down syndrome and certain other defects that may have shown up previously during routine maternal blood screening.

The risk of bearing a child with a nonhereditary genetic defect such as Down syndrome is directly related to a woman's age—the older the woman, the greater the risk. Thirty-five is the recommended age to

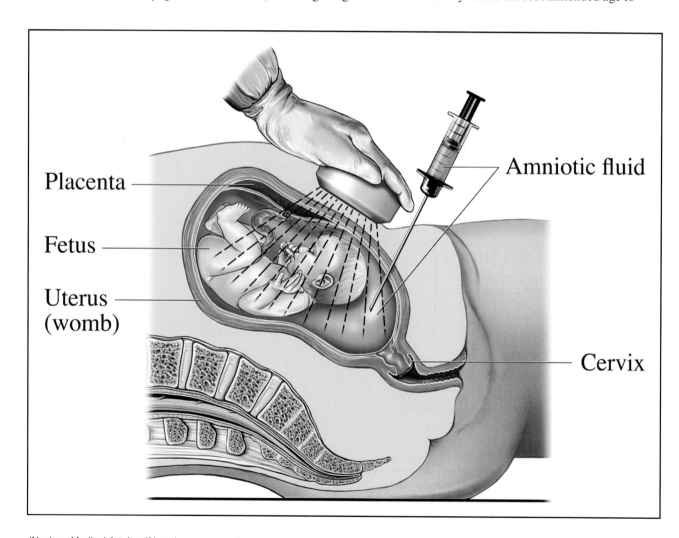

Placenta

Fetus

Uterus (womb)

Amniotic fluid

Cervix

(Nucleus Medical Art, Inc./Alamy)

Alpha-fetoprotein (AFP)—A protein normally produced by the liver of a fetus and detectable in maternal blood samples. AFP screening measures the amount of alpha-fetoprotein in the blood. Levels outside the norm may indicate fetal defects.

Anencephaly—A hereditary defect resulting in the partial to complete absence of a brain and spinal cord. It is fatal.

Chorionic villus sampling (CVS)—A procedure similar to amniocentesis, except that cells are taken from the chorionic membrane for testing. These cells, called chorionic villus cells, eventually become the placenta. The samples are collected either through the abdomen, as in amnio, or through the vagina. CVS can be done earlier in the pregnancy than amnio, but carries a somewhat higher risk.

Chromosomes—Chromosomes are the strands of genetic material in a cell that occur in nearly identical pairs. Normal human cells contain 23 chromosome pairs—one in each pair inherited from the mother, and one from the father. Every human cell contains the exact same set of chromosomes.

Down syndrome—The most prevalent of a class of genetic defects known as trisomies, in which cells contain three copies of certain chromosomes rather than the usual two. Down syndrome, or

trisomy 21, usually results from three copies of chromosome 21.

Genetic—The term refers to genes, the basic units of biological heredity, which are contained on the chromosomes, and contain chemical instructions that direct the development and functioning of an individual.

Hereditary—Something that is inherited or passed down from parents to offspring. In biology and medicine, the word pertains to inherited genetic characteristics.

Maternal blood screening—Maternal blood screening is normally done early in pregnancy to test for a variety of conditions. Abnormal amounts of certain proteins in a pregnant woman's blood raise the probability of fetal defects. Amniocentesis is recommended if such a probability occurs.

Tay-Sachs disease—An inherited disease prevalent among the Ashkenazi Jewish population of the United States. Infants with the disease are unable to process a certain type of fat that accumulates in nerve and brain cells, causing mental and physical retardation, and death by age four.

Ultrasound—A technique that uses high-frequency sound waves to create a visual image (a sonogram) of soft tissues. The technique is routinely used in prenatal care and diagnosis.

begin amnio testing because that is the age at which the risk of carrying a fetus with such a defect roughly equals the risk of miscarriage caused by the procedure, which is about one in 200. At age 25, the risk of giving birth to a child with this type of defect is about one in 1,400; by age 45, it increases to about one in 20. Nearly half of all pregnant women over 35 in the United States undergo amniocentesis, and many younger women also decide to have the procedure. Notably, some 75% of all Down syndrome infants born in the United States each year are to women younger than 35. In January 2007, the American College of Obstetricians and Gynecologists issued a recommendation that all pregnant patients be offered the option of amniocentesis testing, regardless of maternal age.

One of the most common reasons for performing amniocentesis is an abnormal alpha-fetoprotein (AFP) test. Alpha-fetoprotein is a protein produced by the fetus and present in the mother's blood. A

simple blood screening, usually conducted around the fifteenth week of pregnancy, can determine the AFP levels in the mother's blood. Levels that are too high or too low may signal possible fetal defects. Because this test has a high false-positive rate, another test such as amniocentesis is recommended whenever the AFP levels fall outside the normal range.

Amniocentesis is generally performed during the sixteenth week of pregnancy, with results usually available within three weeks. It is possible to perform amnio as early as the eleventh week, but this is not usually recommended because there appears to be an increased risk of miscarriage when done at this time. The advantage of early amnio and speedy results lies in the extra time for decision making if a problem is detected. Potential treatment of the fetus can begin earlier. Important, also, is the fact that elective abortions are safer and less controversial the earlier they are performed.

Precautions

As an invasive surgical procedure, amniocentesis poses a real, although small, risk to the health of a fetus. Parents must weigh the potential value of the knowledge gained, or indeed the reassurance that all is well, against the small risk of miscarriage. The serious emotional and ethical dilemmas that adverse test results can bring must also be considered. The decision to undergo amnio is always a matter of personal choice.

Description

The word amniocentesis literally means "puncture of the amnion," the thin-walled sac of fluid in which a developing fetus is suspended during pregnancy. During the procedure, the obstetrician inserts a very fine needle through the woman's abdomen into the uterus and the amniotic sac and withdraws approximately 1 oz (28.3 g) of amniotic fluid for testing. The relatively painless procedure is performed on an outpatient basis, sometimes using **local anesthesia**.

The physician uses **ultrasound** images to guide needle placement and collect the sample, thereby minimizing the risk of fetal injury and the need for repeated needle insertions. Once the sample is collected, the woman can return home after a brief observation period. She may be instructed to rest for the first 24 hours and to avoid heavy lifting for two days.

The sample of amniotic fluid is sent to a laboratory where fetal cells contained in the fluid are isolated and grown in order to provide enough genetic material for testing. This takes about seven to 14 days. The material is then extracted and treated so that visual examination for defects can be made. For some disorders, like Tay-Sachs, the simple presence of a telltale chemical compound in the amniotic fluid is enough to confirm a diagnosis. Depending on the specific tests ordered, and the skill of the lab conducting them, all the results are available one to four weeks after the sample is taken.

Cost of the procedure depends on the doctor, the lab, and the tests ordered. Most insurers provide coverage for women over 35, as a follow-up to positive maternal blood screening results, and when genetic disorders run in the family.

An alternative to amnio, now in general use, is chorionic villus sampling (CVS), which can be performed as early as the eighth week of pregnancy. While this allows for the possibility of a first-trimester abortion, if warranted, CVS is apparently also riskier and is more expensive. The most promising area of new research in prenatal testing involves expanding the scope and accuracy of maternal blood screening as this poses no risk to the fetus.

Preparation

It is important for a woman to fully understand the procedure and to feel confident in the obstetrician performing it. Evidence suggests that a physician's experience with the procedure reduces the chance of mishap. Almost all obstetricians are experienced in performing amniocentesis. The patient should feel free to ask questions and seek emotional support before, during, and after amniocentesis is performed.

Aftercare

Necessary aftercare falls into two categories, physical and emotional.

Physical aftercare

During and immediately following the sampling procedure, a woman may experience dizziness, nausea, a rapid heartbeat, and cramping. Once past these immediate hurdles, the physician will send the woman home with instructions to rest and to report any complications requiring immediate treatment, including:

- Vaginal bleeding. The appearance of blood could signal a problem.
- Premature labor. Unusual abdominal pain and/or cramping may indicate the onset of premature labor. Mild cramping for the first day or two following the procedure is normal.
- Signs of infection. Leaking of amniotic fluid or unusual vaginal discharge, and fever could signal the onset of infection.

Emotional aftercare

Once the procedure has been safely completed, the anxiety of waiting for the test results can prove to be the worst part of the process. A woman should seek and receive emotional support from family and friends, as well as from her obstetrician and family doctor. Professional counseling may also prove necessary, particularly if a fetal defect is detected.

Risks

Most of the risks and short-term side effects associated with amniocentesis relate to the sampling procedure. A successful amnio sampling results in no long-term side effects. Risks include:

- Maternal/fetal hemorrhaging. While spotting in pregnancy is fairly common, bleeding following amnio should always be investigated.
- Infection. Infection, although rare, can occur after amniocentesis. An unchecked infection can lead to severe complications.
- Fetal injury. A very slight risk of injury to the fetus resulting from contact with the amnio needle does exist.
- Miscarriage. The rate of miscarriage occurring during standard, second-trimester amnio is approximately 0.5%. This compares to a miscarriage rate of 1% for CVS. Many fetuses with severe genetic defects miscarry naturally during the first trimester.
- The trauma of difficult family-planning decisions. The threat posed to parental and family mental health from the trauma accompanying an abnormal test result can not be underestimated.

Normal results

Negative results from an amnio analysis indicate that everything about the fetus appears normal and the pregnancy can continue without undue concern. A negative result for Down syndrome means that it is 99% certain that the disease does not exist.

An overall "normal" result does not, however, guarantee that the pregnancy will come to term, or that the fetus does not suffer from some other defect. Laboratory tests are not 100% accurate at detecting targeted conditions, nor can is there a test for every possible fetal condition.

Abnormal results

Positive results on an amnio analysis indicate the presence of a fetal defect, with an accuracy approaching 100%. With such a diagnosis, prospective parents face emotionally and ethically difficult choices regarding prenatal treatment options, the prospect of treating the defect at birth, and the option of elective abortion. At this point, the parents need expert medical advice and counseling.

Resources

BOOKS

Hassold, Terry and Stuart Schwartz. "Chromosome Disorders." In *Harrison's Principles of Internal Medicine*, edited by Eugene Braunwald, et al. Philadelphia: McGraw-Hill, 2001.

Miesfeldt, Susan and J. Larry Jameson. "Screening, Counseling, and Prevention of Genetic Disorders." In *Harrison's Principles of Internal Medicine*, edited by Eugene Braunwald, et al. Philadelphia: McGraw-Hill, 2001.

Wallach, Jacques. *Interpretation of Diagnostic Tests*. 7th ed. Philadelphia, PA: Lippincott Williams & Wilkens, 2000.

ORGANIZATIONS

American College of Obstetricians and Gynecologists. 409 12th St., S.W., P.O. Box 96920, Washington, DC 20090-6920. http://www.acog.org (accessed March 6, 2008).

OTHER

National Institutes of Health. [cited April 4, 2003]. http://www.nlm.nih.gov/medlineplus/encyclopedia.html (accessed March 6, 2008).

"New Recommendations for Down Syndrome: Screening Should Be Offered to All Pregnant Women." American College of Obstetricians and Gynecologists, Jan. 2, 2007. http://www.acog.org/from_home/publications/press_releases/nr01-02-07-1.cfm (accessed March 10, 2008).

Kurt Richard Sternlof
Mark A. Best
Fran Hodgkins

Amniotic fluid analysis *see* **Amniocentesis**

Amputation

Definition

Amputation is the surgical removal of a limb or body part. It is performed to remove diseased tissue or relieve pain.

Purpose

Arms, legs, hands, feet, fingers, and toes can all be amputated. In the United States, there are approximately 350,000 amputees, with some 135,000 new amputations occurring each year. The number of amputees worldwide is not currently known.

Here in the United States, the most common causes of amputation of the lower extremity are: disease (70%), trauma (22%), congenital or birth defects (4%), and tumors (4%). As for upper extremity amputation, it is usually performed because of trauma or birth defect. Seldom is disease as great a contributing factor. The causes of amputation differ significantly in various countries. For example, countries with a recent history of warfare and civil unrest will have a higher incidence of amputations, due to war itself or its technology (landmines, uncontrolled ordnance, etc).

Amputation

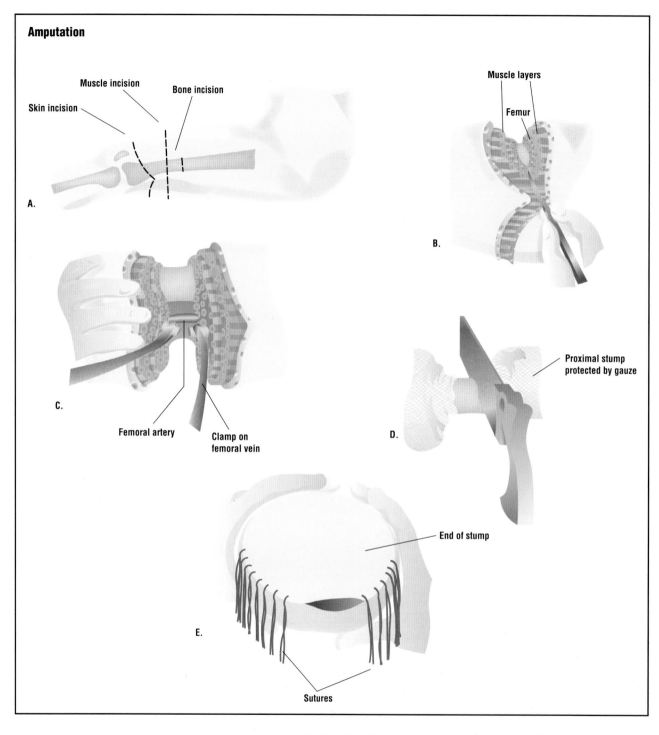

Muscle incision

Bone incision

Skin incision

A.

Muscle layers

Femur

B.

C.

Femoral artery

Clamp on femoral vein

Proximal stump protected by gauze

D.

End of stump

E.

Sutures

In an above-the-knee amputation, three incisions are made (A). First the skin and muscle layers are cut (B). The major blood vessels are clamped and severed (C). The bone is cut with a special saw (D). Finally, the muscles are stitched over the bone, and the skin is closed over the wound (E). *(Illustration by GGS Information Services. Cengage Learning, Gale.)*

Among the diseases and conditions that may lead to amputation of an extremity, the most prevalent are:

- hardening of the arteries

- arterial embolism

- impaired circulation as a complication of diabetes mellitus

- gangrene

- severe frostbite

KEY TERMS

Arterial embolism—A blood clot arising from another location that blocks an artery.

Buerger's disease—An episodic disease that causes inflammation and blockage of the veins and arteries of the limbs. It tends to be present almost exclusively in men under age 40 who smoke, and may require amputation of the hand or foot.

Diabetes mellitus—A disease in which insufficient insulin is made by the body to metabolize sugars.

Raynaud's disease—A disease found mainly in young women that causes decreased circulation to the hands and feet. Its cause is unknown.

- Raynaud's disease
- Buerger's disease

More than 90% of amputations performed in the United States are due to circulatory complications of diabetes. Sixty to eighty percent of these operations involve the legs.

Demographics

Most amputations involve small body parts such as a finger, rather than an entire limb. About 65,000 amputations are performed in the United States each year.

In the United States, there are approximately 350,000 amputees, with some 135,000 new amputations occurring each year. The number of amputees worldwide is not currently known.

Description

Amputations can be either planned or emergency procedures. Injury and arterial embolisms are the main reasons for emergency amputations. The operation is performed under regional or **general anesthesia** by a general or orthopedic surgeon in a hospital **operating room**.

Details of the operation vary slightly depending on what part is to be removed. All amputations consist of a two-fold surgical procedure: to remove diseased tissue so that the wound will heal cleanly, and to construct a stump that will allow the attachment of a prosthesis or artificial replacement part.

The surgeon makes an incision around the part to be amputated. The part is removed, and the bone is smoothed. A flap is constructed of muscle, connective tissue, and skin to cover the raw end of the bone. The flap is closed over the bone with sutures (surgical **stitches**) that remain in place for about one month. Often, a rigid dressing or cast is applied that stays in place for about two weeks.

Diagnosis/Preparation

Before an amputation is performed, extensive testing is done to determine the proper level of amputation. The goal of the surgeon is to find the place where healing is most likely to be complete, while allowing the maximum amount of limb to remain for effective rehabilitation.

The greater the blood flow through an area, the more likely healing is to occur. These tests are designed to measure blood flow through the limb. Several or all of them can be done to help choose the proper level of amputation.

- measurement of blood pressure in different parts of the limb
- xenon 133 studies, which use a radiopharmaceutical to measure blood flow
- oxygen tension measurements in which an oxygen electrode is used to measure oxygen pressure under the skin (If the pressure is 0, the healing will not occur. If the pressure reads higher than 40mm Hg [40 milliliters of mercury], healing of the area is likely to be satisfactory.)
- laser doppler measurements of the microcirculation of the skin
- skin fluorescent studies that also measure skin microcirculation
- skin perfusion measurements using a blood pressure cuff and photoelectric detector
- infrared measurements of skin temperature

No one test is highly predictive of healing, but taken together, the results give the surgeon an excellent idea of the best place to amputate.

Aftercare

After amputation, medication is prescribed for pain, and patients are treated with **antibiotics** to discourage infection. The stump is moved often to encourage good circulation. Physical therapy and rehabilitation are started as soon as possible, usually within 48 hours. Studies have shown that there is a positive relationship between early rehabilitation and effective functioning of the stump and prosthesis. Length of stay in the hospital depends on the severity of the amputation and the general health of the amputee, but ranges from several days to two weeks.

Rehabilitation is a long, arduous process, especially for above the knee amputees. Twice daily physical therapy is not uncommon. In addition, psychological counseling is an important part of rehabilitation. Many people feel a sense of loss and grief when they lose a body part. Others are bothered by phantom limb syndrome, where they feel as if the amputated part is still in place. They may even feel pain in this limb that does not exist. Many amputees benefit from joining self-help groups and meeting others who are also living with amputation. Addressing the emotional aspects of amputation often speeds the physical rehabilitation process.

Risks

Amputation is major surgery. All the risks associated with the administration of anesthesia exist, along with the possibility of heavy blood loss and the development of blood clots. Infection is of special concern to amputees. Infection rates in amputations average 15%. If the stump becomes infected, it is necessary to remove the prosthesis and sometimes to amputate a second time at a higher level.

Failure of the stump to heal is another major complication. Nonhealing is usually due to an inadequate blood supply. The rate of nonhealing varies from 5–30% depending on the facility. Centers that specialize in amputation usually have the lowest rates of complication.

Persistent pain in the stump or pain in the phantom limb is experienced by most amputees to some degree. Treatment of phantom limb pain is difficult. One final complication is that many amputees give up on the rehabilitation process and discard their prosthesis.

Better fitting prosthetics and earlier rehabilitation have decreased the incidence of this problem.

Normal results

The five year survival rate for all lower extremity amputees is less than 50%. For diabetic amputees, the rate is less than 40%. Up to 50% of people who have one leg amputated because of diabetes will lose the other within five years. Amputees who walk using a prosthesis have a less stable gait. Three to five percent of these people fall and break bones because of this instability. Although the fractures can be treated, about half the amputees who suffer them then remain wheelchair bound.

Alternatives

Alternatives to amputation depend on the medical cause underlying the decision to amputate and the degree of medical urgency. In some cases, drug therapy may be considered as an alternative.

For example, one serious complication of diabetes is the development of foot ulcers that often lead to amputation. Some studies have suggested non-surgical treatment of diabetic foot ulcers with a new, recombinant drug (Becaplermin/Regranex). Combined with competent ulcer nursing, the drug leads to fewer amputations compared to the alternative of ulcer nursing on its own.

Resources

BOOKS

Meier, R. H. *Functional Restoration of Adults and Children With Upper Extremity Amputation*. New York: Demos Medical Publishing, 2003.

Murdoch, G. and A. Bennett Wilson. *A Primer on Amputations and Artificial Limbs.* Springfield: Charles C. Thomas Pub. Ltd., 1998.

Watts, H. and M. Williams. *Who Is Amelia?: Caring for Children With Limb Difference.* Rosemont, IL: American Academy of Orthopaedic Surgeons, 1998.

PERIODICALS

Buzato, M. A., E. C. Tribulatto, S. M. Costa, W. G. Zorn, and B. van Bellen. "Major amputations of the lower leg. The patients two years later." *Acta Chirurgica Belgica* 102 (August 2002): 248–252.

Cull, D. L., S. M. Taylor, S. E. Hamontree, E. M. Langan, B. A. Snyder, T. M. Sullivan, and J. R. Youkey. "A reappraisal of a modified through-knee amputation in patients with peripheral vascular disease." *American Journal of Surgery* 182 (July 2001): 44–48.

Gerstein, H. and D. Hunt. "Foot ulcers and amputations in diabetes." *Clinical Evidence* 7 (June 2002): 521–528.

Hagberg, K. and R. Branemark. "Consequences of non-vascular trans-femoral amputation: a survey of quality of life, prosthetic use and problems." *Prosthetic Orthotherapy International* 25 (December 2001): 186–194.

Kazmers, A., A. J. Perkins and L. A. Jacobs. "Major lower extremity amputation in Veterans Affairs medical centers." *Annals of Vascular Surgery* 14 (May 2000): 216–222.

Oyibo, S. O., E. B. Jude, I. Tarawneh, H. C. Nguyen, D. G. Armstrong, L. B. Harkless, and A. J. Boulton. "The effects of ulcer size and site, patient's age, sex and type and duration of diabetes on the outcome of diabetic foot ulcers." *Diabetic Medicine* 18 (February 2001): 133–138.

ORGANIZATIONS

American Academy of Orthopaedic Surgeons. 6300 North River Road, Rosemont, Illinois 60018-4262. (847) 823-7186. www.aaos.org.

American College of Surgeons. 633 N. Saint Clar st., Chicago, IL 60611-3211. (312) 202-5000. www.facs.org.

American Diabetes Association. 1701 North Beauregard Street, Alexandria, VA 22311. (800) 342-2383. www.diabetes.org.

National Amputation Foundation. 40 Church Street, Malverne, NY 11565. (516) 887-3600. www.nationalamputation.org/.

OTHER

The Amputee Newswire. http://www.amputee-online.com/amputation/.

Amputation Prevention Global Resource Center Page. www.diabetesresource.com.

Cripworld Guide to Amputation. http://www.cripworld.com/amputee/ampinfo.htm.

Tish Davidson, AM
Monique Laberge, PhD

Anaerobic bacteria culture

Definition

An anaerobic bacteria culture is a method used to grow anaerobes from a clinical specimen. Obligate anaerobes are bacteria that can live only in the absence of oxygen. Obligate anaerobes are destroyed when exposed to the atmosphere for as briefly as 10 minutes. Some anaerobes are tolerant to small amounts of oxygen. Facultative anaerobes are those organisms that will grow with or without oxygen. The methods of obtaining specimens for anaerobic culture and the culturing procedure are performed to ensure that the organisms are protected from oxygen.

Purpose

Anaerobic bacterial cultures are performed to identify bacteria that grow only in the absence of oxygen and which may cause human infection. If overlooked or killed by exposure to oxygen, anaerobic infections result in such serious consequences as **amputation**, organ failure, sepsis, meningitis, and **death**. Culture is required to correctly identify anaerobic pathogens and institute effective antibiotic treatment.

Precautions

It is crucial that the health care provider obtain the sample for culture via **aseptic technique**. Anaerobes are commonly found on mucous membranes and other sites such as the vagina and oral cavity. Therefore, specimens likely to be contaminated with these organisms should not be submitted for culture (e.g., a throat or vaginal swab). Some types of specimens should always be cultured for anaerobes if an infection is suspected. These include abscesses, bites, blood, cerebrospinal fluid and exudative body fluids, deep wounds, and dead tissues. The specimen must be protected from oxygen during collection and transport, and must be transported to the laboratory immediately.

Description

Anaerobes are normally found within certain areas of the body but result in serious infection when they have access to a normally sterile body fluid or deep tissue that is poorly oxygenated. Some anaerobes normally live in the crevices of the skin, in the nose, mouth, throat, intestine, and vagina. Injury to these tissues (i.e., cuts, puncture wounds, or trauma) especially at or adjacent to the mucous membranes allows anaerobes entry into otherwise sterile areas of the body and is the primary cause of anaerobic infection. A second source of anaerobic infection occurs from the

KEY TERMS

Aerobic bacteria—Bacteria that can grow freely in oxygen-rich environments.

Aseptic—Free from living disease-causing organisms; sterile and without contamination.

Exudative—Pertaining to fluid, cells, or other matter that has escaped from blood vessels and become deposited in or on tissue.

Gram staining—Use of a purple dye to identify pathogens, usually bacteria.

Immunosuppressed—The impaired or nonfuntioning state of the immune system.

Pathogen—An organism capable of causing disease.

Sepsis—The systemic inflammatory response due to an infectious organism circulating throughout the body. Sepsis can progress to severe sepsis and septic shock, where blood pressure drops (hypotension), the blood supply to tissues decreases, and organs fail.

Venipuncture—Puncture of a vein with a needle for the purpose of withdrawing a blood sample for analysis.

introduction of spores into a normally sterile site. Spore-producing anaerobes live in the soil and water, and spores may be introduced via wounds, especially punctures. Anaerobic infections are most likely to be found in persons who are immunosuppressed, those treated recently with broad-spectrum **antibiotics**, and persons who have a decaying tissue injury on or near a mucous membrane, especially if the site is foul-smelling.

Some specimens from which anaerobes are likely to be isolated are:

- blood;
- bile;
- bone marrow;
- cerebrospinal fluid;
- direct lung aspirate;
- tissue biopsy from a normally sterile site;
- fluid from a normally sterile site (like a joint);
- dental abscess;
- abdominal or pelvic abscess;
- knife, gunshot, or surgical wound; and
- severe burn.

Some of the specimens that are not suitable for anaerobic cultures include:

- coughed throat discharge (sputum);
- rectal swab;
- nasal or throat swab;
- urethral swab; and
- voided urine.

Specimen collection

The keys to effective anaerobic bacteria cultures include collecting a contamination-free specimen and protecting it from oxygen exposure. Anaerobic bacteria cultures should be obtained from an appropriate site without the health care professional contaminating the sample with bacteria from the adjacent skin, mucus membrane, or tissue. Swabs should be avoided when collecting specimens for anaerobic culture because cotton fibers may be detrimental to anaerobes. Abscesses or fluids can be aspirated using a sterile syringe that is then tightly capped to prevent entry of air. Tissue samples should be placed into a degassed bag and sealed, or into a gassed out screw top vial that may contain oxygen-free prereduced culture medium and tightly capped. The specimens should be plated as rapidly as possible onto culture media that has been prepared.

Culture

Cultures should be placed in an environment that is free of oxygen, at 95°F (35°C) for at least 48 hours before the plates are examined for growth.

Gram staining is performed on the specimen at the time of culture. While infections can be caused by aerobic or anaerobic bacteria or a mixture of both, some infections have a high probability of being caused by anaerobic bacteria. These infections include brain abscesses, lung abscesses, aspiration pneumonia, and dental infections. Anaerobic organisms can often be suspected because many anaerobes have characteristic microscopic morphology (appearance). For example, *Bacteroides* spp. are gram-negative rods that are pleomorphic (variable in size and shape) and exhibit irregular bipolar staining. *Fusobacterium* spp. are often pale gram-negative spindle-shaped rods having pointed ends. *Clostridium* spp. are large gram-positive rods that form spores. The location of the spore (central, subterminal, terminal, or absent) is a useful differential characteristic. The presence of growth, oxygen tolerance, and Gram stain results are sufficient to establish a diagnosis of an anaerobic infection and begin antibiotic treatment with a drug appropriate for most anaerobes such as clindamycin, metronidazole, or vancomycin.

Gram-negative anaerobes and some of the infections they produce include the following genera:

- *Bacteroides* (the most commonly found anaerobes in cultures; intra-abdominal infections, rectal abscesses, soft tissue infections, liver infection);
- *Fusobacterium* (abscesses, wound infections, pulmonary and intracranial infections);
- *Porphyromonas* (aspiration pneumonia, periodontitis); and
- *Prevotella* (intra-abdominal infections, soft tissue infections).

Gram-positive anaerobes include the following:

- *Actinomyces* (head, neck, pelvic infections; aspiration pneumonia);
- *Bifidobacterium* (ear infections, abdominal infections);
- *Clostridium* (gas, gangrene, food poisoning, tetanus, pseudomembranous colitis);
- *Peptostreptococcus* (oral, respiratory, and intra-abdominal infections); and
- *Propionibacterium* (shunt infections).

The identification of anaerobes is highly complex, and laboratories may use different identification systems. Partial identification is often the goal. For example, there are six species of the *Bacteroides* genus that may be identified as the *Bacteroides fragilis* group rather than identified individually. Organisms are identified by their colonial and microscopic morphology, growth on selective media, oxygen tolerance, and biochemical characteristics. These include sugar fermentation, bile solubility, esculin, starch, and gelatin hydrolysis, casein and gelatin digestion, catalase, lipase, lecithinase, and indole production, nitrate reduction, volatile fatty acids as determined by gas chromatography, and susceptibility to antibiotics. The antibiotic susceptibility profile is determined by the microtube broth dilution method. Many species of anaerobes are resistant to penicillin, and some are resistant to clindamycin and other commonly used antibiotics.

Diagnosis/Preparation

The health care provider should take special care to collect a contamination-free specimen. All procedures must be performed aseptically. The health care professional who collects the specimen should be prepared to take two samples, one for anaerobic culture and one for aerobic culture, since it is unknown whether the pathogen can grow with or without oxygen. In addition, health care professionals should document any antibiotics that the patient is currently taking and any medical conditions that could influence growth of bacteria.

Aftercare

In the case of vein puncture for anaerobic blood cultures, direct pressure should be applied to the vein puncture site for several minutes or until the bleeding has stopped. An adhesive bandage may be applied, if appropriate. If swelling or bruising occurs, ice can be applied to the site. For collection of specimens other than blood, the patient and the collection site should be monitored for any complications after the procedure.

Risks

Special care must be taken by the health care team obtaining, transporting, and preparing the specimen for anaerobic culture. Poor methodology may delay the identification of the bacterium, may allow the patient's condition to deteriorate, and may require the patient to provide more samples than would otherwise be required. Patients may experience bruising, discomfort, or swelling at the collection site when tissue, blood, or other fluids are obtained.

Results

Negative results will show no pathogenic growth in the sample. Positive results will show growth, the identification of each specific bacterium, and its antibiotic susceptibility profile.

Patient education

A health care team member should explain the specimen collection procedure to the patient. If the patient is seriously ill, the team member should explain the procedure to the patient's family members. The patient and his or her family should understand that because bacteria need time to grow in the laboratory, several days may be required for bacterium identification.

Resources

BOOKS

Brook, Itzhak. *Anaerobic Infections: Diagnosis and Management.* New York: Informa Healthcare, 2008.
Fischbach, Frances. "Blood Cultures," in *A Manual of Laboratory and Diagnostic Tests,* 7th ed. Philadelphia: Lippincott Williams & Wilkins, 2003.
McPherson, Richard A. and Matthew R. Pincus, eds. *Henry's Clinical Diagnosis and Management by Laboratory Methods,* 21st ed. Philadelphia: Saunders, 2007.
Wallach, Jacques. *Interpretation of Diagnostic Tests,* 8th ed. Philadelphia: Lippincott Williams & Wilkins, 2006.

PERIODICALS

Song, Y. "PCR-based Diagnostics for Anaerobic Infections." *Anaerobe* 11 (February–April 2005): 79–91.

OTHER

Medical Encyclopedia. Medline Plus. U.S. National Library of Medicine and the National Institutes of Health. January 2, 2008. http://www.nlm.nih.gov/medlineplus/encyclopedia.html (January 10, 2008).

ORGANIZATIONS

American Society for Microbiology, 1752 N Street, NW, Washington, DC, 20036, (202) 737-3600, http://www.asm.org.

National Center for Infectious Disease, Centers for Disease Control and Prevention, Mailstop C-14, 1600 Clifton Road NE, Atlanta, GA, 30333, (800) 232-4636, http://www.cdc.gov/ncidod/.

Linda D. Jones, B.A., P.B.T. (A.S.C.P.)
Mark A. Best, M.D., M.P.H., M.B.A.
Robert Bockstiegel

Analgesia, patient-controlled *see* **Patient-controlled analgesia**

Analgesics

Definition

Analgesics are medicines that relieve pain.

Purpose

The primary classes of analgesics are the narcotics, including additional agents that are chemically based on the morphine molecule but have minimal abuse potential; **nonsteroidal anti-inflammatory drugs** (NSAIDs) including the salicylates; and **acetaminophen**. Other drugs, notably the tricyclic antidepressants and anti-epileptic agents such as gabapentin, have been used to relieve pain, particularly neurologic pain, but are not routinely classified as analgesics. Analgesics provide symptomatic relief, but generally have no effect on causation.

Description

Pain has been classified as "productive" pain and "non-productive" pain. While this distinction has no physiologic meaning, it may serve as a guide to treatment. "Productive" pain has been described as a warning of injury, and so may be both an indication of need for treatment and a guide to diagnosis. "Non-productive" pain by definition serves no purpose either as a warning or diagnostic tool.

Although pain syndromes may be dissimilar, the common factor is a sensory pathway from the affected

---

KEY TERMS

Acute pain—Pain that is usually temporary and results from something specific, such as a surgery, an injury, or an infection.

Chronic pain—Pain that lasts more than three months and threatens to disrupt daily life.

Dose limiting—Case in which the side effects of a drug prevent an increase in dose.

Inflammation—Pain, redness, swelling, and heat that usually develops in response to injury or illness.

Osteoarthritis—Joint pain resulting from damage to the cartilage.

---

organ to the brain. Analgesics work at the level of the nerves, either by blocking the signal from the peripheral nervous system, or by distorting the interpretation by the central nervous system. Selection of an appropriate analgesic is based on consideration of the risk-benefit factors of each class of drugs, based on type of pain, severity of pain, and risk of adverse effects. Traditionally, pain has been divided into two classes, acute and chronic, although severity and projected patient survival are other factors that must be considered in drug selection.

Acute pain

Acute pain is self limiting in duration, and includes post-operative pain, pain of injury, and childbirth. Because pain of these types is expected to be short term, the long-term side effects of analgesic therapy may routinely be ignored. Thus, these patients may safely be treated with narcotic analgesics without concern for their addictive potential, or NSAIDs with only limited concern for their ulcerogenic risks. Drugs and doses should be adjusted based on observation of healing rate, switching patients from high to low doses, and from narcotic analgesics to non-narcotics when circumstances permit.

An important consideration of **pain management** in severe pain is that patients should not be subject to the return of pain. Analgesics should be dosed adequately to assure that the pain is at least tolerable, and frequently enough to avoid the anxiety that accompanies the anticipated return of pain. Analgesics should never be dosed on a "prn" (as needed) basis, but should be administered often enough to assure constant blood levels of analgesic. This applies to both the narcotic and non-narcotic analgesics.

Chronic pain

Chronic pain, pain lasting over three months and severe enough to impair function, is more difficult to treat, since the anticipated side effects of the analgesics are more difficult to manage. In the case of narcotic analgesics this means the addiction potential, as well as respiratory depression and constipation. For the NSAIDs, the risk of gastric ulcers may be dose limiting. While some classes of drugs, such as the narcotic agonist/antagonist drugs bupronophine, nalbuphine and pentazocine, and the selective COX-2 inhibitors celecoxib and rofecoxib represent advances in reduction of adverse effects, they are still not fully suitable for long-term management of severe pain. Generally, chronic pain management requires a combination of drug therapy, life-style modification, and other treatment modalities.

Narcotic analgesics

The narcotic analgesics, also termed opioids, are all derived from opium. The class includes morphine, codeine, and a number of semi-synthetics including meperidine (Demerol), propoxyphen (Darvon), and others. The narcotic analgesics vary in potency, but all are effective in treatment of pain when used in adequate doses. Adverse effects are dose related. Because these drugs are all addictive, they are controlled under federal and state laws. A variety of dosage forms are available, including oral solids, liquids, intravenous and intrathecal injections, and transcutaneous patches.

NSAIDs, non-steroidal anti-inflammatory drugs, are effective analgesics even at doses too low to have any anti-inflammatory effects. There are a number of chemical classes, but all have similar therapeutic effects and side effects. Most are appropriate only for oral administration; however ketorolac (Toradol) is appropriate for injection and may be used for moderate to severe pain for short periods.

Acetaminophen is a non-narcotic analgesic with no anti-inflammatory properties. It is appropriate for mild to moderate pain. Although the drug is well tolerated in normal doses, it may have significant toxicity at high doses. Because acetaminophen is largely free of side effects at therapeutic doses, it has been considered the first choice for mild pain, including that of osteoarthritis.

Recommended dosage

Appropriate dosage varies by drug, and should consider the type of pain, as well as other risks associated with patient age and condition. For example,

narcotic analgesics should usually be avoided in patients with a history of substance abuse, but may be fully appropriate in patients with cancer pain. Similarly, because narcotics are more rapidly metabolized in patients who have used these drugs for a long period, higher than normal doses may be needed to provide adequate pain management. NSAIDs, although comparatively safe in adults, represent an increased risk of gastrointestinal bleeding in patients over the age of 60.

Precautions

Narcotic analgesics may be contraindicated in patients with respiratory depression. NSAIDs may be hazardous to patients with ulcers or an ulcer history. They should be used with care for patients with renal insufficiency or coagulation disorders. NSAIDs are contraindicated in patients allergic to **aspirin**.

Side effects

Adverse effects of each drug vary individually. Drugs within a class may vary in their frequency and severity of adverse effects.

The primary adverse effects of the narcotic analgesics are addiction, constipation, and respiratory depression. Because narcotic analgesics stimulate the production of enzymes that cause the metabolism of these drugs, patients on narcotics for a prolonged period may require increasing doses. This is not the same thing as addiction, and is not a reason for withholding medication from patients in severe pain.

NSAIDs are ulcerogenic and may cause kidney problems. Gastrointestinal discomfort is common, although in some cases, these drugs may cause ulcers without the prior warning of gastrointestinal distress. Platelet aggregation problems may occur, although not to the same extent as if seen with aspirin.

Interactions

Interactions depend on the specific type of analgesic. Patients should see specific drug references or ask their physician.

Resources

BOOKS

Brody, T. M., J. Larner, K. P. Minneman, and H. C. Neu. *Human Pharmacology: Molecular to Clinical, 2nd ed.* St. Louis: Mosby Year-Book, 1998.

Griffith, H. W. and S. Moore. *2001 Complete Guide to Prescription and Nonprescription Drugs*. New York: Berkely Publishing Group, 2001.

OTHER

"Acetaminophen." Federal Drug Administration. Center for Drug Evaluation and Research [cited May 2003]. http://www.fda.gov/cder/foi/nda/2000/75077_Acetaminophen.pdf.

"Acetaminophen." Medline Plus Drug Information [cited May 2003]. http://www.nlm.nih.gov/medlineplus/druginfo/medmaster/a681004.html.

"Anti-inflammatories, nonsteroidal." Medline Plus Drug Information [cited June 25 2003]. http://www.nlm.nih.gov/medlineplus/druginfo/uspdi/202743.html.

"Narcotic analgesics for pain relief." Medline Plus Drug Information [cited June 25 2003]. http://www.nlm.nih.gov/medlineplus/druginfo/uspdi/202390.html.

Samuel Uretsky, PharmD

Analgesics, opioid

Definition

Opioid **analgesics**, also known as narcotic analgesics, are pain relievers that act on the central nervous system. Like all narcotics, they may become habit-forming if used over long periods.

Purpose

Opioid analgesics are used to relieve pain from a variety of conditions. Some are used before or during surgery, including dental surgery, both to relieve pain and to make anesthetics work more effectively. They may also be used for the same purposes during labor and delivery.

Description

Opioid analgesics relieve pain by acting directly on the central nervous system. This can also lead to unwanted side effects, such as drowsiness, dizziness, breathing problems, and physical or mental dependence.

Among the drugs in this category are codeine; propoxyphene (Darvon); propoxyphene and **acetaminophen** (Darvocet N); meperidine (Demerol); hydromorphone (Dilaudid); morphine; oxycodone; oxycodone and acetaminophen (Percocet, Roxicet); and hydrocodone and acetaminophen (Lortab, Anexsia). These drugs come in many forms—tablets, syrups, suppositories, and injections—and are sold only by prescription. For some

---

KEY TERMS

Analgesic—Medicine used to relieve pain.

Central nervous system—The brain, spinal cord, and nerves throughout the body.

Colitis—Inflammation of the colon, or large bowel.

Enzyme—A protein, produced by cells, that causes chemical changes in other substances.

Hallucination—A false or distorted perception of objects, sounds, or events that seem real. Hallucinations usually result from drugs or mental disorders.

Inflammation—Pain, redness, swelling, and heat that usually develop in response to injury or illness.

Metabolize—The chemical changes that occur in the body, including the changes that occur in the liver, converting molecules to forms that are more easily removed from the body.

Narcotic—A drug derived from opium or compounds similar to opium. Such drugs are potent pain relievers and can affect mood and behavior. Long-term use of narcotics can lead to dependence and tolerance.

Tolerance—A decrease in sensitivity to a drug. When tolerance occurs, a person must take more of the drug to get the same effect.

Withdrawal symptoms—A group of physical or mental symptoms that may occur when a person suddenly stops using a drug to which he or she has become dependent.

---

drugs, a new prescription is required for each new supply; refills are prohibited, according to federal regulations.

Recommended dosage

Recommended doses vary depending on the type of opioid analgesic and the form in which it is being used. Doses may be different for different patients. The person should check with the physician who prescribed the drug or the pharmacist who filled the prescription for the correct dosage, and to understand how to take the drug.

A patient should always take opioid analgesics exactly as directed. Larger or more frequent doses should never be taken, and the drug should not be taken for longer than directed. The person should not stop taking the drug suddenly without checking with the physician or dentist who prescribed it.

Gradually tapering the dose may reduce the risk of withdrawal symptoms.

For pain following major surgery, it is common practice to give narcotic analgesics by intravenous injection for the first 24–48 hours. This may be followed by oral narcotics for the next 24–48 hours, and then non-narcotic analgesics.

Many hospitals use patient-controlled analgesia (PCA), a system in which the analgesics are given intravenously, which is in a vein, and the patient can control the dose by pushing a button on a pump. This system lets the patient have more control over the amount of medication needed to relieve pain, and eliminates the anxiety that comes from expecting the return of pain when the dose wears off.

Precautions

Anyone who uses opioid analgesics—or any narcotic—over a long time may become physically or mentally dependent on the drug. Physical dependence may lead to withdrawal symptoms when the person stops taking the medicine. Building tolerance to these drugs is also possible when they are used for a long period. The need for larger and more frequent doses is due to enzyme induction, in which narcotics are metabolized by the liver and changed to a form that can be eliminated from the body. The metabolism of narcotics relies on enzymes that are produced by the liver. As narcotics are used, the liver produces more and more of these enzymes, so that a dose of pain medication is removed from the body more rapidly. This is not a problem when narcotics are used for surgical pain, since this type of pain only lasts for a short time.

Opiod analgesics should be taken exactly as directed. It is not advised to take more than the recommended dose, or more often than directed. If the drugs do not seem to be working, the physician should be consulted. These drugs (or any other prescription drugs) should never be shared with others because the drug may have a completely different effect on different people.

Children and older people are especially sensitive to opioid analgesics and may have serious breathing problems after taking them. Children may also become unusually restless or agitated when given these drugs. These problems can be controlled by adjusting the dose of medication to a safer level.

Opioid analgesics increase the effects of alcohol. Anyone taking these drugs should not drink alcoholic beverages. Some of these drugs may also contain **aspirin**, caffeine, or acetaminophen. A person should refer to the entries on each of these drugs for additional precautions.

Special conditions

People with certain medical conditions or who are taking certain other medicines can have problems if they take opioid analgesics. Before prescribing these drugs, the physician should be informed of any of these conditions.

ALLERGIES. The patient should let the physician know about any allergies to foods, dyes, preservatives, or other substances, and about any previous reactions to opioid analgesics.

PREGNANCY. Women who are pregnant or plan to become pregnant while taking opioid analgesics should let their physicians know. No evidence exists that these drugs cause birth defects in people, but some do cause birth defects and other problems when given to pregnant animals in experiments. Babies can become dependent on opioid analgesics if their mothers use too much during pregnancy. This can cause the baby to go through withdrawal symptoms after birth. If taken just before delivery, some opioid analgesics may cause serious breathing problems in the newborn.

BREAST-FEEDING. Some opioid analgesics can pass into breast milk. Women who are breast-feeding should check with their physicians about the safety of taking these drugs.

OTHER MEDICAL CONDITIONS. These conditions may influence the effects of opioid analgesics:

- head injury—the effects of some opioid analgesics may be stronger and may interfere with recovery in people with head injuries;
- history of convulsions—some of these drugs may trigger convulsions;
- asthma, emphysema, or any chronic lung disease;
- heart disease;
- kidney disease;
- liver disease;
- underactive thyroid—the chance of side effects may be greater;
- Addison's disease, a disease of the adrenal glands;
- colitis;
- gallbladder disease or gallstones—side effects can be dangerous in people with these conditions;
- enlarged prostate or other urinary problems;
- current or past alcohol abuse;
- current or past drug abuse, especially narcotic abuse; or
- current or past emotional problems—the chance of side effects may be greater.

USE OF CERTAIN MEDICINES. Taking opioid narcotics with certain other drugs may increase the chances of serious side effects. In some cases, the physician may combine narcotic analgesics with other drugs that increase the activity of the analgesic. These include some sedatives, tranquilizers, and antihistamines. When these drugs are used together with narcotic analgesics, it may be possible to get the same pain relief with a lower dose of narcotic.

Side effects

Some people experience drowsiness, dizziness, lightheadedness, or a false sense of well-being after taking opioid analgesics. Anyone who takes these drugs should not drive, use machinery, or do anything else that might be dangerous until they know how the drug affects them. Nausea and vomiting are common side effects, especially when first beginning to take the medicine. If these symptoms do not go away after the first few doses, the person should check with the physician or dentist who prescribed the medicine.

Dry mouth is another common side effect, which can be relieved by sucking on sugarless hard candy or ice chips or by chewing sugarless gum. Saliva substitutes, which come in liquid or tablet forms, may also help. Patients who must use opioid analgesics over long periods and who have dry mouth should see their dentists, as the problem can lead to tooth decay and other dental problems.

The following side effects are less common. They usually do not need medical attention and will go away after the first few doses. If they continue or interfere with normal activity, the patient should check with the physician who prescribed the medicine for. The side effects include:

- headache;
- loss of appetite;
- restlessness or nervousness;
- nightmares, unusual dreams, or problems sleeping;
- weakness or tiredness;
- mental sluggishness;
- stomach pain or cramps;
- blurred or double vision or other vision problems;
- problems urinating, such as pain, difficulty urinating, frequent urge to urinate, or decreased amount of urine; and
- constipation.

Other side effects may be more serious and may require quick medical attention. These symptoms could be signs of an overdose. The person should get emergency medical care immediately if he or she experiences:

- cold, clammy skin;
- bluish discoloration of the skin;
- extremely small pupils;
- serious difficulty breathing or extremely slow breathing;
- extreme sleepiness or unresponsiveness;
- severe weakness;
- confusion;
- severe dizziness;
- severe drowsiness;
- slow heartbeat;
- low blood pressure; and/or
- severe nervousness or restlessness.

In addition, the following less-common side effects do not require emergency medical care, but should have medical attention as soon as possible, and include:

- hallucinations, or a sense of unreality;
- depression or other mood changes;
- ringing or buzzing in the ears;
- pounding or unusually fast heartbeat;
- itching, hives, or rash;
- facial swelling;
- trembling or twitching;
- dark urine, pale stools, or yellow eyes or skin (after taking propoxyphene); or
- increased sweating, red or flushed face, which are more common after taking hydrocodone and meperidine.

Interactions

Anyone taking the following drugs should notify his or her physician before taking opioid analgesics:

- central nervous system (CNS) depressants such as antihistamines and other medicines for allergies, hay fever, or colds; tranquilizers; some other prescription pain relievers; seizure medicines; sleeping pills; some anesthetics, including dental anesthetics;
- monoamine oxidase (MAO) inhibitors such as phenelzine (Nardil) and tranylcypromine (Parnate). The combination of the opioid analgesic meperidine (Demerol) and MAO inhibitors is especially dangerous;
- tricyclic antidepressants such as amitriptyline (Elavil);
- anti-seizure medicines such as carbamazepine (Tegretol), which may lead to serious side effects, including

coma, when combined with propoxyphene and acetaminophen (Darvocet-N) or propoxyphene (Darvon);

- muscle relaxants such as cyclobenzaprine (Flexeril);
- sleeping pills such as triazolam (Halcion);
- blood-thinning drugs such as warfarin (Coumadin);
- Naltrexone (Trexan, Revia), which cancels the effects of opioid analgesics;
- Rifampin (Rifadin); or
- Zidovudine (AZT, Retrovir), which causes serious side effects when combined with morphine.

Resources

BOOKS

Drug Facts and Comparisons 2008. Philadelphia: Lippincott Williams & Wilkins, 2007.

McEvoy, Gerald K., Elaine K. Snow, and Linda Kester, eds. *AHFS: Drug Information.* Washington, DC: American Society Healthsystems Pharmaceuticals, 2002.

Sweetman, Sean C., ed. *Martindale: The Complete Drug Reference,* 35th ed. London: The Pharmaceutical Press, 2007.

Nancy Ross-Flanigan
Sam Uretsky, Pharm.D.
Fran Hodgkins

Anesthesia evaluation

Definition

Anesthesia evaluation refers to the series of interviews, physical examinations, and laboratory tests that are generally used in North America and western Europe to assess the general fitness of patients scheduled for surgery and to determine the need for special precautions or additional testing. There is no universally accepted definition of anesthesia evaluation as of 2003; however, the Task Force on Preanesthesia Evaluation of the American Society of Anesthesiologists (ASA) has tentatively defined it as "...the process of clinical assessment that precedes the delivery of anesthesia care for surgery and for non-surgical procedures." Anesthesia evaluation is usually discussed in the context of elective or scheduled surgical procedures rather than **emergency surgery**.

Anesthesia evaluation is a relatively recent development in preoperative patient care. Prior to the 1970s, anesthesiologists were often given only brief notes or outlines of the patient's history and **physical examination** written by the operating surgeon or the patient's internist. This approach became increasingly unsatisfactory as the practice of anesthesiology became more complex. In the last four decades, the introduction of new anesthetics and other medications, laser-assisted surgical procedures, increasingly sophisticated monitoring equipment, and new discoveries in molecular biochemistry and genetics have made the **anesthesiologist's role** more demanding. During the 1980s and 1990s, some departments of anesthesiology in large urban medical centers and major university teaching hospitals began to set up separate clinics for anesthesia evaluation in order to improve the assessment of patients before surgery.

Purpose

Anesthesia evaluation has several different purposes. The information that is obtained during the evaluation may be used to:

- Guide the selection of anesthetics and other medications to be used during surgery.
- Plan for the patient's postoperative recovery and pain management.
- Educate the patient about the operation itself, the possible outcomes, and self-care during recovery at home.
- Determine the need for additional staff during or after surgery.
- Minimize confusion caused by rescheduling operations because of last-minute discoveries about patients' health.
- Improve patient safety and quality of care by collecting data for later review and analysis. The ASA has noted that few controlled trials of different approaches to anesthesia evaluation have been conducted as of 2003, and that further research is needed.

Description

There are several parts or stages in a typical anesthesia evaluation. The evaluation itself may be done in the hospital where the operation is scheduled, or in a separate facility attached to the hospital. The timing of the evaluation is affected by two major variables: the invasiveness of the operation to be performed and the patient's overall physical condition. An invasive operation or procedure is one that requires the surgeon to insert a needle, catheter, or instrument into the body or a part of the body. Surgical procedures are classified as high, medium, or low in invasiveness. Procedures that involve opening the chest, abdomen, or skull are usually considered highly invasive. Examples of less invasive procedures would include **tooth extraction**, most forms of **cosmetic surgery**, and operations on the hands and feet.

The patient's physical condition is classified according to the ASA's six-point system, with the letter E added to the classification if an emergency surgical procedure is performed. The classification system is as follows:

- P1. Normal healthy patient.
- P2. Patient with mild systemic disease.
- P3. Patient with severe systemic disease.
- P4. Patient with severe systemic disease that is life-threatening.
- P5. Moribund (dying) patient who is not expected to survive without an operation.
- P6. Brain-dead patient whose organs are being removed for donation.

As of 2003, the ASA recommends that patients with severe disease be interviewed and have their physical examination before the day of surgery. Patients in good health or with mild systemic disease who are scheduled for a highly invasive procedure should also be interviewed and examined before the day of surgery. Patients in categories P1 and P2 who are scheduled for low- or medium-invasive procedures may be evaluated on the day of surgery or before it.

Patient history and records

The first part of an anesthesia evaluation is the anesthesiologist's review of the patient's medical history and records. This review allows the anesthesiologist to evaluate the patient for risk factors that may increase the patient's sensitivity to the sedatives or other medications given before and during the operation; increase the danger of complications related to heart function and breathing; and increase the difficulty of treating such complications.

These risk factors may include:

- Heart or lung disease. These diseases often require the anesthesiologist to lower the dosages of sedatives and pain-control medications.
- Liver or kidney disease. Disorders of these organs often slow down the rate of medication clearance from the patient's body.
- Present prescription medications. These may interact with the sedatives given before the operation or with the anesthetic agent.
- Herbal preparations and other alternative medicines. Some herbal preparations, particularly those taken for insomnia or anxiety (St. John's wort, valerian, kava kava) may intensify the effects of anesthetics. Others, like ginseng or gingko biloba, may affect blood pressure or blood clotting. It is important for

patients to include alternative health products in the list of medications that they give the doctor.

- Allergies, particularly allergies to medications.
- Alcohol or substance abuse. Substance use typically affects patients' responses to sedatives and anesthetics in one of two ways. If the patient has developed a tolerance for alcohol or another drug of abuse, he or she may require an increased dose of sedatives or pain medications. On the other hand, if the patient has recently consumed a large amount of alcohol or other mood-altering substance, it may interact with the anesthetic by intensifying its effects.
- Smoking. Smoking increases the risk of coughing, bronchospasm, or other airway problems during the operation.
- Previous adverse reactions to sedatives or anesthetics. A family history of anesthesia problems or sudden or unexplained death during surgery should

be included because some adverse reactions to anesthesia can be inherited.

- Age. The elderly and children below the age of puberty do not respond to medications in the same way as adults, and the anesthesiologist must often adjust dosages. In addition, elderly patients often take a number of different prescription medications, each of which may interact with anesthetics in a different way.

Patient interview

During the anesthesia evaluation, the anesthesiologist is responsible for interviewing the patient or the parents or guardians of a minor, or the next of kin, if the patient is unable to communicate. The interview serves in part as additional verification of the patient's identity; cases have been reported in which patients have been scheduled for the wrong procedure because of administrative errors. The anesthesiologist will check the patient's name, date of birth, medical record number, and type or location of scheduled surgery for any inconsistencies. Although the anesthesiologist will ask for some of the same information that is included in the patient's written medical records, he or she may have additional questions. Moreover, it is not unusual for patients to recall significant events or details during the interview that were left out of the written records. The anesthesiologist will explain what will happen during the operation and give instructions about fasting, discontinuing medications, and other precautions that the patient should take before the procedure. The patient will have an opportunity to ask questions about choice of anesthetic and other concerns during the interview.

Physical examination

The physical examination will focus on three primary areas of concern: the heart and circulatory system; the respiratory system; and the patient's airway. Heart and lung function are evaluated because surgery under **general anesthesia** puts these organ systems under considerable stress. The usual tests performed to evaluate heart and lung fitness are an **electrocardiogram (ECG)** and chest x-ray (CXR). These tests may be omitted if the patient was tested within the previous six months and the results were normal. If the patient has an ECG and CXR as part of the anesthesia evaluation and the findings are abnormal, the doctor may order additional tests of heart and lung function. These may include stress or **exercise** tests; **echocardiography**; **angiography**; pulmonary function tests (PFTs); and a computed tomography (CT) scan of the lungs.

Assessment of the airway includes an examination of the patient's teeth, nasal passages, mouth, and throat to check for any signs of disease or structural abnormalities. Certain physical features, such as an abnormally shaped windpipe, prominent upper incisor teeth, an abnormally small mouth opening, a short or inflexible neck, a throat infection, large or swollen tonsils, and a protruding or receding chin can all increase the risk of airway problems during the operation. A commonly used classification scheme rates patients on a four-point scale, with Class I being the least likely to have airway problems under anesthesia and Class IV the most likely.

Laboratory tests

Laboratory tests are categorized as either routine, meaning that they are given to all patients as part of the anesthesia evaluation, or indicated, which means that the test is ordered for a specific reason for a particular patient. Routine preoperative laboratory tests include blood tests and urine tests. Blood samples are taken for white and red blood cell counts and coagulation studies; tests of kidney function, most commonly measurements of **blood urea nitrogen** (BUN) and creatinine; and measurements of blood glucose and electrolyte levels. Urine samples are taken to evaluate the patient's nutritional status, to test for diabetes or the presence of a urinary tract infection, and to determine whether the patient is dehydrated. Some hospitals will accept blood and urine tests performed within six weeks of the operation if the results were within normal ranges. Some facilities also routinely test urine samples from women of childbearing age for pregnancy.

Indicated laboratory tests include platelet counts, certain blood chemistry measurements, and measurements of blood hemoglobin levels. These tests are usually performed for patients with blood or endocrine disorders; persons taking blood-thinning medications; persons who have been treated with some types of alternative therapy; and persons who are known to have kidney or liver disorders.

Consultations

The anesthesiologist may consult other doctors as part of the anesthesia evaluation in order to obtain additional information about the patient's condition. Consultations are often necessary if the patient is very young or very old; is being treated for cancer; or has a rare disease or disorder.

Preparation

Patients can prepare for an anesthesia evaluation by gathering information beforehand to give the hospital or clinic staff. This information includes such matters as insurance cards and documentation; a list of medications presently taken and their dosages; a list of previous operations or hospitalizations, if any; the names and telephone numbers of other physicians who have been consulted within the past two years; information about allergies to medications, if any; the name and telephone number of a designated family member or primary contact; and similar matters.

Resources

BOOKS

Catania, Robert M., MD. *A Patient Guide to Surgery*. January 9, 2006. Available for download without charge at www.preopguide.com [accessed May 5, 2008].

PERIODICALS

American Society of Anesthesiologists Task Force on Preanesthesia Evaluation. "Practice Advisory for Preanesthesia Evaluation." Approved by House of Delegates on October 17, 2001; last amended, October 15, 2003. *Anesthesiology* 96 (February 2002): 485–496.

Larson, Merlin, MD. "Waters, Guedel, and the Pre-Anesthetic Evaluation." *California Society of Anesthesiologists Bulletin* 51 (January-March 2002): 69–75.

Michota, F. A. and F. D. Frost. "Perioperative Management of the Hospitalized Patient." *Medical Clinics of North America* 86 (July 2002): 731–748.

Tobias, J. D. "Anesthesia for Minimally Invasive Surgery in Children." *Best Practice and Research: Clinical Anesthesiology* 16 (March 2002): 115–130.

ORGANIZATIONS

American Association of Nurse Anesthetists (AANA). 222 South Prospect Avenue, Park Ridge, IL 60068-4001. (847) 692-7050. www.aana.com.

American Society of Anesthesiologists (ASA). 520 N. Northwest Highway, Park Ridge, IL 60068-2573. (847) 825-5586. www.asahq.org.

Anesthesia Patient Safety Foundation (APSF). Building One, Suite Two, 8007 South Meridian Street, Indianapolis, IN 46217-2922. www.apsf.org.

OTHER

American Society of Anesthesiologists. *Guidelines for Patient Care in Anesthesiology*. Approved by ASA House of Delegates on October 3, 1967; last amended, October 18, 2006. www.asahq.org/publicationsAndServices/standards/13.pdf.

Hata, Tara, MD, Ellen J. Nickel, Pharm. D., Bradley Hinman, MD, and Douglas Morgan, RPh. *Guidelines, Education, and Testing for Procedural Sedation and Analgesia*. Iowa City, IA: University of Iowa Hospitals and Clinics, 2001.

Shaw, Howard, MD. *Perioperative Management of the Female Patient*. http.www.emedicine.com/med/topic3290.htm.

Rooke, G. Alec, MD, PhD, editor. *Syllabus on Geriatric Anesthesiology*. Park Ridge, IL: American Society of Anesthesiologists, 2001.

Rebecca Frey, Ph.D.
Renee Laux, M.S.

Anesthesia, general

Definition

General anesthesia is the induction of a balanced state of unconsciousness, accompanied by the absence of pain sensation and the paralysis of skeletal muscle over the entire body. It is induced through the administration of anesthetic drugs and is used during major surgery and other invasive surgical procedures.

Purpose

General anesthesia is intended to bring about five distinct states during surgery:

- analgesia, or pain relief;
- amnesia, or loss of memory of the procedure;
- loss of consciousness;
- motionlessness; and
- weakening of autonomic responses.

Precautions

A complete medical history, including a history of allergies in family members, or deaths occurring during surgery is an important precaution. Patients may have a potentially fatal response to anesthesia known

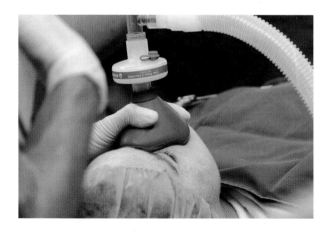

Administering general anesthesia. *(vario images GmbH & Co.KG / Alamy)*

as malignant hyperthermia, even if there is no previous personal history of reaction.

General anesthetics should be administered only by board-certified medical professionals. Anesthesia providers consider many factors, including a patient's age, weight, allergies to medications, medical history, and general health when deciding which anesthetic or combination of anesthetics to use. The American Society of Anesthesiologists has compiled guidelines for classifying patients according to risk levels as follows:

- I: healthy patient
- II: patient with mild systemic disease without functional limitations
- III: patient with severe systemic disease with definite functional limitations
- IV: patient with severe systemic disease that is life-threatening
- V: dying patient not expected to survive for 24 hours without an operation

Equipment for general anesthesia should be thoroughly checked before the operation; all items that might be needed, such as extra tubes or laryngoscope blades, should be available. Staff members should be knowledgeable about the problems that might arise with the specific anesthetic being used, and be able to recognize them and respond appropriately. General anesthetics cause a lowering of the blood pressure (hypotension), a response that requires close monitoring and special drugs to reverse it in emergency situations.

Description

General anesthetics may be gases or volatile liquids that evaporate as they are inhaled through a mask along with oxygen. Other general anesthetics are given intravenously. The amount of anesthesia produced by inhaling a general anesthetic can be adjusted rapidly, if necessary, by adjusting the anesthetic-to-oxygen ratio that is inhaled by the patient. The degree of anesthesia produced by an intravenously injected anesthetic cannot be changed as rapidly and must be reversed by administration of another drug.

The precise mechanism of general anesthesia is not yet fully understood. There are, however, several hypotheses that may explain why general anesthesia occurs. It is known that anesthetics act in several different ways in the central nervous system. They may interfere with the normal release of neurotransmitters or alter the re-uptake of neurotransmitters and disrupt normal synaptic transmission. The Meyer-Overton theory suggests that anesthesia occurs when a sufficient number of molecules of an inhalation anesthetic dissolve

---

KEY TERMS

Analgesia—Relief from pain.

Anticholinergics—Drugs that interfere with impulses from the parasympathetic nervous system. They may be given before general anesthesia to reduce airway secretions or the risk of bronchospasm.

Anxiolytics—Medications given to reduce anxiety; tranquilizers. Benzodiazepines are the anxiolytics most commonly used to premedicate patients before general anesthesia.

Balanced anesthesia—The use of a combination of inhalation and intravenous anesthetics, often with opioids for pain relief and neuromuscular blockers for muscle paralysis.

Clathrates—Substances in which a molecule from one compound fills a space within the crystal lattice of another compound. One theory of general anesthesia proposes that water molecules interact with anesthetic molecules to form clathrates that decrease receptor function.

Laryngoscope—An endoscope equipped for viewing a patient's larynx through the mouth.

Malignant hyperthermia—A type of allergic reaction (probably with a genetic basis) that can occur during general anesthesia in which the patient experiences a high fever, the muscles become rigid, and the heart rate and blood pressure fluctuate.

Volatile anesthetics—Another name for inhalation anesthetics.

---

in the lipid cell membrane. Another theory maintains that protein receptors in the central nervous system are involved, in that inhalation anesthetics inhibit the enzyme activity of proteins. A hypothesis, proposed by Linus Pauling in 1961, suggests that anesthetic molecules interact with water molecules to form clathrates (hydrated microcrystals), which in turn inhibit receptor function. Lastly, another theory describes the activation of gamma-aminobutyric acid (GABA) receptors, hypothesizing that the anesthetics may activate GABA channels and hyperpolarise cell membranes. They also may prevent the release of neurotransmitters by inhibiting certain calcium channels.

Stages of anesthesia

There are four stages of general anesthesia that help providers to better predict the course of events, from anesthesia induction to emergence.

- Stage I begins with the induction of anesthesia, the patient is still conscious and can carry on a conversation, though this stage ends with the patient's loss of consciousness. The patient is able to feel pain in Stage I.
- Stage II, or REM stage, is also known as the excitement stage and may include uninhibited and sometimes dangerous responses to stimuli, including vomiting and uncontrolled movement. The patient may become violent. During this stage, blood pressure rises and may become irregular and breathing rate increases. This stage is typically shortened by administering a barbiturate, such as sodium pentothal, before the anesthetic agent.
- Stage III, or surgical anesthesia, is the stage in which the patient's pupillary gaze is central and the pupils are constricted. This is the target depth of surgical anesthesia. During this stage, the skeletal muscles relax, the patient's breathing becomes regular, and eye movements stop.
- Stage IV, also known as medullary paralysis, occurs if the respiratory centers in the brain stop functioning. This is marked by hypotension or circulatory failure. Death may result if the patient cannot be revived quickly. This stage should never be reached and can be prevented by careful control of the amount of anesthetic that is administered to the patient.

Types of anesthetic agents

There are two major types of anesthetics used for general anesthesia, inhalation and intravenous anesthetics. Inhalation anesthetics, which are sometimes called volatile anesthetics, are compounds that enter the body through the lungs and are carried by the blood to body tissues. Inhalation anesthetics are less often used alone in modern clinical practice; they are usually used together with intravenous anesthetics. A combination of inhalation and intravenous anesthetics, often with opioids added for pain relief and neuromuscular blockers for muscle paralysis, is called balanced anesthesia.

INHALATION ANESTHETICS. The following are the most commonly used inhalation anesthetics:

- Halothane causes unconsciousness but provides little pain relief; often administered with analgesics. It may be toxic to the liver in adults. Halothane, however, has a pleasant smell and is therefore often the anesthetic of choice when mask induction is used with children.
- Enflurane is less potent, but produces a rapid onset of anesthesia and possibly a faster recovery. Enflurane is not used in patients with kidney failure.
- Isoflurane is not toxic to the liver but can induce irregular heart rhythms.

- Nitrous oxide (laughing gas) is used with other such drugs as thiopental to produce surgical anesthesia. It has the fastest induction and recovery time. It is regarded as the safest inhalation anesthetic because it does not slow respiration or blood flow to the brain. Nitrous oxide is a relatively weak anesthetic, therefore it is not suited for use in major surgery. Although it may be used alone for dental anesthesia, it should not be used as a primary agent in more extensive procedures.
- Sevoflurane works quickly and can be administered through a mask since it does not irritate the airway. On the other hand, one of the breakdown products of sevoflurane can cause renal damage.
- Desflurane, a second-generation version of isoflurane, is irritating to the airway and therefore cannot be used for mask (inhalation) inductions, especially not in children. Desflurane causes an increase in heart rate, and so should be avoided for patients with heart problems. Its advantage is that it provides a rapid awakening with few adverse effects.

INTRAVENOUS ANESTHETICS. Commonly administered intravenous general anesthetics include ketamine, thiopental (a barbiturate), methohexital (Brevital), etomidate, and propofol (Diprivan). Ketamine produces a different set of reactions from other intravenous anesthetics. It resembles phencyclidine, which is a street drug that may cause hallucinations. Because patients who have been anesthetized with ketamine often have sensory illusions and vivid dreams during postoperative recovery, ketamine is not often given to adult patients. It is, however, useful in anesthetizing children, patients in shock, and trauma casualties in war zones where anesthesia equipment may be difficult to obtain.

General anesthesia in dental procedures

The use of general anesthesia in dental and oral surgery patients differs from its use in major surgery because the patient's level of fear is usually a more important factor than the nature of the procedure. In 1985, an NIH Consensus Statement reported that high levels of preoperative anxiety, lengthy and complex procedures, and the need for a pain-free operative period may be indications for general anesthesia in healthy adults and very young children. The NIH statement specified that at least three professionals are required when general anesthesia is used during dental procedures: one is the operating dentist; the second is a professional responsible for observing and monitoring the patient; the third person assists the operating dentist.

Although the United States allows general anesthesia for dental procedures to be administered outside hospitals (provided that the facility has the appropriate equipment and emergency drugs), Scotland banned the use of general anesthesia outside hospitals in 2000, after a ten-year-old boy died during a procedure to have a tooth removed.

Preparation

Preparation for general anesthesia includes the taking of a complete medical history and the evaluation of all factors—especially a family history of allergic responses to anesthetics or unexplained deaths during surgery—that might influence the patient's response to specific anesthetic agents.

Patients should not eat or drink before general anesthesia because of the risk of regurgitating food and liquid or aspirating vomitus into the lungs.

Informed consent

Patients should be informed of the risks associated with general anesthesia as part of their **informed consent**. These risks include possible dental injuries from intubation as well as such serious complications as stroke, liver damage, or massive hemorrhage. If **local anesthesia** is an option for some procedures, the patient should be informed of this alternative. In all cases, patients should be given the opportunity to ask questions about the risks and benefits of the procedure requiring anesthesia as well as questions about the anesthesia itself.

Premedication

Depending on the patient's level of anxiety and the procedure to be performed, the patient may be premedicated. Most medications given before general anesthesia are either anxiolytics, usually benzodiazepines; or **analgesics**. Patients in severe pain prior to surgery may be given morphine or fentanyl. Anticholinergics (drugs that block impulses from the parasympathetic nervous system) may be given to patients with a known history of bronchospasm or heavy airway secretions.

Aftercare

The anesthetist and medical personnel provide supplemental oxygen and monitor patients for **vital signs** and monitor their airways. Vital signs include an EKG (unless the patient is hooked up to a monitor), blood pressure, pulse rate, oxygen saturation, respiratory rate, and temperature. The staff also monitors the patient's level of consciousness as well as signs of excess bleeding from the incision.

Risks

Although the risk of serious complications from general anesthesia are low, they can include heart attack, stroke, brain damage, and **death**. The risk of complications depends in part on the patient's age, sex, weight, allergies, general health, and history of smoking, alcohol or drug use.

The overall risk of mortality from general anesthesia is difficult to evaluate, because so many different factors are involved, ranging from the patient's overall health and the circumstances preceding surgery to the type of procedure and the skill of the physicians involved. The risk appears to be somewhere between 1:1,000 and 1:100,000, with infants younger than age one and patients older than 70 being at greater risk.

Awareness during surgery

One possible complication is the patient's waking up during the operation. It is estimated that approximately 1–2 per 1,000 patients in the United States come to be aware or feel pain during surgery. This development is in part the result of the widespread use of short-acting general anesthetics combined with blanket use of neuromuscular blockade. The patients are paralyzed with regard to motion, but otherwise "awake and aware." At present, special devices are available to measure brain wave activity indicating the patient's state of consciousness. The **bispectral index** monitor (BIS) was approved by the FDA in 1996 and the patient state analyzer in 1999. One study has shown that the use of the BIS reduced the frequency of surgical awareness by 82%.

Nausea and vomiting

Post-operative nausea and vomiting is a common problem during recovery from general anesthesia. In addition, patients may feel drowsy, weak, or tired for several days after the operation, a combination of symptoms sometimes called the hangover effect. Fuzzy thinking, blurred vision, and coordination problems are also possible. For these reasons, anyone who has had general anesthesia should not drive, operate machinery, or perform other activities that could endanger themselves or others for at least 24 hours, or longer if necessary.

Anesthetic toxicity

Inhalation anesthetics are sometimes toxic to the liver, the kidney, or to blood cells. Halothane may cause hepatic necrosis or hepatitis. Sevoflurane may react with the carbon dioxide absorbents in anesthesia machines to form compound A, a haloalkene that is toxic to the kidneys. The danger to red blood cells comes from carbon monoxide formed by the breakdown products of inhalation anesthetics in the circuits of anesthesia machines.

Malignant hyperthermia

Malignant hyperthermia is a genetic condition that causes a life-threatening response to general anesthetics due to a biochemical defect. The signs of malignant hyperthermia include rapid, irregular heartbeat; breathing problems; very high fever; and muscle tightness or spasms. These symptoms can occur following the administration of the following general anesthetics, halothane, sevoflurane, desflurane, isoflurane, enflurane, and methoxyflurane or the muscle relaxant, succinylcholine (anectine). This response can be reversed by the quick administration of an antidote drug called dantrolene.

Normal results

General anesthesia is much safer today than it was in the past, thanks to faster-acting anesthetics; improved safety standards in the equipment used to deliver the drugs; and better devices to monitor breathing, heart rate, blood pressure, and brain activity during surgery. Unpleasant side effects are also less common, in part because of developments in equipment that reduces the problems of anesthetizing patients who are difficult to intubate. These developments include the laryngeal mask airway and the McCoy laryngoscope, which has a hinged tip on its blade that allows a better view of the patient's larynx.

Resources

BOOKS

U.S. Pharmacopeia Staff. *Consumer Reports Complete Drug Reference,* 2nd ed. Yonkers, NY: Consumer Reports Books, 2002.

PERIODICALS

Christie, Bryan. "Scotland to Ban General Anaesthesia in Dental Surgeries." *British Medical Journal* 320 (March 4, 2000): 598.

Fox, Andrew J. and David J. Rowbotham. "Recent Advances: Anaesthesia." *British Medical Journal* 319 (August 28, 1999): 557–560.

Marcus, Mary Brophy. "How Does Anesthesia Work? A State That Is Nothing Like Sleep: No Memory, No 'Fight-or-Flight' Response, No Pain." *U.S. News & World Report* 123 (August 10, 1997): 66.

Preboth, Monica A., and Shyla Wright. "Quantum Sufficit: Just Enough." *American Family Physician* (February 15, 1999): 749.

Wenker, Olivier C. "Review of Currently Used Inhalation Anesthetics: Part I." *The Internet Journal of Anesthesiology* 3, no. 2 (1999).

Wenker, Olivier C. "Review of Currently Used Inhalation Anesthetics: Part II." *The Internet Journal of Anesthesiology* 3, no. 3 (1999).

OTHER

"Informed Consent." American Medical Association, Office of the General Counsel. March 20, 2008. http://www.ama-assn.org/ama/pub/category/4608.html (April 12, 2008).

National Institutes of Health. "Anesthesia and Sedation in the Dental Office." *NIH Consensus Statement* 5, no. 10 (April 22–24, 1985): 1–18.

ORGANIZATIONS

American Academy of Anesthesiologist Assistants, 2209 Dickens Road, Richmond, VA, 23230-2005, (804) 565-6353, (866) 328-5858, (804) 822-0090, http://www.anesthetist.org.

American Association of Nurse Anesthetists, 222 South Prospect Avenue, Park Ridge, IL, 60068-4001, (847) 692-7050, (847) 692-6968, info@aana.com, http://www.aana.com.

American Society of Anesthesiologists, 520 N. Northwest Highway, Park Ridge, IL, 60068-2573, (847) 825-5586, (847) 825-1692, mail@asahq.com, http://www.asahq.org.

Lisette Hilton
Sam Uretsky, Pharm.D.
Renee Laux, M.S.

Anesthesia, local

Definition

Anesthesia is used to make it possible for individuals to undergo surgery without pain. Local or regional anesthesia involves the injection or application of an anesthetic, or numbing, drug to a specific area of the body. This is in contrast to **general anesthesia**, which provides anesthesia to the entire body and brain.

Purpose

Local anesthetics are used to prevent patients from feeling pain during medical, surgical, or dental procedures. Over-the-counter local anesthetics are also available to provide temporary relief from pain, irritation, and itching caused by various conditions such as cold sores, canker sores, sore throats, sunburn, insect bites, poison ivy, and minor cuts and scratches.

Regional anesthesia blocks the sensation of pain over a large area of the body. For example, anesthesia is commonly injected into the spinal fluid (an epidural or spinal) to numb sensation in the lower body. Patients who are treated with regional anesthesia remain conscious, but lose feeling in a large part of their body.

Precautions

People who feel strongly that they do not want to be awake and alert during certain procedures may not be good candidates for local or regional anesthesia; however, other medications that have systemic effects may be given in addition to an anesthetic to relieve anxiety and help the patient relax.

Local anesthetics should be used only for the conditions for which they are intended. For example, a topical anesthetic meant to relieve sunburn pain should not be used on cold sores. Anyone who has had an unusual reaction to a local anesthetic in the past should check with a doctor before using any type of local anesthetic again. The doctor should also be told about any allergies to foods, dyes, preservatives, or other substances.

Older people may be more sensitive to the effects of local anesthetics, especially lidocaine. Children may also be especially sensitive to some local anesthetics; certain types should not be used at all on young children. People caring for these groups need to be aware that they are at increased risk of more severe side effects. Package directions should be followed carefully so that the recommended dosage is not exceeded. A doctor or pharmacist should be consulted about any concerns.

Regional anesthetics

Serious and possibly life-threatening side effects may occur when injectable or inhaled anesthetics are given to people who use street drugs. Doctors and nurses should inform patients about the dangers of mixing anesthetics with cocaine, marijuana, amphetamines, **barbiturates**, phencyclidine (also known as PCP or angel dust), heroin, or other street drugs. Some anesthetic drugs may interact with other medicines. When this happens, the effects of one or both of the drugs may change, or the risk of side effects may be greater. In select cases, a **urinalysis** can help identify drug use.

Patients who have a personal or family history of malignant hyperthermia after receiving a general anesthetic must also be cautious when receiving regional or local anesthetics. Malignant hyperthermia is a serious reaction that involves a fast or irregular heartbeat, high

---

KEY TERMS

Canker sore—A painful sore inside the mouth.

Cerebrospinal fluid—A clear fluid that fills the hollow cavity inside the brain and spinal cord. The cerebrospinal fluid has several functions, including providing a cushion for the brain against shock or impact, and removing waste products from the brain.

Cold sore—A small blister on the lips or face, caused by a virus. Also called a fever blister.

Epidural space—The space surrounding the spinal fluid sac.

Malignant hyperthermia—A type of reaction, probably with a genetic basis, that can occur during general anesthesia, in which the patient experiences a high fever, the muscles become rigid, and the heart rate and blood pressure fluctuate.

Subarachnoid space—The space surrounding the spinal cord that is filled with cerebrospinal fluid.

Topical—Not ingested; applied to the outside of the body, for example to the skin, eye, or mouth.

---

fever, breathing problems, and muscle spasms. All patients should be asked if they are aware of such a risk in their family before receiving any kind of anesthetic.

Although problems are rare, some side effects may occur when regional anesthetics are used during labor and delivery. Anesthetics can prolong labor and increase the risk of requiring a Caesarean section. Doctors should discuss the risks and benefits associated with epidural or spinal anesthesia with pregnant patients.

Regional anesthetics should be used only by an experienced anesthesiologist in a properly equipped environment with suitable resuscitative equipment. Although these anesthetics are generally safe when properly selected and administered, severe adverse reactions are still possible. If inadvertent subarachnoid injection occurs, the patient is likely to require resuscitation with oxygen and drug therapy. Careful positioning of the patient is essential to prevent leaking of cerebrospinal fluid.

Patients should not drive or operate machinery immediately following a procedure involving regional anesthesia because numbness or weakness may cause impairment. Doctors and nurses should also warn patients who have had local anesthesia, especially when combined with drugs to make patients sleep or to reduce pain, about operating any type of machinery.

Injectable local anesthetics

Until the anesthetic wears off, patients should be careful not to inadvertently injure the numbed area. If the anesthetic was used in the mouth, patients should not eat or chew gum until feeling returns.

Topical anesthetics

Unless advised by a doctor, topical anesthetics should not be used on or near any part of the body with large sores, broken or scraped skin, severe injury, or infection. They should also not be used on large areas of skin. Some topical anesthetics contain alcohol and should not be used near an open flame or while smoking.

Patients should be careful not to get topical anesthetics in the eyes, nose, or mouth. If a spray-type anesthetic is to be used on the face, it can be applied with a cotton swab or sterile gauze pad. After using a topical anesthetic on a child, the caregiver should make sure the child does not get the medicine in his or her mouth or eyes.

Topical anesthetics are intended for the temporary relief of pain and itching. They should not be used for more than a few days at a time. A doctor should be consulted if:

- discomfort continues for more than seven days;
- the problem gets worse;
- the treated area becomes infected; or
- new signs of irritation such as skin rash, burning, stinging, or swelling appear.

Dental anesthetics

Dental anesthetics should not be used if certain kinds of infections are present. Package directions should be checked or a dentist, pharmacist, or doctor should be consulted if there is any uncertainty. Dental anesthetics should be used only for temporary pain relief. Consult the dentist if problems such as toothache, mouth sores, or pain from dentures or braces continue or if signs of general illness such as fever, rash, or vomiting develop.

Patients should not eat or chew gum while the mouth is numb from a dental anesthetic to avoid accidentally biting the tongue or the inside of the mouth. In addition, the patient should not eat or drink for one hour after applying a dental anesthetic to the back of the mouth or throat because the medicine may interfere with swallowing and could cause choking. If normal feeling does not return to the mouth within a few hours after receiving a dental anesthetic, or if it is difficult to open the mouth, the dentist should be consulted.

Ophthalmic anesthetics

When anesthetics are used in the eye, it is important not to rub or wipe the eye until the effect of the anesthetic has worn off and feeling has returned. Rubbing the eye while it is numb could cause injury.

Description

Medical procedures and situations that regularly make use of local or regional anesthesia include the following:

- biopsies, in which skin or tissue samples are taken for diagnostic procedures;
- childbirth;
- scar repair;
- surgery on the face (including plastic surgery), skin, arms, hands, legs, and feet;
- eye surgery; and
- surgery involving the urinary tract or reproductive organs.

Surgery involving the chest or abdomen is usually performed under general anesthesia; however, **laparoscopy** and hernia repair may be performed under local or regional anesthesia.

Local and regional anesthesia have many advantages over general anesthesia. Most importantly, the risk of unusual and sometimes fatal reactions to general anesthesia is lessened. More minor, but significant, risks of general anesthesia include longer recovery time and the psychological discomfort of losing consciousness.

Regional anesthesia typically affects a larger area than local anesthesia. As a result, regional anesthesia is typically used for more involved or complicated procedures. The duration of action of an anesthetic depends on the type and amount of anesthetic administered.

Regional anesthetics are injected. Local anesthesia involves the injection into the skin or application to the skin surface of an anesthetic directly where pain will occur. Local anesthesia can be divided into four groups: injectable, topical, dental (non-injectable), and regional blockade injection.

Local and regional anesthesia work by altering the flow of sodium molecules into nerve cells (neurons) through the cell membrane. The exact mechanism is not understood, since the drug apparently does not bind to any receptor on the cell surface and does not seem to affect the release of chemicals that transmit nerve impulses (neurotransmitters) from the nerve cells. Experts believe that when the sodium molecules do not get into the neurons, nerve impulses are not generated and pain impulses are not transmitted to the brain.

Regional anesthesia

Types of regional anesthesia include:

- spinal anesthesia, which involves the injection of a small amount of local anesthetic into the cerebrospinal fluid surrounding the spinal cord, known as the subarachnoid space. A drop in blood pressure is a common but easily treated side effect;
- epidural anesthesia, which involves the injection of a large volume of local anesthetic into the space surrounding the spinal fluid sac, or epidural space, and not directly into the spinal fluid. Pain relief occurs more slowly, but is less likely to produce a drop in blood pressure. The block can be maintained for long periods, even for days if necessary; and
- nerve blockades, which involve the injection of an anesthetic into the area around a sensory or motor nerve that supplies a particular region of the body, preventing the nerve from carrying nerve impulses to and from the brain.

Local and regional anesthetics may be administered with other drugs to enhance their action. Examples include vasoconstrictors such as epinephrine (adrenaline) to decrease bleeding, or sodium bicarbonate to lower acidity, which may make a drug work faster. In addition, medications may be administered to help a patient remain calm and more comfortable or to make them sleepy.

Local anesthesia

INJECTABLE LOCAL ANESTHETICS. Injectable local anesthetics provide pain relief for some part of the body during surgery, dental procedures, or other medical procedures. They are given only by a trained health care professional in a doctor's office or a hospital. Some commonly used injectable local anesthetics are lidocaine (Xylocaine), bupivacaine (Marcaine), and mepivacaine (Carbocaine).

TOPICAL ANESTHETICS. Topical anesthetics such as benzocaine, lidocaine (in smaller quantities or doses), dibucaine, and tetracaine relieve pain and itching by blocking the sensory nerve endings in the skin. They are the active ingredients in a variety of nonprescription products that are applied to the skin to relieve the discomfort of sunburn, insect bites or stings, poison ivy, and minor cuts, scratches, and burns. These products are sold as creams, ointments, sprays, lotions, and gels.

Topical dental anesthetics are intended for pain relief in the mouth or throat. They may be used to relieve throat pain, teething pain, painful canker sores, toothaches, or discomfort from dentures, braces, or bridgework. Some dental anesthetics are available only with a doctor's prescription. Others may be purchased over the counter, including products such as Num-Zit, Orajel, Chloraseptic lozenges, and Xylocaine.

Ophthalmic anesthetics are designed for use in the eye. Lidocaine and tetracaine are used to numb the eye before certain eye examinations. Eye doctors may also use these medicines before measuring eye pressure or removing **stitches** or foreign objects from the eye. These drugs are to be given only by a trained health care professional.

The recommended dosage of a topical anesthetic depends on the type of local anesthetic and the purpose for which it is being used. When using a nonprescription local anesthetic, patients are advised to follow the directions on the package. Questions concerning how to use a product should be referred to a doctor, dentist, or pharmacist.

Aftercare

Most patients can return home immediately after a local anesthetic, but some patients might require limited observation. The degree of aftercare needed depends on where the anesthetic was given, how much was given, and other individual circumstances. Patients who have had their eyes numbed should wear a patch after surgery or treatment until full feeling in the eye area has returned. If the throat was anesthetized, the patient cannot drink until the gag reflex returns. If a major extremity was anesthetized, the patient may have to wait until function returns before being discharged. Some local anesthetics can cause cardiac arrhythmia and therefore require monitoring for a time with an EKG. Patients who have had regional anesthesia or larger amounts of local anesthesia usually recover in a post-anesthesia care unit before being discharged. There, medical personnel watch for immediate postoperative problems. These patients need to be driven home after discharge.

Risks

Side effects of regional or local anesthetics vary depending on the type of anesthetic used and the way it is administered. Any unusual symptoms following the use of an anesthetic requires the immediate attention of a doctor.

Paralysis after a regional anesthetic such as an epidural, spinal, or ganglionic blockade is extremely rare, but can occur. Paralysis reportedly occurs even less frequently than deaths due to general anesthesia.

There is also a small risk of developing a severe headache called a spinal headache following a spinal or epidural block. This headache is severe when the patient is upright, even when only elevated 30°, and is hardly felt when the patient lies down. It is treated by increasing fluids to help clear the anesthetic and enhance the flow of spinal fluid.

Finally, blood clots or an abscess can form at the site where an anesthetic is injected. Although these can usually be treated, antibiotic resistance is becoming increasingly common. Such infections must be regarded as potentially dangerous, particularly if they develop at the site of a spinal injection.

A physician should be notified immediately if any of the following symptoms occur:

- symptoms of an allergic reaction such as hives (urticaria), which are itchy swellings on the skin, or swelling in the mouth or throat;
- severe headache;
- blurred vision, double vision, or photophobia, which is sensitivity to light;
- dizziness or lightheadedness;
- drowsiness;
- confusion;
- an irregular, too slow, or rapid heartbeat;
- anxiety, excitement, nervousness, or restlessness;
- convulsions or seizures;
- feeling hot, cold, or numb anywhere other than the anesthetized area;
- ringing or buzzing in the ears;
- shivering or trembling;
- sweating;
- pale skin;
- breathing problems; or
- unusual weakness or tiredness.

Normal results

Local and regional anesthetics help to make many conditions and procedures more comfortable and tolerable with few or no side effects for patients.

Resources

BOOKS

Barash, P. G., B. F. Cullen, and R. K. Stoelting. *Clinical Anesthesia,* 5th ed. Philadelphia: Lippincott, Williams & Williams, 2005.

OTHER

"Anesthesia: A Look at Local, Regional and General Anesthesia." *Mayo Clinic.com.* June 16, 2006. http://www.mayoclinic.com/health/anesthesia/SC00026 (February 6, 2008).
"Anesthesia." *Medline Plus.* January 22, 2008. http://www.nlm.nih.gov/medlineplus/anesthesia.html (February 6, 2008).
Mercandetti, Michael, Adam J. Cohen, and Dedra Hern. "Anesthesia, Local with Sedation." *eMedicine.com.* March 7, 2008. http://www.emedicine.com/plastic/topic112.htm (March 20, 2008).
Virtual Anaesthsia Textbook. December 5, 2004. http://www.virtual-anaesthesia-textbook.com/index.shtml (February 6, 2008).

ORGANIZATIONS

American Academy of Anesthesiologist Assistants, 2209 Dickens Road, Richmond, VA, 23230-2005, (804) 565-6353, (866) 328-5858, (804) 822-0090, http://www.anesthetist.org.
American Association of Nurse Anesthetists, 222 South Prospect Avenue, Park Ridge, IL, 60068-4001, (847) 692-7050, (847) 692-6968, info@aana.com, http://www.aana.com.
American Society of Anesthesiologists, 520 N. Northwest Highway, Park Ridge, IL, 60068-2573, (847) 825-5586, (847) 825-1692, mail@asahq.com, http://www.asahq.org.

Lisette Hilton
Sam Uretsky, Pharm.D.
Tish Davidson, A.M.

Anesthesiologist's role

Definition

The anesthesiologist's role is the practice of medicine dedicated to the relief of pain and total care of the surgical patient before, during, and after surgery.

Training

Anesthesiologists are fully trained physicians. After completing a four-year college program and four years of medical school, anesthesiologists undergo four additional years of specialized residency training. Some will spend one to two more years

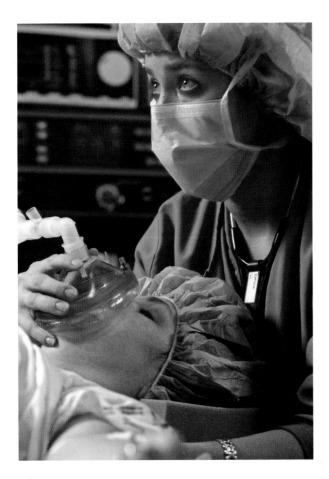

An anesthesiologist monitors a patient. *(Mira/Alamy)*

training in such anesthesiology subspecialty areas as obstetrics, **neurosurgery**, cardiac surgery, pediatrics, or critically ill patients, or to learn more about the treatment of pain. Others may select to work in research laboratories, investigating, for example, how anesthetics work and how they influence disease or recovery.

In the United States, the education of anesthesiologists takes into account their ever-expanding role in offering the best-quality health care available anywhere in the world.

Description

In the twenty-first century, the medical expertise of anesthesiologists has significantly expanded the role of the anesthesiologist. Historically, the anesthesiologist's role was limited to that of the physician who administers anesthesia to suppress pain and consciousness in a patient undergoing surgery. In the twenty-first century, anesthesiologists also provide medical care in settings other than the **operating room**. The American Society of Anesthesiologists

defines the anesthesiologist as the perioperative physician—the "all-around" physician responsible for providing medical care to each patient undergoing surgery at all stages. This includes providing the medical evaluation of the patient before surgery (preoperative), holding consultations with the **surgical team**, providing pain control and support of life functions during surgery (intraoperative), supervising care after surgery (postoperative), and discharging the patient from the recovery unit.

Specifically, the anesthesiologist's role has moved beyond just the operating room and into other areas of care.

- Ninety percent of the approximately 40 million anesthetics used annually in the United States is administered by anesthesiologists. During a surgical procedure, the anesthesiologist continually assesses the medical status of the patient, monitoring and controlling vital life functions, as well as managing pain.

- Postoperatively the anesthesiologist determines when a patient can return home following an outpatient procedure and when a patient can be moved to another ward following a procedure that requires hospitalization.

- The anesthesiologist is also involved in postoperative pain management, prescribing the appropriate pain-relieving medication and therapies.

- The anesthesiologist prescribes individualized drug therapies to patients suffering from acute, chronic, and cancer pain.

- During childbirth, the anesthesiologist must provide pain relief with epidural or spinal blocks for the mother while managing the life functions of both the mother and the baby.

- In critical care and trauma medicine, the anesthesiologist makes immediate diagnoses while supporting respiratory and cardiovascular functions, controlling infection, providing airway management, cardiac and pulmonary resuscitation, advanced life support, and pain control.

- The anesthesiologist is also present during cardiac catheterizations, angioplasties, radiological imaging, gastrointestinal endoscopies, in vitro fertilization, electroshock therapy, lithotripsy, nutritional support, and respiratory therapy.

- The anesthesiologist participates in research and clinical studies, as well as medical education programs and legislative activities.

In the past, complications caused by the use of anesthesia were a medical issue; however, since the 1980s, complications have significantly declined. Despite the growing need for anesthesia and the doubling of the

KEY TERMS

Anesthetic—A drug that causes unconsciousness or a loss of general sensation.

Angioplasty—The surgical repair of a blood vessel.

Catheterization—Placement of a flow-directed catheter for measuring pulmonary arterial pressures.

Endoscopy—The visual inspection of any cavity of the body by means of an endoscope.

Intraoperative—During surgery.

Postoperative—After surgery.

Preoperative—Before surgery.

total number of anesthesiologists practicing within the United States since 1970, patient outcomes have improved. Since 1998, the number of deaths resulting from anesthesia have dropped from an estimated 1 in 10,000 to 1 in 250,000. This drop in deaths has occurred during a time when the neonatal intensive care units are performing complicated procedures on the youngest of premature infants and at the other end of the spectrum, while 100-year-old patients are having major surgeries that at one time were believed to be impossible.

Resources

BOOKS

Ezekiel, Mark. *Handbook of Anesthesiology 2008*. Mission Viejo, CA: Current Clinical Strategies, 2007.

Jaffe, R. A., and S. I. Samuels, eds. *Anesthesiologist's Manual of Surgical Procedures,* 4th ed. Philadelphia: Lippincott Williams & Wilkins, 2003.

Morgan, G. E., M. S. Mikhail, and M. J. Murray. *Clinical Anesthesiology,* 4th ed. New York: McGraw-Hill, 2005.

Stoelting, R. K., and R. D. Miller. *Basics of Anesthesia,* 5th ed. New York: Churchill Livingstone, 2006.

PERIODICALS

Guzzi, L. M. "The Anesthesiologist's Role in Nuclear, Biological and Chemical Warfare: A Response." *ASA Newsletter* 66, no. 3 (March 2002).

White, P. F., H. Kehlet, J. Neal, T. Schricker, D. Carr, F. Carli, and the Fast-Track Surgery Study Group. "The Role of the Anesthesiologist in Fast-Track Surgery: From Multimodal Analgesia to Perioperative Medical Care." *Anesthesia & Analgesia* 104, no. 6 (June 2007): 1380–1396.

Yosaitis, J., J. Manley, L. Johnson, and J. Plotkin. "The role of the anesthesiologist as an integral member of the transplant team." *HBP* 7, no. 3 (2005): 180–182.

ORGANIZATIONS

American Board of Anesthesiology, 4101 Lake Boone Trail, Suite 510, Raleigh, NC, 27607-7506, (919) 881-2570, (919) 881-2575, http://www.theaba.org/.

American Society of Anesthesiologists, 520 N. Northwest Highway, Park Ridge, IL, 60068-2573, (847) 825-5586, (847) 825-1692, mail@asahq.com, http://www.asahq.org.

Monique Laberge, Ph.D.
Renee Laux, M.S.

Aneurysm repair, aortic *see* **Aortic aneurysm repair**

Aneurysm repair, cerebral *see* **Cerebral aneurysm repair**

Angiography

Definition

Angiography is the x-ray (radiographic) study of the blood vessels. An angiogram uses a radiopaque substance, or contrast medium, to make the blood vessels visible under x ray. The key ingredient in most radiographic contrast media is iodine. Arteriography is a type of radiographic examination that involves the study of the arteries.

Purpose

Angiography is used to detect abnormalities, including narrowing (stenosis) or blockages in the blood vessels (called occlusions) throughout the circulatory system and in some organs. The procedure is commonly used to identify atherosclerosis; to diagnose heart disease; to evaluate kidney function and detect kidney cysts or tumors; to map renal anatomy in transplant donors; to detect an aneurysm (an abnormal bulge of an artery that can rupture leading to hemorrhage), tumor, blood clot, or arteriovenous malformations (abnormal tangles of arteries and veins) in the brain; and to diagnose problems with the retina of the eye. It is also used to provide surgeons with an accurate vascular "map" of the heart prior to open-heart surgery, or of the brain prior to **neurosurgery**. Angiography may be used after penetrating trauma, like a gunshot or knife wound, to detect blood vessel injury; it may be used to check the position of shunts and stents placed by physicians into blood vessels.

Arteriosclerosis—A chronic condition characterized by thickening and hardening of the arteries and the build-up of plaque on the arterial walls. Arteriosclerosis can slow or impair blood circulation.

Carotid artery—An artery located in the neck.

Catheter—A long, thin, flexible tube used in angiography to inject contrast material into the arteries.

Cirrhosis—A condition characterized by the destruction of healthy liver tissue. A cirrhotic liver is scarred and cannot break down the proteins in the bloodstream. Cirrhosis is associated with portal hypertension.

Embolism—A blood clot, air bubble, or clot of foreign material that travels and blocks the flow of blood in an artery. When blood supply to a tissue or organ is blocked by an embolism, infarction (death of the tissue the artery feeds) occurs. Without immediate and appropriate treatment, an embolism can be fatal.

Femoral artery—An artery located in the groin area that is the most frequently accessed site for arterial puncture in angiography.

Fluorescein dye—An orange dye used to illuminate the blood vessels of the retina in fluorescein angiography.

Fluoroscope—An imaging device that displays "moving x rays" of the body. Fluoroscopy allows the radiologist to visualize the guide wire and catheter he or she is moving through the patient's artery.

Guide wire—A wire that is inserted into an artery to guide a catheter to a certain location in the body.

Ischemia—A lack of normal blood supply to a organ or body part because of blockages or constriction of the blood vessels.

Necrosis—Cellular or tissue death; skin necrosis may be caused by multiple, consecutive doses of radiation from fluoroscopic or x-ray procedures.

Plaque—Fatty material that is deposited on the inside of the arterial wall.

Portal hypertension—A condition caused by cirrhosis of the liver. It is characterized by impaired or reversed blood flow from the portal vein to the liver, an enlarged spleen, and dilated veins in the esophagus and stomach.

Portal vein thrombosis—The development of a blood clot in the vein that brings blood into the liver. Untreated portal vein thrombosis causes portal hypertension.

Precautions

Patients with kidney disease or injury may suffer further kidney damage from the contrast media used for angiography. Patients who have blood-clotting problems, have a known allergy to contrast media, or are allergic to iodine may also not be suitable candidates for an angiography procedure. Newer types of contrast media classified as non-ionic are less toxic and cause fewer side effects than traditional ionic agents. Because x rays carry risks of ionizing radiation exposure to the fetus, pregnant women are also advised to avoid this procedure.

Description

Angiography requires the injection of a contrast medium that makes the blood vessels visible to x ray. The contrast medium is injected through a procedure known as arterial puncture. The puncture is usually made in the groin area, armpit, inside elbow, or neck.

Patients undergoing an angiogram are advised to stop eating and drinking eight hours prior to the procedure. They must remove all jewelry before the

procedure and change into a hospital gown. If the arterial puncture is to be made in the armpit or groin area, shaving may be required. A sedative may be administered to relax the patient for the procedure. An intravenous (IV) line is also inserted into a vein in the patient's arm before the procedure begins, in case medication or blood products are required during the angiogram or complications arise.

Prior to the angiographic procedure, patients are briefed on the details of the test, the benefits and risks, and the possible complications involved, and asked to sign an **informed consent** form.

The site is cleaned with an antiseptic agent and injected with a local anesthetic. Then, a small incision is made in the skin to help the needle pass. A needle containing a solid inner core called a stylet is inserted through the incision and into the artery. When the radiologist has punctured the artery with the needle, the stylet is removed and replaced with another long wire called a guide wire. It is normal for blood to spurt out of the needle before the guide wire is inserted.

The guide wire is fed through the outer needle into the artery to the area that requires angiographic study.

A fluoroscope displays a view of the patient's vascular system and is used to direct the guide wire to the correct location. Once it is in position, the needle is then removed, and a catheter is threaded over the length of the guide wire until it to reaches the area of study. The guide wire is then removed, and the catheter is left in place in preparation for the injection of the contrast medium.

Depending on the type of angiographic procedure being performed, the contrast medium is either injected by hand with a syringe or is mechanically injected with an automatic injector, sometimes called a power injector, connected to the catheter. An automatic injector is used frequently because it is able to deliver a large volume of contrast medium very quickly to the angiographic site. Usually a small test injection is made by hand to confirm that the catheter is in the correct position. The patient is told that the injection will start, and is instructed to remain very still. The injection causes some mild to moderate discomfort. Possible side effects or reactions include headache, dizziness, irregular heartbeat, nausea, warmth, burning sensation, and chest pain, but they usually last only momentarily. To view the area of study from different angles or perspectives, the patient may be asked to change positions several times, and subsequent contrast medium injections may be administered. During any injection, the patient or the imaging equipment may move.

Throughout the injection procedure, radiographs (x-ray pictures) or fluoroscopic images are obtained. Because of the high pressure of arterial blood flow, the contrast medium dissipates through the patient's system quickly and becomes diluted, so images must be obtained in rapid succession. One or more automatic film changers may be used to capture the required radiographic images. In many imaging departments, angiographic images are captured digitally, obviating the need for film changers. The ability to capture digital images also makes it possible to manipulate the information electronically allowing for a procedure known as digital subtraction angiography (DSA). Because every image captured is comprised of tiny picture elements called pixels, computers can be used to manipulate the information in ways that enhance diagnostic information. One common approach is to electronically remove or (subtract) bony structures that otherwise would be superimposed over the vessels being studied, hence the name digital subtraction angiography.

Once the x rays are complete, the catheter is slowly and carefully removed from the patient. Manual pressure is applied to the site with a sandbag or other weight for 10 to 20 minutes to allow for clotting to take place and the arterial puncture to reseal itself. A pressure bandage is then applied.

Most angiograms follow the general procedures outlined above, but vary slightly depending on the area of the vascular system being studied. A variety of common angiographic procedures are outlined below:

Cerebral angiography

Cerebral angiography is used to detect aneurysms, stenosis, blood clots, and other vascular irregularities in the brain. The catheter is inserted into the femoral or carotid artery, and the injected contrast medium travels through the blood vessels in the brain. Patients frequently experience headache, warmth, or a burning sensation in the head or neck during the injection portion of the procedure. A cerebral angiogram takes two to four hours to complete.

Coronary angiography

Coronary angiography is administered by a cardiologist with training in radiology or, occasionally, by a radiologist. The arterial puncture is typically made in the femoral artery, and the cardiologist uses a guide wire and catheter to perform a contrast injection and x-ray series on the coronary arteries. The catheter may also be placed in the left ventricle to examine the mitral and aortic valves of the heart. If the cardiologist requires a view of the right ventricle of the heart or of the tricuspid or pulmonic valves, the catheter is inserted through a large vein and guided into the right ventricle. The catheter also serves the purpose of monitoring blood pressures in these different locations inside the heart. The angiographic procedure takes several hours, depending on the complexity of the procedure.

Pulmonary angiography

Pulmonary, or lung, angiography is performed to evaluate blood circulation to the lungs. It is also considered the most accurate diagnostic test for detecting a pulmonary embolism. The procedure differs from cerebral and coronary angiography in that the guide wire and catheter are inserted into a vein instead of an artery, and are guided up through the chambers of the heart and into the pulmonary artery. Throughout the procedure, the patient's **vital signs** are monitored to ensure that the catheter doesn't cause arrhythmias, or irregular heartbeats. The contrast medium is then injected into the pulmonary artery where it circulates through the lungs' capillaries. The test typically takes up to 90 minutes and carries more risk than other angiography procedures.

Kidney (renal) angiography

Patients with chronic renal disease or injury can suffer further damage to their kidneys from the contrast medium used in a renal angiogram, yet they often require the test to evaluate kidney function. These patients should be well hydrated with an intravenous saline drip before the procedure, and may benefit from available medications (e.g., dopamine) that help to protect the kidney from further injury associated with contrast agents. During a renal angiogram, the guide wire and catheter are inserted into the femoral artery in the groin area and advanced through the abdominal aorta, the main artery in the abdomen, and into the renal arteries. The procedure takes approximately one hour.

Fluorescein angiography

Fluorescein angiography is used to diagnose retinal problems and circulatory disorders. It is typically conducted as an outpatient procedure. The patient's pupils are dilated with eye drops, and he or she rests the chin and forehead against a bracing apparatus to keep it still. Sodium fluorescein dye is then injected with a syringe into a vein in the patient's arm. The dye travels through the patient's body and into the blood vessels of the eye. The procedure does not require x rays. Instead, a rapid series of close-up photographs of the patient's eyes are taken, one set immediately after the dye is injected, and a second set approximately 20 minutes later once the dye has moved through the patient's vascular system. The entire procedure takes up to one hour.

Celiac and mesenteric angiography

Celiac and mesenteric angiography involves radiographic exploration of the celiac and mesenteric arteries, arterial branches of the abdominal aorta that supply blood to the abdomen and digestive system. The test is commonly used to detect aneurysm, thrombosis, and signs of ischemia in the celiac and mesenteric arteries, and to locate the source of gastrointestinal bleeding. It is also used in the diagnosis of a number of conditions, including portal hypertension and cirrhosis. The procedure can take up to three hours, depending on the number of blood vessels studied.

Splenoportography

A splenoportograph is a variation of an angiogram that involves the injection of contrast medium directly into the spleen to view the splenic and portal veins. It is used to diagnose blockages in the splenic vein and portal-vein thrombosis and to assess the patency and location of the vascular system prior to **liver transplantation**.

Most angiographic procedures are typically paid for by major medical insurance. Patients should check with their individual insurance plans to determine their coverage.

Computerized tomographic angiography (CTA), a new technique, is used in the evaluation of patients with intracranial aneurysms. CTA is particularly useful in delineating the relationship of vascular lesions with bony anatomy close to the skull base. While such lesions can be demonstrated with standard angiography, it often requires studying several projections of the two-dimensional films rendered with standard angiography. CTA is ideal for more anatomically complex skull-base lesions because it clearly demonstrates the exact relationship of the bony anatomy with the vascular pathology. This is not possible using standard angiographic techniques. Once the information has been captured a workstation is used to process and reconstruct images. The approach yields shaded surface displays of the actual vascular anatomy that are three dimensional and clearly show the relationship of the bony anatomy with the vascular pathology.

Angiography can also be performed using MRI (**magnetic resonance imaging**) scanners. The technique is called MRA (magnetic resonance angiography). A contrast medium is not usually used, but may be used in some body applications. The active ingredient in the contrast medium used for MRA is one of the rare earth elements, gadolinium. The contrast agent is injected into an arm vein, and images are acquired with careful attention being paid to the timing of the injection and selection of MRI specific imaging parameters. Once the information has been captured, a workstation is used to process and reconstruct the images. The post-processing capabilities associated with CTA and MRA yield three-dimensional representations of the vascular pathology being studied and can also be used to either enhance or subtract adjacent anatomical structures.

Aftercare

Because life-threatening internal bleeding is a possible complication of an arterial puncture, an overnight stay in the hospital is sometimes recommended following an angiographic procedure, particularly with cerebral and coronary angiography. If the procedure is performed on an outpatient basis, the patient is typically kept under close observation for a period of at six to 12 hours before being released. If the arterial puncture was performed in the femoral artery, the patient is instructed to keep his or her leg straight and relatively immobile during the observation period. The patient's blood pressure and vital signs are monitored, and the puncture site observed closely. Pain medication may be prescribed if the patient is experiencing discomfort from the puncture, and a cold pack is often applied to the site to reduce swelling. It is normal for the puncture site to be sore and bruised for several weeks. The patient may also develop a hematoma at the puncture site, a hard mass created by the blood vessels broken during the procedure. Hematomas should be watched carefully, as they may indicate continued bleeding of the arterial puncture site.

Angiography patients are also advised to have two to three days of rest after the procedure in order to avoid placing any undue stress on the arterial puncture site. Patients who experience continued bleeding or abnormal swelling of the puncture site, sudden dizziness, or chest pain in the days following an angiographic procedure should seek medical attention immediately.

Patients undergoing a fluorescein angiography should not drive or expose their eyes to direct sunlight for 12 hours following the procedure.

Risks

Because angiography involves puncturing an artery, internal bleeding or hemorrhage are possible complications of the test. As with any invasive procedure, infection of the puncture site or bloodstream is also a risk, but this is rare.

A stroke or heart attack may be triggered by an angiogram if blood clots or plaque on the inside of the arterial wall are dislodged by the catheter and form a blockage in the blood vessels, or if the vessel undergoes temporary narrowing or spasm from irritation by the catheter. The heart may also become irritated by the movement of the catheter through its chambers during pulmonary and coronary angiographic procedures, and arrhythmias may develop.

Patients who develop an allergic reaction to the contrast medium used in angiography may experience a variety of symptoms, including swelling, difficulty breathing, heart failure, or a sudden drop in blood pressure. If the patient is aware of the allergy before the test is administered, certain medications can be administered at that time to counteract the reaction.

Angiography involves minor exposure to radiation through the x rays and fluoroscopic guidance used in the procedure. Unless the patient is pregnant, or multiple radiological or fluoroscopic studies are required, the dose of radiation incurred during a single procedure poses little risk. However, multiple studies requiring fluoroscopic exposure that are conducted in a short time period have been known to cause skin necrosis in some individuals. This risk can be minimized by careful monitoring and documentation of cumulative radiation doses administered to these patients, particularly in those who have therapeutic procedures performed along with the diagnostic angiography.

Normal results

The results of an angiogram or arteriogram depend on the artery or organ system being examined. Generally, test results should display a normal and unimpeded flow of blood through the vascular system. Fluorescein angiography should result in no leakage of fluorescein dye through the retinal blood vessels.

Abnormal results of an angiogram may display a narrowed blood vessel with decreased arterial blood flow (ischemia) or an irregular arrangement or location of blood vessels. The results of an angiogram vary widely by the type of procedure performed, and should be interpreted by and explained to the patient by a trained radiologist.

Resources

BOOKS

Baum, Stanley and Michael J. Pentecost, eds. *Abrams' Angiography*. 4th ed. Philadelphia: Lippincott-Raven, 1996.

LaBergem Jeanne, ed. *Interventional Radiology Essentials*. 1st ed. Philadelphia: Lippincott Williams & Wilkins, 2000.

Ziessman, Harvey, ed. *The Radiologic Clinics of North America, Update on Nuclear Medicine* Philadelphia: W. B. Saunders Company, September 2001.

OTHER

Food and Drug Administration. *Public Health Advisory: Avoidance of Serious X-Ray-Induced Skin Injuries to Patients During Fluoroscopically Guided Procedures. September 30, 1994*. Rockville, MD: Center for Devices and Radiological Health, FDA, 1994.

Radiological Society of North America CMEJ. *Renal MR Angiography*. April 1, 1999 [cited June 27, 2003]. <http://ej.rsna.org/ej3/0091-98.fin/mainright.html>.

Stephen John Hage, AAAS, RT(R), FAHRA
Lee Alan Shratter, MD

Angioplasty

Definition

Angioplasty is a procedure used to widen narrowed or partially blocked, or occluded, blood vessels. There are various types of angioplasty. The specific names of these procedures are derived from the type of equipment used and the path of entry to the blood vessel. For example, percutaneous transluminal angioplasty (PTA) means that the vessel is entered through the skin (percutaneous) and that the catheter is moved into the blood vessel of interest through the same vessel or one that communicates with it (transluminal). In the case of an angioplasty involving the coronary arteries, the point of entry might be the femoral artery in the groin, with the catheter/guidewire system passed through the aorta to the heart and the origin of the coronary arteries at the base of the aorta just outside the aortic valve.

Purpose

An angioplasty is done to reopen a partially blocked blood vessel so that blood can flow through it again at a normal rate. In patients with an occlusive vascular disease such as atherosclerosis, the flow of blood to other organs or remote parts of the body is limited by the narrowing (stenosis) of the vessel's lumen due to fatty deposits or patches known as plaque. Once the vessel has been widened, an adequate blood flow is restored, but the vessel may narrow again over time (restenosis) at the same location and the procedure may need to be repeated.

Description

Angioplasties were originally performed by dilating the blood vessel with the introduction of larger and larger stiff catheters through the narrowed space. The complications that resulted from this approach led researchers to develop other ways to open the vessel with smaller devices. An alternative approach was developed in which the catheters used to perform angioplasties contain balloons that are gradually inflated to widen the vessel. Stents, which are thin collapsed tubes made of wire mesh sometimes coated with drugs that help prevent the blood vessel from reclosing can be inserted to provide structural support for the vessel. Lasers may be used to help break up the plaque or fat deposits lining the vessel. Some catheters are equipped with spinning wires or drill tips to clean out the plaque.

Angioplasty may be performed while the patient is either sedated or anesthetized, depending on which vessels are involved. If a percutaneous transluminal coronary angioplasty (PTCA) is to be performed, the patient is sedated so that he or she can report discomfort and cough if asked to do so. PTCA procedures are performed in **cardiac catheterization** laboratories with sophisticated monitoring devices. If angioplasty is performed in the radiology department's angiographic suite, the patient may be sedated for the procedure while a nurse monitors the patient's **vital signs**. Angioplasties performed by vascular surgeons are done in an **operating room** or specially designed vascular procedure suite.

Typically, patients are given anticoagulant, or blood thinning, medications before the procedure to assist in the prevention of thromboses (blood clots), even though these drugs may slow down the sealing of the entry point of the catheter into the vein. Patients may also be given calcium channel blockers and nitrates to reduce the risk of vascular spasm. The angioplasty is performed using fluoroscopic guidance and contrast media. Since the decision to perform angioplasty may have been made following a diagnostic angiogram, the patient's sensitivity to contrast media containing iodine is likely to be known. The procedure may then require the use of an alternative contrast agent.

The patient's skin is cleansed with an antiseptic solution at the site where the surgeon will insert the catheter and other equipment, and the area is protected with a sterile drape. Although many angioplasties are performed by puncturing the vessel through the skin, others are done by surgically exposing the site of entry. Direct view of the vessel's puncture site aids in monitoring damage to the vessel or excessive bleeding at the site. After the vessel has been punctured and the guidewire introduced, a fluoroscope is used to monitor the small amounts of contrast media that have been injected. This technique allows the surgeon to see the guidewire's movement through the vessel. If the fluoroscope has a feature called "roadmap," the amount of contrast media injected is greater in order to define the full route the guidewire will take. The fluoroscopy system then superimposes subsequent images over the roadmap while the physician moves the guidewire along the mapped route to the destination.

When the surgeon reaches the location of the stenosis, he or she inflates the balloon on the catheter that has been passed along the guidewire. The size of the balloon and the duration of its inflation depend on the size and location of the vessel. In some cases, the surgeon may also use a stent, which is opened or expanded inside the blood vessel after it has been guided to the proper location. The blood vessel may be widened before, during, or after the stent has been opened up. In cases where the vessel is tortuous (twisted) or at intersections of vessels, a graft may be necessary to strengthen the walls of the blood vessel. Stents, grafts, and balloon dilation may all be used together or separately. Sometimes radiation is used when a stent is placed.

After the surgeon has widened the blood vessel, he or she verifies its patency by using fluoroscopy and contrast media to produce an angiogram, by using intravascular **ultrasound**, or by using both techniques. After the imaging studies have been completed, the surgeon removes the equipment from the blood vessel and closes the puncture site.

Risks

There is a danger of puncturing the vessel with the guidewire during an angioplasty, although the risk is very small. Patients must be monitored for hematoma or hemorrhage at the puncture site. There is also a small risk of heart attack, stroke, and, although unlikely, death—all related to vessel spasm (transient vessel narrowing from irritation by the catheter), or from emboli (as plaque can be dislodged by the catheter or and travel to the heart or brain). Abrupt closure of the coronary artery occurs in about 4% of patients.

Recurrence of stenosis, known as restenosis, is an additional potential complication. The risk of recurrence is highest in the first six months after angioplasty, with rates as high as 35% reported in some studies.

The length of the patient's hospital stay following an angioplasty depends on his or her overall health, the occurrence of complications, and the availability of **home care**.

Alternatives

For some patients, **thrombolytic therapy** (treatment with drugs that dissolve blood clots) coupled with lifestyle changes is an alternative to angioplasty. Many medical centers, in fact, restrict the use of angioplasty to patients who cannot be treated with thrombolytic therapy.

Health care team roles

Physicians often have specially trained assistants for vascular procedures. These assistants may be nurses, surgical technicians, or X-ray specialists. Cardiac catheterization laboratories will include someone specially trained in monitoring EKG equipment and vital signs. Either a nurse, nurse anesthetist, or anesthesiologist will administer sedation or anesthesia for the procedure.

Resources

BOOKS

Beers, M. H., R. S. Porter, T. V. Jones, J. L. Kaplan, and M. Berkwits, eds. "Diagnostic Cardiovascular Procedures: Invasive Procedures." In *The Merck Manual of Diagnosis and Therapy,* 18th ed. Whitehouse Station, NJ: Merck Research Laboratories, 2006.

Ohman, Magnus. *So You're Having a Heart Cath and Angioplasty.* Hoboken, NJ: Wiley, 2003.

OTHER

"Angioplasty." *MedlinePlus.* February 7, 2008. http://www.nlm.nih.gov/medlineplus/angioplasty.html (February 11, 2008).

"Balloon Angioplasty and Stents." *Texas Heart Institute.* July 2007. http://www.texasheartinstitute.org/HIC/Topics/Proced/angioplasty.cfm (February 11, 2008).

"Coronary Angioplasty and Stenting: Opening Clogged Heart Arteries." *Mayo Clinic.* December 20, 2006. http://www.mayoclinic.com/health/angioplasty/HQ00485 (February 11, 2008).

ORGANIZATIONS

American Heart Association, 7272 Greenville Avenue, Dallas, TX, 75231, (800) 242-8721, http://www.americanheart.org.

National Heart, Lung, and Blood Institute Information Center, P.O. Box 30105, Bethesda, MD, 20824-0105, (301) 592-8573, (240) 629-3246, http://www.nhlbi.nih.gov.

Elaine R. Proseus, M.B.A./T.M., B.S.R.T., R.T.(R)
Lee A. Shratter, M.D.
Tish Davidson, A. M.

Anterior temporal lobectomy

Definition

An anterior temporal lobectomy (ATL) is the complete removal of the anterior portion of the temporal lobe of the brain.

Purpose

ATL surgery has been recognized as an efficient treatment option for certain types of seizures in patients diagnosed with temporal lobe epilepsy (TLE). Characterized by transient disturbances of brain function and seizures, TLE is the most common form of epilepsy. ATL is optimal for patients with seizures that do not respond to medications, patients who are unable to tolerate medication side effects, or patients with seizures caused by structural abnormalities in the brain.

Demographics

Epilepsy is the most common serious neurological condition in the United States. Its incidence is greatest in young chidren and in the elderly, with five to 10 cases diagnosed per 1,000. The lifetime prevalence amounts to 2–5% of the population. Epilepsy is slightly more common in males than females. The frequency of seizure activity in the epileptic population is as follows.

- 33% have less than one seizure per year
- 33% have one to 12 seizures per year
- 33% have more than one seizure per month
- 60% also have other neuropsychiatric problems

Description

ATL surgical procedures involve these steps:

- Anesthesia. The patient is anesthetized with a combination of drugs that achieves a state of unconsciousness.
- Preparation of the surgical field. An antiseptic solution is applied to the patient's scalp, face, and neck. Surgical drapes are placed around the surgical region to maintain a sterile surgical field.
- Temporal incision. Using a scalpel blade, the neurosurgeon makes an incision in the skin and muscle of the temporal region of the head located on the side of the head above the ear, and pulls away the flap of scalp.
- Control of bleeding. Blood obstructing the surgeon's view of the surgical field is irrigated and suctioned away as surgery proceeds.
- Craniotomy. Using a high-speed drill, the neurosurgeon removes a section of bone (bone flap) from the skull and makes an incision through the protective membranes of the brain (dura) in order to expose the temporal lobe.
- Removal of the anterior lobe. Using an operating microscope to enlarge the features of the surgical area, the neurosurgeon removes the temporal anterior lobe.
- Closure. Once bleeding is under control, every layer of tissue cut or divided to reach the surgical site is closed. The cavity is irrigated completely and the dura is closed in a watertight manner using tack-up sutures. The bone flap is returned into place. Muscle and tissues are closed with sutures, while the skin is closed with staples. No drain is needed.

KEY TERMS

Anesthesia—A combination of drugs administered by a variety of techniques by trained professionals that provide sedation, amnesia, analgesia, and immobility adequate for the accomplishment of the surgical procedure with minimal discomfort, and without injury, to the patient.

Cerebral cortex—The outer portion of the brain, consisting of layers of nerve cells and their connections. The cerebral cortex is the part of the brain in which thought processes take place.

Craniotomy—A surgical incision into the skull.

Electroencephalogram (EEG)—A diagnostic test that measures the electrical activity of the brain (brain waves) using highly sensitive recording equipment attached to the scalp by electrodes.

Epilepsy—Chronic medical condition produced by temporary changes in the electrical function of the brain, causing seizures that affect awareness, movement, and/or sensation.

Seizures—Attacks consisting of sudden and abnormal muscle, sensory, or psychic events resulting from transient dysfunction of the brain.

Temporal lobe epilepsy (TLE)—The most common type of epilepsy, with elaborate and multiple sensory, motor, and psychic symptoms. A common feature is the loss of consciousness and amnesia during seizures. Other manifestations may include more complex behaviors like bursts of anger, emotional outbursts, fear, or automatisms.

Diagnosis/Preparation

An ATL pre-surgical diagnosis requires reliable diagnostic levels classified as (1) seizure, (2) epilepsy, and (3) syndrome. The epilepsy and syndromic diagnoses are usually combined. The seizure diagnosis is determined from the physical and neurological manifestations of the condition recorded in the patient's history and from electroencephalogram (EEG) evaluations. Because seizures commonly result from cortical damage, neuroimaging techniques are used to identify and localize the damaged area. They include:

- Magnetic resonance imaging (MRI). Brain MRI is the best structural imaging technique available. Every ATL surgical evaluation usually includes a complete MRI study.
- Positron emission tomography (PET). Unlike MRI, PET provides information on brain metabolism rather than on structure. Typically, the epileptic region's metabolism is lowered unless the scan is obtained during a seizure.

- Single photon emission tomography (SPECT). SPECT scans visualize blood flow through the brain and are used as another method for localizing the epileptic site.

Routinely, all ATL candidates also undergo neuropsychological testing.

To prepare for ATL, the patient discontinues any medication being taken and that has been associated with bleeding disorders at least three weeks prior to ATL surgery. **Antibiotics** may be administered intravenously one hour before surgery. Minimal hair is shaved over the temporal area of the head.

Aftercare

After ATL surgery, the neurosurgeon provides instructions for the nurses, pharmacists, therapists, and other physicians caring for the patient postoperatively. Once the anesthesiologist determines that the patient is stable, the surgeon authorizes transport to the **postoperative care** area. Most patients go to the recovery area, but some critical patients may be taken to an **intensive care unit** (ICU) for close monitoring. As is the case for almost all types of brain surgery, the patient is initially nursed with the head of the bed elevated to 30 degrees.

Risks

All surgical procedures are associated with risks and complications that vary depending on the location of the procedure (the approach and dissection required), the pathology (what has to be done to accomplish the surgical objective), and patient factors (such as age, general medical condition, etc.).

A specific risk associated with ATL is possible injury to the cerebral cortex, the outer portion of the brain that consists of layers of nerve cells and their connections, during the lobectomy procedure.

Normal results

ATL offers a high chance of seizure-free outcome in patients suffering from drug-resistant seizures originating in the temporal lobe of the brain. The procedure is considered to be the most common and rewarding of all the surgeries for epilepsy.

Morbidity and mortality rates

ATL is the most common surgery performed to treat medically refractory epilepsy and, in most cases, will diminish or abolish seizures.

In 1997, Sperling et al. reported in the *Epilepsy Quarterly* the five-year outcomes of 89 patients with uncontrolled seizures who underwent ATL at the Graduate Hospital in Philadelphia, Pennsylvania. The patients in this study underwent ATL as a result of no response (or allergy) to at least three medications. Five years postoperatively, 80 of 89 patients (90%) no longer had seizures or experienced more than 80% seizure reduction. Only five patients (6%) exhibited no worthwhile improvement, although a modest reduction in seizure frequency may have been noted. Among the seizure-free patients, 49 were cured of their epilepsy (i.e., they had no seizures after temporal lobectomy).

Alternatives

Anti-convulsant drug development programs

Once the diagnosis of epilepsy is established, a course of medication is usually prescribed for the control of seizures. ATL only becomes the preferred approach when a patient does not respond to medication. As an alternative to surgery, a patient may elect to become an active participant in an anti-convulsant drug development program that may offer an opportunity to participate in studies of experimental medications.

Other surgical techniques

Other surgical techniques such as **corpus callosotomy** can be performed in selected patients who are

ineligible for ATL. In this procedure, the white matter tract connecting the two halves of the brain is cut to halt the spread of seizures and to limit their severity.

Resources

BOOKS

Chilton, L. *Seizure Free: From Epilepsy to Brain Surgery, I Survived, and You Can, Too!* Dallas: English Press Publications, 2000.

Freeman, J. M., E. P. G. Vining, and D. J. Pillas. *Seizures and Epilepsy in Childhood: A Guide.* Baltimore: Johns Hopkins University Press, 2002.

Hauser, W. A. and D. C. Hesdorffer. *Epilepsy: Frequency, Causes, and Consequences.* New York: Demos Publications, 1990.

Waltz, M. *Partial Seizure Disorders: Help for Patients and Families.* Sebastopol, CA: Patient-Centered Guides, 2001.

PERIODICALS

Clusmann, H., J. Schramm, T. Kral, C. Helmstaedter, B. Ostertun, R. Fimmers, D. Haun, and C. E. Elger. "Prognostic factors and outcome after different types of resection for temporal lobe epilepsy." *Journal of Neurosurgery* 97 (November 2002): 1131–1141.

Crino, P. B. "Outcome Assessment of Anterior Temporal Lobectomy." *Epilepsy Quarterly* 5 (Spring 1997): 1–4.

Elwes, R. D., G. Dunn, C. D. Binnie, and C. E. Polkey. "Outcome following resective surgery for temporal lobe epilepsy: a prospective follow up study of 102 consecutive cases." *Journal of Neurology, Neurosurgery and Psychiatry* 54 (1991): 949–952.

Jarrar, R. G., J. R. Buchhalter, F. B. Meyer, F. W. Sharbrough, and E. Laws. "Long-term follow-up of temporal lobectomy in children." *Neurology* 59 (November 2002): 1635–1637.

Jones, J. E., N. L. Berven, L. Ramirez, A. Woodard, B. P. Hermann. "Long-term psychosocial outcomes of anterior temporal lobectomy." *Epilepsia* 43 (August 2002): 896–903.

Radhakrishnan, K., E. L. So, P. L. Silbert, G. D. Cascino, W. R. Marsh, R. H. Cha, and P. C. O'Brien.

"Prognostic implications of seizure recurrence in the first year after anterior temporal lobectomy." *Epilepsia* 44 (January 2003): 77–80.

Sperling, M. R., M. J. O'Connor, A. J. Saykin, and C. Plummer. "Temporal lobectomy for refractory epilepsy." *Journal of the American Medical Association* 276 (1996): 470–475.

Zimmerman, R. S. and J. I. Sirven. "An overview of surgery for chronic seizures." *Mayo Clinic Proceedings* 78 (January 2003): 109–117.

ORGANIZATIONS

The American Academy of Neurology. 1080 Montreal Avenue, Saint Paul, MN 55116. (800) 879-1960. http://www.aan.com/.

The American Epilepsy Society. 342 North Main Street, West Hartford, CT 06117-2507. (860) 586-7505. http://www.aesnet.org/.

The Epilepsy Foundation. 4351 Garden City Drive Landover, MD 20785-7223. (800) 332-1000. http://www.epilepsyfoundation.org/.

Monique Laberge, Ph.D.

Antianxiety drugs

Definition

Antianxiety drugs are medicines that calm and relax people with excessive anxiety, nervousness, or tension, or for short-term control of social phobia disorder or specific phobia disorder.

Purpose

Antianxiety agents, or anxiolytics, may be used to treat mild transient bouts of anxiety as well as more pronounced episodes of social phobia and specific phobia. Clinically significant anxiety is marked by several symptoms. The patient experiences marked or persistent fear of one or more social or performance situations in which he or she is exposed to unfamiliar people or possible scrutiny by others, and may react in a humiliating or embarrassing way. The exposure to the feared situation produces an anxiety attack. Fear of these episodes of anxiety leads to avoidance behavior, which impairs normal social functioning, including working or attending classes. The patient is aware that these fears are unjustified.

Antianxiety drugs, particularly the injectable benzodiazepines lorazepam (Ativan) and midazolam (Versed) are also used for preoperative sedation in surgery. Used for this purpose, they may induce relaxation, provide sedation, and also reduce memory of an unpleasant experience. They offer the combined benefits of relaxing the patient and reducing the need for other agents including **analgesics**, anesthetics, and **muscle relaxants**. Lorazepam is also used to treat the nausea and vomiting from cancer treatments, epilepsy, irritable bowel syndrome, and insomnia.

Description

In psychiatric practice, treatment of anxiety has largely turned from traditional antianxiety agents, anxiolytics, to antidepressant therapies. The benzodiazepines, the best-known class of anxiolytics, have been largely supplanted by serotonin-specific reuptake inhibitors (SSRIs, including citalopram, fluoxetine, fluvoxamine, and others), which have a milder side effect profile and less risk of dependency. Traditional anxiolytics remain useful for patients who need a rapid onset of action, or whose frequency of exposure to anxiety-provoking stimuli is low enough to eliminate the need for continued treatment. While SSRIs may require three to five weeks to show any effects, and must be taken continuously, benzodiazepines may produce a response within 30 minutes, and may be dosed on an as-needed basis.

The intermediate-action benzodiazepines, alprazolam (Xanax), and lorazepam (Ativan), are the appropriate choice for treatment of mild anxiety and social phobia. Diazepam (Valium) is still widely used for anxiety, but its active metabolite, desmethyldiazepam, has a long half-life, making this a poorer choice than other drugs in its class. There is considerable variation between individuals in the metabolism of benzodiazepines, so patient response may not be predictable. As a class, benzodiazepines are used not only as anxiolytics, but also as sedatives, muscle relaxants (making them useful in the treatment of fibromyalgia and restless leg syndrome), and in treatment of epilepsy and alcoholism. The distinctions between these uses are largely determined by onset and duration of action, and route of administration.

Buspirone (BuSpar), which is not chemically related to other classes of central nervous system drugs, is also a traditional anxiolytic, although it is considered either a third-line or adjunctive agent for use after trials of SSRIs and benzodiazepines. It is appropriate for use in patients who have either failed trials of other treatments, or who should not receive benzodiazepines because of a history of substance abuse problems. Buspirone, in common with antidepressants, requires a two- to three-week

KEY TERMS

Anxiety—Worry or tension in response to real or imagined stress, danger, or dreaded situations. Physical reactions such as fast pulse, sweating, trembling, fatigue, and weakness may accompany anxiety.

Epilepsy—A brain disorder with symptoms that include seizures.

Panic disorder—An disorder in which people have sudden and intense attacks of anxiety in certain situations.

Phobia—An intense, abnormal, or illogical fear of something specific such as heights or open spaces.

Pregnancy category B—Animal studies indicate no fetal risk, but no human studies; or adverse effects in animals, but not in well-controlled human studies.

Pregnancy category C—No adequate human or animal studies; or adverse fetal effects in animal studies, but no available human data.

Seizure—A sudden attack, spasm, or convulsion.

period before there is clinical evidence of improvement, and must be continuously dosed to maintain its effects. Buspirone causes drowsiness, so patients should be careful not to drive or operate machinery until they know how the drug affects them.

In surgery, antianxiety drugs may be used to provide relaxation and reduce fear of surgery. They may reduce the need for anesthetics and muscle relaxants. In addition, some antianxiety drugs may impair memory, which is a benefit since it reduces concern about an unpleasant experience. Short-acting benzodiazepines such as midazolam (Versed) and lorazepam (Ativan) are most often used for this purpose.

Benzodiazepines are controlled drugs under federal law. Buspirone is not a controlled substance and has no established abuse potential.

Recommended dosage

Presurgical dosing of midazolam varies with the route of administration, the age and physical condition of the patient, and the other drugs to be used. For patients under the age of 60 who have not received narcotic analgesics, a dose of 2–3 milligrams (mg) is normally adequate, but some elderly patients may respond to a dose as low as 1 mg. The usual dose of lorazepam is up to 4 mg, administered by intramuscular injection at least two hours prior to surgery. If the drug is given intravenously, a dose of up to 2 mg may be given 15–20 minutes before surgery.

Benzodiazepines should be administered 30–60 minutes before exposure to the anticipated stress. Dosage should be individualized to minimize sedation. The normal dose of alprazolam is 0.25–0.5 mg. The usual dose of lorazepam is 2–3 mg. Doses may be repeated if necessary.

Buspirone is initially dosed at 5 mg three times a day, as a tablet taken by mouth. The dosage should be increased 5 mg/day, at intervals of two to three days, as needed. A dosage of 60 mg/day should not be exceeded. Two to three weeks may be required before a satisfactory response is observed.

Precautions

Precautions and warnings apply to the use of antianxiety agents for use over long periods of time. They are unlikely to occur in patients who have only received a single dose prior to surgery.

Benzodiazepines should not be used in patients with psychosis, acute narrow-angle glaucoma, or liver disease. The drugs can act as respiratory depressants and should be avoided in patients with respiratory conditions. Benzodiazepines are potentially addictive and should not be administered to patients with substance abuse disorders. Benzodiazepines are sedatives and should be avoided in patients who must remain alert. Their use for periods over four months has not been documented. These drugs should not be used during the second and third trimester of pregnancy, although use during the first trimester appears to be safe. They should not be taken while breastfeeding. Specialized references for use in children should be consulted.

Buspirone is metabolized by the liver and excreted by the kidney, and should be used with care in patients with hepatic or renal disease. The drug is classified as schedule B during pregnancy, but should not be taken during breast-feeding. Its use in children under the age of 18 years has not been studied.

Interactions

The metabolism of alprazolam may be increased by cimetidine, oral contraceptives, disulfiram, fluoxetine, isoniazid, ketoconazole, metoprolol, propoxyphene, propranolol, and valproic acid. The absorption of all benzodiazepines is inhibited by concomitant use of antacids. Benzodiazepines may increase blood levels of digoxin, and reduce the efficacy of levodopa. Other drug interactions have been reported.

Buspirone levels will be increased by concomitant use of erythromycin, itraconazole, and nefazadone. Doses should be adjusted based on clinical response. Use of buspirone at the same time as monoamine oxidase inhibitors (MAOIs, including phenelzine and tranycypromine) may cause severe blood pressure elevations. Use of buspirone with MAOIs should be avoided.

Side effects

The most common side effects of benzodiazepines are secondary to their central nervous system (CNS) effects and include sedation and sleepiness, depression, lethargy, apathy, fatigue, hypoactivity, lightheadedness, memory impairment, disorientation, anterograde amnesia, restlessness, confusion, crying or sobbing, delirium, headache, slurred speech, aphonia, dysarthria, stupor, seizures, coma, syncope, rigidity, tremor, dystonia, vertigo, dizziness, euphoria, nervousness, irritability, difficulty in concentration, agitation, inability to perform complex mental functions, akathisia, hemiparesis, hypotonia, unsteadiness, ataxia, incoordination, weakness, vivid dreams, psychomotor retardation, "glassy-eyed" appearance, extrapyramidal symptoms, and paradoxical reactions. Other reactions include changes in heart rate and blood pressure, changes in bowel function, severe skin rash, and changes in genitourinary function. Other adverse effects have been reported.

Buspirone has a low incidence of side effects. Dizziness and drowsiness are the most commonly reported adverse effects. The drug may also cause difficulty sleeping, nervousness, lightheadedness, weakness, excitement, fatigue, depression, headache, fast or irregular heartbeat, blurred vision, and unusual movements of the head or neck muscles. Other CNS effects include dream disturbances, depersonalization, dysphoria, noise intolerance, euphoria, akathisia, fearfulness, loss of interest, disassociative reaction, hallucinations, suicidal ideation, seizures, feelings of claustrophobia, cold intolerance, stupor and slurred speech, and psychosis. Rarely, heart problems, including congestive heart failure and myocardial infarction, have been reported. Other adverse effects have been reported.

Resources

BOOKS

AHFS: Drug Information 2007. Washington, DC: American Society of Health-System Pharmacists, 2007.

Brody, T. M., J. Larner, and K. P. Minneman. *Human Pharmacology: Molecular to Clinical,* 3rd ed. St. Louis: Mosby, 1998.

Karch, A. M. *2008 Lippincott's Nursing Drug Guide.* Philadelphia, PA: Lippincott Williams & Wilkins, 2007.

Racagni, G., C. Massotto, and L. Steardo. *Pharmacology of Anxiolytic Drugs,* WHO Expert Series on Neuroscience, vol. 3. Cambridge, MA: Hogrefe and Huber, 1997.

Sweetman, Sean C., ed. *Martindale: The Complete Drug Reference,* 35th ed. London: The Pharmaceutical Press, 2007.

OTHER

"Busiprone." Medline Plus. April 1, 2003. http://www.nlm.nih.gov/medlineplus/druginfo/medmaster/a688005.html (February 2008).

"Fibromyalgia." National Institute of Arthritis and Musculoskeletal and Skin Diseases. December 1999. http://www.niams.nih.gov/Health_Info/Fibromyalgia/default.asp (February 2008).

"Lorazepam." Medline Plus. April 1, 2003. http://www.nlm.nih.gov/medlineplus/druginfo/medmaster/a68205.html (February 2008).

Sam Uretsky, Pharm.D.
Fran Hodgkins

Antibiotic prophylaxis *see* **Prophylaxis, antibiotic**

Antibiotics

Definition

Antibiotics may be informally defined as the subgroup of anti-infectives derived from bacterial sources and used to treat bacterial infections.

Purpose

Antibiotics are used for treatment or prevention of bacterial infection. Other classes of drugs, most notably the **sulfonamides**, may be effective antibacterials. Similarly, some antibiotics may have secondary uses, such as the use of demeclocycline (Declomycin, a tetracycline derivative) to treat the syndrome of inappropriate antidiuretic hormone (SIADH) secretion. Other antibiotics may be useful in treating protozoal infections.

Description

Although there are several classification schemes for antibiotics, based on bacterial spectrum (broad versus narrow), route of administration (injectable versus oral versus topical), or type of activity (bactericidal versus bacteriostatic), the most useful is based on chemical structure. Antibiotics within a structural class will generally show similar patterns of effectiveness, toxicity, and allergic potential.

Penicillins

The penicillins are the oldest class of antibiotics and have a common chemical structure that they share with the **cephalosporins**. The two groups are classed as the beta-lactam antibiotics, and are generally bacteriocidal—that is, they kill bacteria rather than inhibit growth. The penicillins can be further subdivided. The natural penicillins are based on the original penicillin G structure; penicillinase-resistant penicillins, notably methicillin and oxacillin, are active even in the presence of the bacterial enzyme that inactivates most natural penicillins. Aminopenicillins such as ampicillin and amoxicillin have an extended spectrum of action compared with the natural penicillins; extended spectrum penicillins are effective against a wider range of bacteria. These generally include coverage for *Pseudomonas aeruginosa* and may provide the penicillin in combination with a penicillinase inhibitor.

Cephalosporins

Cephalosporins and the closely related cephamycins and carbapenems, like the penicillins, contain a beta-lactam chemical structure. Consequently, there are patterns of cross-resistance and cross-allergenicity among the drugs in these classes. The "cepha" drugs are among the most diverse classes of antibiotics, and are themselves subgrouped into first, second, and third generations. Each generation has a broader spectrum of activity than the one before. In addition, cefoxitin (Mefoxin), a cephamycin, is highly active against anaerobic bacteria, which makes it useful in prevention and treatment of infections of the intestines. The third generation drugs, cefotaxime, ceftizoxime, ceftriaxone, and others, cross the blood-brain barrier and may be used to treat meningitis and encephalitis. Cephalosporins are the usually preferred agents for prevention of infection during surgery.

Fluoroquinolones

The **fluoroquinolones** are synthetic antibacterial agents, and are not derived from bacteria. They are included here because they can be readily interchanged with traditional antibiotics. An earlier, related class of antibacterial agents, the quinolones, were not well absorbed, and could be used only to treat urinary tract infections. The fluoroquinolones, which are based on the older group, are broad-spectrum bactericidal drugs that are chemically unrelated to the penicillins or the cephalosporins. They are well distributed

---

KEY TERMS

Anaerobic—An organism that lives without oxygen. Anaerobic bacteria are commonly found in the mouth and the intestines.

Bacteria—Tiny, one-celled forms of life that cause many diseases and infections.

Bactericidal—An agent that kills bacteria.

Bacteriostatic—An agent that stops the multiplication of bacteria.

Inflammation—Pain, redness, swelling, and heat that usually develop in response to injury or illness.

Meningitis—Inflammation of tissues that surround the brain and spinal cord.

Microorganism—An independent unit of life that is too small to be seen with the naked eye.

Pregnancy category—A system of classifying drugs according to their established risks for use during pregnancy. Category A: Controlled human studies have demonstrated no fetal risk. Category B: Animal studies indicate no fetal risk, but no human studies; or adverse effects in animals, but not in well-controlled human studies. Category C: No adequate human or animal studies; or adverse fetal effects in animal studies, but no available human data. Category D: Evidence of fetal risk, but benefits outweigh risks. Category X: Evidence of fetal risk. Risks outweigh any benefits.

---

into bone tissue, and so well absorbed that in general they are as effective by the oral route as by intravenous infusion.

Tetracyclines

Tetracyclines got their name because they share a chemical structure having four rings. They are derived from a species of *Streptomyces* bacteria. Broad-spectrum bacteriostatic agents, the tetracyclines may be effective against a wide variety of microorganisms, including rickettsia and amebic parasites.

Macrolides

The macrolide antibiotics are derived from *Streptomyces* bacteria, and got their name because they all have a macrocyclic lactone chemical structure. Erythromycin, the prototype of this class, has a spectrum and use similar to penicillin. Newer members of the group, azithromycin and clarithyromycin, are particularly useful for their high level of lung penetration.

Clarithromycin has been widely used to treat *Helicobacter pylori* infections, the cause of stomach ulcers. For people who are allergic to penicillin, erythromycin is a valuable alternative. But, unlike penicillin, erythromycin can be very irritating both to the stomach when given by mouth, or to veins when given by injection.

Other classes

Other classes of antibiotics include the aminoglycosides, which are particularly useful for their effectiveness in treating *Pseudomonas aeruginosa* infections, and the lincosamindes, clindamycin and lincomycin, which are highly active against anaerobic pathogens. In addition, other individual drugs are available that may have utility in specific infections.

Recommended dosage

Dosage varies with drug, route of administration, pathogen, site of infection, and severity of infection. Additional considerations include renal, or kidney, function, age of patient, and other factors. Patients should consult drug references or ask their physicians.

Side effects

All antibiotics cause risk of overgrowth by nonsusceptible bacteria. Manufacturers list other major hazards by class; however, the health care provider should review each drug individually to assess the degree of risk. Generally, breast-feeding is not recommended while taking antibiotics because of risk of alteration to infant's intestinal flora, and risk of masking infection in the infant. Excessive or inappropriate use may promote growth of resistant pathogens.

- *Penicillins.* Hypersensitivity may be common, and cross allergenicity with cephalosporins has been reported. Penicillins are classed as category B during pregnancy.
- *Cephalosporins.* Several cephalosporins and related compounds have been associated with seizures. Cefmetazole, cefoperazone, cefotetan and ceftriaxone may be associated with a fall in prothrombin activity and coagulation abnormalities. Pseudomembranous colitis (inflammation of the colon) has been reported with cephalosporins and other broad spectrum antibiotics. Some drugs in this class may cause renal toxicity. Pregnancy category B.
- *Fluoroquinolones.* Lomefloxacin has been associated with increased photosensitivity. All drugs in this class have been associated with convulsions. Pregnancy category C.
- *Tetracyclines.* Demeclocycline may cause increased photosensitivity. Minocycline may cause dizziness.

Children under the age of eight should not use tetracyclines, and specifically during periods of tooth development. Oral tetracyclines bind to anions such as calcium and iron. Although doxycycline and minocycline may be taken with meals, patients are advised to take other tetracycline antibiotics on an empty stomach, and not to take the drugs with milk or other calcium-rich foods. Expired tetracycline should never be administered. Pregnancy category D; use during pregnancy may cause alterations in bone development.

- *Macrolides.* Erythromycin may aggravate the weakness of patients with myasthenia gravis. Azithromycin has, rarely, been associated with allergic reactions, including angioedema, anaphylaxis, and dermatologic reactions, including Stevens-Johnson syndrome and toxic epidermal necrolysis. Oral erythromycin may be highly irritating to the stomach and may cause severe phlebitis (inflammation of the vein) when given by injection. These drugs should be used with caution in patients with liver dysfunction. Pregnancy category B: Azithromycin, erythromycin. Pregnancy category C: Clarithromycin, dirithromycin, troleandomycin.
- *Aminoglycosides.* This class of drugs causes kidney and hearing problems. These problems can occur even with normal doses. Dosing should be based on renal function, with periodic testing of both kidney function and hearing. Pregnancy category D.

Interactions

Use of all antibiotics may temporarily reduce the effectiveness of birth control pills; alternative birth control methods should be used while taking these medications. Antacids should be avoided while on tetracyclines as the calcium can impair absorption of this antibiotic class. For this reason, tetracyclines should not be taken just before or after consuming foods rich in calcium or iron. Consult specialized references for additional interactions to specific antibiotics.

Recommended usage

To minimize risk of adverse reactions and development of resistant strains of bacteria, antibiotics should be restricted to use in cases where there is either known or a reasonable presumption of bacterial infection. The use of antibiotics in viral infections is to be avoided. Avoid use of fluoroquinolones for trivial infections.

In severe infections, presumptive therapy with a broad-spectrum antibiotic such as a third generation cephalosporin may be appropriate. Treatment should be changed to a narrow spectrum agent as soon as the pathogen has been identified. After 48 hours of treatment, if there is clinical improvement, an oral antibiotic should be considered.

When the pathogen is known or suspected to be *Pseudomonas*, a suitable beta-lactam drug is often prescribed in combination with an aminoglycoside. A single agent cannot be relied upon for treatment of *Pseudomonas*. When the patient has renal insufficiency, azactam should be considered in place of the aminoglycoside.

In treatment of children with antibiotic suspensions, caregivers should be instructed in use of oral syringes or measuring teaspoons. Household teaspoons are not standardized and will give unreliable doses.

Resources

PERIODICALS

Moellering, R. C., Jr. "Linezolid: The First Oxazolidinone." *Annals of Internal Medicine* 138, no. 2 (January 21, 2003): 1–44.

OTHER

"Antibiotics: Use Them Wisely." *MayoClinic.com.* February 13, 2008. http://www.mayoclinic.com/invoke.cfm?id = FL00075. (March 20, 2008).
"What Is Antibiotic Resistance & Why Is It a Problem?" *Alliance for the Prudent Use of Antibiotics.* 1999. http://www.tufts.edu/med/apua/Patients/patient.html (March 20, 2008).

Sam Uretsky, Pharm.D.
Fran Hodgkins

Antibiotics, topical

Definition

Topical **antibiotics** are medicines applied to the skin to kill or stop the growth of bacteria.

Purpose

Topical antibiotics help prevent infections caused by bacteria that get into minor cuts, scrapes, and burns. Treating minor wounds with antibiotics allows quicker healing. If the wounds are left untreated, the bacteria will multiply, causing pain, redness, swelling,

itching, and oozing. Untreated infections can eventually spread and become much more serious.

Topical antibiotics may also be applied to surgical incision sites to prevent infection; however, when antibiotics are given intravenously, which is in a vein, or during surgery and intravenously, or by mouth following surgery, this may be enough to prevent infection, and antibiotic ointments may not be needed.

Different kinds of topical antibiotics kill different kinds of bacteria. Many antibiotic first-aid products contain combinations of antibiotics to make them effective against a broad range of bacteria.

When treating a wound, it is not enough to simply apply a topical antibiotic. The wound must first be cleaned with soap and water and patted dry. After the antibiotic is applied, the wound should be covered with a dressing such as a bandage or a protective gel or spray. For many years, it was thought that wounds heal best when exposed to the air. Now most experts say it is best to keep wounds clean and moist while they heal, but the covering should still allow some air to reach the wound.

Description

Some topical antibiotics are available without a prescription and are sold in many forms, including creams, ointments, powders, and sprays. Some widely used topical antibiotics are bacitracin, neomycin, mupirocin, and polymyxin B. Among the products that contain one or more of these ingredients are Bactroban (a prescription item), Neosporin, Polysporin, and Triple Antibiotic Ointment or Cream.

Recommended dosage

The recommended dosage depends on the type of topical antibiotic. The patient is advised to follow the directions on the package label or ask a pharmacist for directions.

Only the ointment or cream that actually touches the skin has any benefit, therefore a thin layer of topical antibiotic ointment or cream will usually work just as well as a thick layer.

In general, topical antibiotics should be applied within four hours after injury. It is advised not to use more than the recommended amount and do not apply it more often than three times a day; the medicine should not be applied over large areas of skin or on open wounds.

When topical antibiotics are used for surgical incision sites, a surgeon or nurse should be consulted for instructions.

Precautions

Many public health experts are concerned about antibiotic resistance, a problem that can develop when antibiotics are overused. Over time, bacteria develop new defenses against the antibiotics that once were effective against them. Because bacteria reproduce so quickly, these defenses can be rapidly passed on through generations of bacteria until almost all are immune to the effects of a particular antibiotic. The process happens faster than new antibiotics can be developed. To help control the problem, many experts advise people to use topical antibiotics only for short periods, that is, until the wound heals, and only as directed. For the topical antibiotic to work best, it should be used only to prevent infection in a fresh wound, not to treat an infection that has already started. Wounds that are not fresh may need the attention of a physician to prevent complications such as blood poisoning.

Topical antibiotics are meant to be used only on the skin and for only a few days at a time. If the wound has not healed in five days, the patient is advised to stop using the antibiotic and call a doctor.

It is advised not to use topical antibiotics on large areas of skin or on open wounds. These products should not be used to treat diaper rash in infants or incontinence rash in adults.

Only minor cuts, scrapes, and burns should be treated with topical antibiotics. Certain kinds of injuries may need medical care and should not be self-treated with topical antibiotics. These include:

- large wounds;
- deep cuts;
- cuts that continue bleeding;
- cuts that may need stitches;
- burns any larger than a few inches in diameter;
- scrapes imbedded with particles that will not wash away;
- animal bites;
- deep puncture wounds; or
- eye injuries.

Regular topical antibiotics should never be used in the eyes. Special antibiotic products are available for treating eye infections.

Although topical antibiotics control infections caused by bacteria, they may allow fungal infections to develop. The use of other medicines to treat the fungal infections may be necessary. It is recommended to check with a physician.

Some people may be allergic to one or more ingredients in a topical antibiotic product. If an allergic reaction develops, the person should stop using the product immediately and call a physician.

No harmful or abnormal effects have been reported in babies whose mothers used topical antibiotics while pregnant or nursing; however, pregnant women generally are advised not to use any drugs during the first three months after conception. A woman who is pregnant or breast-feeding or who plans to become pregnant should check with her physician before using a topical antibiotic.

Unless directed by a physician to do so, topical antibiotics should not be used on children under two years of age.

Side effects

The most common minor side effects are itching or burning. These problems usually do not require medical treatment unless they do not go away or they interfere with normal activities.

If any of the following side effects occur, a doctor should be consulted as soon as possible:

- rash;
- swelling of the lips and face;
- sweating;
- tightness or discomfort in the chest;
- breathing problems;
- fainting or dizziness;
- low blood pressure;

- nausea;
- diarrhea; or
- hearing loss or ringing in the ears.

Other rare side effects may occur. Anyone who has unusual symptoms after using a topical antibiotic should get in touch with the physician who prescribed it or the pharmacist who recommended the medication.

Interactions

Using certain topical antibiotics at the same time as hydrocortisone, which is a topical corticosteroid used to treat inflammation, may hide signs of infection or allergic reaction. These two medicines should not be used at the same time unless recommended by a health care provider.

Anyone who is using any other type of prescription or nonprescription (over-the-counter) medicine on the skin should check with a doctor before using a topical antibiotic.

Resources

PERIODICALS
Farley, Dixie. "OTC Options: Help for Cuts, Scrapes and Burns." *FDA Consumer* 30, no. 4 (May 1996): 12.
O'Connor, L. T., and M. Goldstein. "Topical Perioperative Antibiotic Prophylaxis for Minor Clean Inguinal Surgery." *Journal of the American College of Surgeons* 194, no. 4 (April 2002): 407–410.

Nancy Ross-Flanigan
Sam Uretsky, Pharm.D.
Fran Hodgkins

Antibody screening *see* **Type and screen**

Antibody tests, immunoglobulins

Definition

Antibodies, also called immunoglobulins, are proteins produced by the body's immune system that are responsible for fighting off various invaders, such as viruses, bacteria, toxins, and mold spores. They work to clear the body of potentially threatening infections or substances.

The body's immune system is made up of lymphoid organs, including lymph nodes, the bone marrow (located within the center of long bones) and the thymus (located in the chest). These lymphoid organs produce lymphocytes, including T cells and B cells. These lymphocytes circulate within the bloodstream, within the lymph system, and are also positioned in clumps within organs and on mucosal surfaces of the body. When a B cell encounters a foreign invader, it recognized it as foreign by virtue of a chemical identifier on its surface (called an antigen). Once the B cell recognizes an antigen, the B cell gives rise to a large number of plasma cells. These plasma cells are capable of producing antibodies.

Antibodies are made up of units called "chains." All antibodies are composed of two larger chains (called heavy chains) and two smaller chains (called light chains). The tip of the antibody is referred to as the hypervariable region. This hypervariable region is responsible for unique chemical properties possessed by each antibody that allow a specific antibody to "recognize" and match up to a particular antigen. The combination of an antibody with a specific antigen, creates an antibody-antigen complex, marking the invader as foreign and in need of inactivation or destruction by other immune cells in the body.

The first time an antigen is encountered by the immune system, the body's response is slow. Time is required in order to activate the machinery necessary to produce the very specific type of antibody necessary to combat that antigen; however, if that particular antigen is encountered in the future, the needed machinery is already available, and antibody production in response to a "familiar" antigen is quite rapid.

Antibodies are divided into five different specific classes of immunoglobulins, termed IgA, IgG, IgM, IgE, and IgD. Each of these classes of immunoglobulins has different characteristics, including overall percentage of immunoglobulins, location, timing of action, and type of antigen to which it attaches:

- About 80% of all circulating antibodies are IgG. IgG is found in blood and tissue fluids. It coats invading particles, marking them so that they can more easily and rapidly be taken up by other types of immune cells. IgG is the predominant antibody cell in the later or secondary phase of immune response.
- IgM makes up about 13% of all antibodies. IgM is primarily found in the blood. It functions to kill bacteria, and is found in the earlier phases of immune response to bacterial invasion of the bloodstream (bacteremia).
- IgA makes up about 6% of the body's total antibodies. IgA is found in large quantities in a variety of bodily fluids, such as breast milk, tears, saliva, and on the surface mucosal lining of the respiratory and digestive tracts. In these locations, IgA is poised to

protect these areas that serve as entrances to the body.

- IgE is the least prevalent antibody, composing about 0.002% of the body's total antibodies. IgE is found bound to immune cells called basophils and mast cells. It is involved in fighting parasites, and is also the predominant antibody seen in allergic reactions.

- Only about 1% of the body's antibodies are IgD. IgD primarily stays attached to B cells, and helps mediate the B cells' early response to antigen exposure. IgD antibodies are particularly active in newborn babies.

One of the important attributes of a healthy, well-functioning immune system rests on its ability to distinguish between "self" and "other." This means that it's important that the antibodies don't mistakenly identify parts of the body itself as foreign invaders. When this does happen, the body's immune system attacks the body, damaging and destroying it. Conditions in which this occurs are referred to as auto-immune disorders. One example of an autoimmune disorder is the condition called rheumatoid arthritis or RA. In RA, the lining of the joints is mis-recognized by the immune system as foreign, resulting in the immune system creating specific antibodies that repeatedly attack, damage, and destroy the joints' lining, resulting in the severe symptoms that accompany this disease.

Another way that the immune system can accidentally work against the body involves the reaction known as allergy or hypersensitivity reactions. In this situation, the immune system reacts overly strongly to a commonly-encountered substance, such as pollen, animal dander, a food ingredient, or an antibiotic medication. While most people's immune systems do not respond to these substances as antigens, an allergic individual's immune system identifies some aspect of the substance as an antigen, triggering an immune reaction. As a result of the ensuing immune response, the individual experiences symptoms of allergy, which are secondary to the immune system's overly-exuberant response to a substance that is usually ignored by most people's immune systems. Allergic responses can vary from mild reactions to overwhelming, life-threatening (anaphylactic) responses.

Strong activation of the immune system to specific chemical markers on transplanted organs is the phenomenon responsible for organ rejection. In this instance, the individual's immune cells identify the transplanted organ's cells as foreign invaders, and specific antibodies that match the organ's antigens are produced. The organ is attacked by the immune system, and damaged, interfering with the organ's functioning or even destroying it. This same phenomenon is responsible for a **transfusion** reaction; the individual's immune system reacts to the presence of a foreign antigen within the transfused blood, kicking off an immune reaction. The blood cells are attacked by the body's immune cells, and a transfusion reaction ensues.

An understanding of the antibody response is harnessed and used to advantage in the preparation of vaccines or immunizations. In this instance, the vaccine is given in order to "introduce" the body to a particular viral invader that it may encounter in the future. This is done by inactivating the virus (that is, making it unable to actually cause illness). The inactivated virus still has its identifying surface antigen present, allowing the immune system to become acquainted with it. After this introduction, if the individual is actually exposed to that virus, the immune response will be rapid, which will either prevent any illness that occurs due to that virus, or result in a less-severe, shorter course of illness.

Purpose

Immunoglobulin or antibody tests may provide quantitative or qualitative information. Quantitative testing reveals the levels of a particular antibody. Qualitative testing is done to demonstrate the presence or absence of a specific type of antibody.

Immunoglobulin or antibody tests are performed in order to:

- verify that an individual has been exposed to a particular microbial agent or substance (IgG or IgM testing for infectious agents, IgA testing for allergic exposures);

- check to see whether an individual is immune to a particular microbial agent (IgG or IgM testing);

- diagnose and/or monitor an autoimmune disorder;

- ascertain the reason for organ rejection or a transfusion reaction;

- diagnose an allergy (IgE and/or IgA testing);

- verify that you are immune to a particular disease (sometime used to make sure that an immunization was effective);

- monitor treatment for the bacteria that causes stomach ulcers (*Helicobacter pylori*);

- monitor treatment for cancers that affect the functioning of the bone marrow;

- diagnose multiple myeloma or macroglobulinemia (types of cancer that affect immune cells); and

- diagnose and/or monitor the course of an infection (usually IgG and IgM testing). This may require two samples, one during the height of the illness (called the acute sample) and one some weeks later (called the convalescent sample). IgM is usually present in the case of a recent infection; IgG is usually present in the event of an infection that occurred at some point in the past.

Precautions

A number of situations may skew the test results, and should be taken into account when planning an antibody test. These situations include:

- the use of certain medicines, such as birth control pills, antiseizure medications (including phenytoin), corticosteroids, methotrexate, asparaginase, aminophenazone, phenylbutazone, and hydralazine;
- recent cancer treatment (radiation and/or chemotherapy);
- having received a blood transfusion within the previous six months;
- recent (within the previous six months) immunizations, especially those requiring repeat booster doses;
- recent use of alcohol or illegal drugs; and
- recent radioactive scan (within the three days previous to immunoglobulin testing).

Description

This test requires blood to be drawn from a vein (usually one in the forearm), usually by a nurse or phlebotomist (an individual who has been trained to draw blood). A tourniquet is applied to the arm above the area where the needle stick will be performed. The site of the needle stick is cleaned with antiseptic, and the needle is inserted. The blood is collected in vacuum tubes. After collection, the needle is withdrawn, and pressure is kept on the blood draw site to stop any bleeding and decrease bruising. A bandage is then applied.

Preparation

There are no restrictions on diet or physical activity, either before or after the blood test.

Aftercare

As with any blood tests, discomfort, bruising, and/or a very small amount of bleeding is common at the puncture site. Immediately after the needle is withdrawn, it is helpful to put pressure on the puncture site until the bleeding has stopped. This decreases the chance of significant bruising. Warm packs may relieve minor discomfort. Some individuals may feel briefly woozy after a blood test, and they should be encouraged to lie down and rest until they feel better.

Risks

Basic blood tests, such as immunoglobulin or antibody testing, do not carry any significant risks, other than slight bruising and the chance of brief dizziness.

Results

Antibody tests are performed by mixing a sample of the patient's blood with a sample containing a known, identified antigen. If the patient's blood contains antibody to that antigen, then the antibody will bind to the antigen, creating an antibody-antigen complex. This complex can be measured. Depending on the reason for testing, results may be reported very simply as "detected" or "not detected." Alternatively, results may report on whether the amount of complex detected exceed a predetermined level, one which might reflect the individual's immune status to the antigen-containing substance. In this case, the resulting laboratory report might read "immune" or "not-immune." Lastly, the results might be reported as a concentration, in milligrams per deciliter (mg/dL) or grams per liter (g/L).

Normal results for antibody concentrations are as follows:

- Ig: 85–385 mg/dL or 0.85–3085 g/L
- IgG: 565–1765 mg/dL or 5.65–17.65 g/L
- IgM: 55–375 mg/dL or 0.55–3.75 g/L
- IgD: Less than 8 mg/dL or 5–30 micrograms per liter
- IgE: 10–1421 micrograms per liter

High levels

High levels of IgA may indicate a monoclonal gammopathy, the presence of multiple myeloma, autoimmune disease(rheumatoid arthritis or systemic lupus erythematosus, for example), or liver disease (including cirrhosis of the liver or chronic hepatitis).

High levels of IgG may indicate the presence of a chronic infection (including AIDS), or multiple myeloma, chronic hepatitis, or multiple sclerosis.

High levels of IgD may indicate multiple myeloma.

High levels of IgE may indicate the presence of a parasitic infection, as well as an allergic response, asthma, atopic dermatitis, autoimmune disease, cancer or multiple myeloma.

Low levels

Abnormally low levels of IgA may occur in the presence of leukemia, nephritic syndrome, intestinal diseases, rare congenital immune deficiencies of IgA, or a rare genetic disease called ataxia-telangiectasia.

Abnormally low levels of IgG may occur in macroglobulinemia, leukemia, nephritic syndrome, and rare congenital immune deficiencies of IgG.

Abnormally low levels of IgM may occur in the presence of multiple myeloma, leukemia, and some genetic immune disorders.

Abnormally low levels of IgE may occur in the presence of ataxia telangiectasia.

Resources

BOOKS

Harris E., et al. *Kelley's Textbook of Rheumatology,* 7th ed. Philadelphia: Saunders, 2004.

Hoffman R., et al. *Hematology: Basic Principles and Practice,* 4th ed. Philadelphia: Elsevier, 2004.

McPherson R. A., and M. R. Pincus, eds. *Henry's Clinical Diagnosis and Management by Laboratory Methods,* 21st ed. Philadelphia: Saunders, 2006.

OTHER

Medical Encyclopedia. Medline Plus. U.S. National Library of Medicine and the National Institutes of Health. January 2, 2008. http://www.nlm.nih.gov/medlineplus/encyclopedia.html (February 10, 2008).

ORGANIZATIONS

American Association for Clinical Chemistry, 1850 K Street, NW, Suite 625, Washington, DC, 20006, (800) 892-1400, http://www.aacc.org.

Rosalyn Carson-DeWitt, M.D.

Anticlotting drugs *see* **Anticoagulant and antiplatelet drugs**

Anticoagulant and antiplatelet drugs

Definition

Anticoagulants are drugs used to prevent clot formation or to prevent a clot that has formed from enlarging. They inhibit clot formation by blocking the action of clotting factors or platelets. Anticoagulant drugs fall into one of three categories: inhibitors of clotting factor synthesis, inhibitors of thrombin, and antiplatelet drugs.

Purpose

Anticoagulant drugs reduce the ability of the blood to form clots. Although blood clotting is essential to prevent serious bleeding in the case of skin cuts, clots inside the blood vessels block the flow of blood to major organs and cause heart attacks and strokes. Although these drugs are sometimes called blood thinners, they do not actually thin the blood. Furthermore, this type of medication will not dissolve clots that already have formed, although the drug stops an existing clot from worsening. However, another type of drug, used in **thrombolytic therapy**, will dissolve existing clots.

Anticoagulant drugs are used for a number of conditions. For example, they may be given to prevent blood clots from forming after the replacement of a heart valve or to reduce the risk of a stroke or another heart attack after a first heart attack. They are also used to reduce the chance of blood clots forming during open-heart surgery or bypass surgery. Low doses of these drugs may be given to prevent blood clots in patients who must stay in bed for a long time after certain types of surgery. They may also be used to prevent the formation of clots in needles or tubes that are inserted into veins, such as indwelling catheters.

Anticoagulants may be given after major surgery to prevent the formation of clots due to lack of physical activity. Patients who are unable to move around may be at risk of developing clots, particularly in the legs. Anticoagulants are given to prevent this. At the same time, compression stockings may be used to reduce the risk of clots in the legs. Compression stocks are worn on the lower legs, and act by increasing the pressure on the veins of the leg, then relaxing. The compression-relaxation keeps the blood in the veins moving, and reduces the risk of clots following surgery.

Because anticoagulants affect the blood's ability to clot, they can increase the risk of severe bleeding and heavy blood loss. It is thus essential to take these drugs exactly as directed and to see a physician

KEY TERMS

Anticoagulant—Drug used to prevent clot formation or to prevent a clot that has formed from enlarging.

Antiplatelet drug—Drug that inhibits platelets from aggregating to form a plug.

Atherosclerosis—Condition characterized by deposits of fatty plaque in the arteries.

Catheter—A tube for passage of fluid into the body or into a body cavity.

Clot—A soft, semi-solid mass that forms when blood gels.

Platelet—A small, disk-shaped body in the blood that has an important role in blood clotting: they form the initial plug at the rupture site of a blood vessel.

Thrombin—A protein produced by the body that is a specific clotting factor that plays an important role in the blood-clotting process.

Thrombin inhibitor—One type of anticoagulant medication used to help prevent formation of harmful blood clots in the body by blocking the activity of thrombin.

regularly as long as they are prescribed. With some of these drugs, regular blood tests, as often as once a day, may be required.

Description

Most anticoagulant drugs are available only with a physician's prescription. They come in tablet and injectable forms. They fall into three groups:

- Inhibitors of clotting factor synthesis. These anticoagulants inhibit the production of certain clotting factors in the liver. One example is warfarin (brand name: Coumadin).
- Inhibitors of thrombin. These drugs interfere with blood clotting by blocking the activity of thrombin. They include heparin and lepirudin (Refludan).
- Antiplatelet drugs. These drugs interact with platelets, which is a type of blood cell, to block platelets from aggregating into harmful clots. They include aspirin, ticlopidine (Ticlid), clopidogrel (Plavix), tirofiban (Aggrastat), and eptifibatide (Integrilin).

Recommended dosage

The recommended dosage depends on the type of anticoagulant drug and the medical condition for which it is prescribed. The prescribing physician or the pharmacist who fills the prescription can provide information concerning the correct dosage. Usually, the physician will adjust the dose after checking the patient's clotting time.

Anticoagulant drugs must be taken exactly as directed by the physician. Larger or more frequent doses should not be taken, and the drug should also not be taken for longer than prescribed. Taking too much of this medication can cause easy bruising or severe bleeding. Anticoagulants should also be taken on schedule. A record of each dose should be kept as it is taken. If a dose is missed, it should be taken as soon as possible followed by the regular dose schedule. However, a patient who forgets to take a missed dose until the next day should not take the missed dose at all and should not double the next dose, as this could lead to bleeding. A record of all missed doses should be kept for the prescribing physician who should be informed at the scheduled visits.

Precautions

Persons who take anticoagulants should see a physician regularly while taking these drugs, particularly at the beginning of therapy. The physician will order periodic blood tests to check the blood's clotting ability. The results of these tests will help the physician determine the proper amount of medication to be taken each day.

Time is required for normal clotting ability to return after anticoagulant treatment. During this period, patients must observe the same precautions they observed while taking the drug. The length of time needed for the blood to return to normal depends on the type of anticoagulant drug that was taken. The prescribing physician will advise as to how long the precautions should be observed.

People who are taking anticoagulant drugs should tell all physicians, dentists, pharmacists, and other medical professionals who provide them with medical treatments or services that they are taking such a medication. They should also carry identification stating that they are using an anticoagulant drug.

Other prescription drugs or over-the-counter medicine—especially aspirin—should be not be taken without the prescribing physician being informed.

Because of the risk of heavy bleeding, anyone who takes an anticoagulant drug must take care to avoid injuries. Sports and other potentially hazardous activities should be avoided. Any falls, blows to the body or head, or other injuries should be reported to a physician, as internal bleeding may occur without any obvious symptoms. Special care should be taken in shaving and in brushing and flossing the teeth. Soft toothbrushes should be used and the flossing should be very gentle. Electric razors should be used instead of a blade.

Alcohol can change the way anticoagulant drugs affect the body. Anyone who takes this medicine should not have more than one to two alcoholic drinks at any one time, and should not drink alcohol every day.

Special conditions

People with specific medical conditions or who are taking certain other medicines can have problems if they take anticoagulant drugs. Before taking these drugs, the prescribing physician should be informed about any of these conditions.

ALLERGIES. Anyone who has had unusual reactions to anticoagulants in the past should let the physician know before taking the drugs again. The physician should also be told about any allergies to beef, pork, or other foods; dyes; preservatives; or other substances.

PREGNANCY. Anticoagulants may cause many serious problems if taken during pregnancy. Birth defects, severe bleeding in the fetus, and other problems that affect the physical or mental development of the fetus or newborn are possible. The mother may also experience severe bleeding if she takes anticoagulants during pregnancy, during delivery, or even shortly after delivery. Women should not start taking anticoagulants during pregnancy and should not become pregnant while taking the drug. Any woman who becomes pregnant or suspects that she has become pregnant while taking an anticoagulant should check with her physician immediately.

BREASTFEEDING. Some anticoagulant drugs may pass into breast milk. Blood tests can be done on nursing babies to see whether the drug is causing any problems. If it is, other medication may be prescribed to counteract the effects of the anticoagulant drug.

OTHER MEDICAL CONDITIONS. Before using anticoagulant drugs, people should inform their physician about any medical problems they have. They should also let the physician who prescribed the medicine know if they are being treated by any other medical physician or dentist. In addition, people who will be taking anticoagulant drugs should let their physician know if they have recently had any of the following:

- fever lasting more than one to two days
- severe or continuing diarrhea
- childbirth
- heavy or unusual menstrual bleeding
- insertion of an intrauterine contraceptive device (i.e., IUD)
- falls, injuries, or blows to the body or head
- any type of surgery, including dental surgery
- spinal anesthesia
- radiation treatment
- any intestinal condition

Side effects

The most common minor side effects are bloating or gas. These problems usually go away as the body adjusts to the drug and do not require medical treatment.

More serious side effects may occur, especially if excessive anticoagulant is taken. If any of the following side effects occur, a physician should be notified immediately:

- bleeding gums
- sores or white spots in the mouth or throat
- unusual bruises or purplish areas on the skin
- unexplained nosebleeds
- unusually heavy bleeding or oozing from wounds
- unexpected or unusually heavy menstrual bleeding
- blood in the urine
- cloudy or dark urine
- painful or difficult urination or sudden decrease in amount of urine
- black, tarry, or bloody stools
- coughing up blood
- vomiting blood or something that looks like coffee grounds
- constipation
- pain or swelling in the stomach or abdomen
- back pain
- stiff, swollen, or painful joints
- painful, bluish or purplish fingers or toes
- puffy or swollen eyelids, face, feet, or lower legs
- changes in the color of the face
- skin rash, itching, or hives
- yellow eyes or skin
- severe or continuing headache
- sore throat and fever, with or without chills
- breathing problems or wheezing
- tightness in the chest
- dizziness
- unusual tiredness or weakness
- weight gain

In addition, patients taking anticoagulant drugs should check with their physicians as soon as possible if any of these side effects occur:

- nausea or vomiting
- diarrhea
- stomach pain or cramps

Other side effects may occur. Anyone who has unusual symptoms while taking anticoagulant drugs should get in touch with the prescribing physician.

Interactions

Anticoagulants may interact with many other medications. When this happens, the effects of one or both of the drugs may change or the risk of side effects may be increased. Anyone who takes anticoagulants should inform the prescribing physician about other prescription or nonprescription (over-the-counter) medicines he or she is taking—even **aspirin**, **laxatives**, vitamins, and antacids.

Diet also affects the way anticoagulant drugs work in the body. A normal, balanced diet should be followed every day while taking such medication. No dietary changes should be made without informing first the prescribing physician, who should also be told of any illness or other condition interfering with the ability to eat normally. Diet is a very important consideration because the amount of vitamin K in the body affects how anticoagulant drugs work. Dicoumarol and warfarin act by reducing the effects of vitamin K, which is found in meats, dairy products, leafy, green vegetables, and some multiple vitamins and nutritional supplements. For the drugs to work properly, it is best to have the same amount of vitamin K in the body all the time. Foods containing vitamin K should not be increased or decreased without consulting with the prescribing physician. If the patient takes vitamin supplements, he or she should check the label to see if it contains vitamin K. Because vitamin K is also produced by intestinal bacteria, a severe case of diarrhea or the use of laxatives may also alter a person's vitamin K levels.

Resources

BOOKS

AHFS: Drug Information. Washington, DC: American Society Healthsystems Pharmaceuticals, 2002.

Brody, T.M., J. Larner, K.P. Minneman, H.C. Neu. *Human Pharmacology: Molecular to Clinical,* 2nd ed. St. Louis: Mosby Year-Book.

Reynolds, J.E.F., ed. *Martindale: The Extra Pharmacopoeia,* 31st ed. London: The Pharmaceutical Press, 1993.

OTHER

"Abciximab." Medline Plus Drug Information. [cited May 2003]/ http://www.nlm.nih.gov/medlineplus/druginfo/uspdi/500417.html.

"Heparin (Systemic)." Medline Plus Drug Information. [cited May 2003]. http://www.nlm.nih.gov/medlineplus/druginfo/uspdi/202280.html.

"Salicylates (Systemic)." Medline Plus Drug Information. [cited May 2003]. http://www.nlm.nih.gov/medlineplus/druginfo/uspdi/202515.html.

"Warfarin." Medline Plus Drug Information. [cited May 2003]. http://www.nlm.nih.gov/medlineplus/druginfo/medmaster/a682277.html.

Nancy Ross-Flanigan
Sam Uretsky, PharmD

Antiemetic drugs *see* **Antinausea drugs**

Antihypertensive drugs

Definition

Antihypertensive drugs are medicines that help lower blood pressure.

Purpose

All antihypertensive agents lower blood pressure, although the mechanisms of action vary greatly. Within this therapeutic class, there are several subgroups. There are a very large number of drugs used to control hypertension, and the drugs listed below are representatives, but not the only members of their classes.

Description

The calcium channel blocking agents, also called slow channel blockers or calcium antagonists, inhibit the movement of ionic calcium across the cell membrane. This reduces the force of contraction of heart muscles and arteries. Although the calcium channel blockers are treated as a group, there are four different chemical classes, leading to significant variations in the activity of individual drugs. Nifedipine (Adalat, Procardia) has the greatest effect on the blood vessels, while verapamil (Calan, Isoptin) and diltiazem (Cardizem) have a greater effect on the heart muscle itself.

Peripheral vasodilators such as hydralazine (Apresoline), isoxuprine (Vasodilan), and minoxidil (Loniten) act by relaxing blood vessels.

There are several groups of drugs that act by reducing adrenergic nerve stimulation, the excitatory nerve stimulation that causes contraction of the muscles in the arteries, veins, and heart. These drugs include the beta-adrenergic blockers and alpha/beta adrenergic blockers. There are also non-specific adrenergic blocking agents.

Beta-adrenergic blocking agents include propranolol (Inderal), atenolol (Tenormin), and pindolol (Visken). Propranolol acts on the beta-adrenergic receptors anywhere in the body, and has been used as a treatment for emotional anxiety and rapid heart beat. Atenolol and acebutolol (Sectral) act specifically on the nerves of the heart and circulation.

There are two alpha/beta adrenergic blockers, labetalol (Normodyne, Trandate) and carvedilol (Coreg). These work similarly to the beta blockers.

Angiotensin-converting enzyme inhibitors (ACE inhibitors) act by inhibiting the production of angiotensin

II, a substance that induces both constriction of blood vessels and retention of sodium, which leads to water retention and increased blood volume. As of the early 2000s, there are 10 ACE inhibitors marketed in the United States, including captopril (Capoten), benazepril (Lotensin), enalapril (Vasotec), lisinopril (Prinivil, Zestril), and quinapril (Acupril). The primary difference between these drugs is their onset and duration of action.

The ACE II inhibitors, losartan (Cozaar), candesartan (Atacand), irbesartan (Avapro), telmisartan (Micardis), valsartan (Diovan), and eprosartan (Teveten) directly inhibit the effects of ACE II rather than blocking its production. Their actions are similar to the ACE inhibitors, but they appear to have a more favorable side effect and safety profile.

In addition to these drugs, other classes of drugs have been used to lower blood pressure, most notably the thiazide **diuretics**. There are a number of thiazide diuretics marketed in the United States, including hydrochlorothiazide (Hydrodiuril, Esidrex), indapamide (Lozol), polythiazide (Renese), and hydroflumethiazide (Diucardin). The drugs in this class appear to lower blood pressure through several mechanisms. By promoting sodium loss they lower blood volume. At the same time, the pressure of the walls of blood vessels, the peripheral vascular resistance, is lowered. Thiazide diuretics are commonly used as the first choice for reduction of mild hypertension, and may be used in combination with other antihypertensive drugs. These drugs cause a constant loss of potassium from the body; patients should check with their physicians about augmenting their potassium intake.

Sodium nitroprusside (Nitropress) and diazoxide (Hyperstat) are used for rapid treatment of hypertensive emergencies. They are given by vein, often during surgery, to reduce blood pressure that suddenly becomes elevated.

Many classes of antihypertensive drugs have been used before surgery to maintain a low blood pressure during the procedure. There does not appear to be a significant difference between drugs when they are used for blood pressure reduction during surgery.

Recommended dosage

Recommended dosage varies with patient, drug, severity of hypertension, and whether the drug is being used alone or in combination with other drugs. Patients should consult specialized references or ask a physician for further information.

Precautions

The warnings and precautions given below apply to the use of antihypertensive drugs over a long period of time. These adverse effects are generally not a problem when the drugs are given as a single dose prior to surgery.

Because of the large number of classes and individual drugs in this group, patients should ask their physicians about specific drugs.

Peripheral vasodilators may cause dizziness and orthostatic hypotension—a rapid lowering of blood pressure when the patient stands up in the morning. Patients taking these drugs must be instructed to rise from bed slowly. Pregnancy risk factors for this group are generally category C, meaning they may result in adverse affects on the fetus. Hydralazine has been shown to cause cleft palate in animal studies, but there is no human data available. Breast-feeding is not recommended.

ACE inhibitors are generally well tolerated, but may rarely cause dangerous reactions including laryngospasm and angioedema. Persistent cough is a common side effect. ACE inhibitors should not be used in pregnancy. When used in pregnancy during the second and third trimesters, ACE inhibitors can cause injury to and even **death** in the developing fetus. When pregnancy is detected, discontinue the ACE inhibitor as soon as possible. Breast-feeding is not recommended.

ACE II inhibitors are generally well tolerated and do not cause cough. Pregnancy risk factor is category C during the first trimester and category D (known to cause adverse effects in the fetus) during the second and third trimesters. Drugs that act directly on the renin-angiotensin system can cause fetal and neonatal morbidity and death when administered to pregnant women. Several dozen cases have been reported in patients who were taking ACE inhibitors. When pregnancy is detected, discontinue ACE inhibitors as soon as possible. Breast-feeding is not recommended.

Thiazide diuretics commonly cause potassium depletion. Patients should have potassium supplementation either through diet, or potassium supplements. Pregnancy risk factor is category B (chlorothiazide, chlorthalidone, hydrochlorothiazide, indapamide, metolazone) or category C (bendroflumethiazide, benzthiazide, hydroflumethiazide, methyclothiazide, trichlormethiazide). Routine use during normal pregnancy is inappropriate. Thiazides are found in breast milk. Breast-feeding is not recommended.

Beta blockers may cause a large number of adverse reactions including dangerous heart rate abnormalities. Pregnancy risk factor is category B (acebutolol, pindolol, sotalol) or category C (atenolol, labetalol, esmolol, metoprolol, nadolol, timolol, propranolol, penbutolol, carteolol, bisoprolol). Breast-feeding is not recommended.

Interactions

Patients should ask their doctors and consult specific references for food and drug interactions.

Sam Uretsky, Pharm.D.
Fran Hodgkins

Antinausea drugs

Definition

Antinausea drugs are medicines that control nausea—a feeling of sickness or queasiness in the stomach with an urge to vomit. These drugs also prevent or stop vomiting. Drugs that control vomiting are called antiemetic drugs.

Purpose

Prochlorperazine (Compazine or Compro), the medication described in detail in this entry, controls both nausea and vomiting. Prochlorperazine is also sometimes prescribed for symptoms of mental disorders, such as schizophrenia, and psychotic symptoms such as hostility and hallucinations. Prochlorperazine may be used to control the nausea and vomiting that occur during recovery from the general anesthetics used in surgery and is used to treat the nausea and vomiting that follow chemotherapy or radiation therapy for cancer.

Some antihistamines such as dimenhydrate (Dramamine) and meclizine (Antivert, Bonine) are useful for treatment of the nausea and vomiting associated with motion sickness.

A group of drugs called the 5-HT$_3$ receptor antagonists, ondansetron (Zofran) and granisetron (Kytril), are used to control the nausea and vomiting associated with anticancer drugs. Ondansetron and granisetron are also valuable for controlling nausea and vomiting following surgery.

Corticosteroid hormones such as dexamethasone (Decadron, Hexdrol) may also be used as antiemetics.

KEY TERMS

Anesthetic—Medicine that causes a loss of feeling, especially pain. Some anesthetics also cause a loss of consciousness.

Antihistamine—Medicine that prevents or relieves allergy symptoms.

Central nervous system—The brain, spinal cord and the nerves throughout the body.

Corticosteroid—A steroid molecule, produced by the adrenal gland, used in medicine to reduce inflammation. May also apply to synthetic compounds which have structures and uses similar to the natural compounds.

Spasm—Sudden, involuntary tensing of a muscle or a group of muscles.

Tardive dyskinesia—A disorder brought on by certain medications that is characterized by uncontrollable muscle spasms.

Tranquilizer—Medicine that has a calming effect and is used to treat anxiety and mental tension.

Description

Prochlorperazine is available only with a physician's prescription. It is sold in syrup, capsule, tablet, injection, and suppository forms.

Recommended dosage

To control nausea and vomiting in adults, the usual dose is:

- Tablets: one 5-milligram (mg) or 10-mg tablet three to four times a day
- Extended-release capsules: one 15-mg capsule first thing in the morning or one 10-mg capsule every 12 hours
- Suppository: 25 mg, twice a day
- Syrup: 5–10 mg three to four times a day
- Injection: 5–10 mg injected into a muscle three to four times a day

Doses for children must be determined by a physician.

Precautions

Prochlorperazine may cause a movement disorder called tardive dyskinesia (TD), particularly if used for long periods of time. TD may develop in patients who are being treated with antipsychotic drugs. Signs of

this disorder are involuntary twitches and muscle spasms in the face and body and jutting or rolling movements of the tongue. The condition may be permanent; however, it may remit if treatment with the drug is stopped. Older people, especially women, are particularly at risk of developing this problem when they take prochlorperazine.

Antinausea drugs may also cause or worsen the symptoms of the movement disorder known as restless leg syndrome.

Some people feel drowsy, dizzy, lightheaded, or less alert when using this medicine. The drug may also cause blurred vision, and movement problems. For these reasons, people who take this drug should not drive, use machines, or do anything else that might be dangerous until they have found out how the drug affects them.

Prochlorperazine makes some people sweat less, which can allow the body to overheat. The drug may also make the skin and eyes more sensitive to the sun. People who are taking prochlorperazine should try to avoid extreme heat and exposure to the sun. When going outdoors, they should wear protective clothing, a hat, a sunscreen with a skin protection factor (SPF) of at least 15, and sunglasses that block ultraviolet (UV) light. Saunas, sunlamps, tanning booths, tanning beds, hot baths, and hot tubs should be avoided while taking this medicine. Anyone who must be exposed to extreme heat while taking the drug should check with his or her physician.

This medicine adds to the effects of alcohol and other drugs that slow down the central nervous system, such as antihistamines, cold and flu medicines, tranquilizers, sleep aids, anesthetics, some pain medicines, and **muscle relaxants**. People taking prochlorperazine should not drink alcohol, and should check with the physician who prescribed the drug before combining it with any other medicines.

Patients should not stop taking this medicine without checking with the physician who prescribed it. Stopping the drug suddenly can dizziness, nausea, vomiting, tremors, and other side effects. When stopping the medicine, it may be necessary to taper the dose gradually.

Prochlorperazine may cause false pregnancy tests.

Women who are pregnant, planning to become pregnant, or breast-feeding should check with their physicians before using this medicine.

Before using prochlorperazine, people with any of these medical problems should make sure their physicians are aware of their conditions:

- previous sensitivity or allergic reaction to prochlorperazine or any other medicines, including a bad reaction to insulin;
- heart disease;
- glaucoma;
- brain tumor;
- intestinal blockage;
- abnormal blood conditions, such as leukemia;
- exposure to pesticides;
- liver or kidney disease;
- lung disease, including emphysema, chronic bronchitis, or asthma; or
- an enlarged prostate or difficulty urinating.

Side effects

Many side effects are possible with this drug. Drowsiness is most common, so be careful not to drive or operate machinery until you know how it affects you. Patients who experience any of the following side effects should immediately contact their physician: difficulty swallowing, restlessness or pacing, tremors, slow speech, difficulty speaking, spasms of the muscles in the jaw, back, and/or neck, skin rashes, shuffling walk, or a yellowing of the skin or eyes. Anyone who has unusual or troublesome symptoms after taking prochlorperazine should contact his or her physician.

Interactions

Prochlorperazine may interact with other medicines. When this happens, the effects of one or both of the drugs may change or the risk of side effects may be greater. Among the drugs that may interact with prochlorperazine are antiseizure drugs such as phenytoin (Dilantin) and carbamazepine (Tegretol), anticoagulants such as warfarin (Coumadin), and drugs that slow the central nervous system such as alprazolam (Xanax), diazepam (Valium), and secobarbital (Seconal). Not every drug that interacts with prochlorperazine is listed here, and all patients should consult with a physician or pharmacist before taking any other prescription or nonprescription (over-the-counter) drug with prochlorperazine.

Resources

BOOKS

Brody, T. M., J. Larner, and K. P. Minneman. *Human Pharmacology: Molecular to Clinical,* 3rd ed. St. Louis: Mosby, 1998.
Griffith, H. W., and S. Moore. *Complete Guide to Prescription and Nonprescription Drugs 2001*. New York: Berkely Publishing Group, 2001.

OTHER

"Ondansetron." Medline Plus. January 1, 2007. http://www.nlm.nih.gov/medlineplus/druginfo/medmaster/a601209.html (February 27, 2008).
"Prochlorperazine." Medline Plus. April 1, 2003. http://www.nlm.nih.gov/medlineplus/druginfo/medmaster/a682116.html (February 27, 2008).
"Compazine: Warnings and Precautions." RxList.com http:///www.rxlist.com/cgi/generic/compazinespan_wcp.htm (February 27, 2008).
"What Causes Restless Leg Syndrome?" WeMove: Worldwide Education and Awareness for Movement Disorders. January 7, 2008. http://www.wemove.org/rls/rls_cor.html (February 27, 2008).

Nancy Ross-Flanigan
Sam Uretsky, Pharm.D.
Fran Hodgkins

Antiplatelet drugs *see* **Anticoagulant and antiplatelet drugs**

Antiseptics

Definition

An antiseptic is a substance that inhibits the growth and development of microorganisms. For practical purposes, antiseptics are routinely thought of as topical agents, for application to skin, mucous membranes, and inanimate objects, although a formal definition includes agents that are used internally, such as the urinary tract antiseptics.

Purpose

Antiseptics are a diverse class of drugs that are applied to skin surfaces or mucous membranes for their anti-infective effects. This may be either bacteriocidal (kills bacteria) or bacteriostatic (stops the growth of bacteria). Their uses include cleansing of skin and wound surfaces after injury, preparation of skin surfaces prior to injections or surgical procedures, and routine disinfection of the oral cavity as part of a program of oral hygiene. Antiseptics are also used for disinfection of inanimate objects, including instruments and furniture surfaces.

Commonly used antiseptics for skin cleaning include benzalkonium chloride, chlorhexidine, hexachlorophine, iodine compounds, mercury compounds, alcohol, and hydrogen peroxide. Other agents that have been used for this purpose, but have largely been supplanted by more effective or safer agents, include boric acid and volatile oils such as methyl salicylate (oil of wintergreen).

Chlorhexidine shows a high margin of safety when applied to mucous membranes, and has been used in oral rinses and preoperative total body washes.

Benzalkonium chloride and hexachlorophine are used primarily as hand scrubs or face washes. Benzalkonium may also find application as a disinfecting agent for instruments, and in low concentration as a preservative for drugs including ophthalmic solutions. Benzalkonium chloride is inactivated by organic compounds, including soap, and must not be applied to areas that have not been fully rinsed.

Iodine compounds include tincture of iodine and povidone iodine compounds. Iodine compounds have the broadest spectrum of all topical anti-infectives, with action against bacteria, fungi, viruses, spores, protozoa, and yeasts. Iodine tincture is highly effective, but its alcoholic component is drying and extremely irritating when applied to abraded (scraped or rubbed) skin. Povidone iodine, an organic compound, is less irritating and less toxic, but not as effective. Povidone iodine has been used for hand scrubs and disinfection of surgical sites. Aqueous solutions of iodine have also been used as antiseptic agents, but are less effective than alcoholic solutions and less convenient to use than the povidone iodine compounds.

Hydrogen peroxide acts through the liberation of oxygen gas. Although the antibacterial activity of hydrogen peroxide is relatively weak, the liberation of oxygen bubbles produces an effervescent action, which may be useful for wound cleansing through removal of tissue debris. The activity of hydrogen peroxide may be reduced by the presence of blood and pus. The appropriate concentration of hydrogen peroxide for antiseptic use is 3%, although higher concentrations are available.

Thimerosol (Mersol) is a mercury compound with activity against bacteria and yeasts. Prolonged use may result in mercury toxicity.

Recommended dosage

Dosage varies with product and intended use. Patients should ask their physician or a pharmacist.

Precautions

Precautions vary with individual product and use.

Hypersensitivity reactions should be considered with organic compounds such as chlorhexidine, benzalkonium, and hexachlorophine.

Skin dryness and irritation should be considered with all products, but particularly with those containing alcohol.

Systemic toxicity may result from ingestion of iodine-containing compounds or mercury compounds.

Most antiseptics have not been rated according to pregnancy category under the pregnancy risk factor system. Hexachlorophene is category C during pregnancy, and should not be used on newborns due to risk of systemic absorption with potential central nervous system (CNS) effects, including convulsions. Application of hexachlorophene to open wounds, mucous membranes, or areas of thin skin, such as the genitalia, should be avoided, since this may promote systemic absorption.

Chlorhexidine should not be instilled into the ear. There is one anecdotal report of deafness following use of chlorhexidine in a patient with a perforated eardrum. Safety in pregnancy and breast-feeding have not been reported; however, there is one anecdotal report of an infant developing slowed heartbeat apparently related to maternal use of chlorhexidine.

Iodine compounds should be used sparingly during pregnancy and lactation due to risk of infant absorption of iodine with alterations in thyroid function.

Interactions

Antiseptics are not known to interact with any other medicines; however, they should not be used together with any other topical cream, solution, or ointment.

Resources

PERIODICALS

Farley, Dixie. "OTC Options: Help for Cuts, Scrapes and Burns." *FDA Consumer* 30, no. 4 (May 1996): 12.

McDonnell, Gerald and A. Denver Russell. "Antiseptics and Disinfectants: Activity, Action, and Resistance." *Clinical Microbiology Reviews* 12, no. 1 (January 1999): 147–179. http://www.pubmedcentral.nih.gov/articlerender.fcgi?artid=88911 (March 21, 2008).

Waldman, Hilary. "New ways to treat wounds; Doctors abandon failed conventions that focus on caring for bruises at the surface for methods that reach the source." *Los Angeles Times* (May 26, 2003): p F5.

Weber J. et al. "Efficacy of Selected Hand Hygiene Agents Used to Remove *Bacillus atrophaeus* (a Surrogate of *Bacillus anthracis*) from Contaminated Hands." *Journal of the American Medical Association* 289, no. 10 (March 12, 2003): 1274–1277.

OTHER

"Antiseptics and Disinfectants." Ask A Scientist: Molecular Biology Archive. U.S. Department of Energy. December 4, 2002. http://www.newton.dep.anl.gov/askasci/mole00/mole00361.htm (March 21, 2008).

Samuel Uretsky, Pharm.D.
Laura Jean Cataldo, R.N., Ed.D.

Antrectomy

Definition

An antrectomy is the resection, or surgical removal, of a part of the stomach known as the antrum. The antrum is the lower third of the stomach that lies between the body of the stomach and the pyloric canal, which empties into the first part of the small intestine. It is also known as the antrum pyloricum or the gastric antrum. Because an antrectomy is the removal of a portion of the stomach, it is sometimes called a partial or subtotal **gastrectomy**.

Purpose

An antrectomy may be performed to treat several different disorders that affect the digestive system:

- Peptic ulcer disease (PUD). An antrectomy may be done to treat complications from ulcers that have not responded to medical treatment. These complications include uncontrolled or recurrent bleeding and obstructions that prevent food from passing into the small intestine. Because the antrum produces gastrin, which is a hormone that stimulates the production of stomach acid, its removal lowers the level of acid secretions in the stomach.

- Cancers of the digestive tract and nearby organs. An antrectomy may be performed not only to remove a malignant gastric ulcer, but also to relieve pressure on the lower end of the stomach caused by cancers of the pancreas, gallbladder, or liver.

- Arteriovenous malformations (AVMs) of the stomach. AVMs are collections of small blood vessels that may develop in various parts of the digestive system. AVMs can cause bleeding into the gastrointestinal tract, resulting in hematemesis (vomiting blood) or melena (black or tarry stools containing blood). The type of AVM most likely to occur in the antrum is known as gastric antral vascular ectasia (GAVE) syndrome. The dilated blood vessels in GAVE produce reddish streaks on the wall of the antrum that look like the stripes on a watermelon.

- Gastric outlet obstruction (GOO). GOO is not a single disease or disorder but a condition in which the stomach cannot empty because the pylorus is blocked. In about 37% of cases, the cause of the obstruction is benign—most often PUD, gallstones, bezoars, or scarring caused by ingestion of hydrochloric acid or other caustic substance. The other 63% of cases are caused by pancreatic cancer, gastric cancer, or other malignancy that has spread to the digestive tract.

- Penetrating gunshot or stab wounds that have caused severe damage to the duodenum and pancreas. An antrectomy may be done as an emergency measure when the blood vessels supplying the duodenum have been destroyed.

Demographics

Peptic ulcer disease (PUD) is fairly common in the general United States population. According to the Centers for Disease Control (CDC), about 10% of all Americans will develop an ulcer in the stomach or duodenum at some point in their life. About four million adults are diagnosed or treated each year for PUD; one million will be hospitalized for treatment; and 40,000 will have surgery for an ulcer-related condition. About 6,500 Americans die each year from complications related to PUD. The annual costs to the United States economy from peptic ulcer disease are estimated to be over $6 billion.

Peptic ulcers can develop at any age, but in the United States they are very unusual in children and uncommon in adolescents. Adults between the ages of 30 and 50 are most likely to develop duodenal ulcers, while gastric ulcers are most common in those over 60.

KEY TERMS

Antrum—The lower part of the stomach that lies between the pylorus and the body of the stomach. It is also called the gastric antrum or antrum pyloricum.

Bezoar—A collection of foreign material, usually hair or vegetable fibers or a mixture of both, that may occasionally occur in the stomach or intestines and block the passage of food.

Dumping syndrome—A complex physical reaction to food passing too quickly from the stomach into the small intestine, characterized by sweating, nausea, abdominal cramps, dizziness, and other symptoms.

Duodenum—The first portion of the small intestine, lying between the pylorus and the jejunum.

Dysphagia—Difficulty or discomfort in swallowing.

Endoscopy—A technique for looking inside the stomach or esophagus with the help of a flexible instrument containing a light and miniature video camera on one end.

Gastrin—A hormone produced by cells in the antrum that stimulates the production of gastric acid.

Gastroenterology—The branch of medicine that specializes in the diagnosis and treatment of disorders affecting the stomach and intestines.

Helicobacter pylori—A spiral-shaped bacterium that was discovered in 1982 to be the underlying cause of most ulcers in the stomach and duodenum.

Hematemesis—Vomiting blood.

Melena—The passing of blackish-colored stools containing blood pigments or partially digested blood.

Nonsteroidal anti-inflammatory drugs (NSAIDs)—A term used for a group of analgesics that are often given to arthritis patients. About 20% of peptic ulcers are thought to be caused by frequent use of NSAIDs.

Perforation—An opening or hole in the tissues of the stomach caused by a disease process.

Pylorus—The opening at the lower end of the stomach, encircled by a band of muscle. The contents of the stomach are pumped into the duodenum through the pylorus.

Resection—Removal of an organ or structure. An antrectomy is a resection of the antrum.

Vagotomy—Cutting or dividing various parts of the vagus nerve that supply the stomach. A vagotomy is done to reduce acid secretion.

Watermelon stomach—A type of arteriovenous malformation (AVM) that develops in the antrum. The dilated blood vessels in the AVM resemble the stripes of a watermelon. Watermelon stomach is also known as gastric antral vascular ectasia, or GAVE syndrome.

Duodenal ulcers are more common in men, and gastric ulcers are more common in women. Other risk factors for PUD include heavy smoking and a family history of either duodenal or gastric ulcers.

GAVE, or watermelon stomach, is a very rare cause of gastrointestinal bleeding that was first identified in 1952. It has been associated with such disorders as scleroderma, cirrhosis of the liver, familial Mediterranean fever, and heart disease. GAVE affects women slightly more than twice as often as men. It is almost always found in the elderly; the average age at diagnosis is 73 in women and 68 in men.

Gastric cancer is the 14th most common type of malignant tumor in the United States; however, it occurs much more frequently in Japan and other parts of Asia than in western Europe and North America. About 24,000 people in the United States are diagnosed each year with gastric cancer. Risk factors for developing it include infection of the stomach lining by *Helicobacter pylori*; Asian American, Hispanic, or African American heritage; age 60 or older; heavy smoking; a history of pernicious anemia; and a diet heavy in dry salted foods. Men are more likely to develop gastric cancer than women. Some doctors think that exposure to certain toxic chemicals in the workplace is also a risk factor for gastric cancer.

Description

At present almost all antrectomies are performed as open procedures, which means that they are done through a large incision in the patient's abdomen with the patient under **general anesthesia**. After the patient is anesthetized, a urinary catheter is placed to monitor urinary output, and a nasogastric tube is inserted. After the patient's abdomen has been cleansed with an antiseptic, the surgeon makes a large incision from the patient's rib cage to the navel. After separating the overlying layers of tissue, the surgeon exposes the stomach. One clamp is placed at the lower end and another clamp somewhat higher, dividing off the lower third of the stomach. A cutting stapler may be used to remove the lower third (the antrum) and attach the upper portion of the stomach to the small intestine. After the stomach and intestine have been reattached, the area is rinsed with saline solution and the incision closed.

Most antrectomies are performed together with a **vagotomy**. This is a procedure in which the surgeon cuts various branches of the vagus nerve, which carries messages from the brain to the stomach to secrete more stomach acid. The surgeon may choose to perform a selective vagotomy in order to disable the branches of the nerve that govern gastric secretion without cutting the branches that control stomach emptying.

Some surgeons have performed antrectomies with a laparoscope, which is a less invasive type of surgery. However, as of 2003, this technique is still considered experimental.

Diagnosis/Preparation

Diagnosis

Diagnosis of PUD and other stomach disorders begins with taking the patient's history, including a family history. In many cases the patient's primary care physician will order tests in order to narrow the diagnosis. If the patient is older or has lost a large amount of weight recently, the doctor will consider the possibility of gastric cancer. If there is a history of duodenal or gastric ulcers in the patient's family, the doctor may ask questions about the type of discomfort the patient is experiencing. Pain associated with duodenal ulcers often occurs at night, is relieved at mealtimes, but reappears two to three hours after eating. Pain from gastric ulcers, on the other hand, may be made worse by eating and accompanied by nausea and vomiting. Vomiting that occurs repeatedly shortly after eating suggests a gastric obstruction.

The most common diagnostic tests for stomach disorders are:

- Endoscopy. An endoscope is a thin flexible tube with a light source and video camera on one end that can be passed through the mouth and throat in order to look at the inside of the upper digestive tract. The video camera attached to the endoscope projects images on a computer screen that allow the doctor to see ulcers, tissue growths, and other possible problems. The endoscope can be used to collect tissue cells for a cytology analysis, or a small tissue sample for a biopsy. A tissue biopsy can be used to test for the presence of *Helicobacter pylori*, a spiral bacterium that was discovered in 1982 to be the underlying cause of most gastric ulcers, as well as to test for

cancer. Endoscopy is one of the most effective tests for diagnosing AVMs.

- Double-contrast barium x-ray study of the upper gastrointestinal tract. This test is sometimes called an upper GI series. The patient is given a liquid form of barium to take by mouth. The barium coats the tissues lining the esophagus, stomach, and small intestine, allowing them to be seen more clearly on an x ray. The radiologist can also watch the barium as it moves through the digestive system in order to pinpoint the location of blockages.

- Urease breath test. This test can be used to monitor the effects of ulcer treatment as well as to diagnose the presence of *H. pylori*. The patient is given urea labeled with either carbon 13-C or 14-C. *H. pylori* produces urease, which will break down the urea in the test dose to ammonia and carbon dioxide containing the labeled carbon. The carbon dioxide containing the labeled carbon can then be detected in the patient's breath.

Preparation

Preparation for an antrectomy requires tests to evaluate the patient's overall health and fitness for surgery. These tests include an EKG, x rays, blood tests, and a urine test. The patient is asked to discontinue **aspirin** and other blood-thinning medications about a week before surgery. No solid food or liquid should be taken after midnight of the evening before surgery.

In most hospitals the patient will be given a sedative before the operation either intravenously or by injection. The general anesthesia is given in the **operating room**.

Aftercare

Aftercare in the hospital for an antrectomy is similar to the aftercare given for other operations involving the abdomen, in terms of **incision care**, pain medication, and **antibiotics** to minimize the risk of infection. Recuperation at home usually takes several weeks. The patient is given an endoscopic checkup about six to eight weeks after surgery.

The most important aspect of aftercare following an antrectomy is careful attention to diet and eating habits. About 30% of patients who have had an antrectomy or a full gastrectomy develop what is known as dumping syndrome. Dumping syndrome results from food leaving the stomach too quickly after a meal and being "dumped" into the small intestine. There are two types of dumping syndrome, early and late. Early dumping occurs 10–20 minutes after meals and is characterized by feelings of nausea, light-headedness, sweating, heart palpitations, rapid heartbeat, and abdominal cramps. Late dumping occurs one to three hours after meals high in carbohydrates and is accompanied by feelings of weakness, hunger, and mental confusion. Most patients are able to manage dumping syndrome by eating six small meals per day rather than three larger ones; by choosing foods that are high in protein and low in carbohydrate; by chewing the food thoroughly; and by drinking fluids between rather than with meals.

Risks

In addition to early or late dumping syndrome, other risks associated with antrectomies include:

- Diarrhea. This complication is more likely to occur in patients who had a vagotomy as well as an antrectomy.
- Weight loss. About 30–60% of patients who have had a combined antrectomy/vagotomy lose weight after surgery. The most common cause of weight loss is reduced food intake due to the smaller size of the stomach. In some cases, however, the patient loses weight because the nutrients in the food are not being absorbed by the body.
- Malabsorption/malnutrition. Iron-deficiency anemia, folate deficiency, and loss of calcium sometimes occur after an antrectomy because gastric acid is necessary for iron to be absorbed from food.
- Dysphagia. Dysphagia, or discomfort in swallowing, may occur after an antrectomy when digestive juices from the duodenum flow upward into the esophagus and irritate its lining.
- Recurrence of gastric ulcers.
- Bezoar formation. Bezoars are collections of foreign material (usually vegetable fibers or hair) in the stomach that can block the passage of food into the small intestine. They may develop after an antrectomy if the patient is eating foods high in plant fiber or is not chewing them thoroughly.

Normal results

Normal results of an antrectomy depend on the reasons for the surgery. Antrectomies performed to reduce acid secretion in PUD or to remove premalignant tissue to prevent gastric cancer are over 95% successful. The success rate is even higher in treating watermelon stomach. Antrectomies performed to treat gastric cancer or penetrating abdominal trauma are less successful, but this result is related to the severity of the patient's illness or injury rather than the surgical procedure itself.

Morbidity and mortality rates

The mortality rate for antrectomies related to ulcer treatment is about 1–2%; for antrectomies related to gastric cancer, 1–3%.

The rates of complications associated with antrectomies for ulcer treatment are:

- Recurrence of ulcer: 0.5–1%.
- Dumping syndromes: 25–30%.
- Diarrhea: 10%.

Alternatives

As of 2003, antrectomy is no longer the first line of treatment for either peptic ulcer disease or GAVE. It is usually reserved for patients with recurrent bleeding or other conditions such as malignancy, perforation, or obstruction.

Although surgery, including antrectomy, is the most common treatment for stomach cancer, it is almost always necessary to combine it with chemotherapy, radiation treatment, or biological therapy (immunotherapy). The reason for a combination of treatments is that stomach cancer is rarely discovered early. Its first symptoms are often mild and easily mistaken for the symptoms of heartburn or a stomach virus. As a result, the cancer has often spread beyond the stomach by the time it is diagnosed.

Medication

Treatment of peptic ulcers caused by *H. pylori* has changed its focus in recent years from lowering the level of acidity in the stomach to eradicating the bacterium. Since no single antibiotic is effective in curing *H. pylori* infections, so-called triple therapy typically consists of a combination of one or two antibiotics to kill the bacterium plus a medication to lower acid production and a third medication (usually bismuth subsalicylate) to protect the stomach lining.

Specific types of medications that are used as part of triple therapy or for relief of discomfort include:

- H_2 blockers. These are used together with antibiotics in triple therapy to reduce stomach acid secretion. H_2 blockers include cimetidine, ranitidine, famotidine, and nizatidine. Some are available as over-the-counter (OTC) medications.
- Proton pump inhibitors. These medications include drugs such as omeprazole and lansoprazole. They are given to suppress production of stomach acid.
- Prostaglandins. These are given to treat ulcers produced by a group of pain medications known as NSAIDs. Prostaglandins protect the stomach lining

WHO PERFORMS THE PROCEDURE AND WHERE IS IT PERFORMED?

An antrectomy is performed as an inpatient procedure in a hospital. It is usually performed by a specialist in gastrointestinal surgery or surgical oncology.

as well as lower acid secretion. The best-known medication in this category is misoprostol.

- Sucralfate. Sucralfate is a compound of sucrose and aluminum that covers ulcers with a protective coating that allows eroded tissues to heal.

- Antacids. These compounds are available as OTC tablets or liquids.

- Bismuth subsalicylate. Sold as an OTC under the trade name Pepto-Bismol, this medication has some antibacterial effectiveness against *H. pylori* as well as protecting the stomach lining.

Endoscopy

Endoscopy can be used for treatment as well as diagnosis. About 10 different methods are in use as of 2003 for treating bleeding ulcers and AVMs with the help of an endoscope; the most common involve the injection of epinephrine or a sclerosing solution; the application of a thermal probe to the bleeding area; or the use of an Nd:YAG laser to coagulate the open blood vessels. Watermelon stomach is now treated more often with argon plasma coagulation than with an antrectomy. Recurrent bleeding, however, occurs in 15–20% of ulcers treated with endoscopic methods.

Complementary and alternative (CAM) approaches

Complementary and alternative approaches that have been used to treat gastric ulcers related to PUD include acupuncture, Ayurvedic medicine, and herbal preparations. Ayurvedic medicine, which is the traditional medical system of India, classifies people according to metabolic body type. People who belong to the type known as pitta are considered particularly prone to ulcers and treated with a diet that emphasizes "cooling" foods, including large quantities of vegetables. In Japanese medicine, ulcer remedies made from licorice or bupleurum are frequently prescribed. Western herbalists recommend preparations containing fennel, fenugreek, slippery elm, or marshmallow root

QUESTIONS TO ASK THE DOCTOR

- What are the alternatives to an antrectomy for my condition? Which would you recommend and why?
- How many antrectomies have you performed?
- How likely am I to develop dumping syndrome if I have the procedure?
- What is your opinion of laparoscopic antrectomies? Would I be eligible to participate in a clinical study of this procedure?

in addition to licorice to relieve the pain of stomach ulcers.

Resources

BOOKS

"Arteriovenous Malformations." In *The Merck Manual of Diagnosis and Therapy*, edited by Mark H. Beers, MD, and Robert Berkow, MD. Whitehouse Station, NJ: Merck Research Laboratories, 1999.

Pelletier, Kenneth R., MD. *The Best Alternative Medicine*, Part II, "CAM Therapies for Specific Conditions: Ulcers." New York: Simon & Schuster, 2002.

"Peptic Ulcer Disease." In *The Merck Manual of Diagnosis and Therapy*, edited by Mark H. Beers, MD, and Robert Berkow, MD. Whitehouse Station, NJ: Merck Research Laboratories, 1999.

Thomson, A. B. R. and E. A. Shaffer. *First Principles of Gastroenterology*, 3rd ed. Oakville, ON: Canadian Association of Gastroenterology, 2002.

PERIODICALS

Appleyard, M. N. and C. P. Swain. "Endoscopic Difficulties in the Diagnosis of Upper Gastrointestinal Bleeding." *World Journal of Gastroenterology* 7 (2001): 308-12.

Busteed, S., C. Silke, C. Molloy, et al. "Gastric Antral Vascular Ectasia—A Cause of Refractory Anaemia in Systemic Sclerosis." *Irish Medical Journal* 94 (November-December 2001): 310.

Castellanos, Andres, MD, Barry D. Mann, MD, and James de Caestecker, DO. "Gastric Outlet Obstruction." *eMedicine*, February 12, 2002 [cited April 27, 2003]. www.emedicine.com/med/topic2713.htm.

De Caestecker, James, DO. "Upper Gastrointestinal Bleeding: Surgical Perspective." *eMedicine*, October 17, 2002 [cited April 27, 2003]. www.emedicine.com/med/topic3566.htm.

Fowler, Dennis, MD. "Laparoscopic Foregut Surgery: Less Commonly Performed Procedures." *Minimal Access Surgery Center Newsletter, New York-Presbyterian Hospital* 2 (Winter 2002): 7–10.

Komar, Aleksander R., MD and Prem Patel, MD. "Abdominal Trauma, Penetrating." *eMedicine*, April

25, 2002 [cited April 28, 2003]. www.emedicine.com/med/topic2805.htm.

Probst, A., R. Scheubel, and M. Wienbeck. "Treatment of Watermelon Stomach (GAVE Syndrome) by Means of Endoscopic Argon Plasma Coagulation (APC): Long-Term Outcome." *Zeitschrift für Gastroenterologie* 39 (June 2001): 447-52.

Stotzer, P. O., R. Willen, and A. F. Kilander. "Watermelon Stomach: Not Only an Antral Disease." *Gastrointestinal Endoscopy* 55 (June 2002): 897–900.

Tseng, Y. L., M. H. Wu, M. Y. Lin, and W. W. Lai. "Early Surgical Correction for Isolated Gastric Stricture Following Acid Corrosion Injury." *Digestive Surgery* 19 (2002): 276–80.

Yusoff, I., F. Brennan, D. Ormonde, and B. Laurence. "Argon Plasma Coagulation for Treatment of Watermelon Stomach." *Endoscopy* 34 (May 2002): 407–10.

Zarzaur, B. L., K. A. Kudsk, K. Carter, et al. "Stress Ulceration Requiring Definitive Surgery After Severe Trauma." *American Surgeon* 67 (September 2001): 875–79.

ORGANIZATIONS

American Gastroenterological Association (AGA). 4930 Del Ray Avenue, Bethesda, MD 20814. (301) 654-2055. www.gastro.org.

American Society for Gastrointestinal Endoscopy (ASGE). 1520 Kensington Road, Suite 202, Oak Brook, IL 60523 (630) 573-0600. www.asge.org.

Canadian Association of Gastroenterology (CAG). 2902 South Sheridan Way, Oakville, ON L6J 7L6 (888) 780-0007 or (905) 829-2504. www.cag-acg.org.

Centers for Disease Control and Prevention (CDC). 1600 Clifton Road, Atlanta, GA 30333. (888) MY-ULCER or (404) 639-3534. www.cdc.gov.

National Cancer Institute (NCI). NCI Public Inquiries Office, Suite 3036A, 6116 Executive Boulevard, MSC8332, Bethesda, MD 20892-8322. (800) 4-CANCER or (800) 332-8615 (TTY). www.nci.nih.gov.

National Digestive Diseases Information Clearinghouse (NDDIC). 2 Information Way, Bethesda, MD 20892-3570. www.niddk.nih.gov/health/digest/pubs.

OTHER

National Cancer Institute (NCI) Physician Data Query (PDQ). *Gastric Cancer: Treatment*, January 2, 2003 [cited April 28, 2003]. www.nci.nih.gov/cancerinfo/pdq/treatment/gastric/healthprofessional.

National Digestive Diseases Information Clearinghouse (NDDIC). *What I Need to Know About Peptic Ulcers*, August 2002 [cited April 28, 2003]. NIH Publication No. 02-5042. www.niddk.nih.gov/health/digest/pubs/pepticulcers/pepticulcers.htm.

Rebecca Frey, Ph.D.

Anxiolytics *see* **Antianxiety drugs**

Aortic aneurysm repair

Definition

Aortic aneurysm repair involves the removal of a dilated (enlarged) portion of the aorta replaced by a woven or knitted Dacron graft to continue uninterrupted blood flow through the aorta and all branch vessels.

Purpose

Aortic aneurysm repair is performed when a portion of the aorta has become dilated as a result of medionecrosis in the ascending aorta or atherosclerosis in the arch and descending segments. Congenital defects in connective tissue are also a risk factor. A history of blunt trauma may be associated with this disease propagation. Prior to 1950, patients exposed to syphilis were at risk of developing aortic aneurysm. Risk of clot formation and rupture of the aneurysm, seen in 50% of cases, as well as dilation to a size greater than 4 inches (10 centimenters) promote repair of the aneurysm by surgical techniques.

Demographics

The patient population for this procedure is typically male with an average age of 65 and a history of medionecrosis or atherosclerosis of the aorta. Patients with a medical history significant for syphilis or blunt trauma are at risk. Congenital defects associated with Marfan syndrome or Ehlers-Danlos syndrome (disorders resulting in abnormal tissue formation) need to be monitored.

All patients will be monitored until the aneurysm demonstrates consistent enlargement over time, or grows to greater than 2.2 in (5.5 cm) in diameter at which time surgery is suggested. At a diameter of 4 in (10 cm) surgery is the best option, as risk of rupture increases. Many patients live without symptoms, having the aneurysm identified during other medical procedures.

Description

After **general anesthesia** is administered, the surgeon will make an incision through the length of the sternum to repair an ascending, arch, or thoracic aortic aneurysm. Abdominal aneurysms are approached through a vertical incision in the abdominal wall. Depending on the location of the aneurysm, cardiopulmonary bypass with deep hypothermic circulatory arrest (arch), cardiopulmonary bypass (ascending), or left heart bypass (thoracic) may be required. All

Aortic aneurysm repair

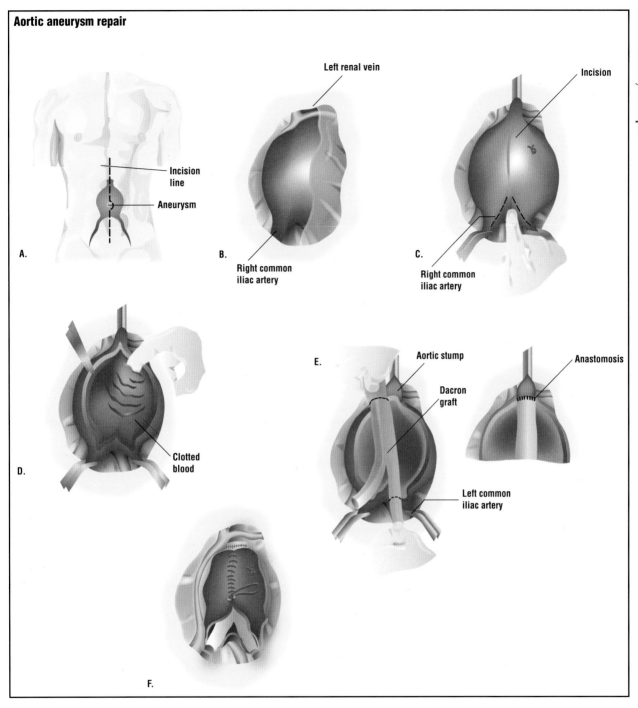

An incision is made in the abdomen (A), and the aneurysm is visualized (B). The aorta is clamped above the aneurysm, and the aorta is cut open (C). The clotted blood is removed (D). A synthetic graft may be used to replace the part of the aorta that had the aneurysm, and it is stitched in place (E). The aorta is then stitched over the graft (F). *(Illustration by GGS Information Services. Cengage Learning, Gale.)*

procedures require some amount of anticoagulation, usually heparin, to be administered to prevent blood clot formation. Clamps will be applied across the aorta to prevent blood flow into the aneurysm. The aneurysm will be opened to an area where the tissue is healthy. The healthy tissue will be sutured to a synthetic fiber fabric graft. The fabric is knit or woven Dacron fibers and may be impregnated with collagen,

KEY TERMS

Abdominal aneurysm—Aneurysm that involves the descending aorta from the diaphragm to the point at which it separates into two iliac arteries.

Hemostatic—Relating to blood clotting and coagulation.

Medionecrosis—Death of the middle layer of tissues in a vessel.

Rupture—Severing of the aorta allowing blood to spill out into the body instead of being carried by the blood vessels.

Systemic circulation—Blood vessels not involved in carrying blood to and from the lungs between the right and left sides of the heart.

Thoracic aneurysm—Aneurysm that involves the ascending, arch, or descending thoracic aorta using the diaphragm as a landmark for transition to abdominal aorta.

gelatin, or other substances. Blood flow is reinstituted to check for a secure seal. Additional sutures will be added to prevent leaking. The incision is then closed at the completion of the procedure with blood drains penetrating the incision during healing.

Ascending aortic aneurysms may involve the aortic valve or coronary arteries. If the aortic valve is damaged, a graft with an integral aortic valve is used. The coronary arteries are reconnected to the graft.

Aortic arch aneurysms require the reattachment of the arch vessels, the innominate artery, the left common carotid artery, and the left subclavian artery. To decrease surgery time, these three vessels can be treated as a single vessel by using part of the patient's native aorta to create an island. This island is then connected to the graft.

Thoracic aneurysms require special care to protect the spinal vessels that supply blood to the spinal cord. Protecting the spinal cord during repair is still an area of intensive research. Some surgeons feel that rapid implant of the graft to restore blood flow is the best method to protect the spinal cord. A bypass graft called a Gott shunt can be used to redirect the blood flow around the area during surgical repair. Left-heart bypass provides the same benefit as a Gott shunt, with the addition of a mechanical pump for more controlled blood flow to the abdomen and lower extremities.

The abdominal aortic aneurysm is repaired by rapid anastomosis of the graft to return blood flow to the circulation. If the renal arteries are involved in the aneurysm, they will be reattached to the graft. Additionally, if the superior celiac, mesenteric, or inferior celiac arteries are involved, they will also be reattached to the graft. Finally, it is common for the bifurcation (separation into two) of the iliac arteries to be involved; this may require a Y-shaped graft to be used to reattach both lower limb vessels.

Diagnosis/Preparation

A simple x ray may provide the initial diagnosis of aortic aneurysm. Initial diagnosis can be made with noninvasive transesophageal **echocardiography** or **ultrasound**. Additional tests such as **magnetic resonance imaging** (MRI) or computed tomography (CT) will allow for additional visualization of the aneurysm. An **angiography** is the preferred method for determining the severity. Blood vessel and aortic valve health can be evaluated.

Aftercare

Following surgery the patient will be cared for in an **intensive care unit**. Cardiac monitoring will be continued for blood pressure and heart function. Intravenous fluids will continue to be given, and may include blood products. Additional medications will be continued to support cardiac function as needed. The ventilator will be removed after the patient is able to breathe on his/her own. The stay in the intensive care unit is approximately two to five days with hospital discharge following a week.

Risks

There are risks associated with general anesthesia not associated with the aortic aneurysm repair. Additional risks of cardiopulmonary bypass are not associated with surgical repair. Depending on the type of aneurysm involved, the risks can differ significantly. Since blood flow to the spinal cord is jeopardized by the surgical repair, thoracic aorta aneurysm repair carries a relatively high rate of paralysis. Ascending arch aneurysms may jeopardize coronary blood flow and aortic valve function. Infection of the sternum can influence recovery time. Renal function can be impacted by abdominal aortic aneurysm repair. Renal function may improve or remain compromised. Long-term complications associated with the abdominal surgery include intra-abdominal adhesions, small bowel obstructions, and incisional hernia. Aortic arch aneurysms carry a risk of brain damage associated with deep hypothermic circulatory arrest.

Cardiothoracic or cardiovascular surgeons or vascular surgeons can perform these procedures. Abdominal and thoracic aortic aneurysm repairs require less sophisticated equipment during the surgical procedure, but do need extensive intensive care postoperatively. Anesthetic management plays a crucial role in the decrease in complications associated with these procedures. Facilities that can also provide cardiovascular surgery are best equipped to manage these patients, but this is not a limitation for all procedures.

- How many of these procedures have been performed by the surgeon?
- What is the mortality rate for this procedure at the institution?
- What side effects are associated with this surgical procedure, and at what rate are they experienced by patients?
- What is the expected length of stay in the hospital?
- Are there any other suitable procedures, such as endovascular grafting?
- How long before normal activities, exercise, work, and driving can be resumed?

Normal results

Repair of the aneurysm will provide normal blood flow to the systemic circulation. Pain associated with the aneurysm will be relieved by the repair. The risk of aneurysm rupture will be eliminated.

Morbidity and mortality rates

During 1999 over 15,000 deaths in the United States were attributed to aortic aneurysm as reported by the American Heart Association. Without treatment, the five-year survival rate is 13%. The Multicentre Aneurysm Screening Group studied nonemergent abdominal aortic aneurysm repair, showing a 2–6% mortality rate at 30 days post surgery. Emergency surgeries demonstrate 37% mortality. In another study, treatment of cardiac disease by open heart surgery, not **cardiac catheterization** intervention, demonstrated a better outcome prior to elective treatment for abdominal aortic aneurysm.

During treatment of thoracic aneurysm repair the incidence of paraplegia is 6–10%. Left vocal cord paralysis is recognized if the laryngeal nerve has been compromised by the procedure. Multiple organ failure is incident in **death**, with respiratory failure being among the most common. If the aneurysm is above or involves the renal arteries, renal failure can occur in 4–9% of patients.

Treatment of the ascending aorta and aortic arch repair carry many of the risks associated with cardiopulmonary bypass, including hemostatic difficulties, left ventricle dysfunction, or myocardial (heart muscle) dysfunction. Irreversible brain damage is also an additional risk.

Cardiac function can be compromised in all patients with thoracic or abdominal aortic aneurysms. Hemorrhage is of frequent concern and is more of a risk as the number of suture lines increases. Forty to seventy percent of all deaths can be contributed to cardiac malfunction and blood loss.

Alternatives

Endovascular graft placement is being used as a suitable option to the open surgical procedure. The endovascular graft can be placed using minimally invasive techniques that reduce or eliminate the stay in the intensive care unit. Light sedation and epidural anesthetic are often adequate.

Resources

BOOKS

Hensley, Frederick A., Donald E. Martin, Glenn P. Gravlee. *A Practical Approach to Cardiac Anesthesia,* 3rd ed. Philadelphia: Lippincott Williams & Wilkins Philadelphia, 2002.

PERIODICALS

Ashton, H. A., M. J. Buxton, N. E. Day, L. G. Kim, et al. "The Multicentre Aneurysm Screening Study (MASS) into the Effect of Abdominal Aortic Aneurysm Screening on Mortality in Men: A Randomized Controlled Trial." *Lancet* 360 (November 16, 2002):1531–1539.

Busch, T., H. Sirbu, I. Aleksic, M. Friedrich, and H. Dalichau. "Importance of Cardiovascular Interventions Before Surgery for Abdominal Aortic Aneurysms." *Cardiovascular Surgery* 8, no. 1 (January 2000): 18–21.

Cooley, D. A. "Aortic Aneurysm Operations: Past, Present, and Future." *Annals of Thoracic Surgery* 67, no. 6 (June 1999): 1959–1962.

Porter, J. M., and A. M. Abou-Zamzam Jr. "Endovascular Aortic Grafting: Current Status." *Cardiovascular Surgery* 7, no. 7 (December 1999): 684–691.

OTHER

American Heart Association. *Heart Disease and Stroke Statistics—2008 Update.* Dallas, TX: American Heart Association, 2007. http://www.americanheart.org/presenter.jhtml?identifier=1928 (March 21, 2008).

Allison Joan Spiwak, M.S.B.M.E.
Tish Davidson, A.M.

Aortic stenting *see* **Endovascular stent surgery**

Aortic valve replacement

Definition

Aortic valve replacement is the insertion of a mechanical or tissue valve in place of the diseased biological aortic valve.

Purpose

Aortic valve replacement is necessary when the aortic valve has become diseased. The aortic valve can suffer from insufficiency (inability to perform adequately) or stenosis (narrowing). An insufficient valve is leaky and allows blood to flow backward from the aorta to the left ventricle during diastole, which occurs when the ventricles fill with blood. A stenotic valve prevents the forward-moving flow of blood from the left ventricle to the aorta, during systole, which is the time period when the heart is contracting.

Either situation can result in heart failure and an enlarged left ventricle. With aortic stenosis, the symptoms of angina pectoris, fainting, and congestive heart failure will develop with the severity of the narrowing. There is an increased rate of sudden **death** of patients with aortic stenosis. Dyspnea (labored breathing), fatigue, and palpitations are late symptoms of aortic insufficiency. Angina pectoris is associated with the latest stages of aortic insufficiency.

Demographics

Congenital birth defects involving a bicuspid aortic valve can develop stenosis. These patients may become symptomatic in mid-teen years through age 65. Patients with a history of rheumatic fever have a disposition for aortic stenosis, but may live symptom

KEY TERMS

Antithrombic—Preventing clot formation.

Biological tissue valve—A replacement heart valve that is harvested from the patient (autograft), a human cadaver (homograft or allograft), or other animal, such as a pig (heterograft).

Diastole—Period between contractions of the heart.

Hemolysis—Separation of hemoglobin from the red blood cells.

Mechanical valve—An artificial device used to replace the patient's heart valve. They include three types: ball valve, disk valve, and bileaflet valve.

Systole—Period while the heart is contracting.

free for more than four decades. Calcification of the aortic valve tends to effect an older population with 30% of patients over age 85 having stenosis at autopsy.

Patients with aortic stenosis who have angina, dyspnea, or fainting are candidates for aortic valve replacement. Asymptomatic patients undergoing coronary artery bypass grafting should be treated with aortic valve replacement, but otherwise are not candidates for preventive aortic valve replacement.

Patients with a history of rheumatic fever or syphilitic aortitis (inflammation of the aorta) face the possibility of developing aortic insufficiency. Successful treatment has decreased this causative relationship. Primary causes of aortic valve disease include bacterial endocarditis, trauma, aortic dissection, and congenital diseases.

Patients showing acute symptoms, including pulmonary edema, heart rhythm problems, or circulatory collapse, are candidates for aortic valve replacement. Chronic pathologies are recommended for surgery when patients appear symptomatic, demonstrating angina and dyspnea. Asymptomatic patients also must be monitored for heart dysfunction. Left ventricular dimensions greater than 2 in (50 mm) at diastole or 3 in (70 mm) at systole are indications for replacement when aortic insufficiency is diagnosed.

Description

While receiving **general anesthesia** in preparation for the surgery, the patient's cardiac function will be monitored. A sternotomy (incision into the sternum) or **thoracotomy** may be used to expose the heart, with the thoracotomy providing a smaller incision through the ribs. Minimally invasive techniques may also be used, utilizing a partial sternotomy or a lateral mini-thoracotomy. These approaches seem to decrease patient recovery time, as well as decreasing potential complications. Anticoagulant is administered in preparation for cardiopulmonary bypass. Cardiopulmonary bypass is instituted by exposing and cannulating (putting tubes into) the great blood vessels of the heart, or by cannulating the femoral artery and vein. A combination of cannulation sites may also be used. The heart is stopped after the aorta is clamped. The base of the aorta root is opened, and the diseased valve is removed. Sutures are placed in the aortic rim and into the replacement valve. The replacement valve can be either mechanical or biological tissue. The replacement valve will be sized prior to implant to ensure that it fits the patient based on the size of the aortic valve annulus. Once seated, the valve is secured by tying the individual sutures. The heart is then deaired. The cross clamp is removed and the heart is allowed to beat as deairing continues by manipulation of the left ventricle. Cardiopulmonary bypass is terminated, the tubes are removed, and drugs to reverse anticoagulation are administered.

A heart valve prevents the flow of blood backward during heartbeats. Replacement heart valves can be mechanical or biological tissue valves. For patients younger than 65 years of age, the mechanical valve offers superior longevity. Anticoagulant medication is required for the life of the patient implanted with a mechanical valve. The biological tissue valve does not require anticoagulation but suffers from deterioration, leading to **reoperation**, particularly in those under age 50. Women considering bearing children should be treated with biological tissue valves because the anticoagulant of choice with mechanical valves, warfarin, is associated with developmental effects in the fetus. **Aspirin** can be substituted in certain circumstances.

Diagnosis/Preparation

Initial diagnosis by auscultation (listening) is done with a **stethoscope**. Additional procedures associated with diagnosis to judge severity of the lesion include **chest x ray**, **echocardiography**, and **angiography** with **cardiac catheterization**. In the absence of angiography, **magnetic resonance imaging** (MRI) or computed tomographic (CT) imaging may be used.

Aftercare

The patient will have continuous cardiac monitoring performed in the **intensive care unit** (ICU) postoperatively. Medications or mechanical circulatory assist may be instituted during the surgery or postoperatively to help the heart provide the necessary cardiac output to sustain the pulmonary and systemic circulations. These will be discontinued as cardiac function improves. As the patient is able to breathe without assistance, ventilatory support will be discontinued. Drainage tubes allow blood to be collected from the chest cavity during healing and are removed as blood flow decreases. Prophylactic **antibiotics** are given. Anticoagulation (warfarin, aspirin, or a combination) therapy is instituted and continued for patients who have received a mechanical valve. The ICU stay is approximately three days with a final hospital discharge occurring within a week after the procedure.

The patient receive **wound care** instructions prior to leaving the hospital. The instructions include how to recognize such adverse conditions as infection or valve malfunction, contact information for the surgeon, and guidelines on when to return to the emergency room.

Risks

There are unassociated risks with general anesthetic and cardiopulmonary bypass. Risks associated with aortic valve replacement include embolism, bleeding, and operative valvular endocarditis. Hemolysis is associated with certain types of mechanical valves, but is not a contraindication for implantation.

Normal results

Myocardial function typically improves rapidly, with decrease in left ventricle enlargement and size of the inner chamber over several months, allowing the heart to return to normal dimensions. Anticoagulation therapy will be continued, depending on the type of mechanical valve implanted. Implantation of biological tissue valves are associated with the formation of blood clots. If non-cardiac surgery or dental care is needed, the anticoagulant medication will be adjusted to prevent bleeding complications.

Morbidity and mortality rates

There is a 3–5% hospital mortality associated with aortic valve replacement. The average survival rate after five years is 85% for patients suffering from aortic stenosis who undergo aortic valve replacement. Structural valve deterioration can occur and is higher in mechanical valves during the first five years; however, biological tissue and mechanical valves have the same failure incidence at 10 years, with a 60% probability of death at 11 years as a result of valve-related complications. Patients with a mechanical valve are more likely to experience bleeding complications. Reoperation is more likely for patients treated with a biological tissue valve, but not significantly different when compared to their mechanical valve counterparts. This combines to an average rate of significant complications of 2–3% per year, with death rate of approximately 1% per year associated directly with the prosthesis.

Alternatives

Balloon valvotomy may provide short-term relief of aortic stenosis, but is considered a temporary treatment until valve replacement can be accomplished. Aortic valve repair by direct commissurotomy may also be successful for some cases of aortic stenosis. Medical treatment for inoperable patients with severe aortic stenosis is used to relive pulmonary congestion and prevent atrial fibrillation.

Severe aortic insufficiency can be treated with medical therapy. Pharmaceuticals to decrease blood pressure, along with **diuretics** and vasodilators, are helpful in patients with aortic insufficiency.

Resources

BOOKS

Khatri, V. P., and J. A. Asensio. *Operative Surgery Manual.* 1st ed. Philadelphia: Saunders, 2003.

Libby, P., et al. *Braunwald's Heart Disease.* 8th ed. Philadelphia: Saunders, 2007.

Townsend, C. M., et al. *Sabiston Textbook of Surgery.* 17th ed. Philadelphia: Saunders, 2004.

PERIODICALS

Walther T, Falk V, and F. Mohr. "Minimally Invasive Surgery for Valve Disease." *Current Problems in Cardiology* 31, No. 6 (June 2006): 399–437.

Allison Joan Spiwak, MSBME
Rosalyn Carson-DeWitt, MD

Aortofemoral bypass *see* **Peripheral vascular bypass surgery**

Apheres *see* **Transfusion**

Apicoectomy *see* **Root canal treatment**

Appendectomy

Definition

Appendectomy is the surgical removal of the appendix. The appendix is a worm-shaped hollow pouch attached to the cecum, the beginning of the large intestine.

Purpose

Appendectomies are performed to treat appendicitis, an inflamed and infected appendix.

Description

After the patient is anesthetized, the surgeon can remove the appendix either by using the traditional open procedure (in which a 2–3 in [5–7.6 cm] incision is made in the abdomen) or via **laparoscopy** (in which four 1-in [2.5-cm] incisions are made in the abdomen).

Appendectomy

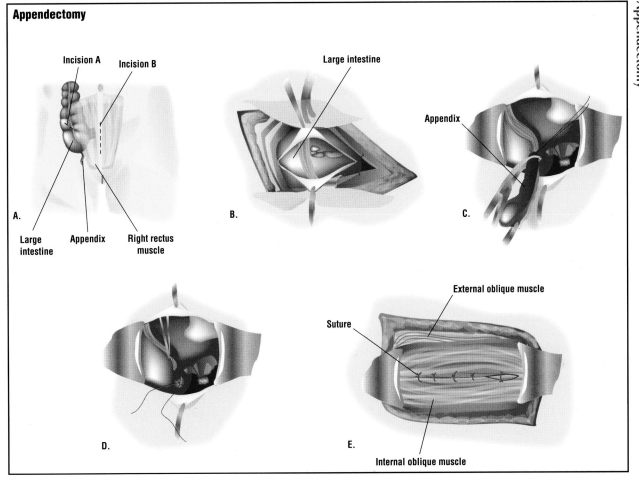

To remove a diseased appendix, an incision is made in the patient's lower abdomen (A). Layers of muscle and tissue are cut, and large intestine, or colon, is visualized (B). The appendix is visualized (C), tied, and removed (D). The muscle and tissue layers are stitched (E). *(Illustration by GGS Information Services. Cengage Learning, Gale.)*

Traditional open appendectomy

When the surgeon uses the open approach, he makes an incision in the lower right section of the abdomen. Most incisions are less than 3 in (7.6 cm) in length. The surgeon then identifies all of the organs in the abdomen and examines them for other disease or abnormalities. The appendix is located and brought up into the wounds. The surgeon separates the appendix from all the surrounding tissue and its attachment to the cecum, and then removes it. The site where the appendix was previously attached, the cecum, is closed and returned to the abdomen. The muscle layers and then the skin are sewn together.

Laparoscopic appendectomy

When the surgeon performs a laparoscopic appendectomy, four incisions, each about 1 in (2.5 cm) in length, are made. One incision is near the umbilicus, or navel, and one is between the umbilicus and the pubis. Two smaller incisions are made on the right side of the lower abdomen. The surgeon then passes a camera and special instruments through these incisions. With the aid of this equipment, the surgeon visually examines the abdominal organs and identifies the appendix. The appendix is then freed from all of its attachments and removed. The place where the appendix was formerly attached, the cecum, is stitched. The appendix is removed through one of the incisions. The instruments are removed and then all of the incisions are closed.

Studies and opinions about the relative advantages and disadvantages of each method are divided. A skilled surgeon can perform either one of these procedures in less than one hour; however, laparoscopic appendectomy (LA) always takes longer than traditional appendectomy (TA). The increased time required to do an LA

KEY TERMS

Abscess—A collection of pus buried deep in the tissues or in a body cavity.

Anesthesia—A combination of drugs administered by a variety of techniques by trained professionals that provide sedation, amnesia, analgesia, and immobility adequate for the accomplishment of the surgical procedure with minimal discomfort to the patient.

Anesthesiologist—A physician who has special training and expertise in anesthesia techniques.

Anesthetics—Drugs used to make a body area free of sensation or pain.

Cecum—The beginning of the large intestine and the place where the appendix attaches to the intestinal tract.

General surgeon—A physician who has special training and expertise in performing a variety of operations.

Pelvic organs— The organs inside of the body that are located within the confines of the pelvis. This includes the bladder and rectum in both sexes, and the uterus, ovaries, and fallopian tubes in females.

Pubis—The front portion of the pelvis located in the anterior abdomen.

Thrombophlebitis—Inflammation of the veins, usually in the legs, which causes swelling and tenderness in the affected area.

Umbilicus—The navel.

increases the patient's exposure to anesthetics, and, therefore, the risk of complications. The longer time requirement also increases the fees charged by the hospital for the **operating room**, and by the anesthesiologist. Since LA also requires specialized equipment, the fees for its use also increase the hospital charges. Patients with either operation have similar pain medication needs, begin eating diets at comparable times, and stay in the hospital equivalent amounts of time. LA is of special benefit to women for whom diagnosis is difficult and gynecological disease (such as endometriosis, pelvic inflammatory disease, ruptured ovarian follicles, ruptured ovarian cysts, and tubal pregnancies) may be the source of pain and not appendicitis. If LA is done in these patients, the pelvic organs can be more thoroughly examined and a definitive diagnosis made prior to removal of the appendix. Most surgeons select either TA or LA based on the individual needs and circumstances of the patient.

Insurance plans do cover the costs of appendectomy. Fees are charged independently by the hospital and the physicians. Hospital charges include fees for operating and **recovery room** use, diagnostic and laboratory testing, as well as the normal hospital room charges. Surgical fees vary from region to region and range between $250–750. The anesthesiologist's fee depends on the health of the patient and the length of the operation.

Preparation

Once the diagnosis of appendicitis is made and the decision has been made to perform an appendectomy, the patient undergoes the standard preparation for an operation. This usually takes only one to two hours and includes signing the operative consents, patient identification procedures, evaluation by the anesthesiologist, and moving the patient to the operating area of the hospital. Occasionally, if the patient has been ill for a prolonged period of time or has had protracted vomiting, a delay of several hours may be necessary to give the patient fluids and **antibiotics**.

Aftercare

Recovery from an appendectomy is similar to other operations. Patients are allowed to eat when the stomach and intestines begin to function again. Usually the first meal is a clear liquid diet—broth, juice, soda, and gelatin. If patients tolerate this meal, the next meal usually is a regular diet. Patients are asked to walk and resume their normal physical activities as soon as possible. If TA was done, work and physical education classes may be restricted for a full three weeks after the operation. If a LA was done, most patients are able to return to work and strenuous activity within one to three weeks after the operation.

Risks

Certain risks are present when any operation is performed under **general anesthesia** and the abdominal cavity is opened. Pneumonia and collapse of the small airways (atelectasis) often occurs. Patients who smoke are at a greater risk for developing these complications. Thrombophlebitis, or inflammation of the veins, is rare but can occur if the patient requires prolonged bed rest. Bleeding can occur but rarely is a blood **transfusion** required. Adhesions (abnormal connections to abdominal organs by thin fibrous tissue) are a known complication of any abdominal surgery such as appendectomy. These adhesions can lead to intestinal obstruction that prevents the normal flow of intestinal contents. Hernia is a complication of any incision; however, they are rarely seen after appendectomy because the abdominal wall is very strong in the area of the standard appendectomy incision.

The overall complication rate of appendectomy depends upon the status of the appendix at the time it is removed. If the appendix has not ruptured, the complication rate is only about 3%. If the appendix has ruptured, the complication rate rises to almost 59%. Wound infections do occur and are more common if the appendicitis was severe, far advanced, or ruptured. An abscess may also form in the abdomen as a complication of appendicitis.

Occasionally, an appendix will rupture prior to its removal, spilling its contents into the abdominal cavity. Peritonitis or a generalized infection in the abdomen will occur. Treatment of peritonitis as a result of a ruptured appendix includes removal of what remains of the appendix, insertion of drains (rubber tubes that promote the flow of infection inside the abdomen to outside of the body), and antibiotics. Fistula formation (an abnormal connection between the cecum and the skin) rarely occurs. It is only seen if the appendix has a broad attachment to the cecum and the appendicitis is far advanced, causing destruction of the cecum itself.

The complications associated with undiagnosed, misdiagnosed, or delayed diagnosis of appendicitis are very significant. This has led surgeons to perform an appendectomy any time that they feel appendicitis is the diagnosis. Most surgeons feel that in approximately 20% of their patients, a normal appendix will be removed. Rates much lower than this would seem to indicate that the diagnosis of appendicitis was being frequently missed.

Normal results

Most patients feel better immediately after an operation for appendicitis. Many patients are discharged from the hospital within 24 hours after the appendectomy. Others may require a longer stay, from three to five days. Almost all patients are back to their normal activities within three weeks.

Morbidity and mortality rates

The mortality rate of appendicitis has dramatically decreased over time. As of 2007, the mortality rate was estimated at one to two per 1,000,000 cases of appendicitis. **Death** is usually due to peritonitis, intra abdominal abscess, or severe infection following rupture.

Alternatives

Appendectomies are usually carried out on an emergency basis to treat appendicitis. There are no alternatives, due to the serious consequence of not removing the inflamed appendix, which is a ruptured appendix and peritonitis, a life-threatening emergency.

Resources

BOOKS

Berger, D. H., and B. M. Jaffe. "The Appendix." In *Schwartz's Principles of Surgery*, 8th ed., edited by F. Charles Brunicardi, et al. New York: McGraw-Hill, 2005.

Silen, William. "Acute Appendicitis and Peritonitis." In *Harrison's Principles of Internal Medicine,* 16th ed., edited by D. L. Kasper, et al. New York: McGraw-Hill, 2004.

PERIODICALS

Eypasch, E., S. Sauerland, R. Lefering, and E. A. Neugebauer. "Laparoscopic versus Open Appendectomy: Between Evidence and Common Sense." *Digestive Surgery* 19, no. 6 (2002): 518–522.

Long, K. H., M. P. Bannon, S. P. Zietlow, E. R. Helgeson, et al. "A prospective randomized comparison of laparoscopic appendectomy with open appendectomy: Clinical and economic analyses." *Surgery* 129, no. 4 (April 2001): 390–400.

Peiser, J. G. and D. Greenberg. "Laparoscopic versus open appendectomy: results of a retrospective comparison in an Israeli hospital." *Israel Medical Association Journal* 4 (February 2002): 91–94.

Piskun, G., D. Kozik, S. Rajpal, G. Shaftan, and R. Fogler. "Comparison of laparoscopic, open, and converted appendectomy for perforated appendicitis." *Surgical Endoscopy* 15, no. 7 (July 2001): 660–662.

Selby, W. S., S. Griffin, N. Abraham, and M. J. Solomon. "Appendectomy protects against the development of ulcerative colitis but does not affect its course." *American Journal of Gastroenterology* 97, no. 11 (November 2002): 2834–2838.

OTHER

"Appendicitis." MayoClinic.com. August 15, 2007. http://www.mayoclinic.com/health/appendicitis/DS00274 (March 21, 2008).

"Appendectomy." Medline Plus. October 16, 2006. http://www.nlm.nih.gov/medlineplus/ency/article/002921.htm (March 21, 2008).

ORGANIZATIONS

American College of Surgeons, 633 N. Saint Clair St., Chicago, IL, 60611-3211, (312) 202-5000, (800) 621-4111, (312) 202-5001, postmaster@facs.org, http://www.facs.org.

Mary Jeanne Krob, M.D., F.A.C.S.
Monique Laberge, Ph.D.
Tish Davidson, A.M.

Appendix removal *see* **Appendectomy**
Arterial anastomasis *see* **Arteriovenous fistula**

Arterial blood gases (ABG)

Definition

An arterial blood gas (ABG test) measures the levels of oxygen and carbon dioxide in the blood. Additionally, it reports the level of acidity or alkalinity of the blood, the pH. An ABG is performed in order to diagnose or monitor respiratory, kidney, or metabolic disorders.

Purpose

An ABG may be ordered to monitor the status of a patient in surgery or after a trauma. The test may also be used to monitor how a patient is responding to **oxygen therapy**. Additionally, an ABG may also help in the evaluation of a variety of symptoms, including shortness of breath.

Precautions

If the patient is on supplemental oxygen, no changes should be made to the setting for a full twenty to thirty minutes prior to drawing the ABG sample. If the sample needs to be drawn with the patient off of supplemental oxygen (that is, on "room air"), then the patient should be removed from oxygen and should be off of oxygen for a full twenty to thirty minutes prior to the blood draw.

If the blood will be drawn from the artery at the wrist, the radial artery, then a simple test (the Allen test) should be performed prior to the blood draw to ascertain that the patient has good blood circulation at the wrist. Pressure is applied to the two main wrist arteries (the radial and ulnar arteries) for several seconds. The pressure is then released from one and then the other, and the patient's hand is observed to verify that if turns a bit red (flushes) as blood returns through those arteries into the hand. If the flushing is not adequate, then the arteries at the other wrist should be tested the same way. If good circulation at either wrist cannot be verified, then the elbow or groin arteries should be considered.

The individual who is drawing the blood should be well-aware if the patient is on any kind of blood thinning medication, since this may make the patient more prone to bleeding or bruising after the blood draw.

Description

Most blood tests involve blood that is drawn from a vein; however, because this test needs to look at the oxygen-carrying capacity of the blood, the sample needs to be drawn from an artery either at the wrist, the elbow crease, or the groin. If the patient has a central line (an intravenous line that goes directly into the heart), the blood sample can be drawn from that. When the radial artery (the artery at the wrist where one checks the pulse rate) is being used for the test, the sample can usually be drawn by a nurse or phlebotomist (an individual who has been trained to draw blood). When an artery at the elbow (the brachial artery), the groin (femoral artery), or a central line is involved, a doctor may be required to

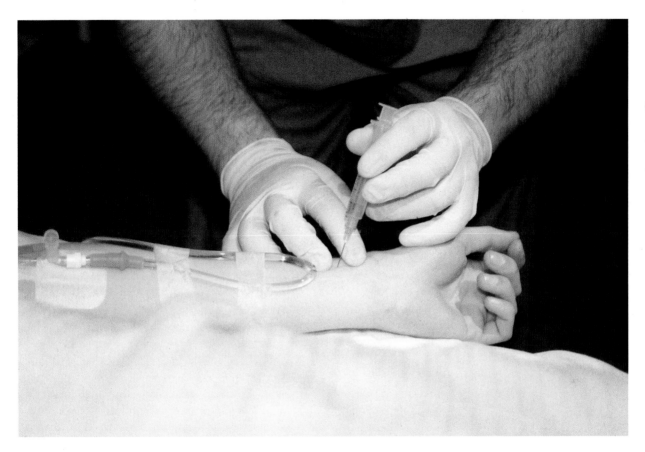

(Medical-on-Line / Alamy)

draw the sample. Because arteries run deeper than veins, the needle stick of an ABG is more painful than other blood tests. In some cases, a local anesthetic may be used to numb the area around the artery to be used. The site of the needle stick is cleaned with antiseptic, and the needle is inserted. The blood is collected in vacuum tubes. After collection, the needle is withdrawn, and a cotton ball is usually pressed onto the blood draw site for about 10 minutes, to stop any bleeding and to decrease bruising. A pressure bandage is then applied over the puncture site, and should be left in place for about an hour to decrease bleeding and bruising.

In newborn babies, blood may be obtained from the umbilical artery and umbilical vein for testing, or whole blood from a heel stick may be utilized.

Preparation

There are no restrictions on diet or physical activity, either before or after the blood test.

Aftercare

As with any blood tests, discomfort, bruising, and/or a very small amount of bleeding is common at the puncture site. Arteries run deeper than veins and the blood pressure within an artery is higher, therefore there is a greater chance for pain, bleeding, and bruising from an ABG than from other blood tests that draw blood from a vein. Immediately after the needle is withdrawn, it is very important to put significant pressure on the puncture site for about 10 minutes, until the bleeding has stopped. This decreases the chance of significant bruising. Warm packs may relieve minor discomfort. Some individuals may feel briefly woozy after a blood test, and they should be encouraged to lie down and rest until they feel better. For about 24 hours after an ABG is drawn, the individual should avoid vigorous **exercise** or heavy lifting.

Risks

Basic blood tests do not carry significant risks, other than slight bruising and the chance of brief dizziness. An arterial blood draw is more painful and more inclined to bleed and bruise, so the risks of these complications are slightly higher after an ABG is drawn.

Results

Results from the ABG include a measurement of the partial pressure of oxygen or paO_2 (how much oxygen is dissolved in the blood), the partial pressure of carbon dioxide or $paCO_2$ (how much carbon dioxide is dissolved in the blood), and pH. The pH is a number that indicates how acidic or alkaline the blood is. It is a measurement involving the concentration of hydrogen ions in the blood. As the $paCO_2$ levels rise, the pH level drops and the blood becomes increasingly acidic; as the paO_2 levels rise, the pH level rises, and the blood becomes increasingly alkaline.

The information obtained from an ABG also allows other important aspects of body chemistry to be evaluated, such as the O_2 saturation (a measurement of the percentage of oxygen that is bound to the hemoglobin in red blood cells) and the amount of bicarbonate in the body. Bicarbonate, or HCO_3- is processed by the kidneys in response to the pH of the body. When the pH goes down (indicating greater acidity), the kidneys excrete HCO_3-, in an effort to counterbalance the acidity. When the pH goes up (indicating greater alkalinity), the kidneys reabsorb more HCO_3-, in an effort to counterbalance the alkalinity. A final calculation can help to measure the patient's base/excess or deficit. This is a measurement of the body's ability to compensate for pH abnormalities through other "buffering" agents in the blood, such as hemoglobin, proteins, phosphates, and bicarbonate.

Normal ABG results

Normal ABG results are as follows:

- paO_2: 75–100 mm Hg (millimeters of mercury
- $paCO_2$: 35–45 mm Hg
- pH: 7.35–7.45
- HCO_3-: 24–28 mEq/L (millequivalents per liter)

Abnormal ABG results

Abnormal ABG results include the following:

- Respiratory acidosis is indicated by a low pH and a high pCO_2, and usually indicates respiratory depression, a situation in which the individual is not breathing in sufficient O_2 and is not breathing out sufficient CO_2. Respiratory acidosis may be caused by pneumonia, emphysema, chronic bronchitis, chronic obstructive pulmonary disease, pulmonary edema, interstitial fibrosis, foreign body obstructing the airway; or slowed, shallow breathing due to disorders of the muscles of respiration (myasthenia gravis, muscular dystrophy), nervous system control of the muscles of respiration (amyotrophic lateral sclerosis, polio, Guillain-Barre syndrome, botulism, tetanus, organophosphate poisoning, spinal cord injury); conditions that depress the respiratory center in the brain (such as narcotic drugs, sedatives, anesthesia, blood clot blocking the vertebral artery or increased intracranial pressure).

- Respiratory alkalosis is indicated by a high pH and a low pCO_2, and may indicate hyperventilation (fast, shallow breathing), brought on by emotional stress, pain, anxiety, problems with the lung that do not allow normal exchange of gases (such as pneumonia, pulmonary embolus, collapsed lung); drugs (salicylates, xanthines, progesterone, epinephrine, thyroxine, nicotine); conditions involving the central nervous system (tumors, strokes, trauma, infections); liver-disease induced encephalopathy; severe infection (gram negative sepsis); low blood sodium.

- Metabolic acidosis is indicated by a low pH and a low HCO_3-, and may indicate diabetes; shock; loss of HCO_3- through severe diarrhea or pancreatic fistula; kidney failure; use of drugs such as amiloride, triamterene, spironolactone, and beta-blockers; exposure to toxins (paraldehyde, methanol, salicylate, ethylene glycol).

- Metabolic alkalosis is indicated by a high pH and a high HCO_3- and may occur with abnormal electrolyte levels, such as low postassium (hypokalemia) or low magnesium (hypomagnesemia); repeated bouts of vomiting or nasogastric suction (which causes a lot of stomach acid to be lost in the vomit); loss through the stool (as in cystic fibrosis, abuse of laxatives); multiple blood transfusions; Cushing's syndrome; or an overdose of sodium bicarbonate.

Resources

BOOKS

Brenner, B. M., and F. C. Rector, eds. *Brenner & Rector's The Kidney*, 7th ed. Philadelphia: Saunders, 2004.

Mason, R. J., V. C. Broaddus, J. F. Murray, and J. A. Nadel. *Murray & Nadel's Textbook of Respiratory Medicine,* 4th ed. Philadelphia: Saunders, 2005.

McPherson R. A., and M. R. Pincus, eds. *Henry's Clinical Diagnosis and Management by Laboratory Methods,* 21st ed. Philadelphia: Saunders, 2006.

OTHER

Medical Encyclopedia. Medline Plus. U.S. National Library of Medicine and the National Institutes of Health. January 2, 2008. http://www.nlm.nih.gov/medlineplus/encyclopedia.html (February 10, 2008).

ORGANIZATIONS

American Association for Clinical Chemistry, 1850 K Street, NW, Suite 625, Washington, DC, 20006, (800) 892-1400, http://www.aacc.org.

Rosalyn Carson-DeWitt, M.D.

Arteriography *see* **Angiography**

Arteriovenous fistula

Definition

An arteriovenous fistula (AV fistula) is an abnormal connection between a vein and an artery. The connection can be congenital (present at birth). Occasionally the connection can develop because of trauma such as a knife or bullet wound. Most often, the AV fistula is created surgically to allow access to the vascular system for hemodialysis. When created surgically, the connection of a vein and an artery is usually done in the forearm.

Purpose

Hemodialysis is the process of mechanically cleansing the blood when the kidneys have failed. The surgical creation of an AV fistula provides a long-lasting site through which blood can be removed and returned during hemodialysis. The fistula, which allows the person to be connected to a dialysis machine, must be prepared by a surgeon weeks or months before dialysis is started. When the vein and artery are joined, blood flow increases and the vein gradually becomes larger and stronger, creating a site that provides vascular access years longer than other types of access and with fewer complications. AV fistulas are for people who will need dialysis for long periods—either until a kidney becomes available for transplantation or for the rest of their life. Short-term access to the vascular system for dialysis can be had by the insertion of a venous catheter.

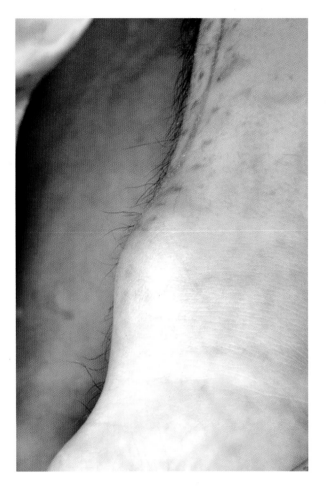

An arteriovenous fistula. *(Medical-on-Line / Alamy)*

Demographics

According to the National Kidney Foundation, at the end of 2005, 336,000 Americans were receiving dialysis for kidney failure. Typically, another condition or disease caused the kidney shutdown. In the United States, kidney failure is disproportionately high among minority populations with the highest rate being found among African Americans, Hispanic Americans, and Native Americans. Among those receiving dialysis, over half will have an AV fistula as vascular access.

Description

The kidneys are paired organs in the mid-abdomen, one on each side of the lower back. Their function is to clean the blood of wastes and to regulate fluid and electrolyte balance in the body. Dialysis performs these functions in place of the failing kidneys. Dialysis cannot restore kidney function, but it can prolong life, often for years, by preventing the build-up of waste products in the body.

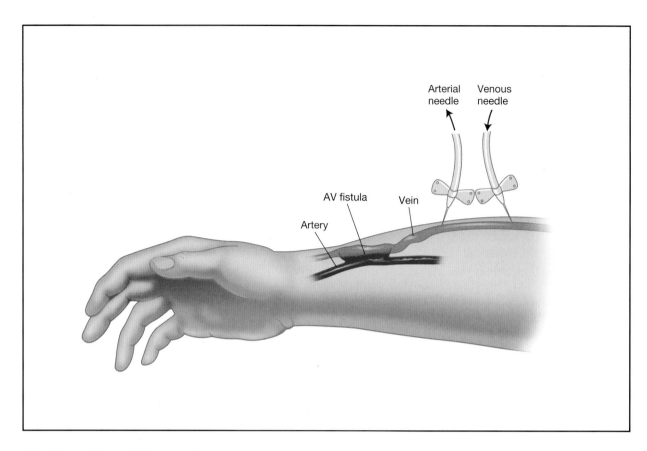

Arterial
needle

Venous
needle

AV fistula

Vein

Artery

(Illustration by Electronic Illustrators Group.)

Acute kidney failure usually happens in circumstances where an extra burden is placed on the renal system. For example, acute kidney failure can occur in advanced liver disease, rapidly progressing terminal illnesses such as cancer and certain severe anemias, after severe allergic reactions, as a reaction to drugs or poisons, in heart and lung diseases, during the formation of blood clots (embolism), and following heart bypass surgery. Diabetes and vascular diseases, especially those with hypertension, are the two most common underlying diseases contributing to chronic kidney failure.

Many advances in the treatment of kidney failure have been made since the first attempts at dialysis treatments in the 1920s. At one time, dialysis was thought of only as a way to keep people alive until kidney function could be restored. Often the treatment for kidney failure had to be discontinued within several days because patients' veins could not endure the trauma that occurred with frequent withdrawing and replacing of blood. The first breakthrough came in 1960 with the introduction of an implantable Teflon tube, called a shunt, that became the first effective vascular access device. Since then, the development of the AV fistula has marked another important advance, allowing effective treatment for longer periods.

Hemodialysis

Dialysis is performed as critical life support when a person experiences acute or chronic kidney failure. It is a mechanical way to cleanse the blood and balance body fluids when the kidneys are not able to perform these essential functions. Kidney failure can, in some cases, be reversible, and dialysis can provide temporary support until renal function is restored. Dialysis may also be used in irreversible or chronic kidney shutdown when transplantation is the medical goal and the patient is waiting for a donated kidney. Some critically ill patients with life-threatening illnesses such as cancer or severe heart disease are not candidates for transplantation and dialysis for them is the only option for treating permanent kidney failure, also called end-stage renal disease (ESRD).

There are two types of dialysis, hemodialysis and peritoneal dialysis. In hemodialysis, the blood circulates through a machine outside the body and is filtered as it circulates. In peritoneal dialysis, the blood is filtered through a membrane that has been placed in the abdomen. Blood remains in the body and waste material is filtered into an exchange fluid through an opening in the abdomen called a port. Only hemodialysis requires an AV fistula or other vascular access.

KEY TERMS

Access—The point where a needle or catheter is inserted for dialysis.

Acute renal (kidney) failure—Abrupt loss of kidney function, possibly temporary.

Artery—Blood vessel that carries blood away from the heart to the body.

Chronic renal (kidney) failure—Progressive loss of kidney function over several years that can result in permanent kidney failure requiring dialysis.

Electrolyte—Ions in the body that participate in metabolic reactions. The major human electrolytes are sodium (Na^+), potassium (K^+), calcium (Ca^{2+}), magnesium (Mg^{2+}), chloride (Cl^-), phosphate (HPO_4^{2-}), bicarbonate (HCO_3^-), and sulfate (SO_4^{2-}).

Hypertension—High blood pressure.

Hemodialysis circulates blood through a dialysis machine that contains a filter membrane. The blood is slowly pumped out of the body and into the machine for cleansing. After being filtered, the blood is returned to the body through the same vascular access. About one cup (235 mL) of blood is outside the body at any given moment during the continuous circulation process.

Hemodialysis is usually done three times a week, taking between three and five hours each time. Healthcare professionals perform the procedure either at independent dialysis centers or in hospitals or medical centers. Dialysis patients must go to the hemodialysis center where they will sit to receive the treatment. Although they cannot walk around, they can watch television, read, or talk to other patients. Dialysis centers offer patient education, including videos and brochures that describe treatment options and self-care. Patients can also receive advice and information about paying for this ongoing treatment through nationally sponsored programs that are available especially for those who need long-term dialysis. Often the dialysis center offers emotional support as well, letting people meet and talk with others who have kidney problems. Some people prefer to perform their own dialysis by having a home dialysis machine. This requires that the dialysis patient and another person, usually a family member, take a three- to six-week training program to learn how to do the treatment.

Vascular access

An access or entry to the vascular system is needed to perform the blood-cleansing role of the kidneys

through hemodialysis. There are three types of vascular access: AV fistula, grafts, and catheters.

ARTERIOVENOUS FISTULA. An AV fistula has proven to be the best kind of vascular access for people whose veins are large enough, not only because it lasts longer, but also because it is less likely than other types of access to form clots or become infected. If the veins are not large enough or there is no time to wait for a fistula to develop, a graft or a catheter must be used.

GRAFT. Grafts are often the access of choice when a hemodialysis patient has small veins that will not likely develop properly into a fistula. This type of access uses a synthetic tube implanted under the skin of the arm that can be used repeatedly for needle placement. Unlike a fistula, which requires time to develop, a graft can be used as soon as two to three weeks after placement. Grafts are known to have more problems than fistulas, such as clots and infection, and will likely need replacement sooner.

CATHETER. A catheter is used to provide temporary vascular access. When kidney disease has progressed quickly, there may not be time to prepare a permanent vascular access site before dialysis treatments are started. The catheter is a tube that is inserted into a vein in the neck, chest, or in the leg near the groin. Two chambers in the tube allow blood to flow in and out. Once the catheter is in place, needle insertion is not necessary. Catheters are effective for dialysis for several weeks or months while surgery is performed and an AV fistula develops. They are not selected for permanent access because they can clog, become infected, or cause the veins to narrow. Long-term catheter access must be used in patients for whom AV fistula or graft surgery has not been successful. If more than three weeks' use is expected, catheters can be made to tunnel under the skin, which increases comfort and reduces complications

Diagnosis/Preparation

Diagnosis

The diagnosis of kidney disease and its progression to kidney failure is typically made by a nephrologist, a specialist in kidney structure and function. The nephrologist will determine whether the patient has acute or chronic kidney failure and if dialysis is appropriate for the patient. If dialysis is recommended, the nephrologist will determine if an AV fistula is the ideal vascular access for the patient. To make these determinations, the nephrologist will need to evaluate the patient's general health, especially the presence of any underlying disease. Kidney function must be evaluated and determined to be seriously impaired before dialysis is recommended. It is typically started when kidney function is down to about 10% of its normal level. Among other tests that will be performed, such as **urinalysis** with microscopic examination of the urine, several blood and urine tests can be used to measure a person's kidney function when chronic or acute kidney failure is suspected. Some of the tests measure electrolytes and other metabolites produced by the body that are normally excreted by the kidneys and passed through urine. The tests can measure effectively if the kidney is filtering out these materials, and how much remains in the blood. These tests include, but are not limited to:

- serum creatinine—found in higher levels in the blood if kidneys fail;
- urinary creatinine—readings are lower in kidney failure;
- urinary output—measuring both fluid intake and all urine produced;
- urinary osmolality—measures the concentration of the urine, an indicator of kidney filtering ability;
- blood urea nitrogen (BUN)—harmful nitrogen waste increases in the blood as kidney function decreases; and
- electrolytes in blood and urine—ions in the blood such as sodium, potassium, magnesium, and chloride are often out of balance when kidneys fail. Potassium, for example, increases in the blood during kidney failure and can cause heart irregularities.

Description

Surgery to create an AV fistula is usually done using a local anesthetic that is injected into the forearm at the site of the proposed fistula. The procedure is performed in a hospital or at an **outpatient surgery** if the patient is not already hospitalized and has no serious underlying disease.

After cleaning and sterilizing the site, the surgeon makes a small incision in the forearm sufficient to allow the permanent uniting of a vein and an artery. The blood vessels will be appropriately blocked to stop blood flow while incisions are made to join them. Silk sutures, just as those used in other types of surgical incisions, are used to close incised areas as needed after the vein and artery have been joined. Once joined, blood flow increases. The vein will become thicker, and over a period of months the connection will become strong and develop into the fistula that will allow permanent vascular access.

Aftercare

The hemodialysis patient should expect needle insertion in the AV fistula at every dialysis session. Patients who prefer to insert their own needles or who perform dialysis at home will need training, and all patients have to learn how to avoid infection and to protect the vascular access. Because vascular access problems can lead to treatment failure, the AV fistula requires regular care to make dialysis easier and to help avoid clots, infection, and other complications.

Patients can help protect the access by:

- making sure the access is checked before each treatment;
- not allowing blood pressure to be taken on the access arm;
- checking the pulse in the access every day;
- keeping the access clean at all times;
- using the access site only for dialysis;
- taking care not to bump or cut the access;
- avoiding wearing tight jewelry or clothing near or over the access site;
- avoiding lifting heavy objects or putting pressure on the access arm; and
- sleeping with the access arm free, not under the head or body.

Risks

The most frequent complications in hemodialysis relate to the vascular access site where needles are inserted. Complications include infection around the access area and formation of clots in the fistula. Usually, because they are in the fistula itself, these clots are not life threatening. The greatest danger is that clots may block the fistula and have to be removed surgically. Frequent clotting may require creating a back-up fistula at another site, to allow dialysis when one access is blocked.

Other complications from dialysis are not directly related to the vascular access. For example, when the kidneys have shut down, they produce very little urine. Because dialysis is the only way people with kidney failure can balance fluid levels in their bodies, hemodialysis can cause bloating and fluid overload, indicating that too much fluid remains in the body. If fluid overload occurs, patients develop swollen ankles, puffy eyes, weight gain, and shortness of breath. Fluid overload can cause heart and circulatory problems and fluctuations in blood pressure. Medications may be prescribed and changes in fluid intake or diet may be made to help balance fluids safely in conjunction with dialysis.

Other problems that can occur during or after hemodialysis include:

- low blood pressure when fluid and wastes are removed from the blood too quickly;
- nausea due to changes in blood pressure;

- muscle cramps from the removal of too much fluid from the blood;

- headaches near the end of a dialysis session resulting from changes in the concentration of fluid and waste in the blood; or

- fatigue after treatment, lasting sometimes into the next day.

Normal results

An AV fistula can usually be created and can function well with no adverse affects in a person whose veins are large enough. The amount of time it takes to develop the fistula after surgery (usually months) depends upon the size and strength of the patient's blood vessels and on the person's health and nutritional status. When the fistula develops, the thickened vein that has been joined to an artery can be seen in the arm and a pulse can be felt in it. The early development of an AV fistula as access for long-term dialysis has been shown to improve the survival of patients with chronic renal failure and to reduce the chances of being hospitalized with complications. It also gives patients a better opportunity to choose self-dialysis as their treatment.

With good nutrition and a fully functioning AV fistula, dialysis patients can be relatively comfortable and free of complications. People may become tired and uncomfortable when it is close to the time for their next dialysis session. This is to be expected because wastes are building up in the blood, and the body senses that it is time to remove them.

Morbidity and mortality rates

Earlier use of dialysis, especially with AV fistula access, has been shown to increase survival in patients with renal failure. The AV fistula is designed to improve the effectiveness of dialysis and is reported to present fewer risks and complications, reduced incidence of clotting and infection, and longer use than other types of vascular access.

Kidney failure is reported to account for 1% of hospital admissions in the United States. It occurs in 2–5% of patients hospitalized for other conditions, surgeries, or diseases. In patients undergoing cardiac bypass surgery, 15% are reported to require dialysis for kidney failure. Overall, deaths in people undergoing dialysis are reported to be about 50% because of the multi-organ dysfunction that has influenced kidney failure.

Resources

BOOKS

Offer, Daniel, Marjorie K. Offer ,and Susan O. Szafir. *Dialysis without Fear: A Guide to Living Well on Dialysis for Patients and Their Families.* New York: Oxford University Press, 2007.

OTHER

"Treatment Methods for Kidney Failure: Hemodialysis." *National Kidney and Urologic Diseases Information Clearinghouse.* December 2006. http://kidney.niddk.nih.gov/kudiseases/pubs/hemodialysis/index.htm (February 1, 2008).

"Vascular Access for Hemodialysis." *National Kidney and Urologic Diseases Information Clearinghouse.* February 2008. http://kidney.niddk.nih.gov/kudiseases/pubs/vascularaccess/ (February 1, 2008).

"Vascular Access for Hemodialysis." *Texas Heart Institute.* July 2007. http://www.texasheartinstitute.org/HIC/Topics/Proced/vascular_access_surgery.cfm (February 1, 2008).

ORGANIZATIONS

National Kidney and Urologic Diseases, 3 Information Way, Bethesda, MD, 20892-3580, (800) 891-5390, http://kidney.niddk.nih.gov.

National Kidney Foundation, 30 East 33rd Street, New York, NY, 10016, (800) 622-9010, http://www.kidney.org.

L. Lee Culvert
Tish Davidson, A. M.

Arthrography

Definition

Arthrograpy is a procedure involving multiple x rays of a joint using a fluoroscope, a special piece of x-ray equipment that shows an immediate x-ray image. A contrast medium (in this case, a contrast iodine solution) injected into the joint area helps highlight structures of the joint.

Purpose

Frequently, arthrography is ordered to determine the cause of unexplained joint pain. This fluoroscopic procedure can show the internal workings of specific joints and outline soft tissue structures. The procedure may also be conducted to identify problems with the ligaments, cartilage, tendons, or the joint capsule of the hip, shoulder, knee, ankle, wrist, or other joints. An arthrography procedure may locate cysts in the joint area, evaluate problems with the joint's arrangement and function, indicate the need for joint replacement, or show problems with existing joint replacement (prostheses). The most commonly studied joints are the knee and shoulder.

Description

Arthrograpy may be referred to as "joint radiography" or "x rays of the joint." The term arthrogram may be used interchangeably with arthrography. The joint area will be cleaned and a local anesthetic will be injected into the tissues around the joint to reduce pain. Next, if fluids are present in the joint, the physician may suction them out (aspirate) with a needle. These fluids may be sent to a laboratory for further study. Contrast agents are then injected into the joint through the same location by attaching the aspirating needle to a syringe containing the contrast medium. The purpose of contrast agents in x-ray procedures is to help highlight details of areas under study by making them opaque. Agents for arthrography are generally air- and water-soluble dyes, the most common containing iodine. Air and iodine may be used together or independently. After the contrast agent is administered, the site of injection will be sealed, and the patient may be asked to bend and flex the joint to distribute the contrast.

Before the contrast medium can be absorbed by the joint itself, several films will be quickly taken under the guidance of the fluoroscope. The patient will be asked to move the joint into a series of positions, keeping still between positioning. Sometimes, the patient will experience some tingling or discomfort during the

procedure, which is normal and due to the contrast. Following fluoroscopic tracking of the contrast, standard x rays of the area may also be taken. The entire procedure will last about one hour.

Generally, a joint is evaluated first by MRI (**magnetic resonance imaging**) instead of an arthrogram, or by MRI combined with the arthrogram. Gadolinium, an MRI contrast agent, is injected if the arthrogram is performed as part of an MRI procedure. If the arthrogram is performed as part of a MRI arthrogram, the MRI scan will then be obtained immediately afterward.

Preparation

It is important to discuss any known sensitivity to local anesthetics or iodine prior to this procedure. A physician should explain the procedure and the risks associated with contrast agents and ask the patient to sign an **informed consent**. If iodine contrast will be administered, the patient may be instructed not to eat or drink anything for a period of hours before the exam. The timeframe of fasting may range from only 90 minutes prior to the exam up to the night before. There is no other preparation necessary.

Aftercare

The affected joint should be rested for approximately 12 hours following the procedure. The joint may be wrapped in an elastic bandage, and the patient should receive instructions on the care and changing of the bandage. Noises in the joint such as cracking or clicking are normal for a few days following arthrography. These noises are the result of liquid in the joints. Swelling may also occur and can be treated with application of ice or cold packs. A mild pain reliever can be used to lessen pain in the first few days. However, if any of these symptoms persist for more than a few days, patients are advised to contact their physician.

Risks

In some patients iodine can cause allergic reactions, ranging from mild nausea to severe cardiovascular or nervous system complications. Since the contrast dye is put into a joint, rather than into a vein, allergic reactions are rare. Facilities licensed to perform contrast exams should meet requirements for equipment, supplies, and staff training to handle a possible severe reaction. Infection or joint damage are possible, although not frequent, complications of arthrography.

Normal results

A normal arthrography exam will show proper placement of the dye or contrast medium throughout the joint structures, joint space, cartilage, and ligaments.

The abnormal placement of dye may indicate rheumatoid arthritis, cysts, joint dislocation, tear of the rotator cuff, tears in the ligament, and other conditions. The entire lining of the joint becomes opaque from the technique, which allows the radiologist to see abnormalities in the intricate workings of the joint. In the case of recurrent shoulder dislocations, arthrography results can be used to evaluate damage. Patients with hip prostheses may receive arthrography to evaluate proper placement or function of their prostheses.

Resources

BOOKS

Juhl, John H., and Andrew B. Crummy. *Paul and Juhl's Essentials of Radiologic Imaging,* 7th edition. Philadelphia: Lippincott Williams & Wilkins, 1998.

ORGANIZATIONS

American College of Radiology. 1891 Preston White Drive, Reston, VA 22091. (800) 227-5463. http://www.acr.org.

Arthritis Foundation. 1300 W. Peachtree St., Atlanta, GA 30309. (800) 283-7800. http://www.arthritis.org.

Teresa Norris, RN
Lee A. Shratter, M. D.
Tish Davidson, A. M.

Arthroplasty

Definition

Arthroplasty is surgery performed to relieve pain and restore range of motion by realigning or reconstructing a dysfunctional joint.

Purpose

The goal of arthroplasty is to relieve pain and restore function in a stiffened joint. This surgery is usually performed when physical therapy or nonsurgical medical treatment have not improved function in the affected joint. There are two types of arthroplastic surgery: joint resection and interpositional reconstruction. Joint resection involves removing a portion of the bone from a stiffened joint. This increases the space between the bones forming the joint and improves the range of motion. Pain is relieved and motion is restored, but the joint is less stable. Scar tissue may eventually develop, filling the space and narrowing the gap between the bones.

Interpositional reconstruction is surgery to reshape the joint and add a prosthetic disk between the bones forming the joint. The prosthesis can be made of plastic, metal, ceramic material, or formed from body tissue such as skin, muscle, or fascia. When interpositional reconstruction fails, total joint replacement may be necessary. Joint replacement is also called total joint arthroplasty.

In recent years, total joint arthroplasty has become the operation of choice for most chronic knee and hip problems because of advances in the type and quality of prostheses (artificial joints). Elbow, shoulder, ankle, and finger joints are more likely to be treated with joint resection or interpositional reconstruction.

Arthroplasty is performed on people experiencing severe pain and disabling joint stiffness. Osteoarthritis (OA), a degenerative joint disease, is the most common condition causing joint destruction with pain and impaired movement. Other causes include rheumatoid arthritis (RA), hemophilia, synovitis, and rare bone diseases, all of which are known to destroy cartilage. Joint resection, rather than joint replacement, is more likely to be performed on people with rheumatoid arthritis, especially when the elbow joint is involved. Joint replacement is usually reserved for older patients, because of the limited life of the replacement joint. The younger the patient, the greater the reliance on nonsurgical treatment.

Arthroplasty

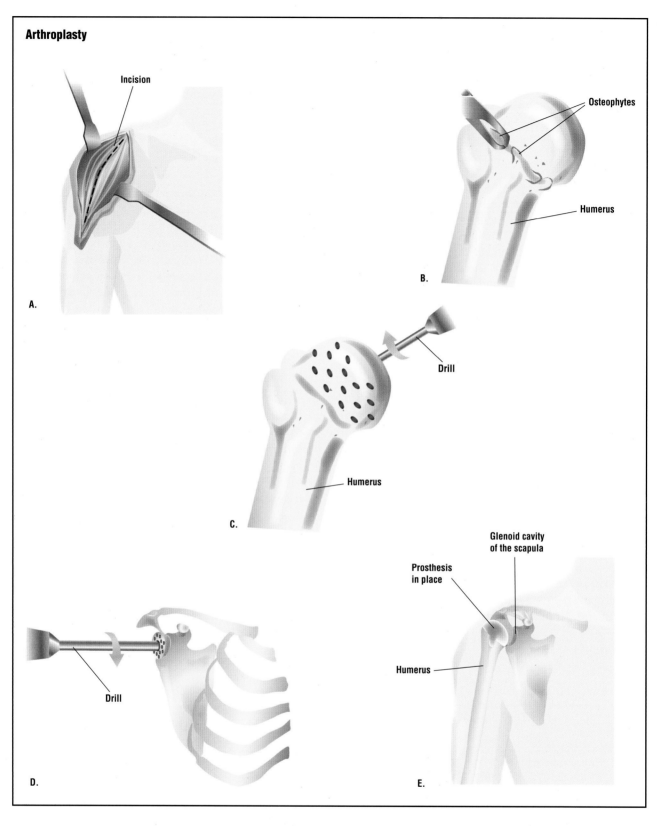

A.

Incision

B.

Osteophytes

Humerus

C.

Drill

Humerus

D.

Drill

E.

Prosthesis
in place

Glenoid cavity
of the scapula

Humerus

In this shoulder arthroplasty procedure, an incision is made into the shoulder (A). The head of the humerus (upper arm bone) is removed from the shoulder joint, and bone growths, or osteophytes, are removed (B). Small holes are drilled into the head to accept the prosthesis (C). Similar holes are drilled in the glenoid cavity (shoulder joint) (D). The final prosthesis improves shoulder function (E). *(Illustration by GGS Information Services. Cengage Learning, Gale.)*

KEY TERMS

Cartilage—The slippery tissue that covers the ends of joint bones.

Fascia—Thin connective tissue covering or separating the muscles and internal organs of the body.

Osteoarthritis—A degenerative "wear-and-tear" joint disease related to aging.

Prosthesis—An artificial joint, part of a joint, or limb.

Rheumatoid arthritis—A chronic autoimmune disease characterized by inflammation of multiple joints and crippling pain and stiffness.

Synovial fluid—A fluid that lubricates the joint and helps prevent wear on the bones.

Synovitis—Inflammation of the synovium, the thin membrane in the joint.

Thrombophlebitis—A condition in which blood clots form in veins near surgery site, causing swelling and pain; clots may travel via veins to the heart or lungs causing serious complications.

Demographics

The American Academy of Orthopaedic Surgeons reports that in 2004 in the United States about 478,000 were total **knee replacement** surgeries and 234,000 were **hip replacement** surgeries were performed. Additional sites for arthroplastic surgery include the ankle, shoulder, elbow, wrist, hand, and big toe. Surgery on smaller joints, such as the toe, have become more common in the 2000s as smaller artificial joints have improved in functionality and reliability.

Because the primary underlying condition in patients undergoing arthroplasty is osteoarthritis, a common cause for disability among older adults, the majority of patients who have arthroplastic surgery fit the demographic profile for osteoarthritis. Osteoarthritis is the most common disease of the elderly worldwide. In the United States in 2006, about 20 million people had diagnosed osteoarthritis. It is estimated that about half of all individuals over age 65 have osteoarthritis. Both men and women develop the disease; under age 45, men are more often affected, although more women than men are affected after age 45. Younger people can have the disease after a traumatic joint injury.

Arthroplasty is reserved for the most severely afflicted—approximately 3% of all patients with osteoarthritis. In addition, approximately 1% of the population worldwide has rheumatoid arthritis, which can strike people of all ages. Few of these people have arthroplastic surgery because this chronic crippling disease affects not only multiple joints but other parts of the body as well, including the immune system. Patients weakened by rheumatoid arthritis (RA) are more subject to infection and less likely to enjoy positive surgical results.

Description

Arthroplasty is performed under **general anesthesia** (affecting the entire body) or regional anesthesia (numbing a specific large area of the body) in a hospital by an orthopedic surgeon. Although many hospitals and medical centers perform common types of joint surgery, orthopedic hospitals that specialize in joint surgery tend to have higher success rates and fewer complications than less specialized centers.

In joint resection, the surgeon makes an incision at the joint, then carefully removes the minimum amount of bone necessary to allow free movement of the joint. The more bone that remains, the more stable the joint. Ligament attachments are preserved as much as possible. In interpositional reconstruction, both bones of the joint are reshaped, and a disk of material is placed between the bones to prevent their rubbing together. **Length of hospital stay** depends on the joint affected. In the absence of complications, a typical stay is brief. For total joint replacement, the entire joint is removed and replaced with an artificial joint. The hospital stay and rehabilitation period for total joint replacement tends to be longer than for joint resection or interpositional reconstruction.

Diagnosis/Preparation

Significant disabling pain, deformity, and reduced quality of life are the primary indications for arthroscopic procedures. Patients at this stage of discomfort and disability will most likely have already been diagnosed with a form of arthritis. Pain and stiffness on weight-bearing joints are the major symptoms that patients report; some experience night pain as well. Other symptoms may include stiffness, swelling, and locking of the joint. The joint may even give way, particularly when the knees or hips are affected.

To determine the extent of disabling, the referring physician and/or the surgeon will ask about walking distance, sporting ability, the need for walking aids, and the ability to perform self-care tasks such as dressing and bathing. Besides evaluation of the joint itself and level of mobility, the clinical examination will include evaluation of the patient's general health, the condition of the ligaments and muscles around the affected joint, and an assessment of the patient's mental outlook and social circumstances to help develop the most effective postoperative rehabilitation plan.

Diagnostic testing will typically include:

- X rays of the affected joint (and often other joints as well) to determine loss of joint space and to differentiate between OA and RA.
- Imaging studies, such as computed tomography (CT) scans, magnetic resonance (MRI), and bone densitometry to assess bone loss or bone infection.
- Cardiac tests, such as an electrocardiogram, to evaluate the heart and circulatory system.
- Blood tests to rule out infection and possibly to confirm arthritis.

Before arthroplastic surgery, standard preoperative blood and urine tests are performed to rule out such conditions as anemia and infection. If a patient has a history of bleeding, the surgeon will ask that clotting tests be performed. The patient will meet with the anesthesiologist to discuss any special conditions that may affect the administration of anesthesia. Surgery will not be performed if infection is present anywhere in the body or if the patient has certain heart or lung diseases. Smokers will be asked to stop smoking. Weight loss may also be recommended for overweight patients. If surgery involves deep tissue and muscle, such as total hip arthroplasty, the surgeon may order units of blood to be prepared in case **transfusion** is needed to replace blood lost during the surgery. Healthy patients may be asked to donate their own blood, which will be returned to them at the time of surgery (autologous transfusion). Certain pain medications may have to be discontinued in the weeks just prior to surgery.

Aftercare

Immediately after surgery, while still in the hospital, patients will be given pain medications for the recovery period and **antibiotics** to prevent infection. When patients are discharged after joint surgery, they must be careful not to overstress or destabilize the joint. Normally, this requires rest at home for a period of days to weeks. Physical therapy will begin almost immediately to improve strength and range of motion. Physical therapy is the most important aid to recovery and may continue for several months. Activity may be resumed gradually, using devices such as walkers or crutches, as recommended by the physical therapist. Lifestyle changes may include the use of special seating or sleeping surfaces and employing **home care** assistance for help with shopping, cooking, and household tasks.

Risks

Joint resection and interpositional reconstruction do not always produce successful results, especially in patients with rheumatoid arthritis, a chronic inflammatory disease that may continue to narrow the joint space and accelerate the formation of scar tissue. Repeat surgery or total joint replacement may be necessary. As with any major surgery, there are always risks of an allergic reaction to anesthesia, postoperative infection, or the formation of blood clots (thrombophlebitis) that may cause pain and swelling near the surgery site and travel through the veins to other parts of the body. A joint that has undergone surgery is less stable than a healthy joint, and dislocation or loosening of the resected joint may occur, especially with inappropriate physical activity.

Normal results

Most patients enjoy an improved range of motion in the joint and relief from pain. Younger people may be able to return to some form of low-impact sports activity. However, people who have degenerative or inflammatory diseases must understand that they will not suddenly have a normal joint, even while they will gain pain relief and improved function.

Morbidity and mortality rates

The number of deaths for all arthroplasty surgeries is less than 1%, with **death** more likely to occur among elderly patients and those with other serious medical conditions.

Alternatives

Pain management alone, particularly with the availability of more effective pain medicines that have fewer side effects, is the primary nonsurgical option when the underlying diagnosis is a form of arthritis. **Nonsteroidal anti-inflammatory drugs** (NSAIDs) are commonly prescribed for patients with arthritis. Those with RA are given drugs that suppress immune system activity, shown to be a factor in this type of arthritis. A range of nutritional supplements and vitamins are reported to offer health benefits to people with OA. Among them, glucosamine and chondroitin sulfate have been shown to offer some relief for pain and stiffness. Weight loss is often recommended as well.

Because immobility of the affected joint can increase pain and stiffness, patients with joint disease are usually encouraged to continue some type of physical activity. Keeping the muscles strong through modest **exercise**, such as stretching or swimming, is often recommended to help support the joint and maintain mobility. Various devices, such as braces or orthopedic shoes, may be recommended, as well as walking aids. Safety rails, special elevated toilet-seat extensions, and bath and shower seats can make the patient more comfortable in daily life. Movement therapy, such as yoga, Pilates, tai chi, and dance, may help maintain joint flexibility and slow chronic arthritis symptoms. Occupational therapy, massage therapy, and physiotherapy may help improve range of motion and overall comfort, as well as patient confidence.

Resources

BOOKS

Grelsamer, Ronald P. *What Your Doctor May Not Tell You about Hip and Knee Replacement Surgery: Everything You Need to Know to Make The Right Decisions.* New York: Warner Books, 2004.

ORGANIZATIONS

American Academy of Orthopaedic Surgeons(AAOS). 6300 North River Rd. Rosemont, Illinois 60018. (847) 823-7186. Fax: (847) 823-8125. http://www.aaos.org (accessed March 6, 2008).

Tish Davidson, AM
Lee Culvert
Tish Davidson, AM

Arthroplasty, shoulder *see* **Shoulder resection arthroplasty**

Arthroscopic knee surgery *see* **Knee arthroscopic surgery**

Arthroscopic surgery

Definition

Arthroscopic surgery is a procedure that allows surgeons to visualize, diagnose, and treat joint problems. The name is derived from the Greek words *arthron*, joint, and *skopein*, to look at. Arthroscopy is performed using an arthroscope, a small fiber-optic instrument that enables a close look at the inside of a joint through a small incision.

Purpose

Arthroscopic surgery is used to diagnose, treat, and monitor joint injuries and diseases that affect the joints. Diagnostic arthroscopic surgery is performed

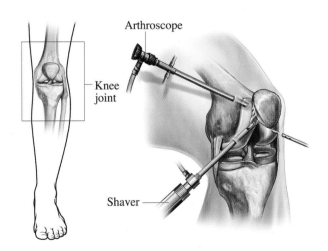

Arthroscopic knee surgery. *(PHOTOTAKE, Inc./Alamy)*

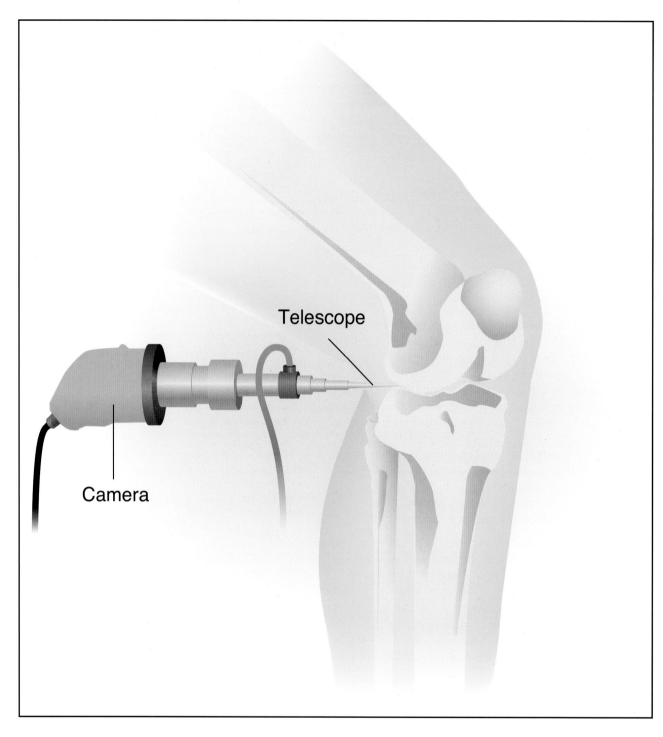

An arthroscope uses optical fibers to form an image of the damaged cartilage, which it sends to a television monitor that helps the surgeon perform surgery. *(Illustration by Argosy Inc. Cengage Learning, Gale.)*

when the medical history, physical exam, x rays, and bone scanning examinations, such as MRI or CT, do not provide a definitive diagnosis. Corrective arthroscopic surgery is used primarily to remove bone or cartilage or repair tendons or ligaments.

Precautions

Diagnostic arthroscopic surgery is not recommended unless nonsurgical treatment does not fix the problem.

Description

Arthroscopic surgery is performed most commonly on the knees, and also on ankles, shoulders, wrists, elbows, and hips. Knee joints are large enough to allow free movement of arthroscopic instruments and therefore are ideal for the benefits of this type of examination and treatment. The technique is valued because it allows surgeons to see inside the joint through incisions as tiny as a quarter of an inch (about 1 cm) rather than the large incisions that open surgery procedures require. The accuracy of arthroscopy is said to be 100% for diagnosis compared to diagnostic imaging such as MRI. Arthroscopic surgery may be used to relieve mechanical joint problems, such as buckling, stiffness, or locking, and can preclude or delay the need for more aggressive surgery such as a joint replacement.

In arthroscopic surgery, an orthopedic surgeon uses a pencil-sized arthroscope—a fiber-optic instrument fitted with a lens, a light source, and a miniature video camera—to see inside a joint. Advanced fiber optics allow even more detail to be seen than in open surgery, often identifying problems that may have been difficult to diagnose with other methods. The arthroscope transmits highlighted images of the structures to a television monitor in the **operating room**. The surgeon is able to view the entire examination, getting a full view of the joint, its cartilage, and surrounding tissue. The type and extent of the injury can be determined and repair or correction can be performed if necessary. Some of the most common joint problems diagnosed and treated with arthroscopic surgery are:

- synovitis (inflamed joint lining) of the knee, shoulder, elbow, wrist, or ankle
- injuries to the shoulder, such as rotator cuff tendon tears, impingement syndrome, and dislocations
- injuries to the knee, such as meniscal (cartilage) tears, wearing down of or injury to the cartilage cushion, and anterior cruciate ligament tears with instability
- injuries to the wrist, such as carpal tunnel syndrome
- loose bodies of bone and/or cartilage in the knee, shoulder, elbow, ankle, or wrist
- joint damage caused by rheumatoid arthritis or osteoarthritis

Arthroscopic procedures are performed in a hospital or outpatient surgical facility by an orthopedic surgeon. The type of anesthesia used (local, spinal, or general) varies, as does the length of the procedure; both depend on the joint that will be operated on, the type and extent of the suspected joint injury, and/or

---

KEY TERMS

Arthroscope—A pencil-sized fiber-optic instrument fitted with a lens, light source, and camera, used for detailed examination of joints.

Cartilage—The slippery tissue that covers the ends of joint bones.

Meniscal—Pertaining to cartilage.

Open surgery—Surgery using a large incision to lay open area for examination or treatment; in joint surgery, the whole joint is exposed.

Osteoarthritis—A degenerative "wear-and-tear" joint disease related to aging.

Rheumatoid arthritis—A chronic autoimmune disease characterized by inflammation of multiple joints and crippling effects.

Synovitis—Inflammation of the synovium, the thin membrane lining the joint.

---

the complexity of the anticipated repair. Arthroscopic surgery rarely takes more than an hour. Most patients who have arthroscopic surgery, whether diagnostic or corrective, are discharged the same day of the procedure; some patients, depending on the complexity of the surgery or their postoperative condition, may stay in the hospital one or two days.

Considered the most important orthopedic development in the twentieth century, arthroscopic surgery is widely used. The American Association of Orthopedic Surgeons reports that it is performed by 80% of all orthopedic surgeons. The use of arthroscopic surgery on famous athletes has been well publicized. Although arthroscopic surgery was initially only a diagnostic tool used prior to open surgery, the availability of better instruments and techniques has encouraged its use to actually treat a variety of joint problems, often avoiding more complicated surgeries with longer recovery times. New techniques under development are likely to lead to other joints being treated with arthroscopic surgery in the future. Laser technology has been introduced as a treatment option in arthroscopic surgery and other advanced technologies are being explored.

Surgical procedure

After making two small incisions about the size of a buttonhole in the skin near the joint, the surgeon injects sterile sodium chloride solution through one incision into the joint to expand it for better viewing and movement of the instruments. The surgeon will

---

also use this access to irrigate (flood with fluid) the joint area during surgery and to suction blood and debris away from the joint. This irrigation, or "washing" part of the procedure, is believed to be of value in itself, improving joint function. The arthroscope is then inserted into the second incision. While looking at the interior of the joint on the television monitor, the surgeon can determine the extent or type of injury and, if necessary, take a biopsy specimen or repair or treat the problem. A third tiny incision may be made in order to see other parts of the joint or to insert additional instruments, such as laser or tiny scalpels, when repairs or corrections need to be made. Arthroscopic surgery can be used to remove floating bits of cartilage, to debride (clean by removing tissue or bone), and to treat minor tears and other disorders. When the procedure is finished, the arthroscope is removed and the joint is once again irrigated. The site of the incision is dressed with compression **bandages** (ace bandages).

Diagnosis/Preparation

Prior to arthroscopy, the patient's medical history will be reviewed and the patient will have a complete **physical examination**. Standard preoperative blood and urine tests will be done as well as scans of the affected joint, such as MRI (**magnetic resonance imaging**), CT (computed tomography), and arthrogram (an x ray using dye). In some cases, an **exercise** regimen or muscle stimulation treatment (TENS) may be recommended to strengthen muscles around the joint prior to surgery. Surgeons may recommend preoperative guidelines, such as:

- Discontinue aspirin and anti-inflammatory medications two weeks before surgery.
- Stop smoking to encourage postoperative healing.
- Inform the surgeon if any fever or other illness occurs, or if cuts, scratches, or bruises appear near the surgical site before the scheduled surgery.
- Do not eat, drink, or chew gum for 12 hours prior to surgery.
- Bring crutches or a walker if hip, knee, or ankle arthroscopy is being performed.
- Wear loose fitting clothing to allow for bulky dressings over the surgical site.

Aftercare

Immediately after the procedure, the patient will spend up to two hours in a recovery area before being discharged. Some patients may be transferred to a hospital room if the surgeon determines overnight care is necessary. The surgical site will be dressed with a compression bandage (ace bandage) or a tightly fitting stocking (support hose). An ice pack will be placed on the joint that was examined or treated by arthroscopy. This treatment may continue for up to 72 hours after surgery to keep swelling down and help prevent the formation of clots. Pain medication will be administered if needed, although most patients require little or no medicine for pain. **Dressings** can usually be removed the morning after surgery and replaced by adhesive strips. The surgeon should be notified if the patient experiences any increase in pain, swelling, redness, drainage or bleeding at the site of the surgery, signs of infection (headache, muscle aches, dizziness, fever), and nausea or vomiting.

It takes several days for the puncture wounds to heal, and several weeks for the joint to fully recover. Many patients can resume their daily activities, including going back to work, within a few days of the procedure. Muscle strength must be regained as soon as possible after surgery to help support the affected joint. A rehabilitation program, including physical therapy, may be suggested to speed recovery and improve the functioning of the joint. The surgeon's recommendations for recovery may include:

- Keep the surgical site and the dressings clean and dry.
- Use ice packs for up to 72 hours to reduce pain and swelling.
- Elevate the affected joint (wrist, elbow, ankle, knee) on pillows; exercise gently to encourage circulation.
- Use a knee brace or shoulder sling temporarily.
- Allow weight-bearing exercise as able.

Risks

Few complications are to be expected with arthroscopy. Those that may occur occasionally (fewer than 1% of all arthroscopies, according to the American Academy of Orthopedic Surgeons) are infection, blood clot formation, swelling or bleeding, or damage to blood vessels or nerves. Rare instrument breakage during procedures has also been reported.

> ## WHO PERFORMS THE PROCEDURE AND WHERE IS IT PERFORMED?
>
> Arthroscopic surgery is performed in a hospital operating room or an outpatient surgical facility by an orthopedic surgeon.

QUESTIONS TO ASK THE DOCTOR

- Why is arthroscopy necessary for me?
- What kind of anesthesia will I have?
- How often do you perform this procedure? What results are typical?
- How much discomfort can I expect short term? Long term?
- Will physical therapy be necessary after the surgery?
- Will this procedure correct my joint problem?

Normal results

Most patients undergo arthroscopic surgery as an outpatient and are home within hours or at most a day or two. Pain and complications are rare, and most patients will enjoy improved mobility as they recover over a period of days, possibly with the aid of physical therapy and gentle exercise.

Some people undergoing arthroscopy may have preexisting conditions and diseases that will affect the surgical result. Recovery times will vary depending on each patient's overall condition. Certain problems may need to be treated with a combination of arthroscopic and open surgical procedures.

Alternatives

Alternatives to arthroscopic surgery include:

- changing activities to those less strenuous or demanding
- anti-inflammatory medications
- physical therapy and appropriate, gentle exercise such as yoga
- wearing a brace or using a walking aid
- glucosamine sulfate and chondroitin to reduce pain and stiffness
- therapeutic massage, acupuncture, or other body work

Resources

BOOKS

Canale, S. T., ed. *Campbell's Operative Orthopaedics*. 10th ed. St. Louis: Mosby, 2003.

DeLee, J. C., and D. Drez. *DeLee and Drez's Orthopaedic Sports Medicine*. 2nd ed. Philadelphia: Saunders, 2005.

PERIODICALS

Committee on Ethics and Standards of the Arthroscopy Association of North America. "Suggested guidelines for the practice of arthroscopic surgery." *Arthroscopy* (June 2005): A3668.

ORGANIZATIONS

American Academy of Orthopedic Surgeons(AAOS). 6300 North River Road, Rosemont, IL 60018. (800) 346-AAOS. http://www.aaos.org (accessed March 6, 2008).

Institute for Bone and Joint Disorders. 2222 East Highland Avenue, Phoenix, AZ 85016; 602-553-3113. http://www.ibjd.com (accessed March 6, 2008).

Cooke, K. V. "Arthroscopy for Rheumatoid Arthritis." September 5, 2002 [cited April 2003]. http://www.laurushealth.com (accessed March 6, 2008).

"Joint Irrigation for Osteoarthritis." Ivanhoe Newswire 5(2003): 20–26 [cited April 2003]. http://www.ivanhoe.com/newsalert (accessed March 6, 2008).

Lori De Milto
L. Lee Culvert
Rosalyn Carson-DeWitt, MD

Artificial sphincter insertion

Definition

Artificial sphincter insertion surgery is the implantation of an artificial valve in the genitourinary tract or in the anal canal to restore continence and psychological well being to individuals with urinary or anal sphincter insufficiency that leads to severe urinary or fecal incontinence.

Purpose

This procedure is useful for adults and children who have severe incontinence due to lack of muscle contraction by either the urethral sphincter or the bowel sphincter. The primary work of the lower urinary tract and the colon is the storage of urine and waste, respectively, until such time as the expulsion of urine or feces is appropriate. These holding and expelling functions in each system require a delicate balance of tension and relaxation of muscles, especially those related to conscious control of the act of urination or defecation through the valve-like sphincter in each system. Both types of incontinence have mechanical causes related to reservoir adequacy and sphincter, or "gatekeeper" control, as well as mixed etiologies in the chemistry, neurology, and psychology of human makeup. The simplest bases of incontinence lie in the mechanical components of reservoir mobility

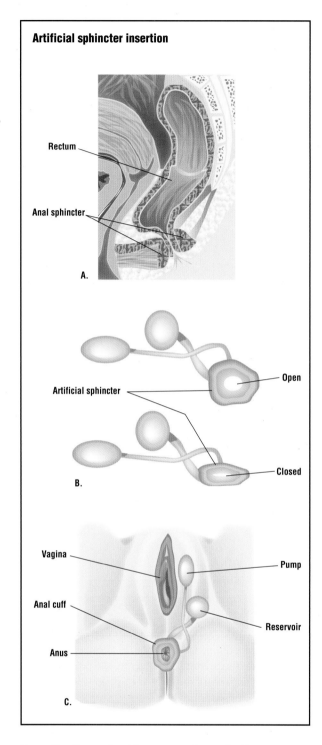

Artificial sphincter insertion

Rectum

Anal sphincter

A.

Artificial sphincter

Open

Closed

B.

Vagina

Pump

Anal cuff

Reservoir

Anus

C.

Normally, the anal sphincter muscles maintain fecal continence (A). In cases of incontinence, an artificial sphincter may be inserted, which can open and close to mimic the function of the natural sphincter (B). Once implanted, the patient uses a pump under the skin to inflate and deflate the anal cuff (C).

(Illustration by GGS Information Services. Cengage Learning, Gale.)

and sphincter muscle tone. These two factors receive the most surgical attention for both urinary and fecal incontinence.

Urinary sphincter surgery

There are four sources of urinary incontinence related primarily to issues of tone in pelvic, urethral, and sphincter muscles. Most urinary incontinence is caused by leakage when stress is applied to the abdominal muscles by coughing, sneezing, or exercising. Stress incontinence results from reduced sphincter adequacy in the ability to keep the bladder closed during movement. Stress incontinence can also be related to the mobility of the urethra and whether this reservoir for urine tilts, causing spilling of urine. The urethral cause of stress incontinence is treated with other surgical procedures. A second form of incontinence is urge incontinence. It relates to sphincter overactivity, or sphincter hyperflexia, in which the sphincter contracts uncontrollably, causing the patient to urinate, often many times a day. Finally, there is urinary incontinence due to an inadequately small urethra that causes urine overflow. This is known as overflow incontinence and can often be treated with augmentation to the urethra to increase its size.

Only severe stress incontinence related to sphincter adequacy can benefit from the artificial urinary sphincter. This includes conditions that result in the removal of the sphincter. Sphincter deficiency can result directly from pelvic fracture; urethral reconstruction; prostate surgeries; spinal cord injury; neurogenic bladder conditions that include sphincter dysfunction; and some congenital conditions. Each can warrant consideration for a sphincter implant.

Implantation surgery related to urinary sphincter incompetence is also called artificial sphincter insertion or inflatable sphincter insertion. The artificial urinary sphincter (AUS) is a small device placed under the skin that keeps pressure on the urethra until there is a decision to urinate, at which point a pump allows the urethra to open and urination commences. Since the 1990s, advances in prostate cancer diagnosis and surgery have resulted in radical prostatectomies being performed, with urinary incontinence rates ranging from 3–60%. The AUS has become a reliable treatment for this main source of urinary incontinence in men. Women with intrinsic sphincter deficiency, or weakened muscles of the sphincter, also benefit from the AUS. However, the use of AUS with women has declined with advances in the use of the sub-urethral sling due to its useful "hammock" effect on the sphincter and its high rates of continence success. Women with neurologenic incontinence can benefit from the AUS.

Artificial anal sphincter surgery

Fecal incontinence is the inability to control bowel function. The condition can be the result of a difficult childbirth, colorectal disease such as Crohn's disease, accidents involving neurological injuries, surgical resection for localized cancer, or by other neurological disorders. Severe fecal incontinence may, depending upon the underlying disease, require surgical intervention that can include repair of the anal sphincter, **colostomy**, or replacement of the anal sphincter. Artificial anal sphincter is a very easy-to-use device implanted under the skin that mimics the function of the anal sphincter.

Demographics

Artificial urinary sphincter surgery

According to the Agency for Health Care Policy and Research, urinary incontinence affects approximately 13 million adults. Men have incontinence rates that are much lower than women, with a range of 1.5–5%, compared to women over 65 with rates of almost 50%. In older men, prostate problems and their treatments are the most common sources of incontinence. Incontinence is a complication in nearly all male patients for the first three to six months after radical prostatectomy. A year after the procedure, most men regain continence. Stress incontinence occurs in 1–5% of men after the standard treatment for severe benign prostatic hyperplasia.

Artificial anal sphincter surgery

According to the National Institute of Diabetes & Digestive & Kidney Diseases (NIDDK), more than 6.5 million Americans have fecal incontinence. Fecal incontinence affects people of all ages. It is estimated that over 2% of the population is affected by fecal incontinence. Many cases are never reported. Community-based studies reveal that 30% of patients are over the age of 65, and 63% are female. According to one study published in the *American Journal of Gasteronology,* only 34% of incontinent patients have ever mentioned their problem to a physician, even though 23% wear absorbent pads, 12% are on medications, and 11% lead lives restricted by their incontinence. Women are more than five times as likely as men to have fecal incontinence, primarily due to obstetric injury, especially with forceps delivery and anal sphincter laceration. Fecal incontinence is frequent in men who have total and subtotal prostatectomies. Fecal incontinence is not a part of aging, even though it affects people over 65 in higher numbers than other populations.

Description

Artificial urinary sphincter surgery

The artificial urinary sphincter is an implantable device that has three components:

- an inflatable cuff
- a fluid reservoir (balloon)
- a semiautomatic pump that connects the cuff and balloon

Open surgery is the major form of surgery for the implant. Infections are minimized by sterilization of the urine preoperatively and preoperative bowel preparation. The pelvic space is entered from the abdomen or from the vagina, with **general anesthesia** for the patient. Broad-spectrum **antibiotics** are given intravenously and at the site of small incisions for the device. A urinary catheter is put into place. The cuff is implanted around the bladder neck and secured and passed through the rectus muscle and anterior fascia to be connected later to the pump. A space is fashioned to hold the balloon in the pubic region, and a pump is placed in a pouch below the abdomen. The artificial urinary sphincter is activated only after six to eight weeks to allow healing from the surgery. The patient is trained in the use of the device by understanding that the cuff remains inflated in its "resting state," and keeps the urethra closed by pressure, allowing continence. Upon the decision to urinate, the patient temporarily deflates the cuff by pressing the pump. The urethra opens and the bladder empties. The cuff closes automatically.

Artificial anal sphincter surgery

The artificial anal sphincter is an implantable device that has three components:

- an inflatable cuff
- a fluid reservoir (balloon)
- a semiautomatic pump that connects the cuff and balloon

In open abdominal surgery, the implant device is placed beneath the skin through small incisions within the pelvic space. One incision is placed between the anus and the vagina or scrotum, and the inflatable cuff is put around the neck of the anal sphincter. A second incision at the lower end of the abdomen is used to make a space behind the pubic bone for placement of the balloon. The pump is placed in a small pocket beneath the labia or scrotum, using two incisions. The artificial anal sphincter is activated only after six to eight weeks to allow healing from the surgery. The patient is trained in the use of the device by understanding that the anal cuff remains inflated in its "resting state," and keeps the anal canal closed by pressure, allowing continence. Upon the decision to have a bowel movement, the patient temporarily deflates the cuff by pressing the pump and fecal matter is released. The balloon re-inflates after the movement.

Diagnosis/Preparation

Artificial urinary sphincter surgery

Patients must be chosen carefully, exhibit isolated sphincter deficiency, and be motivated and able to work with the device and its exigencies. To characterize the condition to be treated and to determine outcomes, full clinical, urodynamic, and radiographic evaluations are necessary. The ability to distinguish mobility of the urethra as the cause of incontinence from sphincter insufficiency is difficult, but very important in the decision for surgery. A combination of pelvic examination for urethral hypermobility and a leak-point pressure as measured by coughing or other abdominal straining has been shown to be very effective in identifying the patient who needs the surgical implant. Visual examination of the bladder with a cystoscope is very important in the preoperative evaluation for placement of the sphincter. Urethral and bladder conditions found by the examination should be addressed before implantation. Previous reconstruction or repair of the urethra may prevent implantation of the cuff. In open abdominal surgery, the implant surgery uses preventive infection measures that are very important, including sterilization of the urine preoperatively with antibiotics, the cleansing of the intestines from fecal matter and

secretions through **laxatives** immediately prior to surgery, and antibiotic treatment and vigorous irrigation of the wound sites.

Artificial anal sphincter surgery

Since only a limited number of patients with fecal incontinence would benefit from an artificial sphincter, it is very important that a thorough examination be performed to distinguish the causes of the incontinence. A medical history and physical, as well as documented entries or an incontinence diary are crucial to the diagnosis of fecal incontinence. The physical exam usually includes a visual inspection of the anus and the area lying between the anus and genitals for hemorrhoids, infections, and other conditions. The strength of the sphincter is tested by the doctor probing with a finger to test muscle strength.

Medical tests usually include:

- Anorectal manometry. This is a long tube with a balloon on the end that is inserted in the anus and rectum to measure the tightness of the anal sphincter and the ability to respond to nerve firings.
- Anorectal ultrasonography. This test also includes an insertion of a small instrument into the anus with a video screen that produces sound waves, picturing the rectum and anus.
- X rays. A substance called barium is used to make the rectum walls visible to x ray. This liquid is swallowed by the patient before the test.
- Anal electromyography. This test uses the insertion of tiny needle electrodes into muscles around the anus and tests for nerve damage.

Aftercare

Artificial urinary sphincter surgery

Surgery requires a few days of hospitalization. Oral and intravenous pain medications are administered, along with postoperative antibiotics. A general diet is available, usually on the evening of surgery. When the patient is able to walk, the urethral catheter is removed. Patients are discharged on the second day postoperatively, unless they have had other procedures and need extra recovery time. Patients may not lift heavy objects or engage in strenuous activity for approximately six weeks. After six to eight weeks, the patient returns to the physician for training in the use of the implant device.

Artificial anal sphincter surgery

Surgery hospitalization requires a few days with dietary restrictions and anti-diarrheal medicine to bind the bowels. Antibiotics are administered to lower the risk of infection, and skin incisions are cleaned frequently. Patients may not lift heavy objects or engage in strenuous activity for approximately six weeks. After the body has had time to heal over six to eight weeks, the patient returns to the physician for training in the use of the pump. Two or three sessions are required and after the training, the patient is encouraged to lead as normal a life as possible.

Normal results

Artificial urinary sphincter surgery

One problem with the urinary sphincter implant is failure. If the device fails, or the cuff erodes, the surgery must be repeated. In a study published in 2001, 37% of women had the implant after an average of seven years, but 70% had the original or a replacement and 82% were continent. Studies on men report similar findings. Malfunction has improved with advances in using a narrower cuff. In one large study encompassing one surgeon over 11 years, the re-operative rate of AUS related to malfunction in men was 21%. Over 90% of patients were alive with a properly functioning device.

Another problem with the surgery is urinary voiding. This may be difficult initially due to postoperative edema caused by bruising of the tissue. In the majority of cases, urination occurs after swelling has receded.

AUS is a good alternative for children. The results of AUS in children range from 62–90%, with similar rates for both girls and boys.

Artificial anal sphincter surgery

Anal sphincter implant surgery has been successfully performed for many years. The device most often used has a cumulative failure rate of 5% over 2.5 years. The long-term functional outcome of artificial anal sphincter implantation for severe fecal incontinence has not been determined. However, adequate sphincter function is recovered in most cases, and the removal rate of the device is low. Most of the good results are dependent upon careful patient selection and appropriate surgical and operative management with a highly experienced **surgical team**.

Morbidity and mortality rates

Artificial urinary sphincter surgery

Infection has been a frequent and serious complication of surgery, not only because of the infection per

se, but also because infection can cause erosion of the urethra or bladder neck under the implant. The infection may actually worsen the incontinence. The overall infection rate with AUS implants is 1–3%. Because of interactions between the host and the foreign body represented by the implant, infections can occur soon after the surgery, or months and even years later. New techniques using antibiotics and skin preparations have improved infection rates considerably.

Artificial anal sphincter surgery

This surgery is for a limited number of patients who have isolated sphincter deficiency. Patients must be chosen who have little co-morbidity (serious illnesses) and can be trained in the use of the pump. Although it is a fairly simple operation, some researchers report a 30% infection rate.

Alternatives

Artificial urinary sphincter surgery

Milder forms of urinary incompetence can be treated with changes in diet, evaluation of medications, and the use of antidepressants and estrogen replacement, as well as bladder training and pelvic muscle strengthening. However, sphincter deficiency, unlike incontinence caused by urethral mobility, requires a substitute for the sphincter contraction by implant or by auxiliary tissue. If AUS cannot treat sphincter deficiency, the sling or "hammock" procedure is a good second choice. It brings tightness to the sphincter by using tissue under the urethra to increase contractual function. The **sling procedure** is already preferred over the AUS for women.

Artificial anal sphincter surgery

Milder forms of fecal incontinence are being treated by changes in diet and the use of certain bowel-binding medications. For some forms of mild fecal incontinence, special forms of **exercise** can help to strengthen and tone the pelvic floor muscles, along with providing **biofeedback** to train the muscles to work with an appropriate schedule. Only after these measures have been tried, including the use of pads, is the patient counseled on the benefits of an anal sphincter implant.

Resources

BOOKS

Walsh, P., et al. Campbell's Urology, 9th Edition. St. Louis: Elsevier Science, 2006.

PERIODICALS

Michot, F. "Artificial Anal Sphincter in Severe Fecal Incontinence: Outcome of Prospective Experience with 37 Patients in One Institution." Annals of Surgery, 237, no. 1 (January 1, 2003): 52–56.

Rotholtz, N. A., and S. D. Wexner. "Surgical Treatment of Constipation and Fecal Incontinence." Gastroenterology Clinics, 30, no. 01 (March 2001).

ORGANIZATIONS

American Society of Colon and Rectal Surgeons. 85 W. Algonquin Rd., Suite 550, Arlington Heights, IL 60005. <http://fascrs.org.>.

National Institute of Diabetes and Digestive and Kidney Diseases. (800) 891-5390 (kidney); (800) 860-8747 (diabetes); (800) 891-5389 (digestive diseases). http://www2.niddk.nih.gov.

National Association of Incontinence. www.nafc.org.

OTHER

Fecal Incontinence. National Institute of Diabetes & Digestive & Kidney Diseases (NIDDK). www.niddk.nih.gov/health/digest/pubs/fecalincon/fecalincon.htm.

Incontinence in Men. Health and Age. http://www.healthandage.com/Home/%21gm%3D20%21gsq%3Dincontinence%2Bin%2Bmen%21gid2=816.

Urinary Incontinence. WebMD Patient Handout. www.MDconsult.com.

Urinary Incontinence in Women. National Institute of Diabetes & Digestive & Kidney Diseases (NIDDK). http://kidney.niddk.nih.gov/kudiseases/pubs/uiwomen/.

Nancy McKenzie, PhD
Laura Jean Cataldo, RN, EdD

Ascending contrast phlebography *see* **Phlebography**

Ascites shunt *see* **Peritoneovenous shunt**

Aseptic technique

Definition

Aseptic technique is a set of specific practices and procedures performed by health-care personnel under carefully controlled conditions with the goal of minimizing contamination by pathogens.

Purpose

Aseptic technique is employed to maximize and maintain asepsis, the absence of pathogenic organisms, in the clinical setting. The goals of aseptic technique are to protect the patient from infection and to prevent the spread of pathogens. Often, practices that clean (remove dirt and other impurities), sanitize (reduce the number of microorganisms to safe levels), or disinfect (remove most microorganisms but not highly resistant ones) are not sufficient to prevent infection.

The Centers for Disease Control and Prevention (CDC) estimates that over 27 million surgical procedures are performed in the United States each year. Surgical site infections are the third most common nosocomial (hospital-acquired) infection and are responsible for longer hospital stays and increased costs to the patient and hospital. Aseptic technique is vital in reducing the morbidity and mortality associated with surgical infections.

Description

Aseptic technique can be applied in any clinical setting. Pathogens may introduce infection to the patient through contact with the environment, personnel, or equipment. All patients are potentially vulnerable to infection, although certain situations further increase vulnerability, such as extensive burns or immune disorders that disturb the body's natural

KEY TERMS

Clean—To remove dirt and other impurities.

Contamination—A breach in the preservation of a clean or sterile object or environment.

Disinfect—To remove most microorganisms but not highly resistant ones.

Host—A living organism that harbors or potentially harbors infection.

Immunocompromised—Lacking or deficient in defenses provided by the immune system, usually due to disease state or a side effect of treatment.

Invasive—Involving entry into the body.

Nosocomial—Occurring in the hospital or clinical setting.

Pathogen—A disease-causing organism.

Resistant organisms—Organisms that are difficult to eradicate with antibiotics.

Sanitize—To reduce the number of microorganisms to safe levels.

Sterile—Completely free of pathogens.

defenses. Typical situations that call for aseptic measures include surgery and the insertion of intravenous lines, urinary catheters, and drains.

Asepsis in the operating room

Aseptic technique is most strictly applied in the **operating room** because of the direct and often extensive disruption of skin and underlying tissue. Aseptic technique helps to prevent or minimize postoperative infection.

PREOPERATIVE PRACTICES AND PROCEDURES. The most common source of pathogens that cause surgical site infections is the patient. While microorganisms normally colonize parts in or on the human body without causing disease, infection may result when this endogenous flora is introduced to tissues exposed during surgical procedures. In order to reduce this risk, the patient is prepared or prepped by shaving hair from the surgical site; cleansing with a disinfectant containing such chemicals as iodine, alcohol, or chlorhexidine gluconate; and applying sterile drapes around the surgical site.

In all clinical settings, handwashing is an important step in asepsis. The "2002 Standards, Recommended Practices, and Guidelines" of the Association of Perioperative Registered Nurses (AORN) states that proper handwashing can be "the single most important measure to reduce the spread of microorganisms." In general settings, hands are to be washed when visibly soiled, before and after contact with the patient, after contact with other potential sources of microorganisms, before invasive procedures, and after removal of gloves. Proper handwashing for most clinical settings involves removal of jewelry, avoidance of clothing contact with the sink, and a minimum of 10–15 seconds of hand scrubbing with soap, warm water, and vigorous friction.

A surgical scrub is performed by members of the **surgical team** who will come into contact with the sterile field or sterile instruments and equipment. This procedure requires use of a long-acting, powerful, antimicrobial soap on the hands and forearms for a longer period of time than used for typical handwashing. Institutional policy usually designates an acceptable minimum length of time required; the CDC recommends at least two to five minutes of scrubbing. Thorough drying is essential, as moist surfaces invite the presence of pathogens. Contact with the faucet or other potential contaminants should be avoided. The faucet can be turned off with a dry paper towel, or, in many cases, through use of a foot pedal. An important principle of aseptic technique is that fluid (a potential mode of pathogen transmission) flows in the direction of gravity. With this in mind, hands are held below elbows during the surgical scrub and above elbows following the surgical scrub. Despite this careful scrub, bare hands are always considered potential sources of infection.

Sterile surgical clothing or protective devices such as gloves, face masks, goggles, and transparent eye/face shields serve as barriers against microorganisms and are donned to maintain asepsis in the operating room. This practice includes covering facial hair, tucking hair out of sight, and removing jewelry or other dangling objects that may harbor unwanted organisms. This garb must be put on with deliberate care to avoid touching external, sterile surfaces with nonsterile objects including the skin. This ensures that potentially contaminated items such as hands and clothing remain behind protective barriers, thus prohibiting inadvertent entry of microorganisms into sterile areas. Personnel assist the surgeon to don gloves and garb and arrange equipment to minimize the risk of contamination.

Donning sterile gloves requires specific technique so that the outer glove is not touched by the hand. A large cuff exposing the inner glove is created so that the glove may be grasped during donning. It is essential to avoid touching nonsterile items once sterile gloves are applied; the hands may be kept interlaced to avoid inadvertent contamination. Any break in the glove or touching the glove to a nonsterile surface requires immediate removal and application of new gloves.

Asepsis in the operating room or for other invasive procedures is also maintained by creating sterile surgical fields with drapes. Sterile drapes are sterilized linens placed on the patient or around the field to delineate sterile areas. Drapes or wrapped kits of equipment are opened in such a way that the contents do not touch nonsterile items or surfaces. Aspects of this method include opening the furthest areas of a package first, avoiding leaning over the contents, and preventing opened flaps from falling back onto contents.

Equipment and supplies also need careful attention. Medical equipment such as **surgical instruments** can be sterilized by chemical treatment, radiation, gas, or heat. Personnel can take steps to ensure sterility by assessing that sterile packages are dry and intact and checking sterility indicators such as dates or colored tape that changes color when sterile.

INTRAOPERATIVE PRACTICES AND PROCEDURES. In the operating room, staff have assignments so that those who have undergone surgical scrub and donning of sterile garb are positioned closer to the patient. Only scrubbed personnel are allowed into the sterile field. Arms of scrubbed staff are to remain within the field at all times, and reaching below the level of the patient or turning away from the sterile field are considered breaches in asepsis.

Other "unscrubbed" staff members are assigned to the perimeter and remain on hand to obtain supplies, acquire assistance, and facilitate communication with outside personnel. Unscrubbed personnel may relay equipment to scrubbed personnel only in a way that preserves the sterile field. For example, an unscrubbed nurse may open a package of forceps in a sterile fashion so that he or she never touches the sterilized inside portion, the scrubbed staff, or the sterile field. The uncontaminated item may either be picked up by a scrubbed staff member or carefully placed on to the sterile field.

The environment contains potential hazards that may spread pathogens through movement, touch, or proximity. Interventions such as restricting traffic in the operating room, maintaining positive-pressure airflow (to prevent air from contaminated areas from entering the operating room), or using low-particle generating garb help to minimize environmental hazards.

Other principles that are applied to maintain asepsis in the operating room include:

- All items in a sterile field must be sterile.
- Sterile packages or fields are opened or created as close as possible to time of actual use.
- Moist areas are not considered sterile.
- Contaminated items must be removed immediately from the sterile field.
- Only areas that can be seen by the clinician are considered sterile (i.e., the back of the clinician is not sterile).
- Gowns are considered sterile only in the front, from chest to waist and from the hands to slightly above the elbow.
- Tables are considered sterile only at or above the level of the table.
- Nonsterile items should not cross above a sterile field.
- There should be no talking, laughing, coughing, or sneezing across a sterile field.
- Personnel with colds should avoid working while ill or apply a double mask.
- Edges of sterile areas or fields (generally the outer inch) are not considered sterile.
- When in doubt about sterility, discard the potentially contaminated item and begin again.
- A safe space or margin of safety is maintained between sterile and nonsterile objects and areas.
- When pouring fluids, only the lip and inner cap of the pouring container is considered sterile; the pouring container should not touch the receiving container, and splashing should be avoided.
- Tears in barriers and expired sterilization dates are considered breaks in sterility.

Other clinical settings

A key difference between the operating room and other clinical environments is that the operating area has high standards of asepsis at all times, while most other settings are not designed to meet such standards. While clinical areas outside of the operating room generally do not allow for the same strict level of asepsis, avoiding potential infection remains the goal in every clinical setting. Observation of medical aseptic practices will help to avoid nosocomial infections. The application of aseptic technique in such settings is termed medical asepsis or clean technique (rather than surgical asepsis or sterile technique required in the operating room).

Specific situations outside of the operating room require a strict application of aseptic technique. Some of these situations include:

- wound care
- drain removal and drain care
- intravascular procedures
- vaginal exams during labor
- insertion of urinary catheters
- respiratory suction

For example, a surgical dressing change at the bedside, though in a much less controlled environment than the operating room, will still involve thorough handwashing, use of gloves and other protective garb, creation of a sterile field, opening and introducing packages and fluids in such a way as to avoid contamination, and constant avoidance of contact with nonsterile items.

General habits that help to preserve a clean medical environment include:

- safe removal of hazardous waste, i.e., prompt disposal of contaminated needles or blood-soaked bandages to containers reserved for such purposes
- prompt removal of wet or soiled dressings
- prevention of accumulation of bodily fluid drainage, i.e., regular checks and emptying of receptacles such as surgical drains or nasogastric suction containers
- avoidance of backward drainage flow toward patient, i.e., keeping drainage tubing below patient level at all times
- immediate clean-up of soiled or moist areas
- labeling of all fluid containers with date, time, and timely disposal per institutional policy
- maintaining seals on all fluids when not in use

The isolation unit is another clinical setting that requires a high level of attention to aseptic technique. Isolation is the use of physical separation and strict aseptic technique for a patient who either has a contagious disease or is immunocompromised. For the patient with a contagious disease, the goal of isolation is to prevent the spread of infection to others. In the case of respiratory infections (i.e., tuberculosis), the isolation room is especially designed with a negative pressure system that prevents airborne flow of pathogens outside the room. The severely immunocompromised patient is placed in reverse isolation, where the goal is to avoid introducing any microorganisms to the patient. In these cases, attention to aseptic technique is especially important to avoid spread of infection in the hospital or injury to the patient unprotected by sufficient immune defenses. Entry and exit from the isolation unit involves careful handwashing, use of protective barriers like gowns and gloves, and care not to introduce or remove potentially contaminated items. Institutions supply specific guidelines that direct practices for different types of isolation, i.e., respiratory versus body fluid isolation precautions.

In a multidisciplinary setting, all personnel must constantly monitor their own movements and practices, those of others, and the status of the overall field to prevent inadvertent breaks in sterile or clean technique. It is expected that personnel will alert other staff when the field or objects are potentially contaminated. Health care workers can also promote asepsis by evaluating, creating, and periodically updating policies and procedures that relate to this principle.

Resources

PERIODICALS

Mangram, Alicia, Teresa Horan, Michele Pearson, Leah Christine Silver, and William Jarvis. "Guideline for Prevention of Surgical Site Infection, 1999." Infection Control and Hospital Epidemiology 20 (April 1999): 247–78.

Pittet, Didier. "Improving Adherence to Hand Hygiene Practice: A Multidisciplinary Approach." Emerging Infectious Diseases 7 (March/April 2001).

ORGANIZATIONS

Association of Perioperative Registered Nurses (AORN). 2170 South Parker Road, Suite 300, Denver, CO 80231-5711. (303) 755-6300 or (800) 755-2676. http://www.aorn.org.

Centers for Disease Control and Prevention (CDC). 1600 Clifton Road, Atlanta, GA 30333. (404) 639-3534 or (800) 311-3435. http://www.cdc.gov.

OTHER

Pyrek, Kelly. "2008 Industry Report: Infection Prevention Industry Update." Infection Control Today December 2007. http://www.infectioncontroltoday.com/articles/2008-industry-report.html.

Bjerke, Nancy. "Hand Hygiene in Healthcare: Playing by the New Rules." Infection Control Today February 2003 [cited February 2008]. http://www.infectioncontroltoday.com/articles/400/400_321bpract.html.

Dix, Kathy. "Observing Standard Precautions in the OR." Infection Control Today October 2002 [cited February 2008]. http://www.infectioncontroltoday.com/articles/2a1topics.html.

Osman, Cathy. "Asepsis and Aseptic Practices in the Operating Room." Infection Control Today July 2000 [cited February 2008]. http://www.infectioncontroltoday.com/articles/071best.html.

Katherine Hauswirth, APRN
Stephanie Dionne Sherk
Laura Jean Cataldo, RN, EdD

Aspartate aminotransferase test

Definition

The aspartate aminotransferase test measures levels of AST, an enzyme released into the blood when certain organs or tissues, particularly the liver and heart, are injured. Aspartate aminotransferase (AST) is also known as serum glutamic oxaloacetic transaminase (SGOT).

Purpose

The determination of AST levels aids primarily in the diagnosis of liver disease. In the past, the AST test was used to diagnose heart attack (myocardial infarction or MI) but more accurate blood tests have largely replaced it for cardiac purposes.

Demographics

The number of AST tests administered each year can only be estimated. Since statins are the most prescribed drugs in the United States and standards of care call for quarterly **liver function tests**, the number of ASTs can easily exceed 500 million per year.

Description

AST is determined by analysis of a blood sample, usually taken from a venipuncture site at the bend of the elbow.

AST is found in the heart, liver, skeletal muscle, kidney, pancreas, spleen, lung, red blood cells, and brain tissue. When disease or injury affects these tissues, the cells are destroyed and AST is released into the bloodstream. The amount of AST is directly related to the number of cells affected by the disease or injury, but the level of elevation depends on the length of time that the blood is tested after the injury. Serum AST levels become elevated eight hours after cell injury, peak at 24–36 hours, and return to normal in three to seven days. If the cellular injury is chronic (ongoing), AST levels will remain elevated.

One of the most important uses for AST determination has formerly been in the diagnosis of a heart attack, or MI. AST can assist in determining the timing and extent of a recent MI, although it is less specific than **creatine phosphokinase (CPK)**, CK-MB, myoglobin, troponin, and lactic dehydrogenase (LDH). Assuming no further cardiac injury occurs, the AST level rises within 6–10 hours after an acute attack, peaks at 12–48 hours, and returns to normal in three to four days.

Myocardial injuries such as angina (chest pain) or pericarditis (inflammation of the pericardium, the membrane around the heart) do not increase AST levels.

AST is also a valuable aid in the diagnosis of liver disease. Although not specific for liver disease, it can be used in combination with other enzymes to monitor the course of various liver disorders. Chronic, silent hepatitis (hepatitis C) is sometimes the cause of elevated AST. In alcoholic hepatitis, caused by excessive alcohol ingestion, AST values are moderately elevated; in acute viral hepatitis, AST levels can rise to over 20 times normal. Acute extrahepatic (outside the liver) obstruction, such as gallstones, produces AST levels that can quickly rise to 10 times normal, and then rapidly fall. In cases of cirrhosis, the AST level is related to the amount of active inflammation of the liver. Determination of AST also assists in early recognition of toxic hepatitis that results from exposure to drugs toxic to the liver, like **acetaminophen** and cholesterol-lowering medications.

Other disorders or diseases in which the AST determination can be valuable include acute pancreatitis, muscle disease, trauma, severe burn, and infectious mononucleosis.

Preparation

The physician may require discontinuation of any drugs that might affect the test. These types include such drugs as antihypertensives (for treatment of high blood pressure), coumarin-type anticoagulants (blood-thinning drugs), digitalis, erythromycin (an antibiotic), oral contraceptives, and opiates, among others. The patient may also need to cut back on strenuous activities temporarily, because **exercise** can also elevate AST for a day or two.

Aftercare

This test involves blood being drawn, usually from a vein in the elbow. The person being tested should keep the wound from the needle puncture covered (with a bandage) until the bleeding stops. Individuals should report any unusual symptoms to their physician.

Risks

Risks for this test are minimal, but may include slight bleeding from the blood-drawing site, fainting or feeling lightheaded after venipuncture, or hematoma (blood accumulating under the puncture site).

Normal results

Normal ranges for the AST are laboratory-specific, but can range from 3–45 units/L (units per liter).

Abnormal results

Striking elevations of AST (400–4000 units/L) are found in almost all forms of acute hepatic necrosis, such as viral hepatitis and carbon tetrachloride poisoning. In alcoholics, even moderate doses of the analgesic acetaminophen have caused extreme elevations (1,960–29,700 units/L). Moderate rises of AST are seen in jaundice, cirrhosis, and metastatic carcinoma. Approximately 80% of patients with infectious mononucleosis show elevations in the range of 100–600 units/L.

Morbidity and mortality rates

Morbidity rates are excessively miniscule. The most common problems are minor bleeding and bruising. Since neither are reportable events, morbidity can only be estimated. Mortality is essentially zero.

Alternatives Resources

There are no alternatives to an aspartate aminotransferase test.

Precautions

The only precaution needed is to clean the venipuncture site with alcohol.

Side effects

The most common side effects of an AST test are minor bleeding and bruising.

Interactions

There are no known interactions with an AST test.

Resources

BOOKS

Fischbach, F. T. and M. B. Dunning. *A Manual of Laboratory and Diagnostic Tests,* 8th ed. Philadelphia: Lippincott Williams & Wilkins, 2008.

McGhee, M. *A Guide to Laboratory Investigations,* 5th ed. Oxford, UK: Radcliffe Publishing Ltd., 2008.

Price, C. P. *Evidence-Based Laboratory Medicine: Principles, Practice, and Outcomes,* 2nd ed. Washington, DC: AACC Press, 2007.

Scott, M. G., A. M. Gronowski, and C. S. Eby. *Tietz's Applied Laboratory Medicine,* 2nd ed. New York: Wiley-Liss, 2007.

Springhouse Corp. *Diagnostic Tests Made Incredibly Easy!,* 2nd ed. Philadelphia: Lippincott Williams & Wilkins, 2008.

PERIODICALS

Inoue, K., M. Matsumoto, Y. Miyoshi, and Y. Kobayashi. "Elevated liver enzymes in women with a family history of diabetes." *Diabetes Research in Clinical Practice* 79, no. 3 (February 2008): e4–e7.

Kansu, A. "Treatment of chronic hepatitis B in children." *Recent Patents on Anti-Infectious Drug Discoveries* 3, no. 1 (January 2008): 64–69.

Lampe, E., C. F. Yoshida, R. V. De Oliveira, G. M. Lauer, and L. L. Lewis-Ximenez. "Molecular analysis and patterns of ALT and hepatitis C virus seroconversion in haemodialysis patients with acute hepatitis." *Nephrology (Carlton)* 13, no. 3 (June 2008): 186–192.

Lazo, M., E. Selvin, and J. M. Clark. "Brief communication: clinical implications of short-term variability in liver function test results." *Annals of Internal Medicine* 148, no. 5 (March 2008): 348–352.

OTHER

American Clinical Laboratory Association. Information about clinical chemistry. http://www.clinical-labs.org/ (February 24, 2008).

Clinical Laboratory Management Association. Information about clinical chemistry. http://www.clma.org/ (February 22, 2008).

Lab Tests Online. Information about lab tests. http://www.labtestsonline.org/ (February 24, 2008).

National Accreditation Agency for Clinical Laboratory Sciences. Information about laboratory tests. http://www.naacls.org/ (February 25, 2008).

ORGANIZATIONS

American Association for Clinical Chemistry, 1850 K Street, NW, Suite 625, Washington, DC, 20006, (800) 892-1400, http://www.aacc.org/AACC/.

American Society for Clinical Laboratory Science, 6701 Democracy Blvd., Suite 300, Bethesda, MD, 20817, (301) 657-2768, http://www.ascls.org/.

American Society for Clinical Pathology, 1225 New York Ave., NW, Suite 250, Washington, DC, 20005, (202) 347-4450, http://www.ascp.org/.

College of American Pathologists, 325 Waukegan Rd., Northfield, IL, 60093-2750, (800) 323-4040, http://www.cap.org/apps/cap.portal.

L. Fleming Fallon, Jr., M.D., Dr.P.H.

Aspirin

Definition

Aspirin is a medication given to relieve pain and reduce fever. The name "aspirin" was originally a trademark, first used when the drug was introduced in Europe in 1899. Aspirin was developed by a German chemist named Felix Hoffman as a treatment for his father's arthritis.

Purpose

Aspirin is still used to relieve many kinds of minor aches and pains—headaches, toothaches, muscle pain, menstrual cramps, joint pains associated with arthritis, and the general achiness that many people experience with colds and flu. Some people take aspirin daily to reduce the risk of stroke, heart attack, or other heart problems.

Description

Aspirin, also known as acetylsalicylic acid, is not a prescription drug. It is sold over the counter in many forms, from the familiar white tablets to chewing gum and rectal suppositories. Coated, chewable, buffered, and extended-release forms are available. Many other over-the-counter (OTC) medications contain aspirin. Alka-Seltzer Original Effervescent Antacid Pain Reliever (R), for example, contains aspirin for pain relief as well as sodium bicarbonate to relieve acid indigestion, heartburn, and sour stomach.

Aspirin belongs to a group of drugs called salicylates. Other members of this group include sodium salicylate, choline salicylate, and magnesium salicylate. These drugs are more expensive and no more effective than aspirin; however, they are preferred by some patients who find that aspirin upsets their stomach. Aspirin is quickly absorbed into the bloodstream and provides rapid and relatively long-lasting pain relief. Aspirin in high doses also reduces inflammation. Researchers believe these effects are due to aspirin's ability to block the production of pain-producing chemicals called prostaglandins.

In addition to relieving pain and reducing inflammation, aspirin also lowers fever by acting on the

---

KEY TERMS

Diuretic—A type of medication that increases the amount of urine produced and relieves excess fluid buildup in body tissues. Diuretics may be used in treating high blood pressure, lung disease, premenstrual syndrome, and other conditions.

Inflammation—A response to injury or illness characterized by pain, redness, swelling, and warmth.

Nonsteroidal anti-inflammatory drugs (NSAIDs)—Drugs that relieve pain and reduce inflammation but are not related chemically to cortisone. Common drugs in this class are aspirin, ibuprofen (Advil, Motrin), naproxen (Aleve, Naprosyn), ketoprofen (Orudis), and several others.

Polyp—Any mass of tissue that grows out of a mucous membrane in the digestive tract, uterus, or elsewhere in the body.

Prostaglandin—A hormonelike chemical produced in the body that has a variety of effects. Prostaglandins may be responsible for the production of some types of pain and inflammation.

Reye's syndrome—A life-threatening disease that affects the liver and the brain and sometimes occurs after a viral infection, such as flu or chickenpox. Children or teenagers who are given aspirin for flu or chickenpox are at increased risk of developing Reye's syndrome.

Rhinitis—Inflammation of the membranes inside the nose.

Salicylates—A group of drugs that includes aspirin and related compounds. Salicylates are used to relieve pain, reduce inflammation, and lower fever.

Stroke—An event that impairs the circulation of the brain. Ischemic stroke is caused by a blood clot in the brain. Hemorrhagic stroke is caused by bleeding into the brain.

---

hypothalamus, which is the part of the brain that regulates temperature. The brain then signals the blood vessels to dilate (widen), which allows heat to leave the body more quickly.

Recommended dosage

Adults

PAIN RELIEF OR FEVER REDUCTION. The usual dosage is one to two tablets every three to four hours, up to six times per day.

RISK REDUCTION FOR STROKE. One tablet four times a day or two tablets twice a day.

RISK REDUCTION FOR HEART ATTACK. Aspirin may be used as a first-line treatment for a heart attack. The patient should chew a single uncoated aspirin tablet, since chewing makes it easier for the body to absorb the medication rapidly. Aspirin will not stop a heart attack, and proper emergency care is essential; however, an aspirin tablet may reduce the amount of damage done by the heart attack.

Patients should check with a physician for the proper dose and number of times per week they should take aspirin to reduce the risk of a heart attack. The most common dose for this purpose is a single baby aspirin tablet taken daily. Enteric-coated aspirin is often used, since it reduces the risk of stomach irritation.

Children

Parents should consult the child's physician about the proper dosage for their child's condition.

Precautions

Aspirin—even children's aspirin—should never be given to children or teenagers with flu-like symptoms or chickenpox. Aspirin can cause Reye's syndrome, a life-threatening condition that affects the nervous system and liver. As many as 30% of children and teenagers who develop Reye's syndrome die. Those who survive may have permanent brain damage.

Parents should consult a physician before giving aspirin to a child under 12 years of age for arthritis, rheumatism, or any condition that requires long-term use of the drug.

No one should take aspirin for more than 10 days in a row unless instructed to do so by a physician. Anyone with fever should not take aspirin for more than three days without a physician's advice. In addition, no one should take more than the recommended daily dosage.

People in the following categories should not use aspirin without first checking with their physician:

- Pregnant women. Aspirin can cause bleeding problems in both the mother and the developing fetus. Aspirin can also cause the infant's weight to be too low at birth.
- Women who are breastfeeding. Aspirin can pass into breast milk and affect the baby.
- People with a history of bleeding problems.

- People who are taking such blood-thinning drugs as warfarin (Coumadin).
- People who have had recent surgery. Aspirin increases the risk of bleeding from an incompletely healed incision.
- People with a history of stomach ulcers.
- People with a history of asthma, nasal polyps, or both. Patients with these disorders are more likely to be allergic to aspirin.
- People who are allergic to fenoprofen, ibuprofen, indomethacin, ketoprofen, meclofenamate sodium, naproxen, sulindac, tolmetin, or an orange food coloring known as tartrazine. They may also be allergic to aspirin.
- People with AIDS or AIDS-related complex who are taking AZT (zidovudine). Aspirin can increase the risk of bleeding in these patients.
- People taking any of the drugs listed below under Interactions.
- People with liver damage or severe kidney failure.

Aspirin should not be taken before a surgical procedure, as it can increase the risk of excessive bleeding during surgery. People scheduled for an operation should check with their surgeon to find out when they should discontinue taking aspirin.

Aspirin can cause stomach irritation. Taking aspirin with food or milk, or drinking an eight-ounce glass of water with it may help to prevent damage to the stomach lining. Some patients find that using coated or buffered aspirin reduces the risk of stomach upset. Patients should be aware, however, that drinking alcoholic beverages can make the stomach irritation worse.

Patients with any of the following symptoms should stop taking aspirin immediately and call their physician:

- a sensation of ringing or buzzing in the ears
- hearing loss
- dizziness
- stomach pain that does not go away

Patients should discard any aspirin that has developed a vinegary smell. That is a sign that the medication is too old and ineffective.

Side effects

The most common side effects of aspirin include upset stomach, heartburn, loss of appetite, and small amounts of blood in the stool. Less common side effects are rashes, hives, fever, vision problems, liver damage, thirst, stomach ulcers, and bleeding. People with asthma, rhinitis, polyps in the nose, or allergies to aspirin may have trouble breathing after taking the drug.

Interactions

Aspirin may increase, decrease, or change the effects of many drugs. Aspirin can increase the toxicity of such drugs as methotrexate (Rheumatrex) and valproic acid (Depakote, Depakene). Taken with such blood-thinning drugs as warfarin (Coumadin) and dicumarol, aspirin can increase the risk of excessive bleeding. Aspirin counteracts the effects of certain other drugs, including angiotensin-converting enzyme (ACE) inhibitors and beta blockers, which lower blood pressure, and medicines used to treat gout (probenecid and sulfinpyrazone). Blood pressure may drop unexpectedly and cause fainting or dizziness if aspirin is taken along with nitroglycerin tablets. Aspirin may also interact with **diuretics**, diabetes medications, other **nonsteroidal anti-inflammatory drugs** (NSAIDs), seizure medications, and steroids. Anyone who is taking these drugs should ask his or her physician whether they can safely take aspirin.

Resources

BOOKS

"Factors Affecting Drug Response: Drug Interactions." Section 22, Chapter 301 in The Merck Manual of Diagnosis and Therapy, edited by Mark H. Beers, MD, and Robert Berkow, MD. Whitehouse Station, NJ: Merck Research Laboratories, 1999.

Wilson, Billie Ann, RN, PhD, Carolyn L. Stang, PharmD, and Margaret T. Shannon, RN, PhD. Nurses Drug Guide 2000. Stamford, CT: Appleton and Lange, 1999.

PERIODICALS

Cryer, B. "Gastrointestinal Safety of Low-Dose Aspirin." American Journal of Managed Care 8 (December 2002) (22 Suppl): S701-S708.

Grattan. C. E. "Aspirin Sensitivity and Urticaria." Clinical and Experimental Dermatology 28 (March 2003): 123-127.

MacDonald, T. M., and L. Wei. "Effect of Ibuprofen on Cardioprotective Effect of Aspirin." Lancet 361 (February 15, 2003): 573-574.

Nordenberg, Tamar. "'An Aspirin a Day'— Just Another Cliché?" FDA Consumer (March-April 1999): 2-4.

ORGANIZATIONS

American Society of Health-System Pharmacists (ASHP). 7272 Wisconsin Avenue, Bethesda, MD 20814. (301) 657-3000. www.ashp.org.

Aspirin Foundation of America. (800) 432-3247; fax (202) 737-8406. www.aspirin.org.

United States Food and Drug Administration (FDA). 5600 Fishers Lane, Rockville, MD 20857-0001. (888) INFO-FDA. www.fda.gov.

Nancy Ross-Flanigan
Sam Uretsky, PharmD
Fran Hodgkins

Atrial fibrillation surgery *see* **Maze procedure for atrial fibrillation**

Atrial septal defect surgery *see* **Heart surgery for congenital defects**

Autograft *see* **Skin grafting**

Autologous blood donation

Definition

Autologous **blood donation** is the process of donating one's own blood prior to an elective surgical or medical procedure to avoid or reduce the need for an allogeneic blood **transfusion** (from a volunteer blood donor).

Purpose

Blood transfusions are given to restore lost blood, to improve clotting time, and to improve the ability of the blood to deliver oxygen to the body's tissues. There are some disadvantages to traditional allogeneic blood transfusions. Although strict regulations are in place to ensure correct matching by blood type, errors in this process can lead to the transfusion of mismatched blood, which can cause a serious and sometimes fatal adverse reaction called transfusion reaction. In addition, while donated blood is rigorously tested for infectious agents such as human immunodeficiency virus (HIV) and hepatitis, there is always a chance that an infectious disease may be transmitted via allogeneic transfusion.

The donation and transfusion of autologous blood has arisen as an alternative to allogeneic blood transfusion. Autologous donation is indicated for an elective surgical or medical procedure in which the likelihood of a blood transfusion is high. Such procedures include surgery on the heart, blood vessels, bones, and chest.

Some of the advantages of autologous blood donation include:

KEY TERMS

Allogeneic blood transfusion—Blood that has originated from volunteer blood donor (i.e., not the patient).

Directed donation—Blood donated by a patient's family member or friend, to be used by the patient.

Vasovagal reaction—A collection of symptoms that includes dizziness, fainting, profuse sweating, hyperventilation, and/or low blood pressure that occurs in a small percentage of individuals who donate blood.

- The patient is assured that the blood is an exact match to his or her blood type, thereby avoiding transfusion reaction.
- There is no risk of inadvertently transmitting infectious agents.
- Autologous blood donations supplement the community blood supply.
- The process of donating blood promotes blood cell production by bone marrow.
- The patient is often reassured by the knowledge that his or her own blood will be used if a blood transfusion becomes necessary.

Some disadvantages to autologous blood donation do exist, which include:

- Contamination of autologous blood with infectious agents is possible during the donation process.
- There is a possibility that a patient's blood will be mislabeled or that allogeneic blood will be inadvertently transfused.
- Autologous blood donation costs more to process and store.
- Blood may be transfused unnecessarily because an autologous blood supply exists.
- Unused units of autologous blood are usually disposed of; approximately 44% of autologous donations remain unused after surgery.

Demographics

Autologous blood donations account for approximately 5% of all blood donated in the United States each year.

Description

The most common form of autologous donation is called preoperative autologous blood donation (PABD). PABD is generally indicated when there is a

reasonable chance that a blood transfusion will become necessary, when the patient is in adequate health to donate blood, and when there is sufficient preoperative time for the patient to donate. As the shelf life of liquid blood is approximately 42 days, the patient may begin donating up to six weeks before the scheduled procedure. It is generally recommended that a patient donate no more than once or twice a week, and no later than 72 hours before surgery.

The PABD process is similar to the process of donating allogeneic blood. A tourniquet is placed on the upper arm to increase the pressure in the arm veins and make them swell and become more accessible. Once a suitable vein is identified, the area where the needle will be inserted is sterilized by washing with soap solution or an iodine-containing antiseptic. The donor lies on a bed or cot during the procedure, which takes about 10 minutes. Blood is collected in sterile plastic bags that hold one pint (450 ml). The bags contain an anticoagulant to prevent clotting and preservatives to keep the blood cells alive.

The collected blood may then be transfused during and/or after surgery in a similar manner to allogeneic blood. If the amount transfused is less than anticipated or if no blood was necessary, then the autologous blood is generally disposed of (since the restrictions placed on volunteer donors are stricter than those on autologous donors). If the patient's surgery is postponed, the donated blood may be frozen and stored until the procedure is rescheduled.

Acute normo-volemic hemodilution (ANH) is a variant of autologous donation in which a volume of the patient's blood is removed directly before surgery and replaced with fluids so that any blood lost during surgery has a lower red blood cell count (i.e., the red blood cells have been diluted). The removed blood is then reinfused after surgery. Advantages to ANH are that no processing and storage costs are necessary and the risk of contamination during processing is reduced.

Blood may also be collected during surgery (intraoperative **blood salvage**, or IBS) or after surgery (postoperative blood salvage, PBS). IBS is commonly used during cardiac, bone, transplant, and trauma surgery and involves the use of specialized equipment to collect and process the blood before reinfusion. PBS involves the collection of blood from drainage tubes, although generally this volume is small.

Diagnosis/Preparation

Patients must meet certain selection criteria before donating their own blood for future use. In the case of

WHO PERFORMS THE PROCEDURE AND WHERE IS IT PERFORMED?

Blood may be donated at a hospital or a blood donor center. The procedure of blood donation is generally performed by a nurse or phlebotomist (a person trained to draw blood).

QUESTIONS TO ASK THE DOCTOR

- What is the chance that I will require a blood transfusion for my upcoming surgical procedure?
- Do I qualify to be an autologous blood donor?
- Where will blood collection take place and how many units should I donate?
- What will happen to my donated blood if my surgery is postponed or cancelled?

PABD, there must be sufficient time before the procedure to safely collect enough blood. A patient must be medically stable, have no active infection, and have a close-to-normal red blood cell count to quality for PABD.

Aftercare

Individuals who donate blood are generally given fluids and/or light refreshments to prevent possible side effects such as dizziness and nausea. Iron supplements may be prescribed to prevent or treat anemia (low red blood cell count).

Risks

Complications associated with autologous blood donation are similar to those associated with allogeneic blood donation. These include dizziness, fainting, profuse sweating, hyperventilation, and/or low blood pressure. (This collection of symptoms is called a vaso-vagal response.) Among patients with heart disease, there is an increased risk of cardiac complications after donating blood.

Risks associated with autologous blood transfusion include transfusion reaction if an allogeneic blood transfusion was inadvertently given and transmission of infectious agents if the blood became contaminated. Symptoms of transfusion reaction include general discomfort, anxiety, breathing difficulties, dizziness, itching, fever, headache, rash, and swelling. Patients who are given too much blood can develop high blood pressure, which is a concern for people who have heart disease. Very rarely, an air embolism is created when air is introduced into a patient's veins through the tubing used for intravenous infusion.

Normal results

If a patient loses enough blood during a surgical or medical procedure to warrant a blood transfusion, a transfusion of autologous blood will under normal circumstances confer the same benefits as a transfusion of allogeneic blood with none of the associated risks (i.e., transfusion reaction or transmission of infectious agents).

Morbidity and mortality rates

One study found the risk of a complication requiring hospitalization to be one in approximately 17,000 among autologous blood donors, and one in approximately 200,000 among volunteer blood donors. The most common complication is a vasovagal reaction, although approximately 12% of patients requiring hospitalization have angina (chest pain resulting from inadequate supply of oxygen to the heart). There is a higher chance of a vasovagal reaction with autologous blood donation than with allogeneic blood donation.

Alternatives

Allogeneic blood is a more commonly used alternative to autologous blood and accounts for 95% of all blood donations in the United States. Patients may also choose to have blood donated by family or friends, a process called directed donation. For patients who are interested in avoiding a blood transfusion, alternatives include:

- Volume expanders. Certain fluids (saline, Ringer's lactate solution, dextran, etc.) may be used to increase the volume of blood.
- Blood substitutes. Much research is currently being done into compounds that can replace some or all of the functions of blood components. One such compound, called HBOC-201, or Hemopure, is derived from bovine (cow) blood and is showing promise as a substitute for red blood cell transfusion.
- Bloodless surgery. It may be possible to avoid excessive blood loss through careful planning prior to surgery. Specialized instruments can minimize the amount of blood lost during a procedure.

Resources

BOOKS

AABB Perioperative Standards Unit.Standards for Perioperative Autologous Blood Collection and Administration, 3rd Edition. Amer Assn of Blood Banks, 2007.

PERIODICALS

Henry, D. A., et al. "Pre-operative Autologous Donation for Minimizing Perioperative Allogeneic Blood Transfusion." Cochrane Review, Issue 1 (January 20, 2003).

Vanderlinde, Elizabeth S., Joanna M. Heal, and Neil Blumberg. "Autologous Transfusion." British Medical Journal, 324 (March 30, 2002): 772–5.

ORGANIZATIONS

American Association of Blood Banks. 8101 Glenbrook Rd., Bethesda, MD 20814. (301) 907-6977. http://www.aabb.org/content.

American Red Cross. 431 18th St., NW, Washington, DC 20006. (202) 639-3520. http://www.redcross.org.

OTHER

"Autologous Blood as an Alternative to Allogeneic Blood Transfusion." American Association of Blood Banks, January 2002 [cited March 19, 2003]. http://www.aabb.org/Content/About_Blood/FAQ/.

"Preoperative Autologous Blood Donation (PABD)." Health Technology Advisory Committee, September 2000 [cited March 19, 2003]. http://www.health.state.mn.us/htac/pabd.htm.

"Transfusion Alert: Use of Autologous Blood." National Heart, Lung, and Blood Institute, [cited March 19, 2003]. http://www.nhlbi.nih.gov/health/prof/blood/transfusion/logo.htm.

Stephanie Dionne Sherk
Laura Jean Cataldo, RN, EdD

Automatic implantable cardioverter-defibrillator *see* **Implantable cardioverter-defibrillator**

Axillary dissection

Definition

Axillary dissection is a surgical procedure that incises (opens) the armpit (axilla or axillary) to identify, examine, or remove lymph nodes (small glands, part of the lymphatic system, which filters cellular fluids).

Purpose

Axillary dissection is utilized to stage breast cancer in order to determine the necessity of further treatment based on cancer cell spread. Additionally, axillary dissection includes removal and pathological examination of axillary lymph nodes for persons having operable breast cancer. The anatomy of the axilla is complex and composed of several critical nerves, arteries, and muscles. Because of this complex anatomy and connection with the breast, the axilla is a common route for possible metastatic (cancer cell spread to distant areas within the body) involvement from breast cancer. The absence or presence of cancer cells in axillary lymph nodes is the most power prognostic (outcome) indicator for breast cancer. Axillary dissection is an accurate procedure for axillary node assessment (removal and pathological examination). Clinical examination of the breast (more specifically palpation, or feeling the affected area for lumps) for the axillary region is inaccurate and unreliable. The only method to identify whether or not a lymph node has cancer cells, is to surgically remove the node and perform examination with a microscope to detect abnormal cancer cells.

Demographics

If axillary dissection is not performed, recurrence of cancer in the armpit is common even after breast surgery. Recent evidence suggests that persons who underwent **lumpectomy** alone without axillary dissection had a 10-year average recurrence rate of 28% in the axilla. Generally, recent evidence also suggests that the more nodes and tissues removed in the axilla, the lower the risk of recurrence of cancer. Research also indicates that 10-year axillary cancer recurrence rates are low (10% for node negative and 3% for node positive) for women who have **mastectomy** and axillary node removal. The recurrence rate for breast cancer is approximately 17% for women who did not have axillary node removal.

Description

Lymph nodes (or lymph glands) are filtering centers for the lymphatic system (a system of vessels that collects fluids from cells for filtration and reentry into the blood). Additionally, there is a complex arrangement of muscles, tissues, nerves and blood vessels. Axillary dissection is surgically explained in terms of three levels. Level I axillary dissection is also called lower axillary dissection because it is the removal of all tissue below the axillary vein and extending to the side where the axillary vein crosses the tendon of a muscle called the latissimus dorsi. Level II dissection is continuous—it includes the removal of level tissues and further extensive removal of

Axillary dissection

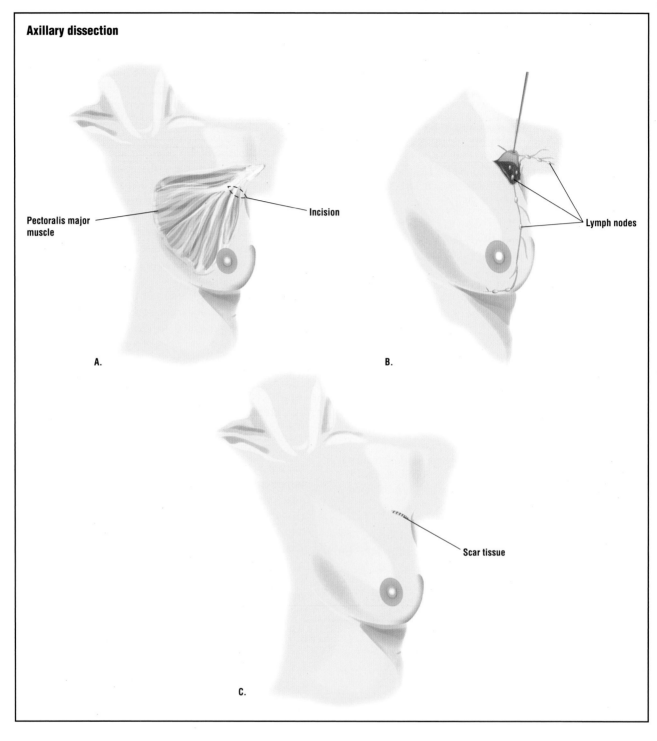

Pectoralis major
muscle

Incision

A.

Lymph nodes

B.

Scar tissue

C.

To determine the advancement of breast cancer, lymph nodes in the armpit are removed. An incision is made (A), and lymph nodes are removed and tested (B), leaving a small scar (C). *(Illustration by GGS Information Services. Cengage Learning, Gale.)*

cancerous tissues. Level II dissection removes diseased tissues deeper in the middle (medial) area of another muscle called the pectoralis minor. Level III dissection is the most aggressive breast cancer axillary surgery, and it entails the removal of all nodal tissue (tissues related to the lymphatic system) from the axilla.

KEY TERMS

Axillary vein—A blood vessel that takes blood from tissues back to the heart to receive oxygenated blood.

Latissimus dorsi—In Latin, this muscle literally means "widest of the back." This is a large fan-shaped muscle that covers a wide area of the back.

Lymph nodes—Small masses of lymphoid tissue that are connected to lymphatic vessels.

Lymphatic system—Part of the cardiovascular system, lymphatic vessels will bring fluids from cells (cellular debris) for filtration in lymph nodes. Filtered fluid is returned back to the blood circulation.

Lymphedema—Retention of lymph fluid in an affected (affected by surgery or disease) area.

Pectoralis minor—A triangular-shaped muscle in front of (anterior) the axilla.

Tendon—Connective tissue that attaches muscle to bone.

Diagnosis/Preparation

Operable breast cancer is the primary indication for axillary dissection. Persons receiving this surgery have been diagnosed with breast cancer and are undergoing surgical removal of the breast. Diagnosis of breast cancer typically involves palpation of a lump (mass), and other tests such as **mammography** (special type of x ray used to visualize deep into breast tissues) and biopsy. The specific diagnosis to estimate the extent of axillary (cancerous) involvement can be made by performing a sentinel node biopsy. The sentinel node is the first lymph node that drains fluid from the primary tumor site. If there is no presence of cancerous cells in the sentinel node, the likelihood that higher echelon lymph nodes have cancer is very small. Conversely, if cancerous cells are detected in the sentinel node, then axillary dissection is recommended.

Preparation for axillary dissection is the same as that for **modified radical mastectomy**. This includes but is not limited to preoperative assessments (special tests and blood analysis), patient education, **postoperative care**, and follow-up consultations with surgeon and cancer specialist (medical hematologist/oncologist). Psychotherapy and/or community-centered support group meetings may also be beneficial to treatment.

WHO PERFORMS THE PROCEDURE AND WHERE IS IT PERFORMED?

The procedure is performed in a hospital equipped to perform major surgery. A general surgeon usually performs the operation with specialized formal training in surgical oncology (the specialty of surgery that provides surgical treatment for operable cancers).

Aftercare

One of the major problems that can result from axillary lymph node removal is lymphedema (fluid accumulation in the arm). Postoperative aftercare should include the use of compression garments, pneumatic compression pumps, and massage to combat fluid retention. Additionally, persons may have pain and should discuss this with the attending surgeon. Other surgical measures for aftercare should be followed similar to persons receiving a modified radical mastectomy. Skin care is important and caution should be exercised to avoid cuts, bites, and skin infections in the affected area. Further measures to control lymphedema can include arm exercises and maintenance of normal weight.

Risks

There are several direct risks associated with axillary surgery. A recent study indicated that approximately 31% of persons may have numbness and tingling of the hand and 10% develop carpal tunnel syndrome. In females who have had a previous breast surgery before the axillary surgery, recurrent wound infections and progression of lymphedema can occur. Additionally, persons may also feel tightness and heaviness in the arm as a result of lymphedema.

Normal results

Normal results can include limited but controlled lymphedema and adequate wound healing. Persons receiving axillary dissection due to breast cancer require several weeks of postoperative recovery to regain full strength.

Morbidity and mortality rates

Sickness and/or **death** are not necessarily related to axillary surgery per se. Rather, breast cancer outcome is related to breast cancer staging. Staging determined by axillary surgery can yield valuable information concerning

QUESTIONS TO ASK THE DOCTOR

- How do I prepare for the procedure?
- How long does it take to know the results?
- What postoperative care will be needed?
- What are the possible risks involved in this procedure?

disease progression. Early stage (stage I) breast cancer usually has a better outcome, whereas advance stage cancer (stage 4) is correlated with a 10-year survival rate.

Alternatives

Currently research does not support other therapies. Further study is required but other therapies are currently not recommended. There are no adequate alternatives to axillary surgery in breast cancer persons. The most recent evidence suggests that removal of lymph nodes and tissues in the armpit is correlated with elevated survival rates.

Resources

BOOKS

Hanna, L., Crosby, T., and Macbeth, F. Practical Clinical Oncology. 1st ed. Cambridge, UK: Cambridge University Press., 2008.

Noble, J. Textbook of Primary Care Medicine. 3rd ed. St. Louis, MO: Mosby, Inc., 2001.

Townsend, C., Beauchamp, D., Evers, B., and Mattox, K. Sabiston Textbook of Surgery. 18th ed. St. Louis: W. B. Saunders Company, 2007.

PERIODICALS

Cantin, J., H. Scarth, M. Levine, and M. Hugi. "Clinical practice guidelines for the care and treatment of breast cancer." Canadian Medical Association Journal 165 (July 24, 2001).

Fiorica, James. "Prevention and Treatment of Breast Cancer." Obstetrics and Gynecology Clinics 28 (December 2001).

Hugi,M. R., I. A. Olivotto, and S. R. Harris. "Clinical practice guidelines for the care and treatment of breast cancer:11.Lymphedema." Canadian Medical Association Journal 164 (January 23,2001).

ORGANIZATIONS

American Cancer Society. (800) ACS-2345. http://www.cancer.org.

Y-ME National Breast Cancer Organization. 212 W. Van Buren, Suite 500 Chicago, IL 60607. (312) 986-8338. Fax: (312) 294-8597. (800) 221-2141 (English). (800) 986-9505 (Español). <http:// http://www.y-me.org.

OTHER

Cancernews. [cited May 15, 2003]. http://www.cancernews.com.

Laith Farid Gulli, MD, MS
Nicole Mallory, MS, PA-C
Bilal Nasser, MD, MS
Laura Jean Cataldo, RN, EdD

B

Balloon angioplasty *see* **Angioplasty**

Balloon valvuloplasty

Definition

Balloon valvuloplasty, also called percutaneous balloon valvuloplasty, is a surgical procedure used to open a narrowed heart valve. The procedure is sometimes described as balloon enlargement of a narrowed heart valve.

Purpose

Balloon valvuloplasty is performed on children and adults who have a narrowed heart valve, a condition called stenosis. The goal of the procedure is to improve valve function and blood flow by enlarging the valve opening. It is sometimes used to avoid or delay open heart surgery and valve replacement.

There are four valves in the heart: aortic valve, pulmonary valve, mitral valve, and tricuspid valve. Each is located at the exit of one of the heart's four chambers. These valves open and close to regulate the blood flow from one chamber to the next and are vital to the efficient functioning of the heart and circulatory system. Balloon valvuloplasty is used primarily to treat pulmonary, mitral, and aortic valves when narrowing is present and medical treatment has not corrected or relieved the related problems. With mitral stenosis, for example, medical solutions are typically tried first, such as diuretic therapy (reducing excess fluid), anticoagulant therapy (thinning the blood and preventing blood clots), or blood pressure medications. Valvuloplasty is recommended for those patients whose symptoms continue to progress even after taking such medications for a period of time.

Valvular stenosis can be a congenital defect (develops in the fetus and is present at birth) or can be acquired, that is, it stems from other conditions. Mitral valve stenosis in adults, for example, is rarely congenital and is usually acquired, either a result of having rheumatic fever as a child or developing calcium obstruction in the valve later in life. Pulmonary stenosis is almost entirely congenital. Aortic stenosis usually does not produce symptoms until the valve is 75% blocked; this occurs over time and is consequently found in people between the ages of 40 and 70. Tricuspid stenosis is usually the result of rheumatic fever; it occurs less frequently than other valve defects.

Childhood symptoms of valve narrowing may include heart dysfunction, heart failure, blood pressure abnormalities, or a murmur. Adult symptoms will likely mimic heart disease and may include blood pressure abnormalities, shortness of breath, chest pain (angina), irregular heart beat (arrhythmia), or fainting spells (syncope). **Electrocardiogram** (EKG), x ray, and **angiography** (a special x-ray examination using dye in the vascular system) may be performed to identify valvular heart problems. Depending on the severity of symptoms, **cardiac catheterization** may also be performed to examine heart valve function prior to recommending a surgical procedure. Valvular **angioplasty** is performed in children and adults to relieve stenosis. While it offers relief, it does not always cure the problem, particularly in adults, and often valvotomy (cutting the valve leaflets to correct the opening) or valve replacement is necessary at a later date.

Demographics

Congenital heart-valve disease occurs in one of every 1,000 newborns and is thought to be caused by inherited factors. In 2–4% of valve problems, health or environmental factors affecting the mother during pregnancy are believed to contribute to the defect. Pulmonary valve stenosis represents about 10% of all congenital heart problems. About 5% of all cardiac defects is stenosis of the aortic valve. Valve abnormalities are diagnosed in children and adults of both sexes;

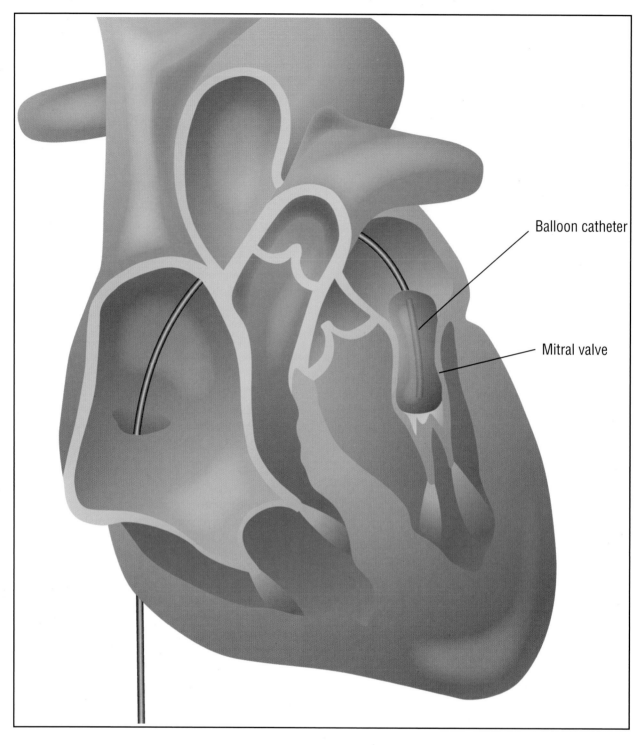

Balloon catheter

Mitral valve

The balloon at the end of the catheter spreads open the mitral valve, relieving the obstruction. *(Illustration by GGS Information Services. Cengage Learning, Gale.)*

80% of adult patients with stenosis are male, while most adults with mitral stenosis are women who had rheumatic fever as a child. Tricuspid stenosis is rarely found in North America or Europe.

Description

In balloon valvuloplasty, a thin tube (catheter) with a small deflated balloon at its tip (balloon-tipped

KEY TERMS

Cardiac catheterization—A minimally invasive technique that runs a catheter through veins into the heart to evaluate heart function. Fluoroscopy is used to observe the catheterization.

Dilate—To expand or open a valve or blood vessel.

Electrocardiography (EKG)—A method to measure the variations in the actions of the heart. An EKG machine produces wave-like patterns either on paper or on a monitor that can be used to diagnose irregularities in rhythm.

Stenosis—The narrowing of any valve, especially one of the heart valves or the opening into the pulmonary artery from the right ventricle.

Valve—Flaps (leaflets) of tissue in the passageways between the heart's upper and lower chambers.

catheter) is inserted through an incision in the skin in the groin area into a vein, and then is threaded up to the opening of the narrowed heart valve. The balloon is inflated to stretch the valve open and relieve the valve obstruction.

The procedure, which takes up to four hours, is performed in a cardiac catheterization laboratory that has a special x-ray machine and an x-ray monitor that looks like a regular TV screen. The patient will be placed on an x-ray table and covered with a sterile sheet. An area on the inside of the upper leg will be washed and treated with an antibacterial solution to prepare for the insertion of a catheter. The patient is given **local anesthesia** to numb the insertion site and will usually remain awake, able to watch the procedure on the monitor. After the insertion site is prepared and anesthetized, the cardiologist inserts a catheter into the appropriate blood vessel, and then passes the smaller balloon-tipped catheter through the first catheter. Guided by the x-ray monitor that allows visualization of the catheter in the blood vessel, the physician slowly threads the catheter up into the coronary artery to the heart. The deflated balloon is carefully positioned in the opening of the valve that is being treated, and then is inflated repeatedly, which applies pressure to dilate the valve. The inflated balloon widens the valve opening by splitting the valve leaflets apart. Once the valve is widened, the balloon-tipped catheter is removed. The other catheter remains in place for 6–12 hours because, in some cases, the procedure must be repeated. A double-balloon valvuloplasty procedure is often performed on certain high-

risk patients because it is considered more effective in restoring blood flow.

Preparation

For at least six hours before balloon valvuloplasty, the patient will have to avoid eating or drinking anything. An intravenous line is inserted so that medications (anticoagulants to prevent clot formation and radioactive dye for x rays) can be administered. The patient's groin area is shaved and cleaned with an antiseptic. About an hour before the procedure, the patient is given an oral sedative such as diazepam (Valium) to ensure that he or she will relax sufficiently for the procedure.

Aftercare

After balloon valvuloplasty, the patient will spend several hours in the **recovery room** to be monitored for **vital signs** (such as heart rate and breathing) and heart sounds. During this time, electrical leads attached to an EKG machine will be placed on the patient's chest and limbs, and a monitor will display the electrical impulses of the heart continuously, alerting nurses quickly if any abnormality occurs. For at least 30 minutes after removal of the catheter, direct pressure is applied to the site of insertion; after this, a pressure dressing will be applied. The skin condition is monitored. The insertion site will be observed for bleeding until the catheter is removed. The leg in which the catheter was inserted is temporarily prevented from moving. Intravenous fluids will be given to help eliminate the x-ray dye; intravenous anticoagulants or other medications may be administered to improve blood flow and to keep coronary arteries open. Pain medication is administered as needed. Some patients will continue to take anticoagulant medications for months or years after the surgery and will have regular blood tests to monitor the effectiveness of the medication.

Following **discharge from the hospital**, the patient can usually resume normal activities. After balloon valvuloplasty, lifelong follow-up is necessary because valves sometimes degenerate or narrowing recurs, a condition called restenosis, which will likely require repeat valvuloplasty, valvotomy, or valve replacement.

Risks

Balloon valvuloplasty can have serious complications. For example, the valve can become misshapen so that it does not close completely, which makes the condition worse. Embolism, where either clots or pieces of valve tissue break off and travel to the brain or the lungs causing blockage, is another possible risk. If the procedure causes severe damage to the valve leaflets, immediate valve replacement is required. Less frequent complications are bleeding and hematoma (a local collection of clotted blood) at the puncture site, abnormal heart rhythms, reduced blood flow, heart attack, heart puncture, infection, and circulatory problems. Because restenosis is frequent in adult patients with valvular disease, particularly when underlying heart disease or other conditions are present, the procedure is recommended only as an emergency rescue for high-risk patients who are not candidates for valve replacement.

Normal results

Balloon valvuloplasty is considered a safe, effective treatment in children with congenital stenosis, improving heart function and blood flow. In adults, balloon valvuloplasty may give temporary relief and improve heart function and blood flow, but underlying coronary artery disease or other disease conditions may encourage restenosis, making valve replacement eventually necessary. The most successful valvuloplasty results are achieved in treating narrowed pulmonary valves, although the treatment of mitral valve stenosis is also generally good. The aortic valve procedure is more difficult to perform and is generally less successful.

Resources

BOOKS

Khatri, V. P., and J. A. Asensio. *Operative Surgery Manual.* 1st ed. Philadelphia: Saunders, 2003.

Libby, P., et al. *Braunwald's Heart Disease.* 8th ed. Philadelphia: Saunders, 2007.

Townsend, C. M., et al. *Sabiston Textbook of Surgery.* 17th ed. Philadelphia: Saunders, 2004.

ORGANIZATIONS

American Heart Association. 7320 Greenville Ave. Dallas, TX 75231. (214) 373-6300. http://www.americanheart.org (accessed March 7, 2008).

Lori De Milto
L. Lee Culvert
Rosalyn Carson-DeWitt, MD

Bandages and dressings

Definition

Bandages and dressings are both used in wound management. A bandage is a piece of cloth or other material used to bind or wrap a diseased or injured part of the body. Usually shaped as a strip or pad, bandages are either placed directly against the wound or used to bind a dressing to the wound. A dressing can consist of a wide range of materials, sometimes containing medication, placed directly against the wound.

Purpose

The purposes served by dressings include protecting wounds; promoting healing; and providing, retaining, or removing moisture. Bandages can be used to hold dressings in place, to relieve pain, and generally to make the patient comfortable. Elastic bandages are useful to provide ongoing pressure on wounds such as varicose veins, fractured ribs, and swollen joints.

Description

In recent years, there have been tremendous advances in the design and composition of bandages and dressings. The field is becoming increasingly complex, and there are numerous reports of health care workers applying inappropriate products. Wound-care materials come in a wide variety of product classes, including the following:

- Alginate dressings. These are derived from brown seaweed and contain calcium alginate, which turns into a sodium alginate gel when it comes in contact with wound fluid. They are available as pads or ropes.

- Biosynthetic dressings. These are composites of biological (often animal-derived) and synthetic materials such as polymers.

- Collagen dressings. These are made from collagen, a protein obtained from cowhide, cattle tendons, or birds. They are available as particles or gels.

- Composite dressings. These are similar to plastic adhesive strips and include an adhesive border, a non-adhesive or semi-adhesive surface that is applied to the wound, an absorbent layer, and a bacterial barrier.

- Contact layers. A low-adherent layer of perforated or woven polymer material designed to stop a secondary absorbent dressing from sticking to the surface of a wound.

- Gauze. This woven fabric of absorbent cotton is available in a number of formats and materials, including cotton or synthetic, non-impregnated, and impregnated with water, saline, or other substances. Gauze is sold as surgical swabs, sheets, rolls, pads, sponges, and ribbon.

- Growth factors. These short-chain proteins affect specific target cells. They exist naturally in humans, and can be transplanted from one part of the body to another or manufactured outside the body.

- Hydrocolloid dressings. Used for leg ulcers, minor burns, pressure sores and traumatic injuries, these self-adhesive dressings form a gel as they absorb fluid from the wound. They consist of materials such as sodium carboxymethylcellulose (an absorbent), pectin, and gelatin that are attached to a foam sheet or a thin polyurethane film.

- Hydrofibers. Similar in appearance to cotton, carboxymethylcellulose fibers turn into a gel when they come into contact with wound fluid. They are available as ribbons or pads and are highly absorbent.

- Hydrogels. These are sold as sheets and in gel form, and are primarily used to supply moisture to wounds. Depending on the state of the tissue, they can either absorb fluid or moisten the wound. An electrically conductive aloe vera gel is available to provide electrotherapy to wounds.

- Hydropolymers. These foamed-gel products consist of multiple layers. The surface layer is designed to expand to fill the contours of a wound and, at the same time, draw away fluids.

- Leg compression/wrapping products. These are designed to apply external pressure to improve blood flow and resolve chronic edema in the feet and legs. They are available in a broad range of formats, including stockings, compression bandages, or pneumatic pump.

- Polyurethane foam dressings. These are sheets of foamed polymer solutions with small open chambers that draw fluids away from the wound. Some of these foam products offer adhesive surfaces. They are available as sheets and rolls, as well as in various other formats suitable for packing wounds.

- Skin substitutes. Also known as allografts or skin equivalents, these are obtained from human cells cultured and expanded in vitro from neonatal foreskins.

- Superabsorbents. These are particles, hydropolymers, or foams that act like the material inside diapers, with a high capacity for rapid absorption.

- Transparent films. These consist of a thin, clear polyurethane sheet that, on one side, has a special adhesive that does not stick to moist surfaces like those found on a wound. They prevent bacteria and fluids from entering the wound through the dressing, but allow limited circulation of oxygen.

- Wound fillers. These can be bought as powders or pastes, or in strands or beads. They are used to fill wounds and also absorb wound fluid.

- Wound pouches. Equipped with a special collection system for wounds that have a high flow of secretion, they are designed to contain odors and to be easily drained.

- Other assorted wound-care products. These include adhesive bandages, surgical tapes, adhesive skin closures, surgical swabs, paste bandages, specialty absorptive dressings, support bandages, retention bandages, elasticized tubular bandages, lightweight elasticized tubular bandages, foam-padded elasticized tubular bandages, and plain stockinettes.

Just as there is a large selection of bandage and dressing products to choose from, there is also a broad range of applications for these products:

- Alginate dressings are used on wounds that exude moderate to heavy amounts of fluid. They are useful for packing wounds, although strip-packing gauze may be preferable for deeper wounds because it is easier to retrieve. Common applications of alginate dressings include treatment of acute surgical wounds, leg ulcers, sinuses, and pressure sores. These dressings should not be used on third-degree burns. Neither are they advisable for wounds that are dry or are secreting only small amounts of fluid, because their powerful absorbing capability may dry out the wound. These are primary dressings that need be covered by a secondary dressing.

- Biosynthetic dressings are used on burns and other wounds. Another application is as a temporary dressing for skin autograft sites. Some persons may be allergic to these dressing materials.

- Collagen dressings are believed to hasten wound repair and are often used on stubborn wounds. They are most effective on wounds that contain no dead tissue. Collagen dressings should not be used in dry wounds, third-degree burns, or on any patient who is sensitive to bovine (cow) products.

- Composite dressings are sometimes used alone, sometimes in combination with other dressings. Deep wounds should first be packed with wound-filler material. These dressings should not be cut, and are not recommended for use on third-degree burns.

- Contact layers are designed for use in clean wounds that contain no dead tissue. They are not recommended for infected, shallow, dry, or infected wounds, or on third-degree burns.

- Gauze is used to pack wounds, and also for debridement and wicking. It is especially desirable for packing deep wounds. When using gauze to pack wounds, a loose packing technique is preferred.

- Growth factors. These have highly specific applications against such conditions as diabetic foot ulcers involving disease of the peripheral nerves. Growth factors are heat sensitive and often require refrigeration. These are not recommended for persons with benign or malignant tumors.

- Hydrocolloid dressings are used for leg ulcers, minor burns, pressure sores, and traumatic injuries. Because they are not painful to remove, hydrocolloid dressings are often employed in pediatric wound management. Because of their absorbent capabilities, they are used on wounds that are secreting light to moderate amounts of fluid.

- Hydrofibers are highly absorbent, so they are particularly useful for wounds that are draining heavily. For this reason, they are not recommended for dry wounds or wounds with little secretion, because they may result in dehydration. Hydrofibers should not be used as surgical sponges or on third-degree burns.

- Hydrogels are often used on wounds that contain dead tissue, on infected surgical wounds, and on painful wounds. They should not be used on wounds with moderate to heavy secretions. As with all dressings, it is important to check and follow the directions of the manufacturer. In the case of hydrogels, directions on some products indicate they are not to be used on third-degree burns.

- Hydropolymers are typically used on wounds with minimal to moderate drainage. They are not indicated for dry wounds or third-degree burns.

- Leg compression/wrapping products are used to increase blood flow and reduce edema in the lower extremities of the body. A medical doctor should be consulted before using these products on people with edema. In many cases, topical dressings are used under these products.

- Polyurethane foam dressings are very absorbent and are typically used on wounds with moderate to heavy secretions. They should not be used on third-degree burns or on wounds that are not draining or that have sinuses or tunneling.

- Skin substitutes are a relatively new product category, approved for treating venous leg ulcers. It is often advisable to cut slits in the artificial skin, so that wound secretions underneath do not lift the newly applied skin.

- Superabsorbents are employed on wounds that are secreting heavily, or in applications requiring extended wear. A packing material is commonly employed under this product. Superabsorbents should not be used on third-degree burns or wounds that are either dry or have minimal secretions.

- Transparent films are often employed as a secondary cover for another, primary dressing. They are used on superficial wounds and on intact skin at risk of infection. It is important to remove transparent films very carefully to avoid damaging fragile skin.

- Wound fillers are primary dressings that are usually used in conjunction with other, secondary dressings. Wound fillers are considered appropriate for shallow wounds with little or moderate secretions. They are not appropriate for use in third-degree burns or in dry wounds. They are similarly not recommended for wounds with tunnels or sinuses.

- Wound pouches are useful in treating wounds with high volumes of secretion. They are not suitable for dry wounds.

Recommended intervals between dressing changes vary widely among product classes. The materials used in some dressings require that they be changed several times a day. Others can remain in place for one week. Manufacturer's directions should be consulted and followed.

KEY TERMS

Debridement—Removing dead or non-viable tissue from a wound.

Edema—Swelling of body tissues, caused by collection of excess fluid.

Electrotherapy—The treatment of body tissues by passing electrical currents through them, stimulating the nerves and muscles.

Sinus—In the context of wound management, a narrow hollow in the body extending from an infected area to the surface of the skin.

Stockinette—A soft elastic material used for bandages and clothing for infants.

Preparation

Wounds require appropriate cleaning, **debridement**, closure, and medication before bandages and dressings are applied.

Determining the cause of wounds is often very important, especially the cause of chronic wounds such as skin ulcers. A physician should be advised of any signs of infection or other changes in a wound. Signs of infection may include redness around the wound site, fever, red streaks extending from the wound, yellow drainage from the wound, or a mal odor noted at the wound site.

Wound-care nursing is a rapidly advancing field that requires considerable training, clinical experience, and judgment, causing some observers to predict that it will eventually develop into an advanced practice nursing or a specialty-based practice. Increasingly, the demands on wound-care nurses are expected to require that they undertake graduate studies. For all nurses working in the field, ongoing education is a must to keep up with new knowledge, technologies, and techniques. Numerous organizations and institutions offer continuing education courses in **wound care** management.

Results

Wounds that receive appropriate and timely care are most likely to heal in an acceptable manner.

Resources

BOOKS

Brown, P., D. Oddo, and J. P. Maloy. Quick Reference to Wound Care. Boston: Jones & Bartlett Publishers, 2003.

Hodgetts, T., and Turner, L. Trauma Rules 2. Malden, MA: Blackwell Publishing Ltd, 2006.

Mani, Raj. Chronic Wound Management: The Evidence for Change. Boca Raton, FL: CRC Press, 2002.

Milne, C. T., L. Q. Corbett, and D. Duboc. Wound, Ostomy, and Continence Nursing Secrets.Philadelphia: Hanley & Belfus, 2002.

Peitzman, Andrew B. The Trauma Manual, 2nd Edition. Philadelphia: Lippincott Williams & Wilkins, 2002.

PERIODICALS

Atiyeh, B. S., K. A. El-Musa, and R. Dham. "Scar Quality and Physiologic Barrier Function Restoration after Moist and Moist-exposed Dressings of Partial-thickness Wounds." Dermatolic Surgery 29, no. 1 (2003): 14–20.

King, B. "Pain at First Dressing Change after Toenail Avulsion: The Experience of Nurses, Patients and an Observer: 1." Journal of Wound Care 12, no. 1 (2003): 5–10.

Ovington, Liza G., PhD. "Know Your Options for Secondary Dressings." Wound Care Newsletter 2, no. 4 (July 1997)[cited March 24, 2003]. <http://wwww.woundcare.org/newsvol2n4/prtpt2.htm.

Skelhorne, G., and H. Munro. "Hydrogel Adhesives for Wound-care Applications." Medical Device Technology 13, no. 9 (2002): 19–23.

St. Clair, K., and J. H. Larrabee. "Clean versus Sterile Gloves: Which to Use for Postoperative Dressing Changes?" Outcomes Management 6, no. 1 (2002): 17–21.

ORGANIZATIONS

American Academy of Family Physicians. 11400 Tomahawk Creek Parkway, Leawood, KS 66211-2672. (913) 906-6000. Email: fp@aafp.org. http://www.aafp.org.

American College of Physicians. 190 N. Independence Mall West, Philadelphia, PA 19106-1572. (800) 523-1546, x2600, or (215) 351-2600. http://www.acponline.org.

American Medical Association. 515 N. State Street, Chicago, IL 60610. (312) 464-5000. http://www.ama-assn.org.

American Nurses Association. 600 Maryland Avenue, SW, Suite 100 West, Washington, DC 20024. (800) 274-4262. http://www.nursingworld.org.

American Red Cross National Headquarters. 2025 E St. NW, Washington DC 20006. (202) 303-4498. http://www.redcross.org.

Wound, Ostomy, and Continence Nurses Society. 1550 South Coast Highway, Suite #201, Laguna Beach, CA 92651. (888) 224-9626. http://www.wocn.org.

OTHER

National Library of Medicine. http://www.nlm.nih.gov/medlineplus/firstaidemergencies.html.

Woundcare.com http://www.woundcare.com/.

L. Fleming Fallon, Jr, MD, DrPH
Laura Jean Cataldo, RN, Ed.D.

Bankart procedure

Definition

A Bankart procedure, also known as a Broca-Perthes-Bankart procedure, is a surgical technique for the repair of recurrent shoulder joint dislocations. In the procedure, the torn ligaments are re-attached to the proper place in the shoulder joint, with the goal of restoring normal function.

Purpose

The shoulder is the junction of three bones: the upper arm bone (humerus), the collarbone (clavicle), and the shoulder blade (scapula). The shoulder joint (glenohumeral joint) is the result of the head of the humerus bone fitting in the cavity of the shoulder blade (glenoid cavity), the joint being held together by the labrum, a rim of soft tissue that surrounds the glenoid. As a result of excessive force being applied to the arm, the head of the humerus may be forced out of the glenoid cavity (dislocation), and the supporting ligaments of the shoulder joint may be torn. These ligaments may heal so that the shoulder regains its stability. However, sometimes the ligaments do not heal, making the shoulder unstable and painful. This condition is referred to as traumatic instability of the shoulder, traumatic glenohumeral instability, or a Bankart lesion.

The goal of a Bankart procedure for traumatic glenohumeral instability is the safe and secure re-attachment of the torn ligaments to the tip of the glenoid from which they were detached. The surgery has the advantage of allowing patients to resume many of their activities of daily living while the repair is healing. The surgery also minimizes the unwanted joint stiffness associated with such injuries.

Demographics

The shoulder is the most commonly dislocated major joint following severe trauma, such as an auto collision or a fall onto an outstretched arm. Some 96% of dislocations involve the front of the shoulder (anterior), with 1–3% occurring in the back (posterior). Falls and car accidents are common causes of first-time dislocations, but recurrent dislocations are often due to seemingly inoffensive activities such as raising the arm over the head, or combing hair. Shoulder dislocations are more common in males than females, and in young adults.

Description

In general, shoulder surgery can be performed in two fundamentally different ways: either using closed surgical techniques (**arthroscopic surgery**) or using open surgical techniques.

An open surgery Bankart procedure is performed under **general anesthesia**. The patient is placed in a 30-degree inclined chair position with the arm free over the edge of the operating table. A bag is placed under the center of the shoulder blade of the shoulder being operated on to support the shoulder and to push the shoulder blade forward. Prepping and draping allow the arm to be freely moveable and allow a good view of the surgical field.

The whole upper limb is prepared with antiseptic. An examination under anesthesia is performed to confirm the exact nature of the instability. The surgeon makes a long incision to gain access to the joint, often cutting through the deltoid muscle to operate on the internal structures of the shoulder, and proceeds to sew the joint capsule to the detached labrum tissues.

The arthroscopic Bankart procedure tries to imitate the open Bankart procedure. Arthroscopy is a microsurgical technique by which the surgeon can use an endoscope to look through a small hole into the shoulder joint. The endoscope is an instrument the size of a pen, consisting of a tube fitted with a light and a miniature video camera, which transmits an image of the joint interior to a television monitor. The detached part of the labrum and the associated ligaments are reattached to bone along the rim of the glenohumeral cavity through a small "keyhole" incision. This is done with little disruption to the other shoulder structures and without the need to detach and reattach the overlying shoulder muscle (subscapularis).

Diagnosis/Preparation

The physician diagnoses a Bankart lesion from the patient's history, by performing a thorough **physical examination** of the joint, and taking the proper x rays. The examination often reveals that the head of the humerus slips easily out of the joint socket, even when it is pressed into it. This is called the "load and shift test." X rays may also reveal that the bony lip of the glenoid socket is rounded or deficient, or that the head of the humerus is not centered in the glenoid cavity.

A diagnostic arthroscopy is also often used to confirm the presence and extent of the shoulder instability. In this procedure, a thin fiberoptic scope is inserted into the shoulder joint space to allow direct visualization of its internal structures. An electromyogram may also be obtained if the treating physician suspects the possibility of nerve injury.

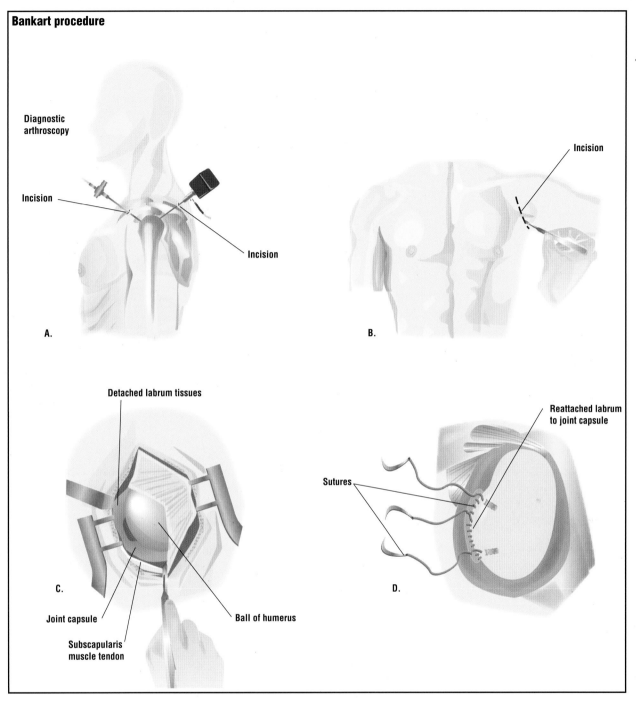

Bankart procedure

Diagnostic arthroscopy

Incision

Incision

A.

Incision

B.

Detached labrum tissues

Joint capsule

Ball of humerus

Subscapularis muscle tendon

C.

Reattached labrum to joint capsule

Sutures

D.

A Bankart procedure may be performed laparoscopically (A), or through an open incision in the shoulder (B). In the open procedure, the surgeon exposes the joint capsule and labrum, a rim of soft tissue that surrounds the cavity, which has become detached (C). Sutures reattach the labrum to the joint capsule (D). *(Illustration by GGS Information Services. Cengage Learning, Gale.)*

Patients should attend to any health problem so as to be in the best possible condition for this procedure. Smoking should be stopped a month before surgery and not resumed for at least three months afterwards. Any heart, lung, kidney, bladder, tooth, or gum problems should be managed before surgery. The orthopedic surgeon needs to be informed of all health issues, including allergies and the non-prescription and prescription medications being used by the patient.

KEY TERMS

Arthroscopy—The introduction of a thin fiberoptic scope (arthroscope) into a joint space to allow direct visualization of internal structures. In some cases, surgical repair can also be performed using the arthroscope.

Coracoid process—A long curved projection from the scapula overhanging the glenoid cavity; it provides attachment to muscles and ligaments of the shoulder and back region.

Electromyography—A test that measures muscle response to nerve stimulation. It is used to evaluate muscle weakness and to determine if the weakness is related to the muscles themselves or to a problem with the nerves that supply the muscles.

General anesthesia—A form of anesthesia that results in putting the patient to sleep.

Glenoid cavity—The hollow cavity in the head of the scapula that receives the head of the humerus to make the glenohumeral or shoulder joint.

Glenohumeral joint—A ball-and-socket synovial joint between the head of the humerus and the glenoid cavity of the scapula. Also called the glenohumeral articulation or shoulder joint.

Humerus—The bone of the upper part of the arm.

Scapula—A large, flat, triangular bone that forms the back portion of the shoulder. It articulates with the clavicle (at the acromion process) and the humerus (at the glenoid). Also called the shoulder blade.

Aftercare

Exercises are usually started on the day following surgery with instructions from a physical therapist, five times daily, including assisted flexion and external rotation of the arm. The other arm is used to support the arm that underwent surgery until it can perform the exercises alone. The patient is allowed to perform many activities of daily living as tolerated, but without lifting anything heavier than a glass or plate. If a patient can not comply with restricted use of the shoulder, the arm is kept in a sling for three weeks. Otherwise, a sling is used only for comfort between **exercise** sessions and to protect the arm when the patient is out in public and at night while sleeping. Driving is allowed as early as two weeks after surgery, if the shoulder can be used comfortably, especially if the patient's car has automatic transmission. At eight

to 10 weeks, the patient can usually resume light, low-risk activities, such as swimming and jogging. If involved in sports, the patient may return to training at three months. Hospital physiotherapy is rarely prescribed and only in cases of delayed rehabilitation or shoulder stiffness.

Risks

The following risks are associated with a Bankart procedure:

- Perioperative: Nerve damage during surgery and poor placement of anchor sutures.
- Within six weeks after surgery: Wound infection and rupture of the repair.
- Between six weeks and six months: Shoulder stiffness, recurrence of instability, failure of the repair resulting in shoulder weakness, failure of the anchor sutures.

Normal results

Normal results for a Bankart procedure include:

- good control of pain and inflammation
- normal upper arm strength and endurance
- normal shoulder range of motion

According to the American Academy of Family Physicians, the classic treatment of recurrent shoulder dislocations remains open surgical Bankart repair. This approach has a success rate as high as 95% in effectively removing shoulder instabilities. In a recent study of young athletes, Bankart repair was compared with three weeks of immobilization for the treatment of an initial anterior shoulder dislocation. The group treated surgically had fewer episodes of recurrent instability than the group managed with immobilization.

Morbidity and mortality rates

Surgery for anterior dislocation of the shoulder fails in one out of 10 to one out of 20 cases, with a higher incidence of failure in arthroscopic Bankart procedures when compared to the open surgical approach. There is also a higher incidence of failure in patients who smoke, those who start using their shoulder vigorously very early after the repair, and those with very loose ligaments.

Alternatives

Surgical

The Bristow procedure is an alternative surgical procedure used to treat shoulder instability. In this technique, the coracoid process (a long, curved projection

WHO PERFORMS THE PROCEDURE AND WHERE IS IT PERFORMED?

A Bankart procedure is performed in a hospital setting by an orthopedic surgeon specializing in shoulder instability problems.

from the scapula) with its muscle attachments is transferred to the neck of the scapula and creates a muscle sling at the front of the glenohumeral joint.

Non-surgical

Shoulders can be stabilized and strengthened with special exercises. During the early phases of such physical therapy programs, the patient is taught to use the shoulder only in the most stable positions—those in which the humerus is elevated in the plane of the scapula. As coordination and confidence improve, progressively less stable positions are attempted.

Resources

BOOKS

Neumann, L., and W. A. Wallace. "Open Repair of Instability." In *Shoulder Surgery*. Ed. By S. Copeland. London: WB Saunders, 1997.

Parker, J. N., ed. *The Official Patient's Sourcebook on Shoulder Dislocation*. San Diego, CA: ICON Health Publications, 2002.

Warren, R. F., E. V. Craig, and D. W. Altcheck, eds. *The Unstable Shoulder*. Philadelphia: Lippincott Williams & Wilkins Publishers, 1999.

PERIODICALS

Itoi, E., S. B. Lee, K. K. Amrami, D. E. Wenger, and K. N. An. "Quantitative assessment of classic anteroinferior bony Bankart lesions by radiography and computed tomography." *American Journal of Sports Medicine* 31 (January-February 2003): 112–118.

Kim, S. H., K. I. Ha, and S. H. Kim. "Bankart repair in traumatic anterior shoulder instability: open versus arthroscopic technique." *Arthroscopy* 18 (September 2002): 755–763.

Magnusson, L., J. Kartus, L. Ejerhed, I. Hultenheim, N. Sernert, and J. Karlsson. "Revisiting the open Bankart experience: a four- to nine-year follow-up." *American Journal of Sports Medicine* 30 (November-December 2002): 778–782.

Massoud, S. N., O. Levy, and S. A. Copeland. " The vertical-apical suture Bankart lesion repair for anteroinferior glenohumeral instability." *Journal of Shoulder and Elbow Surgery* 11 (September-October 2002): 481–485.

QUESTIONS TO ASK THE DOCTOR

- How long will it take to recover from the surgery?
- What are the different types of surgery available for shoulder instability?
- Specifically, how will my shoulder be improved by a Bankart procedure?
- Will surgery cure my shoulder condition so that I may resume my activities?
- Can medications help?
- Are there any alternatives to surgery?
- How many Bankart procedures do you perform each year?

Porcellini, G., F. Campi, and P. Paladini. "Arthroscopic approach to acute bony Bankart lesion." *Arthroscopy* 18 (September 2002): 764–769.

ORGANIZATIONS

American Academy of Orthopedic Surgeons. 6300 North River Road, Rosemont, IL 60018-4262. (847) 823-7186; (800) 346-AAOS. www.aaos.org.

OTHER

McNeal, Melanie, and David Lintner, M.D. "Traumatic Instability: ACLR or Bankart Procedure." *Dr. Lintner*. Copyright 2003 [cited June 7, 2003]. www.drlintner.com/aclr.htm.

Monique Laberge, PhD

Barbiturates

Definition

Barbiturates are medicines that act on the central nervous system. They cause drowsiness and can control seizures.

Purpose

Barbiturates are in the group of medicines known as central nervous system depressants (CNS). Also known as sedative-hypnotic drugs, barbiturates make people very relaxed, calm, and sleepy. These drugs are sometimes used to help patients relax before surgery. Some may also be used to control seizures (convulsions). Although barbiturates have been used to treat nervousness and sleep problems, they have generally been replaced by other medicines for these purposes.

KEY TERMS

Adrenal glands—Two glands located next to the kidneys. The adrenal glands produce the hormones epinephrine and norepinephrine and the corticosteroid (cortisone-like) hormones.

Anemia—A lack of hemoglobin. Hemoglobin is the compound in blood that carries oxygen from the lungs throughout the body and brings waste carbon dioxide from the cells to the lungs, where it is released.

Central nervous system—The brain, spinal cord, and nerves throughout the body.

Hallucination—A false or distorted perception of objects, sounds, or events that seems real. Hallucinations usually result from drugs or mental disorders.

Hypnotic—A medicine that causes sleep.

Porphyria—A disorder in which porphyrins build up in the blood and urine.

Porphyrin—A type of pigment found in living things, such as chlorophyll which makes plants green and hemoglobin which makes blood red.

Sedative—Medicine that has a calming effect and may be used to treat nervousness or restlessness.

Seizure—A sudden attack, spasm, or convulsion.

Withdrawal symptoms—A group of physical or mental symptoms that may occur when a person suddenly stops using a drug on which he or she has become dependent.

Although barbiturates have largely been replaced by other classes of drugs, some are still used in anesthesiology to induce anesthesia and lower the dose of inhaled anesthetics required for surgical procedures. Barbiturates used for anesthesia may be classified as ultrashort, short, intermediate, and long-acting. Ultrashort-acting barbiturates such as methohexital (Brevital) and thiopental (Pentothal) produce anesthesia within about one minute after intravenous administration. Short and intermediate acting barbituates include amobarbital (Amytal), secobarbital (Seconal), and butabarbital (Butisol). They are taken orally and may begin their effects in about 15 to 45 minutes after administration and last for about 6 hours. Long-acting barbiturates such as phenobarbital (Luminal) may last for up to 12 hours and are used primarily for treatment of seizure disorders.

Pentobarbital (Nembutal) has been used in **neurosurgery** to reduce blood flow to the brain. This reduces swelling and pressure in the brain, making brain surgery safer.

Secobarbital (Seconal) may be given by mouth or as a suppository to induce sleepiness and relaxation before **local anesthesia** or the insertion of a tube into the nose or throat.

These medicines may become habit-forming and should not be used to relieve everyday anxiety and tension or to treat sleeplessness over long periods.

Description

Barbiturates are available only with a physician's prescription and are sold in capsule, tablet, liquid, and injectable forms. Some commonly used barbiturates are phenobarbital (Barbita) and secobarbital (Seconal).

Recommended dosage

Recommended dosage depends on the type of barbiturate and other factors such as the patient's age and the condition for which the medicine is being taken. The patient should consult with the physician who prescribed the drug or the pharmacist who filled the prescription for the correct dosage.

The following recommendations do not apply when barbiturates are given as a single oral or intravenous dose prior to or during surgery. The recommendations should be considered if the drugs are used for treatment of anxiety or seizures.

Patients should always take barbiturates exactly as directed. Larger or more frequent doses should never be taken, and the drug should not be taken for longer than directed. If the medicine does not seem to be working, even after taking it for several weeks, the patient should *not* increase the dosage. Instead, the physician who prescribed the medicine should be consulted.

People taking barbiturates should not stop taking them suddenly without first checking with the physician who prescribed the medication. It may be necessary to taper the dose gradually to reduce the chance of withdrawal symptoms. If it is necessary to stop taking the drug, the patient should check with the physician for instructions on how to stop.

Precautions

People taking barbiturates must see a physician regularly. The physician will check to make sure the medicine is working as it should and will note unwanted side effects.

Because barbiturates work on the central nervous system, they may add to the effects of alcohol and other drugs that slow the central nervous system, such as antihistamines, cold medicine, allergy medicine, sleep aids, medicine for seizures, tranquilizers, some pain relievers, and **muscle relaxants**. They may also add to the effects of anesthetics, including those used for dental procedures. The combined effects of barbiturates and alcohol or other CNS depressants (drugs that slow the central nervous system) can be very dangerous, leading to unconsciousness or even **death**. Anyone taking barbiturates should not drink alcohol and should check with his or her physician before taking any medicines classified as CNS depressants.

Taking an overdose of barbiturates or combining barbiturates with alcohol or other central nervous system depressants can cause unconsciousness and even death. Anyone who shows signs of an overdose or a reaction to combining barbiturates with alcohol or other drugs should get emergency medical help immediately. Signs include:

- severe drowsiness
- breathing problems
- slurred speech
- staggering
- slow heartbeat
- severe confusion
- severe weakness

Barbiturates may change the results of certain medical tests. Before having medical tests, anyone taking this medicine should alert the health care professional in charge.

People may feel drowsy, dizzy, lightheaded, or less alert when using these drugs. These effects may even occur the morning after taking a barbiturate at bedtime. Because of these possible effects, anyone who takes these drugs should not drive, use machines or do anything else that might be dangerous until they have found out how the drugs affect him or her.

Barbiturates may cause physical or mental dependence when taken over long periods. Anyone who shows these signs of dependence should check with his or her physician right away:

- the need to take larger and larger doses of the medicine to get the same effect
- a strong desire to keep taking the medicine
- withdrawal symptoms, such as anxiety, nausea or vomiting, convulsions, trembling, or sleep problems, when the medicine is stopped

Children may be especially sensitive to barbiturates. This sensitivity may increase the chance of side effects such as unusual excitement.

Older people may also be more sensitive than others to the effects of this medicine. In older people, barbiturates may be more likely to cause confusion, depression, and unusual excitement. These effects are also more likely in people who are very ill.

Special conditions

People with certain medical conditions or who are taking certain other medicines can have problems if they take barbiturates. Before taking these drugs, be sure to let the physician know about any of these conditions:

ALLERGIES. Anyone who has had unusual reactions to barbiturates in the past should let his or her physician know before taking the drugs again. The physician should also be told about any allergies to foods, dyes, preservatives, or other substances.

PREGNANCY. Taking barbiturates during pregnancy increases the chance of birth defects and may cause other problems such as prolonged labor and withdrawal effects in the baby after birth. Pregnant women who must take barbiturates for serious or life-threatening conditions should thoroughly discuss with their physicians the benefits and risks of taking this medicine.

BREASTFEEDING. Barbiturates pass into breast milk and may cause problems such as drowsiness, breathing problems, or slow heartbeat in nursing babies whose mothers take the medicine. Women who are breastfeeding should check with their physicians before using barbiturates.

OTHER MEDICAL CONDITIONS. Before using barbiturates, people with any of these medical problems should make sure their physicians are aware of their conditions:

- alcohol or drug abuse
- depression
- hyperactivity (in children)
- pain
- kidney disease
- liver disease
- diabetes
- overactive thyroid
- underactive adrenal gland
- chronic lung diseases such as asthma or emphysema
- severe anemia
- porphyria

USE OF CERTAIN MEDICINES. Taking barbiturates with certain other drugs may affect the way the drugs work or may increase the chance of side effects.

Side effects

The most common side effects are dizziness, light-headedness, drowsiness, and clumsiness or unsteadiness. These problems usually go away as the body adjusts to the drug and do not require medical treatment unless they persist or interfere with normal activities.

More serious side effects are not common, but may occur. If any of the following side effects occur, the physician who prescribed the medicine should be contacted immediately:

- fever
- muscle or joint pain
- sore throat
- chest pain or tightness in the chest
- wheezing
- skin problems, such as rash, hives, or red, thickened, or scaly skin
- bleeding sores on the lips
- sores or painful white spots in the mouth
- swollen eyelids, face, or lips

In addition, if confusion, depression, or unusual excitement occur after taking barbiturates, a physician should be contacted as soon as possible.

Patients who take barbiturates for a long time or at high doses may notice side effects for some time after they stop taking the drug. These effects usually appear within eight to 16 hours after the patient stops taking the medicine. If these or other troublesome symptoms occur after stopping treatment with barbiturates, a physician should be contacted:

- dizziness, lightheadedness or faintness
- anxiety or restlessness
- hallucinations
- vision problems
- nausea and vomiting
- seizures (convulsions)
- muscle twitches or trembling hands
- weakness
- sleep problems, nightmares, or increased dreaming

Other side effects may occur. Anyone who has unusual symptoms during or after treatment with barbiturates should consult with his or her physician.

Interactions

Birth control pills may not work properly when taken while barbiturates are being taken. To prevent pregnancy, additional methods of birth control are advised while taking barbiturates.

Barbiturates may also interact with other medicines. When this happens, the effects of one or both of the drugs may change or the risk of side effects may be greater. Anyone who takes barbiturates should let the physician know all other medicines he or she is taking. Among the drugs that may interact with barbiturates are:

- other central nervous system (CNS) depressants such as medicine for allergies, colds, hay fever, and asthma; sedatives; tranquilizers; prescription pain medicine; muscle relaxants; medicine for seizures; sleep aids; barbiturates; and anesthetics
- blood thinners
- adrenocorticoids (cortisone-like medicines)
- antiseizure medicines such as valproic acid (Depakote and Depakene), and carbamazepine (Tegretol)

The list above does not include every drug that may interact with barbiturates. A physician or pharmacist should be consulted before combining barbiturates with any other prescription or nonprescription (over-the-counter) medicine.

Resources

BOOKS

AHFS: Drug Information. Washington, DC: American Society of Healthsystems Pharmaceuticals, 2003.

Brody, T. M., Larner, J., and Minneman, K P.*Human Pharmacology: Molecular to Clinical* 2nd edition. St. Louis: Mosby Year-Book, 1998.

Karch, A. M. *Lippincott's Nursing Drug Guide* Springhouse, Penn: Lippincott Williams & Wilkins, 2007.

Reynolds, J. E. F., ed. *Martindale The Extra Pharmacopoeia* 31st ed. London: The Pharmaceutical Press, 1993.

Preston, J., O'Neal, J, and Talaga, M.*Handbook of Clinical Psychopharmacology for Therapists*Oakland: New Harbinger Publications, 2008.

OTHER

Drugs Information Training, 2008.http://www.drugstraining. co.uk/DrugsInfo/info-barbiturate.html [Accessed April 7, 2008].

Nancy Ross-Flanigan
Samuel Uretsky, PharmD
Laura Jean Cataldo, RN, EdD.

Barium enema

Definition

A barium enema, also known as a lower GI (gastrointestinal) exam, is a test that uses x-ray examination to view the large intestine. There are two types of tests: the single-contrast technique, where barium sulfate is injected into the rectum to gain a profile view of the large intestine, and the double-contrast (or "air contrast") technique, where air and barium are inserted into the rectum.

Purpose

A barium enema may be performed for a variety of reasons. One reason may be to help in the diagnosis of colon and rectal cancer (or colorectal cancer), and inflammatory disease. Detection of polyps (benign growths in the tissue lining the colon and rectum), diverticula (pouches pushing out from the colon), and structural changes in the large intestine can also be confirmed by the barium enema. The double-contrast barium enema is the best method for detecting small tumors (such as polyps), early inflammatory disease, and bleeding caused by ulcers.

A doctor's decision to perform a barium enema is based on a patient's history of altered bowel habits. These can include diarrhea, constipation, lower abdominal pain, or patient reports of blood, mucus, or pus in the stools. It is recommended that healthy people have a colorectal cancer screening **colonoscopy** every five to 10 years, because this form of cancer is the second most deadly type in the United States. Those who have a close relative with colorectal cancer, or who have had a pre-cancerous polyp, are considered to be at an increased risk for the disease and should be screened more frequently by their doctor for possible abnormalities.

Description

To begin a barium enema, the doctor will have the patient lie with their back down on a tilting radiographic table so that x rays can of the abdomen can be taken. The film is then reviewed by a radiologist, who assesses if the colon has been adequately cleansed of stool during the prep process. After being assisted into a different position, a well-lubricated rectal tube is inserted through the anus. This tube allows the physician or the assisting health care provider to slowly administer the barium into the intestine. While this filling process is closely monitored, the patient must keep the anus tightly contracted against the rectal tube

Barium sulfate—A barium compound used during a barium enema to block the passage of x rays during the exam.

Bowel lumen—The space within the intestine.

Colonoscopy—An examination of the colon performed with a colonoscope.

Diverticula—A diverticulum of the colon is a sac or pouch in the colon wall which is usually asymptomatic (without symptoms) but may cause difficulty if it becomes inflamed. Diverticula is the plural of diverticulum.

Diverticulitis—A condition of the diverticulum of the intestinal tract, especially in the colon, where inflammation may cause distended sacs extending from the colon and pain.

Diverticulosis—The development of diverticula.

Megacolon—Abnormally large colon associated with some chronic intestine disorders.

Proctosigmoidoscopy—A visual examination of the rectum and sigmoid colon using a sigmoidoscope, also known as sigmoidoscopy.

Sigmoidoscopy—Endoscopic examination of the lower colon.

Ulcerative colitis—An ulceration or erosion of the lining of the colon.

so that the position is maintained and the barium is prevented from leaking. This step is emphasized to the patient because inaccuracy may occur if the barium leaks. A rectal balloon may also be inflated to help the patient retain the barium. The table may be tilted or the patient may be moved to different positions to aid in the filling process.

As the barium fills the intestine, x rays of the abdomen are taken to distinguish significant findings. There are many ways to perform a barium enema. One way is that shortly after filling, the rectal tube is removed and the patient expels as much of the barium as possible. Alternatively, the tube will remain in place, and the barium will move through that tube. A thin film of barium remains in the intestine, and air is then slowly injected through the rectum and to expand the bowel lumen. Usually no films will be taken until after the air is injected. Multiple films are generally obtained by a radiologist; then, additional films are made by a technologist.

Preparation

To conduct the most accurate barium enema test, the patient must follow a prescribed diet and bowel preparation instructions prior to the test. This preparation commonly includes restricted intake of diary products and a liquid diet for 24 hours prior to the test, in addition to drinking large amounts of water or clear liquids 12–24 hours before the test. Patients may also be given **laxatives**, and asked to give themselves a cleansing enema.

In addition to the prescribed diet and bowel preparation prior to the test, the patient can expect the following during a barium enema:

- They will be well draped with a gown as they are placed on a tilting x-ray table.
- As the barium or air is injected into the intestine, they may experience cramping pains or the urge to defecate.
- The patient will be instructed to take slow, deep breaths through the mouth to ease any discomfort.

Aftercare

Patients should follow several steps immediately after undergoing a barium enema, including:

- Drinking plenty of fluids to help counteract the dehydrating effects of bowel preparation and the test.
- Taking time to rest. A barium enema and the bowel preparation taken before it can be exhausting.
- A cleansing enema may be given to eliminate any remaining barium. Lightly colored stools will be prevalent for the next 24–72 hours following the test.

Risks

While a barium enema is considered a safe screening test used on a routine basis, it can cause complications in certain people. The following indications should be kept in mind before a barium enema is performed:

- Those who have a rapid heart rate, severe ulcerative colitis, toxic megacolon, or a presumed perforation in the intestine should not undergo a barium enema.
- The test can be performed cautiously if the patient has a blocked intestine, ulcerative colitis, diverticulitis, or severe bloody diarrhea.
- Complications that may be caused by the test include perforation of the colon, water intoxication, barium granulomas (inflamed nodules), and allergic reaction. However, these conditions are all very rare.

Normal results

When patients undergo single-contrast enemas, their intestines are steadily filled with barium to differentiate markings of the colon markings. Normal results display uniform filling of the colon.

As the barium is expelled, the intestinal walls collapse. A normal result on the x ray after defecation will show the intestinal lining as having a standard, feathery appearance.

The double-contrast enema expands the intestine, which is already lined with a thin layer of barium, using air to display a detailed image of the mucosal pattern. Varying positions taken by the patient allow the barium to collect on the dependent walls of the intestine by way of gravity.

A barium enema allows abnormalities to appear on an x ray that may aid in the diagnosis of several different conditions. Most colon cancers occur in the rectosigmoid region, or on the upper part of the rectum and adjoining portion of the sigmoid colon. However, they can also be detected with a proctosigmoidoscopy (usually referred to as a **sigmoidoscopy**). Further, an enema can identify other early signs of cancer.

Identification of polyps, diverticulosis, and inflammatory disease (such as **diverticulitis** and ulcerative colitis) is attainable through a barium x ray. Some cases of acute appendicitis may also be apparent by viewing this x ray, though acute appendicitis is usually diagnosed clinically, or by CT scan.

Resources

BOOKS
PERIODICALS

Gazelle, G. "Screening for Colorectal Cancer." *Radiology* 327 (May 2000)

Rubesin, S. "Double Contrast Barium Enema Examination Technique." *Radiology* 642 (June 2000).

ORGANIZATIONS

American Cancer Society. 1599 Clifton Rd., NE, Atlanta, GA 30329-4251. (800) 227-2345. http://www.cancer.org.

Beth A. Kapes
Lee A. Shratter, M.D.

Barium swallow *see* **Upper GI exam**

Beating heart surgery *see* **Minimally invasive heart surgery**

Beclomethasone *see* **Corticosteroids**

Bedside monitors *see* **Cardiac monitor**

Bedsores

Definition

Bedsores are also called decubitus ulcers, pressure ulcers, or pressure sores. They begin as tender, inflamed patches that develop when a person's weight rests against a hard surface, exerting pressure on the skin and soft tissue over bony parts of the body. For example, bedsores are common when skin covering a weight-bearing part of the body, such as a knee or hip, is pressed between a bone and a bed, chair, another body part, splint, or other hard object. This is most likely to happen when the person is confined to a bed or wheelchair for long periods and is relatively immobile. Usually, mobile individuals receive pain signals from the compressed part of the body and will automatically move to relieve the pressure, thus bedsores do not usually develop in people with normal mobility and mental alertness. However, people compromised through spinal cord injury, acute illness, heavy sedation, unconsciousness, or diminished mental functioning, may not receive signals to move, and as a result of the constant pressure, tissue damage often progresses to bedsores in these individuals.

Demographics

Each year, about 1.8 million people in the United States develop bedsores at a treatment cost of $1.3 billion. In 2004, 17,000 lawsuits resulted from treatment related to bedsores. Pressure sores are most common in elderly patients; records show that 70% of all bedsores occur in people over age 70. People who are neurologically impaired, such as those with spinal injuries or paralysis, have a 5–8% chance annually of developing a bedsore. This translates into a 25–85% lifetime risk. Complications from pressure sores are the direct cause of **death** in about 8% of nursing home residents.

The National Pressure Ulcer Advisory Panel (NPUAP) estimates that bedsores afflict:

- 9–13% of all hospital patients
- up to 23.9% of nursing home residents
- at least 60% of elderly individuals with hip and femur (thigh bone) fractures

Description

Bedsores range from mild inflammation to ulceration (breakdown of tissue) and deep wounds that involve muscle and bone. This painful condition usually starts with shiny red skin that quickly blisters and

deteriorates into open sores. These sores leave the body open to bacterial and fungal contamination and can harbor life-threatening infection. Bedsores are not contagious or cancerous, although the most serious complication of chronic bedsores is the development of malignant degeneration, which is a type of cancer.

Bedsores develop because of pressure that cuts off the flow of blood and oxygen to tissue. Constant pressure pinches off capillaries, the tiny blood vessels that deliver oxygen and nutrients to the skin. If the skin is deprived of oxygen and essential nutrients (a condition known as ischemia) for as little as one hour, tissue cells can die (anoxia) and bedsores can form. Even the slightest rubbing or friction between a hard surface and skin stretched over bones can cause minor pressure ulcers. They can also develop when a patient stretches or bends blood vessels by slipping into a different position in a bed or chair.

Urine, feces, or other moisture increase the risk of skin infection, so people who are incontinent (unable to control bladder or bowel movements), as well as those who are immobile or have nerve damage that prevents them from feeling pain, have a high risk of developing bedsores.

Bedsores are difficult to successfully treat and recurrence is common. People who have experienced bedsores have a 90% chance of developing them again, even when the bedsores have been successfully treated. While mild pressure sores themselves can usually be cured, complications from pressure ulcers are the direct cause of death in about 8% of paraplegic individuals. Pressure sores can be slow to heal, particularly when the patient's overall physical status may be weakened. Without proper treatment, bedsores can lead to:

- gangrene (tissue death)
- osteomyelitis (infection of the bone beneath the bedsore)
- sepsis (a poisoning of tissue or the whole body from bacterial infection)
- other localized or systemic infections that slow the healing process, increase the cost of treatment, lengthen hospital or nursing home stays, or cause death

About 93% of bedsores develop below the waist. Bedsores are most apt to develop on bony parts of the body, including:

- ankles
- heels
- hips and buttocks
- knees
- lower back
- shoulder blades
- back of the head

Although impaired mobility is a leading factor in the development of pressure sores, the risk is also increased by illnesses and conditions that weaken muscle and soft tissue or that affect blood circulation and the delivery of oxygen to body tissue, leaving skin thinner and more vulnerable to breakdown and subsequent infection. These conditions include:

- atherosclerosis (hardening of arteries) that restricts blood flow
- diabetes
- diminished sensation or lack of feeling or inability to feel pain
- heart problems
- incontinence
- malnutrition
- obesity
- paralysis
- poor circulation
- infection
- prolonged bed rest, especially in unsanitary conditions or with wet or wrinkled sheets
- spinal cord injury

Diagnosis/Preparation

Physical examination, medical history, and patient and caregiver observations are the basis of diagnosis. Special attention must be paid to physical or mental problems, such as an underlying disease, incontinence, or confusion that could complicate a patient's recovery. Nutritional status and smoking history should also be noted.

The National Pressure Ulcer Advisory Panel recommends classification of bedsores in four stages of ulceration based primarily on the depth of a sore at the time of examination. This helps to create standardized descriptive language and encourages effective communication of medical personnel caring for patients with bedsores. The NPUAP advises that not all bedsores follow the stages directly from I to IV. The four most widely accepted stages are described as:

- Stage I: intact skin with redness (erythema) and sometimes with warmth. In people with dark skin, rather than appearing red, the area may appear blue or purple or sometimes lighter than the rest of the skin.
- Stage II: tissue damage has occurred. The outermost layer of skin has been lost and the sore shows abrasion, swelling, and possible blistering or peeling.
- Stage III: all skin has been lost; damage has reached the tissue below the skin. The bedsore appears as a deep open wound (crater).
- Stage IV: extensive skin loss with damage to the underlying tissue that extends into muscle, bone, tendon, or joint. These bedsores can be fatal.

In addition to observing the depth of the wound, the caregiver should note the presence or absence of wound drainage, foul odors, or any debris in the wound, such as pieces of dead skin tissue or other material. Any condition that could likely contaminate the wound and cause infection, such as the presence of urine or feces from incontinence, should be noted as well.

A physician should be notified whenever a person:

- will be bedridden or immobilized for an extended time period.
- is very weak or unable to move.
- develops redness (inflammation) and warmth or peeling on any area of skin.

Immediate medical attention is required whenever:

- skin turns black or becomes inflamed, tender, swollen, or warm to the touch.
- the patient develops a fever during treatment.
- a bedsore contains pus or has a foul-smelling discharge.

Prompt medical attention can prevent surface pressure sores from deepening into more serious infections. The first step is always to reduce or eliminate the pressure that is causing bedsores. For minor bedsores, stages I and II, treatment involves relieving pressure, keeping the wound clean and moist, and keeping the area around the ulcer clean and dry. This is often accomplished with saline (salt water) washes and the use of sterile medicated gauze **dressings** that both absorb the wound drainage and fight infection-causing bacteria. **Antiseptics**, harsh soaps, and other skin cleansers can damage new tissue and should be avoided. Only sterile saline solution should be used to cleanse bedsores whenever fresh non-stick dressings are applied.

The patient's doctor may prescribe infection-fighting **antibiotics**, special dressings or drying agents, and/or lotions or ointments to be applied to the wound in a thin film three or four times a day. Warm whirlpool treatments are sometimes recommended for sores on the arm, hand, foot, or leg.

Typically, with the removal or reduction of pressure in conjunction with proper treatment and attention to the patient's general health, including good nutrition, bedsores should begin to heal two to four weeks after treatment begins.

A 2006 peer-reviewed clinical trial of 89 residents in 23 **nursing homes** reinforced the concept that good nutrition will aid in treatment. The trial reported that patients receiving the protein supplement, Pro-Stat, along with standard pressure sore care, showed a 96% improvement in healing over patients receiving a placebo (supplement with no protein) and standard care.

Surgical options are often considered for non-healing wounds. When deep wounds are not responding well to standard medical procedures, consultation with a plastic surgeon may be needed to determine if **reconstructive surgery** is the best possible treatment. In a procedure called debriding, a scalpel may be used to remove dead tissue or other debris from stage III and IV wounds. A surgical procedure called urinary (or fecal) diversion may also be used with incontinent patients to divert the flow of urinary or fecal material. This keeps the wound clean and encourages wound healing. Reconstruction involves the complete removal of the ulcerated area and surrounding damaged tissue (excision), debriding the bone, and reducing the amount of bacteria in the area with vigorous flushing (lavage) with saline solution. The surgical wound is then drained for a period of days until it is clear that no infection is present and that healing has begun. **Plastic surgery** may follow to close the wound with a flap (skin from another part of the body), providing a new tissue surface over the bone. For surgery to succeed, infection must not be present. High rates of complications tend to occur after reconstructive surgery. These include bleeding under the skin (hematoma), wound infection, and the recurrence of pressure

sores. Infection in deep wounds can progress to life-threatening systemic infection. **Amputation** may be required when a wound will not heal or when reconstructive surgery is not an option for a particular patient.

Alternatives

Zinc and vitamins A, C, E, and B complex provide necessary nutrients for the skin and help it to repair injuries and stay healthy. Large doses of vitamins or minerals should not be used without a doctor's approval.

A poultice made of equal parts of powdered slippery elm (*Ulmus fulva*), marsh mallow (*Althaea officinalis*), and echinacea blended with a small amount of hot water can relieve minor inflammation. An infection-fighting rinse of two drops of essential tea tree oil (Melaleuca) to every 8 oz (0.23 g) of water can also be administered. An herbal tea made from calendula (*Calendula officinalis*) is also an effective antiseptic and wound-healing agent. Calendula cream can also be used.

Contrasting hot and cold compresses applied to the bedsore site can increase circulation to the area and help flush out waste products, speeding the healing process. The temperatures should be extreme (very hot and ice cold), yet tolerable to the skin. Hot compresses should be applied for three minutes, followed by 30 seconds of cold compress application, repeating the cycle three times. The cycle should always end with a cold compress.

Prevention

It is easier to prevent bedsores from developing than to cure them once they have occurred. Good nutrition plays an important role in keeping the skin intact and in promoting wound healing; the diet of bedridden individuals should not be ignored. All patients recovering from illness or surgery or confined to a bed or wheelchair long term should be inspected at least daily, but preferably more often. They should be bathed or should shower every day using warm water and mild soap, and should avoid cold or dry air. Bedridden patients who are either mentally unaware or physically unable to turn themselves must be repositioned regularly by caregivers at minimum once every two hours while awake and preferably more frequently. People who use a wheelchair should be encouraged to shift their weight every 10–15 minutes or be repositioned by caregivers at least once an hour.

It is important to lift, rather than to drag, a person being repositioned. Bony parts of the body should not be massaged. Even slight friction can remove the weakened top layer of skin and damage blood vessels beneath it. Sensitive body parts can be protected by:

- sheepskin pads
- special cushions placed on top of a mattress
- a water-filled mattress
- a variable-pressure mattress with individually inflatable sections to redistribute pressure

Pillows or foam wedges can prevent the ankles of a bedridden patient from rubbing on each other, and pillows placed under the legs from mid-calf to ankle can raise the heels off the bed. Raising the head of the bed slightly and briefly can provide relief, but raising the head of the bed more than 30° can cause the patient to slide, thereby causing damage to skin and tiny blood vessels.

A person who uses a wheelchair should be encouraged to sit up as straight as possible. Pillows behind the head and between the legs can help prevent bedsores, as can a special cushion placed on the chair seat. Donut-shaped cushions should not be used because they restrict blood flow and cause tissues to swell.

Special support surfaces are manufactured and readily available for care in medical facilities or at home, including air-filled mattresses and cushions, low-air loss beds, and air-fluidized beds. These devices give adequate support while reducing pressure on vulnerable skin. They have been shown to exert less pressure on the skin of compromised patients than do regular mattresses. Patients using these devices and beds must still be repositioned every two hours.

Resources

ORGANIZATIONS

National Pressure Ulcer Advisory Panel. 12100 Sunset Hills Road, Suite 130, Reston, VA 20190. (703)464-4849. http://www.npuap.org (accessed March 7, 2008).

OTHER

"Bedsores." MoonDragon's Health and Wellness. August 23, 2006. [cited January 1, 2008]. http://www.moondragon. org/health/disorders/bedsores.html (accessed March 7, 2008).

"Bedsores (Pressure sores)." Mayo Clinic. March 19, 2007. [cited January 1, 2008]. http://www.mayoclinic.com/ health/bedsores/DS00570 (accessed March 7, 2008).

"Pressure Sores." American Academy of Family Physicians. December 2006/ [cited January 1, 2008]. http://family doctor.org/online/famdocen/home/seniors/endoflife/ 039.html (accessed March 7, 2008).

"Pressure Ulcers." American Medical Association.August 23, 2006. [cited January 1, 2008]. http://jama.ama-

assn.org/cgi/reprint/296/8/1020.pdf (accessed March 7, 2008).

Maureen Haggerty
L. Lee Culvert
Tish Davidson, AM

Betamethasone *see* **Corticosteroids**

Bicarbonate test *see* **Electrolyte tests**

Bile duct stone removal *see* **Endoscopic retrograde cholangiopancreatography**

Biliary stenting

Definition

A biliary stent is a plastic or metal tube that is inserted into a bile duct to relieve narrowing of the duct (also called bile duct stricture).

Purpose

Biliary stenting is used to treat obstructions that occur in the bile ducts. Bile is a substance that helps to digest fats and is produced by the liver, secreted through the bile ducts, and stored in the gallbladder. It is released into the small intestine after a fat-containing meal has been eaten. The release of bile is controlled by a muscle called the sphincter of Oddi found at the junction of the bile ducts and the small intestine.

There are a number of conditions, malignant or benign, that can cause strictures of the bile duct. Pancreatic cancer is the most common malignant cause, followed by cancers of the gallbladder, bile duct, liver, and large intestine. Noncancerous causes of bile duct stricture include:

- injury to the bile ducts during surgery for gallbladder removal (accounting for 80% of nonmalignant strictures)
- pancreatitis (inflammation of the pancreas)
- primary sclerosing cholangitis (an inflammation of the bile ducts that may cause pain, jaundice, itching, or other symptoms)
- gallstones
- radiation therapy
- blunt trauma to the abdomen

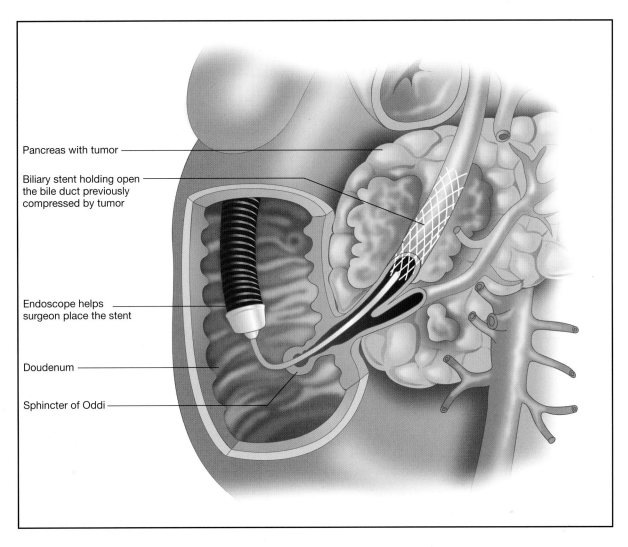

Pancreas with tumor

Biliary stent holding open
the bile duct previously
compressed by tumor

Endoscope helps
surgeon place the stent

Doudenum

Sphincter of Oddi

(Illustration by Electronic Illustrators Group.)

Demographics

The overall incidence of bile duct stricture is not known. Approximately 0.2–0.5% of patients undergoing gallbladder surgery or other operations affecting the bile duct develop biliary stricture.

Description

A biliary stent is a thin, tube-like structure that is used to support a narrowed part of the bile duct and prevent the reformation of the stricture. Stents may be made of plastic or metal. The two most common methods that are used to place a biliary stent are **endoscopic retrograde cholangiopancreatography** (ERCP) and percutaneous transhepatic cholangiography (PTC).

ERCP

ERCP is an imaging technique used to diagnose diseases of the pancreas, liver, gallbladder, and bile ducts that also has the advantage of being used as a therapeutic device. The endoscope (a thin, lighted, hollow tube attached to a viewing screen) is inserted into a patient's mouth, down the esophagus, through the stomach, and into the upper part of the small intestine, until it reaches the spot where the bile ducts empty. At this point a small tube called a cannula is inserted through the endoscope and used to inject a contrast dye into the ducts; the term retrograde refers to the backward direction of the dye. A series of x rays are then taken as the dye moves through the ducts.

If the x rays show that a biliary stricture exists, a stent may be placed into a duct to relieve the obstruction.

In order to do this, special instruments are inserted into the endoscope and a sphincterotomy (a cut into the sphincter of Oddi) is performed to provide access to the bile ducts. In some cases, the biliary stricture may first be dilated (expanded) using a thin, flexible tube called a catheter, followed by a balloon-type device that is inflated. The stent is then inserted into the bile duct.

PTC

PTC is similar to ERCP in that the test is used to diagnose and treat obstructions affecting the flow of bile from the liver to the gastrointestinal tract. The procedure is generally reserved for patients who have undergone unsuccessful ERCP. A thin needle is used to inject a contrast dye through the skin and into the liver or gallbladder; x rays are taken while the dye moves through the bile ducts. If a biliary stricture becomes evident, a stent may then be placed. A hollow needle is introduced into the bile duct, and a thin guide wire inserted into the needle. The wire is guided to the area of obstruction; the stent is advanced over the wire and placed in the obstructed duct.

Diagnosis/Preparation

Prior to ERCP or PTC, the patient will be instructed to refrain from eating or drinking for at least six hours to ensure that the stomach and upper part of the intestine are free of food. The physician should be notified as to what medications the patient takes and if the patient has an allergy to iodine, which is found in the contrast dye. **Antibiotics** will be started prior to surgery and continued for several days afterward.

Aftercare

After the procedure, the patient is monitored for signs of complications. In the case of ERCP, the patient generally remains at the hospital or outpatient facility until the effects of the sedative wear off and to ensure no complications occur. After PTC, the patient is instructed to lie on his or her right side for at least six

hours to reduce the risk of bleeding from the injection site. To ensure that the stent is functioning properly, the patient will be frequently assessed for symptoms that indicate the recurrence of biliary stricture. These symptoms include changes in stool or urine color, jaundice (yellowing of the skin), itching, and abnormal **liver function tests**.

Risks

Complications associated with ERCP include excessive bleeding, infection, pancreatitis, cholangitis (inflammation of the bile ducts), cholecystitis (inflammation of the gallbladder), and injury to the intestine. PTC may result in bleeding, infection of the injection site, sepsis (spread of infection to the blood), or leakage of the dye into the abdomen. Complications specific to the stent include migration (movement of the stent out of the area in which it was placed), occlusion (blockage), and intestinal perforation.

Normal results

In more than 90% of patients, the placement of a biliary stent relieves the obstruction and allows the bile duct to drain properly.

Morbidity and mortality rates

The rate of serious complications with ERCP is approximately 11%, and 5–10% with PTC. Stent occlusion occurs in up to 25% of patients, and stent migration in up to 6%. Recurrence of biliary stricture occurs in 15–45% of patients after an average time of four to nine years.

Alternatives

The major alternative to biliary stenting is surgical repair of the stricture. The most common method is resection (removal) of the narrowed area followed by the creation of a connection between the bile duct and the middle portion of the small intestine (called a choledochojejunostomy) or the hepatic duct and the small intestine (called a hepaticojejunostomy). Surgical stricture repair results in a cure for 85–98% of patients and is associated with a low risk of complications.

Resources

BOOKS

Feldman, Mark, et al. *Sleisenger & Fordtran's Gastrointestinal and Liver Disease.* 7th ed. Philadelphia: Elsevier Science, 2002.

Clavien, Pierre Alain., Michael G. Sarr, and Yuman Fong. *Atlas of Upper Gastrointestinal and Hepato Pancreato Biliary Surgery.* 1st ed. New York: Spinger, 2007.

Poston, Graeme J., Daniel Beauchamp, and Theo Rue. *Textbook of Surgical Oncology.* London: Informa Healthcare, 2007.

ORGANIZATIONS

American Gastroenterological Association. 7910 Woodmont Ave., 7th Floor, Bethesda, MD 20814. (301) 654–2055. http://www.gastro.org.

American Society for Gastrointestinal Endoscopy. 1520 Kensington Rd., Suite 202, Oak Brook, IL 60523. (630) 573–0600. http://www.asge.org.

Society of Interventional Radiology. 10201 Lee Highway, Suite 500, Fairfax, VA 22030. (800) 488–7284. http://www.sirweb.org.

OTHER

Pande, Hemant, Parviz Nikoomanesh, and Lawrence Cheskin. "Bile Duct Strictures." eMedicine. June 20, 2006. http://www.emedicine.com/med/topic3425.htm [Accessed April 7, 2008].

Yakshe, Paul. "Biliary Disease." eMedicine. July 21, 2006. http://www.emedicine.com/MED/topic225.htm [Accessed April 7, 2008].

Stephanie Dionne Sherk
Laura Jean Cataldo, RN, EdD

Biliopancreatic diversion *see* **Gastric bypass**
Bilirubin test *see* **Liver function tests**

Biofeedback

Definition

Biofeedback, or applied psychophysiological feedback, is a patient-guided treatment that teaches an individual to control muscle tension, pain, **body temperature**, brain waves, and other bodily functions and processes through relaxation, visualization, and other cognitive control techniques. The name biofeedback refers to the biological signals that are fed back, or returned, to the patient in order for the patient to develop techniques of manipulating them.

Purpose

Biofeedback has been used to successfully treat a number of disorders and their symptoms, including temporomandibular joint disorder (TMJ), chronic pain, irritable bowel syndrome (IBS), Raynaud's syndrome, epilepsy, attention-deficit hyperactivity disorder (ADHD), migraine headaches, anxiety, depression, traumatic brain injury, and sleep disorders.

Illnesses that may be triggered at least in part by stress are also targeted by biofeedback therapy. Certain types of headaches, high blood pressure, bruxism (teeth grinding), post-traumatic stress disorder, eating disorders, substance abuse, and some anxiety disorders may be treated successfully by teaching patients the ability to relax and release both muscle and mental tension. Biofeedback is often just one part of a comprehensive treatment program for some of these disorders.

The U.S. National Aeronautics and Space Administration (NASA) has used biofeedback techniques to treat astronauts who suffer from severe space sickness, during which the autonomic nervous system is disrupted. Scientists at the University of Tennessee have adapted these techniques to treat individuals suffering from severe nausea and vomiting that is also rooted in autonomic nervous system dysfunction.

Recent research also indicates that biofeedback may be a useful tool in helping patients with urinary incontinence regain bladder control. Individuals learning pelvic-floor muscle strengthening exercises can gain better control over these muscles by using biofeedback. Sensors are placed on the muscles to help the patient learn where they are and when proper contractions are taking place.

Description

Origins

In 1961, Neal Miller, an experimental psychologist, suggested that autonomic nervous system responses (for instance, heart rate, blood pressure, gastrointestinal activity, regional blood flow) could be under voluntary control. As a result of his experiments, he showed that such autonomic processes were controllable. This work led to the creation of biofeedback therapy. Miller's work was expanded by other researchers. Research performed in the 1970s by UCLA researcher Dr. Barry Sterman established that both cats and monkeys could be trained to control their brain wave patterns. Sterman then used his research techniques on human patients with epilepsy; he was able to reduce seizures by 60% with the use of biofeedback techniques. Throughout the 1970s, other researchers published reports of their use of biofeedback in the treatment of cardiac arrhythmias, headaches, Raynaud's syndrome, excess stomach acid, and as a tool for teaching deep relaxation. Since the early work of Miller and Sterman, biofeedback has developed into a front-line behavioral treatment for an even wider range of disorders and symptoms.

During biofeedback, special sensors are placed on the body. These sensors measure the bodily function that is causing the patient problem symptoms, such as heart rate, blood pressure, muscle tension (EMG or electromyographic feedback), brain waves (EEC or electroencephalographic feedback), respiration, and body temperature (thermal feedback), and translates the information into a visual and/or audible readout, such as a paper tracing, a light display, or a series of beeps.

While the patient views the instantaneous feedback from the biofeedback monitors, he or she begins to recognize what thoughts, fears, and mental images influence his or her physical reactions. By monitoring this relationship between mind and body, the patient can then use these same thoughts and mental images as subtle cues, as these act as reminders to become deeply relaxed, instead of anxious. These reminders also work to manipulate heart beat, brain wave patterns, body temperature, and other bodily functions. This is achieved through relaxation exercises, mental imagery, and other cognitive therapy techniques.

As the biofeedback response takes place, patients can actually see or hear the results of their efforts instantly through the sensor readout on the biofeedback equipment. Once these techniques are learned and the patient is able to recognize the state of relaxation or visualization necessary to alleviate symptoms, the biofeedback equipment itself is no longer needed. The patient then has a powerful, portable, and self-administered treatment tool to deal with problem symptoms.

Biofeedback that specializes in reading and altering brain waves is sometimes called neurofeedback. The brain produces four distinct types of brain waves—beta, alpha, theta, and delta—that all operate at a different frequency. Delta, the slowest frequency wave, is the brain wave pattern associated with deep sleep. Beta waves, the fastest frequency wave, occur in a normal, waking state and can range from 12–35 Hertz (Hz). Problems begin to develop when beta wave averages fall in the low end (underarousal) or the high end (overarousal) of that spectrum. Underarousal might be present in conditions such as depression or attention deficit disorder, and overarousal may be indicative of an anxiety disorder, obsessive compulsive disorder, or excessive stress. Beta wave neurofeedback focuses on normalizing that beta wave pattern to an optimum value of around 14 Hz. A second type of neurofeedback, alpha-theta, focuses on developing the more relaxing alpha (8–13 Hz) and theta waves (4–9 Hz) that are usually associated with deep, meditative states, and has been used with some success in substance abuse treatment.

Through brain-wave manipulation, neurofeedback can be useful in treating a variety of disorders that are suspected or proven to impact brain-wave patterns, such as epilepsy, attention deficit disorder, migraine headaches, anxiety, depression, traumatic brain injury, and sleep disorders. The equipment used for neurofeedback usually uses a monitor as an output device. The monitor displays specific patterns that the patient attempts to change by producing the appropriate type of brain wave. Or, the monitor may reward the patient for producing the appropriate brain wave by producing a positive reinforcer, or reward. For example, children may be rewarded with a series of successful moves in a displayed video game.

Depending on the type of biofeedback, individuals may need up to 30 sessions with a trained professional to learn the techniques required to control their symptoms on a long-term basis. Therapists usually recommend that their patients practice both biofeedback and relaxation techniques on their own at home.

Preparations

Before initiating biofeedback treatment, the therapist and patient will have an initial consultation to record the patient's medical history and treatment background and discuss goals for therapy.

Before a neurofeedback session, an EEG is taken to determine the patient's baseline brainwave pattern.

Biofeedback typically is performed in a quiet and relaxed atmosphere with comfortable seating for the patient. Depending on the type and goals of biofeedback being performed, one or more sensors will be attached to the patient's body with conductive gel and/or adhesives. These may include:

- Electromyographic (EMG) sensors—EMG sensors measure electrical activity in the muscles, specifically muscle tension. In treating TMJ or bruxism, these sensors would be placed along the muscles of the jaw. Chronic pain might be treated by monitoring electrical energy in other muscle groups.
- Galvanic skin response (GSR) sensors—These are electrodes placed on the fingers that monitor perspiration, or sweat gland, activity. These may also be called skin conductance level (SCL).
- Temperature sensors—Temperature, or thermal, sensors measure body temperature and changes in blood flow.
- Electroencephalography (EEG) sensors—These electrodes are applied to the scalp to measure the electrical activity of the brain, or brain waves.
- Heart rate sensors—A pulse monitor placed on the finger tip can monitor pulse rate.
- Respiratory sensors—Respiratory sensors monitor oxygen intake and carbon dioxide output.

Precautions

Individuals who use a pacemaker or other implantable electrical devices should inform their biofeedback therapist before starting treatments, as certain types of biofeedback sensors have the potential to interfere with these devices.

Biofeedback may not be suitable for some patients. Patients must be willing to take a very active role in the treatment process. And because biofeedback focuses strictly on behavioral change, those patients who wish to gain insight into their symptoms by examining their past might be better served by psychodynamic therapy.

Biofeedback may also be inappropriate for cognitively impaired individuals, such as those patients with organic brain disease or a traumatic brain injury, depending on their function level.

Patients with specific pain symptoms of unknown origin should undergo a thorough medical examination before starting biofeedback treatments to rule out any serious underlying disease. Once a diagnosis has been made, biofeedback can be used concurrently with conventional treatment.

Biofeedback may only be one component of a comprehensive treatment plan. For illnesses and symptoms that are manifested from an organic disease process, such as cancer or diabetes, biofeedback should be an adjunct to (complementary to), and not a replacement for, conventional medical treatment.

Side effects

There are no known side effects to properly administered biofeedback or neurofeedback sessions.

Research and general acceptance

Preliminary research published in late 1999 indicated that neurofeedback may be a promising new tool in the treatment of schizophrenia. Researchers reported that schizophrenic patients had used neurofeedback to simulate brain wave patterns that antipsychotic medications produce in the brain. Further research is needed to determine what impact this may have on treatment for schizophrenia.

The use of biofeedback techniques to treat an array of disorders has been extensively described in the medical literature. Controlled studies for some applications are limited, such as for the treatment of menopausal symptoms and premenstrual disorder (PMS). There is also some debate over the effectiveness of biofeedback in ADHD treatment, and the lack of controlled studies on that application. While many therapists, counselors, and mental health professionals have reported great success with treating their ADHD patients with neurofeedback techniques, some critics attribute this positive therapeutic impact to a placebo effect.

There is also be some debate among mental health professionals as to whether biofeedback should be considered a first line treatment for some mental illnesses, and to what degree other treatments, such as medication, should be employed as an adjunct therapy.

Interactions

There are no known interactions with biofeedback.

Resources

BOOKS

Demos, J. N. *Getting Started with Neurofeedback*. New York: W. W. Norton & Company, 2004.

Robbins, J. *A Symphony in the Brain: The Evolution of the New Brain Wave Biofeedback*. New York: Grove Press, 2001.

Schwartz, M. S., and F. Andrasik. *Biofeedback: A Practitioner's Guide*, 3rd ed. New York: Guilford Press, 2003.

Swingle, P. G. *Biofeedback for the Brain: How Neurotherapy Effectively Treats Depression, ADHD, Autism, and More*. New Brunswick, NJ: Rutgers University Press, 2008.

PERIODICALS

Conde-Pastor, M., F. Javier-Menendez, M. T. Sanz, and E. Vila-Abad. "The influence of respiration on biofeedback techniques." *Applied Psychophysiology and Biofeedback* 33, no. 1 (March 2008): 49–54.

Lourencao, M. I., L. R. Battistella, C. M. de Brito, G. R. Tsukimoto, and M. H. Miyazaki. "Effect of biofeedback accompanying occupational therapy and functional electrical stimulation in hemiplegic patients." *International Journal of Rehabilitation and Research* 31, no. 1 (March 2008): 33–41.

Reiner, R. "Integrating a portable biofeedback device into clinical practice for patients with anxiety disorders: results of a pilot study." *Applied Psychophysiology and Biofeedback* 33, no. 1 (March 2008): 55–61.

Roach, M., and J. A. Christie. "Fecal incontinence in the elderly." *Geriatrics* 63, no. 2 (2008): 13–22.

OTHER

Association for Applied Psychophysiology and Biofeedback. Information about biofeedback. http://www.aapb.org/i4a/pages/index.cfm?pageid = 1 (February 25, 2008).

Biofeedback Network. Information about biofeedback. http://www.biofeedback.net/ (February 22, 2008).

"Biofeedback: Using Your Mind to Improve Your Health." Mayo Clinic. January 25, 2008. http://www.mayoclinic.com/health/biofeedback/SA00083 (February 24, 2008).

"What is Biofeedback?" American Cancer Society. February 12, 2000. http://www.cancer.org/docroot/NWS/content/NWS_2_1x_What_is_Biofeedback_.asp (February 24, 2008).

ORGANIZATIONS

Association for Applied Psychotherapy and Biofeedback, 10200 W. 44th Avenue, Suite 304, Wheat Ridge, CO, 80033, (303) 422-8436, http://www.aapb.org..

Biofeedback Certification Institute of America, 10200 W. 44th Avenue, Suite 310, Wheat Ridge, CO, 80033, (303) 420-2902, http://www.bcia.org..

L. Fleming Fallon, Jr., M.D., Dr.P.H.

Birthmark excision *see* **Hemangioma excision**

Bispectral index

Definition

The bispectral index (BIS) is one of several systems used in anesthesiology as of 2003 to measure the effects of specific anesthetic drugs on the brain and to track changes in the patient's level of sedation or hypnosis. In technical terms, the bispectral index itself is a complex mathematical algorithm that allows a computer inside an anesthesia monitor to analyze data from a patient's electroencephalogram (EEG) during surgery. BIS, which has been in use since 1997, is a type of automated direct measurement of the patient's condition, in comparison to the Glasgow Coma Scale and similar scoring systems, which are indirect assessments of sedation.

Purpose

Anesthetic depth

A brief discussion of anesthetic depth may be helpful in understanding people's interest in monitoring the brain's responses to anesthesia. Ever since the first modern anesthetics (ether, chloroform, and nitrous oxide) were used in the 1840s, doctors have been searching for a reliable method of measuring the depth of the patient's unconsciousness in order to guarantee the safety as well as the painlessness of surgery. Anesthetic drugs, whether inhaled or given intravenously, are toxic in high doses; too high a dose can stop the patient's breathing. On the other hand, too small a dose can result in the patient's coming to various degrees of awareness during surgery. Events of this type occur frequently enough to be publicized in general medical news sources as well as the professional literature. One Australian medical journal reports that postoperative recall of operations, including the patient's overhearing conversations among members of the **surgical team** as well as feeling helpless and experiencing physical pain, occurs in one of every 1,000 patients undergoing non-cardiac surgery and three of every 1,000 cardiac patients. An Israeli researcher gives the rate of accidental awareness during surgery as between 0.2% and 1.2% of patients. According to an American news account, "An estimated 40,000 to 200,000 mid-operative awakenings may occur each year in the United States alone." Research has indicated that patients' attitudes toward undergoing surgery are affected by the possibility of awakening during the procedure. A group of Australian researchers found that 56% of a group of 200 patients awaiting surgery had heard about awareness during operations, mostly from the mass media; 42.5% of the group expressed anxiety about it. Post-traumatic stress disorder (PTSD) is a common result of awareness episodes; a 2001 study done at Boston University reported that 56.3% of a group of patients who had awakened during surgery met the diagnostic criteria for PTSD—as late as 17 years after their operation.

There are several reasons for anesthesiologists' difficulty in evaluating dosages of anesthetic agents:

- The lack of a universally accepted definition of "consciousness." There are a number of scientific periodicals devoted solely to the study of human consciousness, as it concerns philosophers, psychologists, psychiatrists, and lawyers, as well as doctors involved in anesthesiology and critical care medicine. Some researchers emphasize the emotional or psychological dimensions of consciousness while others focus on physiological definitions—for example, the response of skin or muscle tissue to painful stimuli.

- The complex effects of anesthesia on the human organism. Scholarly debates about the nature of human consciousness are reflected in the variety of different goals that surgical anesthesia is expected to achieve. These goals are usually listed as blocking the nervous system's responses to pain (analgesia), inducing muscular relaxation and blocking reflexes (areflexia), keeping the patient asleep during the procedure (hypnosis), and preventing conscious recall of the procedure afterwards (amnesia). It is not always possible, however, to meet all four goals with the same degree of accuracy, since some patients suffer from health conditions that require the anesthesiologist to keep them under lighter sedation in order to lower the risk of heart or circulation problems.

- The increased use of combinations of anesthetic agents rather than single drugs. At present, anesthesiologists rarely use inhaled anesthetics by themselves; most prefer what is known as balanced anesthesia, which combines inhaled and intravenous anesthetics. When different agents are used together, however, they are often synergistic, which means that they intensify each other's effects. This characteristic makes it more difficult for the anesthesiologist to predict how much of each drug will be needed during the operation.

- Changes in the patient's response to anesthesia over the course of the operation.

- Age- and sex-related differences in responsiveness to specific anesthetics. Anesthesiologists have become increasingly aware of the special needs of elderly patients, for example; they are more likely than younger patients to develop cardiovascular complications under anesthesia. With regard to sex, several studies have reported that women appear to emerge from anesthesia more rapidly than men after standardized anesthetic administration with the same agents.

- Large differences among individuals apart from age or sex groupings in regard to sensitivity to anesthesia.

Indirect measurements of consciousness

Indirect methods that allow an observer to assess a person's level of awareness have been used since the early 1970s. The earliest and most widely used instrument for evaluating impaired consciousness is the Glasgow Coma Scale (GCS), first published in the *Lancet* in 1974. The GCS evaluates the patient's responsiveness under three headings: eye response (four levels of responsiveness), verbal response (five levels), and motor (movement) response (six levels). A normally conscious individual would score 15, the maximum score. In practice, however, the total score on the GCS is usually broken down into three subscores for the three types of response measured; thus E2V2M3 would represent a total GCS score of 7. Total scores on the Glasgow Coma Scale are interpreted as follows: 13–14 indicates mild impairment of consciousness; 9–12 indicates moderate impairment; 8 or lower indicates coma.

There are about a dozen other scales that have been devised to measure consciousness in addition to the GCS; the two that are the most important in this context are the Ramsay Sedation Score, first published in 1974 as a measurement of sedation in patients receiving intravenous sedatives prior to surgery; and the Observer's Assessment of Alertness/Sedation Scale (OAA/SS), first used in 1990 for the same purpose as the Ramsay. These two instruments are significant because they are commonly used in research evaluations of the bispectral index and similar monitoring systems. The Ramsay Score is a six-point scale ranging from one ("patient agitated or restless") through six ("patient asleep; has no response to firm nailbed pressure or other noxious stimuli"). A score of 1 indicates inadequate sedation; 2–4, an acceptable level of sedation; and 5–6, oversedation.

The OAA/SS resembles the Glasgow Coma Scale in that it evaluates different categories of responsiveness, although the categories are different. The OAA/SS measures the patient's responsiveness to his or her name, quality of speech, degree of facial relaxation, and ability to focus the eyes.

KEY TERMS

Algorithm—A procedure or formula for solving a problem. It is often used to refer to a sequence of steps used to program a computer to solve a specific problem.

Analgesia—Absence of the ability to feel pain. The term is also sometimes used to refer to pain relief without loss of consciousness. An analgesic is a drug that is given to relieve pain.

Anesthesia—Loss of the ability to feel pain, brought about by administration of a drug or such other medical interventions as hypnosis or acupuncture.

Anesthesiology—The branch of medicine that specializes in the study of anesthetic agents, their effects on patients, and their proper use and administration.

Areflexia—A condition in which the body's normal reflexes are absent. It is one of the objectives of general anesthesia.

Balanced anesthesia—The use of a combination of inhaled and intravenous drugs in anesthetizing patients.

Coma—A state of unconsciousness from which a person cannot be aroused, even by strong or painful stimuli.

Electroencephalogram (EEG)—A recording of the electrical activity of the nerve cells in the brain. The first such recording was made in 1929 by Hans Berger, an Austrian psychiatrist.

Hemodynamics—Measurement of the movements involved in the circulation of the blood; it usually includes blood pressure and heart rate.

Hypnosis—The term is used to refer to a specific verbal technique for refocusing a person's attention in order to change their perceptions, judgment, control of movements, and memory. A hypnotic medication is one that induces sleep.

Proprietary—Referring to a drug, device, or formula that is secret or sold only by the holder of the patent, trademark, or copyright. The algorithm used in BIS systems is proprietary information.

Sedation—A condition of calm or relaxation, brought about by the use of a drug or medication.

Sequela (plural, sequelae)—An abnormal condition or event resulting from a previous disease or disorder.

Synergistic—Enhancing the effects of another drug. Anesthetics given in combination are often synergistic.

Direct measurements of consciousness

A variety of different physiological responses have been used in attempts to measure the depth of a patient's unconsciousness under anesthesia. Most anesthesiologists use hemodynamic responses—the patient's blood pressure and heart rate—as basic guidelines for adjusting the amount of anesthetic delivered to the patient during surgery. Other direct measurements have been based on movements of the patient's body during surgery, hormonal responses, sweating, eye movement, and the reactivity of the eyes to light. One difficulty that has emerged from these attempts at direct measurement is that that they are not good predictors of the likelihood of awareness during surgery or recall of the procedure after surgery.

Another measurement that researchers have explored in their attempts to measure depth of anesthesia directly is the electroencephalogram, or EEG. The EEG is a complex recording of the electrical activity of the nerve cells in the brain. The first published paper on the EEG was written in 1929 by Dr. Hans Berger, an Austrian psychiatrist, on 73 recordings of

brain waves using his son Klaus as the subject. Berger was the first to distinguish between alpha and beta brain waves, and to use the term EEG to describe the technique of **electroencephalography**. In 1931 Berger discovered that brain waves change in amplitude and frequency when a person is asleep or anesthetized; they slow down, shift to lower frequencies, and become more closely synchronized with one another. He also noted that such diseases as multiple sclerosis and Alzheimer disease affect a person's EEG.

Several attempts were made in the late 1980s and early 1990s to make use of what is known about changes in the EEG in order to monitor anesthetic depth. One attempt is known as spectral edge frequency, or SEF. SEF is the frequency just above 95% of the total power spectrum of electrical energy recorded on an EEG. It was thought that the spectral edge frequency would be useful in guiding adjustments of anesthetics administered during surgery. Unfortunately, SEF is difficult to use with balanced anesthesia; it is also difficult to correlate with such other measures of anesthetic depth as movement or memory of the procedure. Another method that has been tried is median frequency, which is based on the median frequency of the complex EEG electrical signal at any given moment. This method proved to have the same drawbacks as spectral edge frequency. The bispectral index can be understood historically as a slightly later and more sophisticated attempt to use EEG signals to monitor patients' responses to anesthesia.

Development of the bispectral index

The bispectral index was first developed in the early 1990s by applying bispectral analysis to EEG recordings. Bispectral analysis is a method of analyzing the mathematical relationships among the various components of an EEG signal (phase couplings) as well as measuring amplitudes and frequencies. To compile a database for the index, researchers recorded EEGs from several thousand patients and volunteers anesthetized with a range of commonly used anesthetics and anesthetic combinations. Each subject's depth of unconsciousness was evaluated on the basis of a modified version of the OAA/SS described earlier (in the volunteers) or the amount of drug concentration in blood serum (in the patients). Segments of the recorded EEGs were used to draw up a set of EEG features that were then tested for their ability to distinguish between different levels of sedation or unconsciousness. The index that resulted from this process was then tested on different EEG recordings from the researchers' larger database. It is scaled from 100 to 0 so that the BIS value decreases linearly with increasing doses of anesthesia.

It should be noted that the bispectral index is a work in progress. As new anesthetic agents are developed and used, the BIS algorithm is continually retested and refined. In addition, the algorithm is proprietary information, which means that it is kept secret by the company that developed it.

Description

When a patient is brought into the **operating room**, special BIS sensors are applied to his or her forehead. No additional gels or electrodes are required. The anesthesiologist can attach the sensors to the patient in less than 30 seconds, since preparing the patient's skin requires no more than an alcohol wipe to provide good electrical contact. The BIS system itself is integrated into patient monitoring devices produced by a number of different manufacturers that use enhanced EEG monitors. The BIS system displays both raw data from the EEG and a single number between 100 (indicating an awake patient) and 0

(indicating the absence of brain activity) that represents the patient's degree of sedation. The target number for most anesthetized patients is between 50 and 60.

Results

Current applications of BIS

BIS is presently used in intensive care units (ICUs) and some emergency departments as well as in operating rooms. According to company information, the bispectral index is used in about 26% of all hospital operating rooms in the United States as of late 2002. It is claimed that BIS reduces the risk of patient awareness during surgery as well as lowering hospital costs by speeding patient recovery and reducing the overuse of anesthetic agents.

Limitations of BIS

As of 2003, published studies of the bispectral index and other anesthetic monitoring systems presently available indicate that none of them can be considered a "gold standard" for preventing instances of patient awareness under anesthesia or for predicting the depth of anesthesia in a specific patient. Researchers have noted several specific limitations of the BIS system:

- BIS values are affected by the choice of anesthetic agent. This finding means that a patient with a BIS score of 60 anesthetized with one combination of agents may be more deeply sedated than another patient with the same score but anesthetized with a different combination of drugs. In addition, the BIS monitor appears unable to accurately track changes in consciousness produced by certain anesthetics, specifically ketamine and nitrous oxide.
- The changes in the BIS algorithm resulting from updating and refinement of the producer's database make it difficult to compare results obtained by different investigators using different versions of the BIS monitor. This fact also leaves hospital-based anesthesiologists uncertain as to whether findings based on earlier versions of the BIS system are still valid.
- BIS values are difficult to correlate with other measurements of anesthetic depth or altered consciousness. One group of Norwegian researchers found that BIS values had little relationship to serum blood concentrations of anesthetic agents. Other researchers in the United States have found that BIS scores showed wide variability when compared with Glasgow Coma Scores for emergency room patients.

• Standard BIS scores are not useful in monitoring special patient populations, particularly critically ill patients with unstable body temperatures and patients with dementia.

Alternatives

Other anesthesia monitoring systems that are in use as of 2003 include the Patient State Analyzer, or PSA 4000, which is also based on EEG data; and the A-Line (R) monitor, which processes signals derived from auditory stimuli. Current opinion among anesthesiologists appears to be that none of the present monitoring systems are sufficiently sensitive to guarantee that patients will not awaken during surgery while simultaneously preventing undesirable cardiovascular reactions, other stress responses, or overuse of anesthetic agents.

Resources

PERIODICALS

Baars, Bernard J. "The Brain Basis of a 'Consciousness Monitor.' A Breakthrough in Testing Unconsciousness During Anesthesia." *Science and Consciousness Review* 1 May 2002 [cited May 13, 2003]. http://www.psych.pomona.edu/scr/news/articles/20020401.html.

Blanchard, Amy R. "Sedation and Analgesia in Critical Care." *Postgraduate Medicine* 111 (February 2002): 59–60, 63–64, 67–70.

Drover, D. R., H. J. Lemmens, E. T. Pierce, et al. "Patient State Index: Titration of Delivery and Recovery from Propofol, Alfentanil, and Nitrous Oxide Anesthesia." *Anesthesiology* 97 (July 2002): 82–89.

Drummond, John C. "Monitoring Depth of Anesthesia: With Emphasis on the Application of the Bispectral Index and the Middle Latency Auditory Evoked Response to the Prevention of Recall." *Anesthesiology* 93 (September 2000): 876–882.

Frenzel, D., C. A. Greim, C. Sommer, et al. "Is the Bispectral Index Appropriate for Monitoring the Sedation Level of Mechanically Ventilated ICU Patients?" *Intensive Care Medicine* 28 (February 2002): 178–183.

Gill, M., S. M. Green, and B. Krauss. "Can the Bispectral Index Monitor Quantify Altered Level of Consciousness in Emergency Department Patients?" *Academic Emergency Medicine* 10 (February 2003): 175–179.

Hameroff, Stuart, MD. "Anesthesia: The 'Other Side' of Consciousness." *Consciousness and Cognition* 10 (June 2001): 217–229.

Hoymork, S. C., J. Raeder, B. Grimsmo, and P. A. Steen. "Bispectral Index, Predicted and Measured Drug Levels of Target-Controlled Infusions of Remifentanil and Propofol During Laparoscopic Cholecystectomy and Emergence." *Acta Anaesthesiological Scandinavica* 44 (October 2000): 1138–1144.

Kalkman, Cor J., and John C. Drummond. "Monitors of Depth of Anesthesia, Quo Vadis?" *Anesthesiology* 96 (April 2002): 784–787.

Leslie, K., and P. S. Myles. "Awareness During General Anesthesia: Is It Worth Worrying About?" *Medical Journal of Australia* 174 (March 5, 2001): 212–213.

Leslie, K., L. Lee, P. S. Myles, et al. "Patients' Knowledge of and Attitudes Toward Awareness and Depth of Anesthesia Monitoring." *Anaesthesia and Intensive Care* 31 (February 2003): 63–68.

Muncaster, A. R., J. W. Sleigh, and M. Williams. "Changes in Consciousness, Conceptual Memory, and Quantitative Electroencephalographical Measures During Recovery from Sevoflurane- and Remifentanil-Based Anesthesia." *Anesthesia and Analgesia* 96 (March 2003): 720–725.

Osterman, J. E., J. Hopper, W. J. Heran, et al. "Awareness Under Anesthesia and the Development of Posttraumatic Stress Disorder." *General Hospital Psychiatry* 23 (July-August 2001): 198–204.

Renna, M., J. Handy, and A. Shah. "Low Baseline Bispectral Index of the Electroencephalogram in Patients with Dementia." *Anesthesia and Analgesia* 96 (May 2003): 1380–1385.

Riess, M. L., U. A. Graefe, C. Goeters, et al. "Sedation Assessment in Critically Ill Patients with Bispectral Index." *European Journal of Anaesthesiology* 19 (January 2002): 18–22.

Tassi, P., and A. Muzet. "Defining the States of Consciousness." *Neuroscience and Biobehavioral Reviews* 25 (March 2001): 175–191.

Welsby, Ian J., J. Mark Ryan, John V. Booth, et al. "The Bispectral Index in the Diagnosis of Perioperative Stroke: A Case Report and Discussion." *Anesthesia and Analgesia* 96 (February 2003): 435–437.

Wong, C. S. "What's the Matter of Depth of Anesthesia?" *Acta Anaesthesiologica Sinica* 39 (March 2001): 1–2.

ORGANIZATIONS

American Academy of Emergency Medicine (AAEM). 611 East Wells Street, Milwaukee, WI 53202. (800) 884-2236. http://www.aaem.org.

American Association of Nurse Anesthetists (AANA). 222 South Prospect Avenue, Park Ridge, IL 60068-4001. (847) 692-7050. http://www.aana.com.

American Society of Anesthesiologists (ASA). 520 N. Northwest Highway, Park Ridge, IL 60068-2573. (847) 825-5586. http://www.asahq.org.

American Society of Perianesthesia Nurses (ASPAN). 10 Melrose Avenue, Suite 110, Cherry Hill, NJ 08003. (877) 737-9696 or (856) 616-9600. http://www.aspan.org.

Center for Emergency Medicine. 230 McKee Place, Suite 500, Pittsburgh, PA 15213. (412) 647-5300. http://www.centerem.com.

Society for Technology in Anesthesia (STA). PMB 300, 223 North Guadalupe, Santa Fe, NM 87501. (505) 983-4923. http://www.anestech.org.

OTHER

Aspect Medical Systems White Paper. *Technology Overview: Bispectral Index*. Natick, MA: Aspect Medical Systems, 1997.

Greenwald, Scott D., Ph.D., Charles P. Smith, Jeffrey C. Sigl, Ph.D., et al. *Development of the EEG Bispectral Index (R) (BIS(R))*. Abstract presented at the first annual meeting of the Society for Technology in Anesthesia (STA), January 2000 [cited May 12, 2003]. http://www.anestech.org/Publications/Annual_2000/Greenwald.html.

Vuyk, Jaap, MD. *Does Bispectral Index Monitoring Optimize Intravenous Anaesthetic Drug Delivery?* Paper delivered on April 5, 2002 at the fifth annual meeting of the European Society for Intravenous Anaesthesia (Eurosiva) in Nice, France. http://www.eurosiva.org/Archive/Nice/SpeakerAbstracts/Vuyk.htm.

Rebecca Frey, PhD

Bladder augmentation

Definition

Bladder augmentation, also known as augmentation cystoplasty, is **reconstructive surgery** to increase the reservoir capacity of the bladder. The procedure is very common and involves tissue grafts (anastomosis) from a section of the small intestine (bowel), stomach, or other substitutes that are attached to the urinary bladder by sewing or stapling. Whether due to chronic obstructive bladder damage, birth defects that resulted in small reservoir capacity, or dysfunction due to nerve innervation of the bladder muscle (sphincter), surgery is chosen only after a thorough medical work-up that involves assessment of the lower urinary tract, functional physiological evaluation, and anatomic assessment. Some laparoscopic methods (surgery with a fiber-optic instrument inserted through the abdomen) of bladder augmentation have been tried, but reports indicate that these are technically arduous and may not have the long-lasting effects of open surgery.

Purpose

Bladder dysfunction and incontinence may be due to problems with the reservoir capacity of the bladder or with the "gatekeeping" muscle (the sphincter), which, instructed by the brain, allows urine to build up or to be released. Bladder augmentation is used to treat serious and irreversible forms of incontinence and to protect the upper urinary tract (kidney function) from reflexia (urine back up to the kidneys).

Many candidates for the surgery are highly compromised individuals with other serious conditions like spinal cord injuries and multiple sclerosis, as well as patients likely to undergo **kidney transplantation**. Patients who undergo bladder augmentation must be free of bowel and urethral disease and be able to perform self-catheterization (place a urinary tube into their urethra).

Description

Standard augmentation involves segments of the bowel used to create a pouch or wider wall for the bladder in order to enhance its reservoir capacity. Often this reconstruction surgery is accompanied by procedures that tighten the neck of the bladder as well. Until the 1970s it was thought that those with bladder dysfunction could be treated with bladder diversion, and that this procedure offered a simple and safe means of emptying the bladder. However, it was soon discovered that pressure from the bladder caused irreparable damage to the kidneys, with 50% of patients exhibiting such deterioration. The new diagnostic assessment of the bladder as well as the need for a new medical intervention for patients with severe bladder dysfunction opened the way for urinary tract reconstruction. Today, many techniques are available, along with new types of grafting substitutions.

The basic procedure involves open abdominal surgery with removal of a 10–12-in (25–30-cm) segment of ileum (part of the small intestine), cecum (first part of the large intestine), or the ileocecum (the junction of small and large intestines) cut down the middle (detubularized), and shaped into a U-configuration with a pouch at the bottom. This opening or pouch will be the "patch" for the bladder. During surgery, the bladder itself is also opened at the dome and cut at right angles to create a clam-like shape. The open bowel "patch" is then attached to the bladder with sutures or stapling.

Diagnosis/Preparation

Patients selected for bladder augmentation are chosen after they undergo a thorough physical exam, x-ray tests, and bladder physiology tests, as well as a renal and bladder **ultrasound** for any dilation of the kidneys or ureters or kidney obstruction. A VCUG (holding and voiding urine) test is performed to assess the contour of the bladder and to assess for ureteral reflux (back up of urine to the kidneys). Finally, a cystometrogram (CMG) is performed in the physician's office to judge the pressure and volume levels

Bladder augmentation

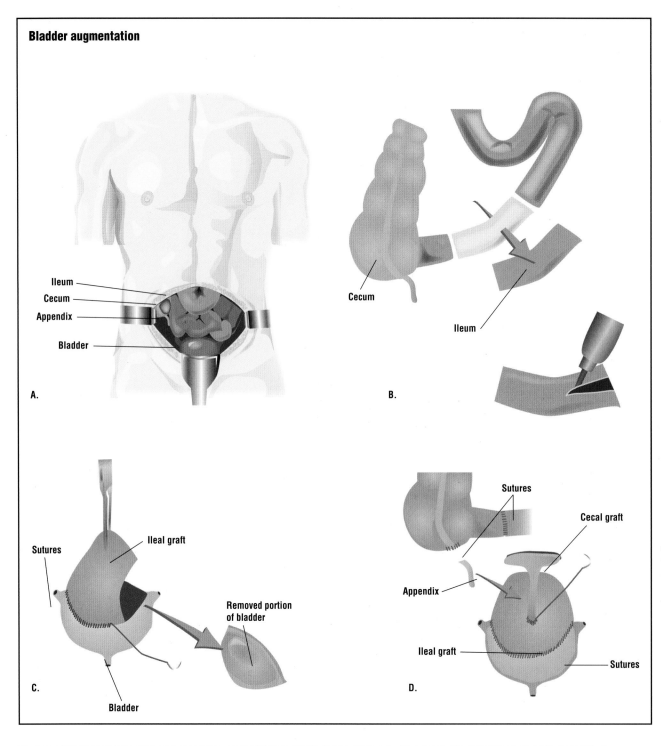

A.

B.

C.

D.

Ileum
Cecum
Appendix
Bladder

Cecum

Ileum

Sutures

Ileal graft

Removed portion
of bladder

Bladder

Sutures

Cecal graft

Appendix

Ileal graft

Sutures

During a bladder augmentation procedure, an incision is made in the abdomen to expose the intestines and bladder **(A)**. A section of ileum (small intestine) is removed and opened **(B)**. After being sterilized, it is grafted onto the bladder to increase its capacity **(C)**. The appendix and cecum (large intestine) may also be used **(D)**. *(Illustration by GGS Information Services. Cengage Learning, Gale.)*

at which the urine leakage occurs. Once the tests, patient history, and physical exam are completed, a treatment plans commence.

The patient should plan for up to two weeks in the hospital. The patient will have been on a low-residue diet for a few days before admission. Surgery will take

KEY TERMS

Anastomosis—The surgical union of parts and especially hollow tubular parts.

Catherization— the use of or insertion of a catheter (as in or into the bladder, trachea, or heart).

Cystoplasty—Reconstructive surgery of the urinary bladder.

Neurogenic bladder—A urinary problem of neurological origin in which there is abnormal emptying of the bladder with subsequent retention or incontinence of urine.

Ureter—Either of the paired channels that carry urine from a kidney to the bladder.

place two to three days after hospital admittance. In the hospital, a general examination will be performed and blood taken. The bowel will need to be cleaned in preparation. Clear fluids will be given, as well as a strong laxative prior to surgery.

Aftercare

Early complications of surgery include cardiovascular, thrombo-embolic (blood clot), gastrointestinal, and respiratory complications associated with major abdominal surgery. Many patients require three months after surgery to allow their augmented bladder to establish itself. This involves a special diet for a few months. The patient also should be aware that the augmented bladder empties after their own (native) bladder. Two weeks after surgery, tests are performed to ensure that the patch is leak proof. Once a watertight reservoir is demonstrated, the catheters and drains that were introduced for surgery are removed.

Risks

Long term risks of the procedure include peptic ulceration of the bladder and perforation of the gastric segment. Spontaneous perforation is rare but it is life threatening and has a 25% mortality rate. Other risks include bacterial infections, metabolic changes, urinary tract infections, and urinary tract stones. Nocturnal incontinence is sometimes a problem after the surgery.

Normal results

Although some patients recover spontaneous voiding function, this does not occur with reliable predictability. Preoperatively, patients should be prepared for

the likelihood that they will have to perform lifelong intermittent catherization and irrigation of the augmented bladder. Other effects are a special diet for up to three months and pain after surgery.

Morbidity and mortality rates

Reported surgical risks include 3–5.7% rate of adhesive small bowel obstruction requiring operative intervention; 5–6% incidence of wound infection; and up to 3% **reoperation** rate for bleeding. Long term complications include a 50% unchanged bladder compliance and renal deterioration. No reduction in growth in children has been reported, but the procedure is not recommended for children who have not reached puberty unless there is the threat of kidney damage without surgery.

Alternatives

Bladder augmentation is a medical treatment of last resort for those patients unable to avoid incontinence through medical alternatives. Other surgeries may be indicated if the individual is not a candidate for self-catherization or has other medical or psychological conditions that would rule out bladder augmentation.

Resources

BOOKS

Dewan, P., and M. E. Mitchell, eds. *Bladder Augmentation.* Oxford Press, 2000.

PERIODICALS

Abrams, P., S. K. Lowry, et al. "Assessment and Treatment of Urinary Incontinence." *Lancet* 355 (June 2000): 2153–58

Fantl, J. A., D. K. Newman, J. Colling, et al. "Urinary Incontinence in Adults: Acute and Chronic Management. Clinical Practice Guideline, Number 2, 1996." *Agency for Health Policy and Research Publications* (March 1996).

Greenwell, T. J., S. N. Venn, and A. R. Mundy. "Augmentation Cystoplasty." *British Journal of Urology International* 88, no. 6 (October 2001): 511–534.

Qucek, M. I., and D. A. Ginsberg. "Long-term Urodynamics Follow-up of Bladder Augmentation for Neurogenic Bladder." *Urology* 169 (January 2003): 195–198.

Rackley, R. R., and J. B. Abdelmalak. "Radical Prostatectomy: Laparoscopic Augmentation Cystoplasty." *Urological Clinics of America* 28 (August 2001).

ORGANIZATIONS

National Association for Continence. P.O. Box 8310 Spartanburg, SC 29305. (800) BLADDER, (252-3337). http://www.nafc.org.

National Kidney and Urologic Diseases Information Clearinghouse. 3 Information Way, Bethesda, MD 20892-3580. (301) 654-4415. http://www.niddk.nih.gov.

The Simon Foundation for Continence. P.O. Box 835 Wilmette, IL 60091. (800) 23SIMON (237-4666). http://www.simonfoundation.org.

OTHER

"Bladder Augmentation." Dr. Rajhttp. [cited April 2003]. http://www.drrajmd.com/treatments/treatments.htm.

Carr, Michael, and M. E. Mitchell. "Bladder Augmentation." *Digital Urological Journal* [cited April 2003]. http://www.duj.com/Article/Carr/Carr.html.

"Neurogenic Bladder." [cited April 2003]. http://www.med.wayne.edu/urology/DISEASES/neurogenicbladder.html.

Nancy McKenzie, Ph.D.

Bladder removal *see* **Cystectomy**

Bladder resection *see* **Transurethral bladder resection**

Bladder tumor antigen test *see* **Tumor marker tests**

Blepharoplasty

Definition

Blepharoplasty is a cosmetic surgical procedure that removes fat deposits, excess tissue, or muscle from the eyelids to improve the appearance of the eyes.

Purpose

The primary use of blepharoplasty is for improving the cosmetic appearance of the eyes. In some older persons, however, sagging and excess skin surrounding the eyes can be so extensive that it limits the range of vision. In those cases, blepharoplasty serves a more functional purpose.

Demographics

Approximately 100,000 blepharoplasty procedures are performed each year in the United States. The procedure is more common among women than men.

Description

Blepharoplasty can be performed on the upper or lower eyelid. It can involve the removal of excess skin and fat deposits and the tightening of selected muscles surrounding the eyelids. The goal is to provide a more youthful appearance and/or to improve eyesight.

The surgeon begins by deciding whether excess skin, fat deposits, or muscle looseness are at fault. While a person is sitting upright, the surgeon marks where incisions will be made on the skin. Care is taken to hide the incision lines in the natural skin folds above and below the eye. The surgeon then injects a local anesthetic to numb the pain. Many surgeons also administer a sedative intravenously during the procedure.

After a small, crescent-shaped section of eyelid skin is removed, the surgeon works to tease out small pockets of fat that have collected in the lids. If muscle looseness is also a problem, the surgeon may trim tissue or add a stitch to pull muscle tissue tighter. Then the incision is closed with **stitches**.

In some persons, fat deposits in the lower eyelid may be the only or primary problem. Such people may be good candidates for transconjunctival blepharoplasty. In this procedure the surgeon makes no incision on the surface of the eyelid, but instead enters from behind, through the inner surface of the lid, to tease out the fat deposits from a small incision. The advantage of this procedure is that there is no visible scar.

Ectropion—A complication of blepharoplasty, in which the lower lid is pulled downward, exposing the inner surface.

Intravenous sedation—A method of injecting a fluid sedative into the blood through the vein.

Retrobulbar hematoma—A rare complication of blepharoplasty, in which a pocket of blood forms behind the eyeball.

Transconjuctival blepharoplasty—A type of blepharoplasty in which the surgeon makes no incision on the surface of the eyelid, but, instead, enters from behind to tease out the fat deposits.

Diagnosis/Preparation

Before performing blepharoplasty, the surgeon assesses whether a person is a good candidate for the treatment. A thorough medical history is important. The surgeon requires knowledge of any history of thyroid disease, hypertension, or eye problems, which may increase the risk of complications.

Prior to surgery, surgeons and their candidates meet to discuss the procedure, clarify the results that can be achieved, and discuss potential problems that might occur. Having realistic expectations is important in any cosmetic procedure. Candidates learn, for example, that although blepharoplasty can improve the appearance of the eyelid, other procedures, such as a chemical peel, may be necessary to reduce the appearance of wrinkles around the eye. Some surgeons prescribe vitamin C and vitamin K for 10 days prior to surgery in the belief that this helps the healing process. Candidates are also told to stop smoking in the weeks before and after the procedure, and to refrain from using alcohol or **aspirin**.

Aftercare

An antibiotic ointment is applied to the line of stitches each day for several days after surgery. Patients also take an antibiotic several times a day to prevent infection. Ice-cold compresses are applied to the eyes continuously for the first day following surgery, and several times a day for the next week or so, to reduce swelling. Some swelling and discoloration around the eyes is expected with the procedure. Persons should avoid aspirin or alcoholic beverages for one week and should limit their activities, including bending, straining, and lifting. The stitches are removed a

Blepharoplasty procedures are performed by surgeons with specialized training in plastic and reconstructive surgery. They are most commonly performed in outpatient facilities or in private professional offices. The procedure may also be performed in a hospital.

In 2003, the average price of blepharoplasty for both upper lids was approximately $4,000. For both lower lids, the cost may be slightly higher. The cost for both upper and lower blepharoplasty was approximately $6,000. These prices usually include anesthesia and surgeon fees. Medications and lab work, as well as any revisionary work, are not included.

few days after surgery. People can generally return to their usual activities within a week to 10 days.

Risks

As with any surgical procedure, blepharoplasty can lead to infection and scarring. Good care of the wound following surgery can minimize these risks. In cases where too much skin is removed from the eyelids, people may experience difficulty closing their eyes. Dry eye syndrome may develop, requiring the use of artificial tears to lubricate the eye. In a rare complication, called retrobulbar hematoma, a pocket of blood forms behind the eyeball.

Normal results

Most people can expect good results from blepharoplasty, with the removal of excess eyelid skin and fat producing a more youthful appearance. Some swelling and discoloration is expected immediately following the procedure, but this clears in time. Small scars will be left where the surgeon has made incisions; but these generally lighten in appearance over several months, and, if placed correctly, will not be readily noticeable.

Morbidity and mortality rates

If too much excess skin is removed from the upper eyelid, persons may be unable to close their eyes completely. Another surgery to correct the defect may be required. Similarly, too much skin can be removed from the lower eyelid, allowing too much of the white of the eye (the sclera) to show. In extreme cases, the lower lid may be pulled down too far, revealing the underlying tissue. This is called an ectropion and also may require a second, corrective surgery. The eye's ability to make tears may also be compromised, leading to dry eye syndrome. Dry eye syndrome can be dangerous; in rare cases it leads to damage to the cornea of the eye and vision loss.

Alternatives

Some of the alternatives to blepharoplasty include losing some excess body fat through diet and **exercise**, accepting one's body and appearance as it is, or using makeup to de-emphasize the area.

Resources

BOOKS

Engler, Alan M. *BodySculpture: Plastic Surgery of the Body for Men and Women,* 2nd ed. Hudson Pub, 2000.

Irwin, Brandith and Mark McPherson. *Your Best Face: Looking Your Best without Plastic Surgery.* Carlsbad, CA: Hay House, Inc, 2002.

Man, Daniel, and L. C. Faye. *New Art of Man: Faces of Plastic Surgery: Your Guide to the Latest Cosmetic Surgery Procedures, 3rd ed.* New York: BeautyArt Press, 2003.

Papel, I. D., and S. S. Park. *Facial Plastic and Reconstructive Surgery,* 2nd ed. New York: Thieme Medical Publishers, 2000.

PERIODICALS

Byrd, H. S. and J. D. Burt. "Achieving Aesthetic Balance in the Brow, Eyelids, and Midface." *Plastic and Reconstructive Surgery* 110 (2002): 926–939.

Cather, J. C., and A. Menter. "Update on Botulinum Toxin for Facial Aesthetics." *Dermatology Clinics of North America* 20 (2002): 749–761.

Oliva, M. S., A. J. Ahmadi, R. Mudumbai, J. L. Hargiss, and B. S. Sires. "Transient Impaired Vision, External Ophthalmoplegia, and Internal Ophthalmoplegia after Blepharoplasty under Local Anesthesia." *American Journal of Ophthalmology* 135 (2003): 410–412.

Yaremchuk, M. J. "Restoring Palpebral Fissure Shape after Previous Lower Blepharoplasty." *Plastic and Reconstructive Surgery* 111 (2003): 441–450.

ORGANIZATIONS

American Academy of Facial Plastic and Reconstructive Surgery. 310 S. Henry Street, Alexandria, VA 22314. (703) 299-9291. Fax: (703) 299-8898. http://www.facial-plastic-surgery.org.

American Board of Plastic Surgery. Seven Penn Center, Suite 400, 1635 Market Street, Philadelphia, PA 19103-2204. (215) 587-9322. http://www.abplsurg.org.

American College of Plastic and Reconstructive Surgery. http://www.breast-implant.org.

American College of Surgeons. 633 North Saint Claire Street, Chicago, IL, 60611. (312) 202-5000. http://www.facs.org.

American Society for Aesthetic Plastic Surgery. 11081 Winners Circle, Los Alamitos, CA 90720. (800) 364-2147 or (562) 799-2356. http://www.surgery.org.

American Society for Dermatologic Surgery. 930 N. Meacham Road, P.O. Box 4014, Schaumburg, IL 60168-4014. (847) 330-9830. http://www.asds-net.org.

American Society of Plastic and Reconstructive Surgeons. 44 E. Algonquin Rd., Arlington Heights, IL 60005. (847) 228-9900. http://www.plasticsurgery.org.

American Society of Plastic Surgeons. 444 E. Algonquin Rd., Arlington Heights, IL 60005. (888) 475-2784. http://www.plasticsurgery.org.

OTHER

"Blepharoplasty." *American Society of Ophthalmic Plastic and Reconstructive Surgery.* [cited April 2003]. http://www.asoprs.org/blepharoplasty.html.

"Blepharoplasy." *Facial Plastic Surgery Network.* [cited March 2003]. http://www.facialplasticsurgery.net/blepharoplasty.htm.

"Eyelid Surgery (Blepharoplasty)." *Department of Otolaryngology/Head and Neck Surgery at Columbia University and New York Presbyterian Hospital.* 2002 [cited April 2003]. http://www.entcolumbia.org/bleph.htm.

Galli, Suzanne K. Doud, and Phillip J. Miller. "Blepharoplasty, Transconjunctival Approach." *emedicine.* September 11, 2001 [cited April 2003]. http://www.emedicine.com/ent/topic95.htm.

L. Fleming Fallon, Jr., MD, DrPH

Blood Ca (calcium) level

Definition

Calcium is the most prevalent mineral in the body. It is a major component of bones and teeth, and is also important in the functioning of the muscles, nervous system, heart, and the blood clotting system.

Vorbefund / Prior Analysis	Element	Normalbereich / Normal Range	Ergebnis / Result
	Na	1900-2000	1848
	K	1750-1850	1859
	Ca	59.0-61.0	56.24
	Mg	34.0-36.0	31.21
	Cu	1.10-1.20	0.98
	Fe	440-480	500.6
	Zn	7.30-7.70	7.42
	P	350-390	348.8
	Pb	bis 0.10	
	Li	0.010-0.050	

Alle Werte beziehen sich auf mg/l. – All values refer to mg/l.

Blood calcium level results. (blickwinkel / Alamy)

The bones are the body's major storage compartment for calcium. About 99% of the body's total calcium is located in bone. In the blood, calcium is either free or bound to the protein albumin. The bound calcium is essentially inactive; the free calcium is considered biologically active. Calcium is obtained through the diet, and requires the presence of a normal quantity of vitamin D for efficient absorption from the intestine into the bloodstream.

Hormones involved in calcium metabolism include parathyroid hormone and calcitonin. Parathyroid hormone is released by the parathyroid glands, which are located behind the thyroid gland in the mid-neck. When blood calcium levels are low, the parathyroid glands are stimulated to produce and release parathyroid hormone. Parathyroid hormone acts to induce the release of calcium from bone. Parathyroid hormone is also active in the kidney, and is involved in keeping calcium from being excreted out of the body. Parathyroid hormone also stimulates the kidney to convert vitamin D into its active form, calcitriol, which is paramount to the intestinal absorption of calcium. Calcitonin is produced by special cells (parafollicular cells) in the thyroid gland. Calcitonin is involved in prompting bone to resorb calcium from the bloodstream.

Purpose

A blood calcium level may be drawn as part of a general metabolic panel, during a routine **physical examination**. A blood calcium level may also be ordered if there are concerns regarding arrhythmias of the heart; problems with the muscles or nervous system; kidney stone; pancreatitis; infection; evidence of kidney disease; concerns about intestinal absorption; or problems with blood clotting. The test may also be useful if the patient has signs of too much blood calcium (hypercalcemia) or low blood calcium (hypocalcemia). Signs of hypercalcemia can include abnormal tiredness, weakness, decreased appetite, nausea and vomiting, constipation, excessive thirstiness, increased urination. Signs of hypocalcemia can include numbness or a tingling sensation in the hands and feet and around the mouth, muscle spasms, or abdominal cramps. Blood calcium levels may also be monitored regularly in patients who have conditions that may cause abnormal calcium levels, such as cancers of the breast, lung, head and neck, kidney, and multiple myeloma; malnutrition (including due to anorexia or other eating disorders); thyroid disease; intestinal disorders; kidney disease; history of kidney transplant; treatment with calcium or vitamin D supplements.

Precautions

Patients who use calcium supplements or vitamin D should stop taking them for the twenty-four hours prior to their blood test.

Description

This test requires blood to be drawn from a vein (usually one in the forearm), generally by a nurse or phlebotomist (an individual who has been trained to draw blood). A tourniquet is applied to the arm above the area where the needle stick will be performed. The site of the needle stick is cleaned with antiseptic, and the needle is inserted. The blood is collected in vacuum tubes. After collection, the needle is withdrawn, and pressure is kept on the blood draw site to stop any bleeding and decrease bruising. A bandage is then applied.

Preparation

There are no restrictions on diet or physical activity, either before or after the blood test.

Aftercare

As with any blood tests, discomfort, bruising, and/or a very small amount of bleeding is common at the puncture site. Immediately after the needle is withdrawn, it is helpful to put pressure on the puncture site until the bleeding has stopped. This decreases the chance of significant bruising. Warm packs may relieve minor discomfort. Some individuals may feel briefly woozy after a blood test, and they should be encouraged to lie down and rest until they feel better.

KEY TERMS

Calcitonin—A hormone made by the thyroid gland. Calcitonin is involved in regulating levels of calcium and phophorus in the blood.

Hypercalcemia—High levels of blood calcium.

Hypocalcemia—Low levels of blood calcium.

Pancreatitis—Inflammation of the pancreas.

Parathyroid hormone—A hormone that is secreted by the parathyroid glands. Parathyroid hormone is involved in the regulation of calcium levels in the blood.

Risks

Basic blood tests, such as blood calcium levels, do not carry any significant risks, other than slight bruising and the chance of brief dizziness.

Results

The blood calcium level can be determined by measuring the total blood calcium (the calcium that is bound to the protein albumin and the calcium that is free in the blood serum), or by measuring the free (ionized) calcium. Although measuring the total blood calcium is generally easier and usually sufficient in most patients, some patients have conditions that will affect these results; in these patients, it is important to measure the free calcium. Such patients include those who are extremely, critically ill, patients who are getting blood transfusions or large quantities of intravenous fluids or nutrition; patients who will undergo or have recently undergone major surgery, and patients who do not have normal levels of blood protein (albumin).

Normal results for a total blood calcium level in adults ranges from 0.0–103.5 milligrams per deciliter (mg/dL) or 2.25–2.75 millimoles per liter (mmol/L). Children have higher calcium levels, because their bones are in such a high-growth phase. Normal total blood calcium levels in children range from 7.6–10.8 mg/dL or 1.9–2.7 mmol/L. A normal free or ionized calcium level in adults is 4.65–5.28 mg/dL.

High levels

High blood calcium levels may be due to:

• prolonged bedrest;
• hyperparathyroidism (overactive parathyroid glands);
• kidney disease;

• tuberculosis;
• cancer in the bones;
• too much calcium, vitamin D, or vitamin A in the diet; excessive intake of dairy products; excessive intake of antacids or supplements;
• dehydration;
• sarcoidosis;
• Paget's disease;
• Addison's disease; or
• chronic kidney or liver diseases.

Low levels

Low blood calcium levels may be due to:

• hypoparathyroidism (underactive parathyroid glands);
• intestinal problems that interfere with appropriate absorption of nutrients;
• bone disorders;
• kidney disease;
• pancreatitis;
• low serum albumin (hypoalbuminemia);
• low magnesium;
• pregnancy; or
• advanced age in men.

Resources

BOOKS

Brenner, B. M., and F. C. Rector, eds. *Brenner & Rector's The Kidney,* 7th ed. Philadelphia: Saunders, 2004.

Goldman L., D. Ausiello, eds. *Cecil Textbook of Internal Medicine,* 23rd ed. Philadelphia: Saunders, 2007.

McPherson R. A., and M. R. Pincus, eds. *Henry's Clinical Diagnosis and Management by Laboratory Methods,* 21st ed. Philadelphia: Saunders, 2006.

OTHER

Medical Encyclopedia. Medline Plus. U.S. National Library of Medicine and the National Institutes of Health. January 2, 2008. http://www.nlm.nih.gov/medlineplus/encyclopedia.html (February 10, 2008).

ORGANIZATIONS

American Association for Clinical Chemistry, 1850 K Street, NW, Suite 625, Washington, DC, 20006, (800) 892-1400, http://www.aacc.org.

Rosalyn Carson-DeWitt, M.D.

Blood carbon dioxide level

Definition

Carbon dioxide is the waste product of the respiratory system. It is a gas that is exchanged for oxygen in the body's tissues, transported to the lungs, and then breathed off during exhalation.

Carbon dioxide travels throughout the body in the form of bicarbonate, or HCO_3-. Bicarbonate levels are involved in keeping the body in appropriate acid-base balance (pH level). When the kidneys sense that the body's acid-base balance is tending towards the acidic, the kidneys secrete more bicarbonate, in order to neutralize the acid. When the kidneys sense that the body's acid-base balance is tending towards the more alkaline, the kidneys reabsorb bicarbonate from the bloodstream, in order to decrease the body's alkalinity.

On a cellular level, bicarbonate works in concert with sodium, chloride, and potassium to attain and maintain appropriate pH balance within cells.

A blood carbon dioxide level reflects the presence of all three forms of carbon dioxide in the blood, including bicarbonate (HCO_3-), carbonic acid (H_2CO_3) and dissolved CO_2. The level of bicarbonate present, therefore, is extrapolated from the overall blood carbon dioxide level; it is not an exact measurement, but an estimate based on the total blood carbon dioxide level measured.

Purpose

A blood carbon dioxide level is usually drawn as part of a larger panel of electrolytes. Other measurements in the electrolyte panel include chloride, potassium, and sodium. Sometimes the blood carbon dioxide level is drawn along with an **arterial blood gas**, and the results are correlated with each other to help determine whether the acid-base imbalance is due to respiratory causes or metabolic causes. Respiratory acid-base imbalances are due to an imbalance in the intake of oxygen relative to the output of carbon dioxide. Metabolic acid-base imbalances are due to inappropriate amounts of bicarbonate in the blood. Excess bicarbonate results in metabolic alkalosis; a shortage of bicarbonate results in metabolic acidosis.

Precautions

There are no precautions necessary prior to having a blood carbon dioxide level drawn. Patients can continue their usual diet, activities, and medications.

Patients who are taking anticoagulant medications should inform their healthcare practitioner, since this may increase their chance of bleeding or bruising after a blood test.

Description

This test requires blood to be drawn from a vein (usually one in the forearm), generally by a nurse or phlebotomist (an individual who has been trained to draw blood). A tourniquet is applied to the arm above the area where the needle stick will be performed. The site of the needle stick is cleaned with antiseptic, and the needle is inserted. The blood is collected in vacuum tubes. After collection, the needle is withdrawn, and pressure is kept on the blood draw site to stop any bleeding and decrease bruising. A bandage is then applied.

Preparation

There are no restrictions on diet or physical activity, either before or after the blood test.

Aftercare

As with any blood tests, discomfort, bruising, and/or a very small amount of bleeding is common at the puncture site. Immediately after the needle is withdrawn, it is helpful to put pressure on the puncture site until the bleeding has stopped. This decreases the chance of significant bruising. Warm packs may relieve minor discomfort. Some individuals may feel briefly woozy after a blood test, and they should be encouraged to lie down and rest until they feel better.

Risks

Basic blood tests, such as blood carbon dioxide levels, do not carry any significant risks, other than slight bruising and the chance of brief dizziness.

Results

In adults, a normal blood carbon dioxide level is 23–29 millimoles per liter (mmol/L). In children a normal blood carbon dioxide level is 20–28 mmol/L. In infants, a normal blood carbon dioxide level is 13–22 mmol/L.

A number of drugs may affect the results of the test. Blood carbon dioxide levels may be elevated in patients who are using steroid medications, **barbiturates**, bicarbonates, and loop **diuretics**. Blood carbon dioxide levels may be decreased in patients who are using methicillin, nitrofurantoin, tetracycline, thiazide diuretics, and triamterene. It is important that the healthcare provider take into consideration the effects that these drugs may have on the blood carbon dioxide level.

High levels

High blood carbon dioxide levels may be due to:

- chronic obstructive pulmonary disease;
- emphysema;
- pneumonia;
- Cushing's disease;
- Conn's syndrome;
- alcoholism; or
- vomiting.

Low levels

Low blood carbon dioxide levels may be due to:

- pneumonia;
- cirrhosis of the liver;
- liver failure;
- hyperventilation (fast, shallow breathing);
- diabetes;
- kidney failure;
- liver failure;

- salicylate (aspirin) overdose;
- shock states;
- chronic diarrhea;
- dehydration;
- chronic severe malnutrition; or
- ingestion of toxins such as antifreeze (ethylene glycol) or wood alcohol (methanol).

Resources

BOOKS

Brenner, B. M., and F. C. Rector, eds. *Brenner & Rector's The Kidney,* 7th ed. Philadelphia: Saunders, 2004.

Goldman L., D. Ausiello, eds. *Cecil Textbook of Internal Medicine,* 23rd ed. Philadelphia: Saunders, 2007.

Mason, R. J., V. C. Broaddus, J. F. Murray, and J. A. Nadel. *Murray & Nadel's Textbook of Respiratory Medicine,* 4th ed. Philadelphia: Saunders, 2005.

McPherson R. A., and M. R. Pincus, eds. *Henry's Clinical Diagnosis and Management by Laboratory Methods,* 21st ed. Philadelphia: Saunders, 2006.

OTHER

Medical Encyclopedia. Medline Plus. U.S. National Library of Medicine and the National Institutes of Health. January 2, 2008. http://www.nlm.nih.gov/medlineplus/encyclopedia.html (February 10, 2008).

ORGANIZATIONS

American Association for Clinical Chemistry, 1850 K Street, NW, Suite 625, Washington, DC, 20006, (800) 892-1400, http://www.aacc.org.

Rosalyn Carson-DeWitt, M.D.

Blood clot prevention *see* **Venous thrombosis prevention**

Blood count *see* **Complete blood count**

Blood crossmatching *see* **Type and screen**

Blood culture

Definition

A blood culture is done when a person has symptoms of a blood infection, also called bacteremia. Blood is drawn from the person one or more times and is tested in a laboratory to find and identify any microorganism present and growing in the blood. If a microorganism is found, more testing is done to determine the **antibiotics** that will be effective in treating the infection.

Description

Culture strategies

There are many variables involved in performing a blood culture. Before the person's blood is drawn, the physician must make several decisions based on a knowledge of infections and the person's clinical condition and medical history.

Several groups of microorganisms, including bacteria, viruses, mold, and yeast, can cause blood infections. The bacteria group can be further broken down into aerobes and anaerobes. Most microbes do not need oxygen to live. They can grow with oxygen (aerobic microbes) or without oxygen (anaerobic microbes).

Based on the clinical condition of the patient, the physician determines what group of microorganisms is likely to be causing the infection and then orders one or more specific types of blood culture, including aerobic, anaerobic, viral, or fungal (for yeasts and molds). Each specific type of culture is handled differently by the laboratory. Most blood cultures test for both aerobic and anaerobic microbes. Fungal, viral, and mycobacterial blood cultures can also be done, but are less common.

The physician must also decide how many blood cultures should be done. One culture is rarely enough; two to three are usually adequate. Four cultures are occasionally required. Some factors influencing this decision are the specific microorganisms the physician expects to find based on the person's symptoms or previous culture results, and whether or not the person has had recent antibiotic therapy.

The time at which the cultures are to be drawn is another decision made by the physician. During most blood infections (called intermittent bacteremia) microorganisms enter the blood at various time intervals. Blood drawn randomly may miss the microorganisms. Since microorganisms enter the blood 30–90 minutes before the person's fever spikes, collecting the culture just after the fever spike offers the best likelihood of finding the microorganism. The second and third cultures may be collected at the same time, but from different places on the person, or spaced at 30-minute or one-hour intervals, as the physician chooses. During continuous bacteremia, such as infective endocarditis, microorganisms are always in the blood and the timing of culture collection is less important. Blood cultures should always be collected before antibiotic treatment has begun.

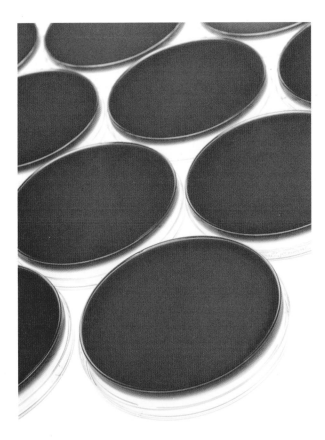

Blood in agar growth medium. (Andrew Paterson / Alamy)

Purpose

Bacteremia is a serious clinical condition and can lead to **death**. To give the best chance for effective treatment and survival, a blood culture is done as soon as an infection is suspected.

Symptoms of bacteremia are fever, chills, mental confusion, anxiety, rapid heart beat, hyperventilation, blood clotting problems, and shock. These symptoms are especially significant in a person who already has another illness or infection, is hospitalized, or has trouble fighting infections because of a weak immune system. Often, the blood infection results from an infection somewhere else in the body that has spread.

Additionally, blood cultures are done to find the causes of other infections. These include bacterial pneumonia (an infection of the lung), and infectious endocarditis (an infection of the inner layer of the heart). Both of these infections leak bacteria into the blood.

After a blood infection has been diagnosed, confirmed by culture, and treated, an additional blood culture may be done to make sure the infection is gone.

Laboratory analysis

Bacteria are the most common microorganisms found in blood infections. Laboratory analysis of a bacterial blood culture differs slightly from that of a fungal culture and significantly from that of a viral culture.

Blood is drawn from a person and put directly into a blood culture bottle containing a nutritional broth. After the laboratory receives the blood culture bottle, several processes must be completed:

- provide an environment for the bacteria to grow;
- detect the growth when it occurs;
- identify the bacteria that grow; and
- test the bacteria against certain antibiotics to determine which antibiotic will be effective.

There are several types of systems, both manual and automated, available to laboratories to carry out these processes.

The broth in the blood culture bottle is the first step in creating an environment in which bacteria will grow. It contains all the nutrients that bacteria need to grow. If the physician expects anaerobic bacteria to grow, oxygen will be kept out of the blood culture bottle; if aerobes are expected, oxygen will be allowed in the bottle.

The bottles are placed in an incubator and kept at **body temperature**. They are watched daily for signs of growth, including cloudiness or a color change in the broth, gas bubbles, or clumps of bacteria. When there is evidence of growth, the laboratory does a gram stain and a subculture. To do the gram stain, a drop of blood is removed from the bottle and placed on a microscope slide. The blood is allowed to dry and then is stained with purple and red stains and examined under the microscope. If bacteria are seen, the color of stain they picked up (purple or red), their shape (such as round or rectangular), and their size provide valuable clues as to what type of microorganism they are and what antibiotics might work best. To do the subculture, a drop of blood is placed on a culture plate, spread over the surface, and placed in an incubator.

If there is no immediate visible evidence of growth in the bottles, the laboratory looks for bacteria by doing gram stains and subcultures. These steps are repeated daily for the first several days and periodically after that.

When bacteria grows, the laboratory identifies it using biochemical tests and the gram stain. Sensitivity testing, also called antibiotic susceptibility testing, is also done. The bacteria are tested against many different antibiotics to see which antibiotics can effectively kill it.

All information is passed on to the physician as soon as it is known. An early report, known as a preliminary report, is usually available after one day. This report will tell if any bacteria have been found yet and, if so, the results of the gram stain. The next preliminary report may include a description of the bacteria growing on the subculture. The laboratory notifies the physician immediately when an organism is found and as soon as sensitivity tests are complete. Sensitivity tests may be complete before the bacteria is completely identified. The final report may not be available for five to seven days. If bacteria was found, the report will include its complete identification and a list of the antibiotics to which the bacteria is sensitive.

One automated system is considered one of the most important technical advances in blood cultures. It is called continuous-monitoring blood culture systems (CMBCS). The instruments automatically monitor the bottles containing the patient blood for evidence of microorganisms, usually every 10 minutes. Many data points are collected daily for each bottle, and fed into a computer for analysis. Sophisticated mathematical calculations can determine when microorganisms have grown. This, combined with more frequent blood tests, make it possible to detect microbial growth earlier. In addition, all CMBCS instruments have the detection system, incubator, and agitation device in one unit.

Preparation

Ten ml (milliliter) of blood is usually needed for each blood culture bottle. First a healthcare worker locates a vein in the inner elbow region. The area of skin where the blood will be drawn must be disinfected to prevent any microorganisms on a person's skin from entering the blood culture bottle and contaminating it. The area is disinfected by wiping the area with alcohol in a circular fashion, starting with tiny circles at the spot where the needle will puncture the skin and enlarging the size of the circles while wiping away from the puncture site. The same pattern of wiping is repeated using an iodine or iodophor solution. The top of the bottle is disinfected using alcohol. After the person's skin has been disinfected, the healthcare worker draws the blood and about 10 ml of blood is injected into each blood culture bottle. The type of bottles used will vary based on whether the physician is looking for bacteria (aerobes or anaerobes), yeast, mold, or viruses.

Aftercare

Discomfort or bruising may occur at the puncture site or the person may feel dizzy or faint. Pressure to the puncture site until the bleeding stops reduces bruising. Warm packs relieve discomfort.

Normal results

Normal results will be negative. A single negative culture does not rule out a blood infection. False negatives can occur if the person was started on antibiotics before the blood was drawn, if the environment for growth was not right, the timing was off, or for some unknown reason the microorganism just didn't grow. Three negative cultures may be enough to rule out bacteremia in the case of endocarditis.

Abnormal results

The physician's skill in interpreting the culture results and assessing the person's clinical condition is essential in distinguishing a blood culture that is truly positive from a culture that is positive because it became contaminated. In true bacteremia, the patient's clinical condition should be consistent with a blood infection caused by the microorganism that was found. The microorganism is usually found in more than one culture, it usually grows soon after the bottles are incubated, and it is often the cause of an infection somewhere else in the person's body.

When the culture is positive because of contamination, the patient's clinical condition usually is not consistent with an infection from the identified microorganism. In addition, the microorganism is often one commonly found on skin, it rarely causes infection, it is found in only one bottle, and it may appear after several days of incubation. More than one microorganism often grow in contaminated cultures.

Morbidity and mortality rates

Morbidity rates are miniscule. The most common problems are minor bleeding and bruising. Since neither are reportable events, morbidity can only be estimated. Mortality is essentially zero.

Precautions

The only precaution needed is to clean the venipuncture site with alcohol.

Side effects

The most common side effects of a blood culture are minor bleeding and bruising.

Resources

BOOKS

Fischbach, F. T. and M. B. Dunning. *A Manual of Laboratory and Diagnostic Tests,* 8th ed. Philadelphia: Lippincott Williams & Wilkins, 2008.

McGhee, M. *A Guide to Laboratory Investigations,* 5th ed. Oxford, UK: Radcliffe Publishing Ltd., 2008.

Price, C. P. *Evidence-Based Laboratory Medicine: Principles, Practice, and Outcomes,* 2nd ed. Washington, DC: AACC Press, 2007.

Scott, M. G., A. M. Gronowski, and C. S. Eby. *Tietz's Applied Laboratory Medicine,* 2nd ed. New York: Wiley-Liss, 2007.

Springhouse Corp. *Diagnostic Tests Made Incredibly Easy!,* 2nd ed. Philadelphia: Lippincott Williams & Wilkins, 2008.

PERIODICALS

Dagogo-Jack, S., M. M. Funnell, and J. Davidson. "Barriers to achieving optimal glycemic control in a multi-ethnic society: a US focus." *Current Diabetes Reviews* 2, no. 3 (August 2006): 285–293.

Dosanjh, D. P., T. S. Hinks, J. A. Innes, et al. "Improved diagnostic evaluation of suspected tuberculosis." *Annals of Internal Medicine* 148, no. 5 (March 2008): 325–336.

Haylock, D. N., and S. K. Nilsson. "Expansion of umbilical cord blood for clinical transplantation." *Current Stem Cell Research and Therapy* 2, no. 4 (December 2007): 324–335.

Tavil, B., Y. I. Balci, I. Yildirim, G. Secmeer, M. Ceyhan, and M. Turncer. "Linezolid-induced reversible bicytopenia in a 4-year-old boy with methicillin-resistant Staphylococcus aureus bacteremia." *Pediatric Hematology and Oncology* 25, no. 1 (January 2008): 67–71.

OTHER

American Clinical Laboratory Association. Information about clinical chemistry. http://www.clinical-labs.org/ (February 24, 2008).

Clinical Laboratory Management Association. Information about clinical chemistry. http://www.clma.org/ (February 22, 2008).

Lab Tests Online. Information about lab tests. http://www.labtestsonline.org/ (February 24, 2008).

National Accreditation Agency for Clinical Laboratory Sciences. Information about laboratory tests. http://www.naacls.org/ (February 25, 2008).

ORGANIZATIONS

American Association for Clinical Chemistry, 1850 K Street, NW, Suite 625, Washington, DC, 20006, (800) 892-1400, http://www.aacc.org/AACC/.

American Society for Clinical Laboratory Science, 6701 Democracy Blvd., Suite 300, Bethesda, MD, 20817, (301) 657-2768, http://www.ascls.org/.

American Society for Clinical Pathology, 1225 New York Ave., NW, Suite 250, Washington, DC, 20005, (202) 347-4450, http://www.ascp.org/.

College of American Pathologists, 325 Waukegan Rd., Northfield, IL, 60093-2750, (800) 323-4040, http://www.cap.org/apps/cap.portal.

L. Fleming Fallon, Jr., M.D., Dr.P.H.

Blood donation and registry

Definition

Blood donation, also called blood banking, refers to the process of collecting, testing, preparing, and storing whole blood and blood components intended primarily for **transfusion**. Blood donors are typically unpaid volunteers, but they may also be paid by commercial blood donation and processing enterprises, such as independent blood banks and donor centers. Blood registry refers to the collection and sharing of data about donated blood and donors. Donors who have been determined to be temporarily or permanently ineligible to donate blood are listed in a confidential national data base known as the Donor Deferral Register. The quality and safety of the U.S. blood supply is governed by physician-established guidelines for the practice of blood banking as found in the Standards of the American Association of Blood Banks (AABB) and through the organization's inspection and accreditation program. The Food and Drug Administration (FDA) controls federal licensure of blood banks. Hospital blood banks are also inspected by The College of American Pathologists (CAP) and the Joint Commission on Accreditation of Healthcare Organizations (JCAHC).

Purpose

Blood is collected, processed, stored, and distributed to maintain an adequate supply of whole blood and blood components for transfusion as needed. Blood replacement may be needed by people who have lost blood through accidents, burns, hemorrhage, or surgery. Blood or blood components are also used in the treatment of certain types of anemia, various disease conditions, and for medical research.

Healthy donors may be called upon to donate periodically to help maintain the overall blood supply or when their specific blood type is needed. People may sometimes donate blood to benefit a specific person. Directed donor blood is reserved for an intended recipient, such as a family member or friend; it is tested and processed as all other donated blood to ensure that it is appropriate for the recipient. People

---

KEY TERMS

Apheresis—Extraction of a specific component from donated blood, with the remainder returned to the donor.

Autologous donation—Blood donated for the donor's own use.

Granulocytes—White blood cells.

Plasma—The liquid part of anticoagulated blood. (Serum is the term for the liquid in a clotted blood sample.)

Platelets—Tiny, disk-like elements of plasma that promote clotting.

---

preparing for **elective surgery** may have their blood collected and held, and then returned to them if needed during their surgery. This process is known as **autologous blood donation**. Donors are advised to give blood only once in an eight-week period to maintain the iron stores in their blood. Autologous donors may donate more often if it is determined by their physician to be to their benefit.

The National Blood Data Resource Center reports that about 13.9 million units of whole blood (one unit of whole blood equals 450 ml, or about 1 pt) are donated annually in the United States, of which about 695,000 are autologous donations for elective surgery. The country's blood supply is donated by about eight million people, representing a broad cross section of the population, although fewer than 5% of those eligible donate. About half of the total amount needed is processed, stored, and delivered by the 36 regional blood centers of the American Red Cross; hospital blood banks, community blood centers, mobile blood drives, and independent blood banks collect, process, and distribute the other half.

Blood is donated as whole blood, collected in a plastic bag containing an anticoagulant that will keep the blood from clotting and allow it to be separated into multiple components. By dividing blood into components that each offer different clinical benefits, one unit of donated blood can meet the transfusion needs for more than one person. This practice is essential to meet the constant demand for blood; every year in the United States, more than four million people require blood transfusions. About 26 million transfusions are administered either as whole blood or components that have been prepared from whole blood. About 34,000 units per day, for example, are transfused as red cells.

Whole blood and blood components are used in various ways to meet the clinical needs of recipients. Whole blood is sometimes used to replace blood volume when a significant amount of blood has been lost through accidents or surgery. Red blood cells, which carry oxygen, are used to treat certain anemias and are often the preferred component when multiple transfusions are being administered to one person, as in open heart surgery or organ transplants. Platelets, part of the complex coagulation (clotting) system that helps control bleeding, are commonly used in the treatment of acute leukemia and some types of cancer. Fresh frozen plasma, which contains critical coagulation factors, is used to control bleeding in people who lack these factors. Cryoprecipitated (prepared from frozen plasma) antihemophilic factor (AHF) is transfused to provide a specific coagulation factor that is deficient in hemophilia and other diseases. Blood for transfusion is requested by physicians. Pre-transfusion testing and issuance of blood and components to the recipients is performed by a transfusion service, which is commonly provided or supervised by a hospital blood bank.

Description

The actual process of donating whole blood takes about 20 minutes. The donor will either lie down or will sit in a special donor chair that elevates the lower body and legs. After selecting an appropriate vein, the phlebotomist (an individual trained in blood collection technique) will clean the arm well at the site of the needle puncture (venipuncture). With a tourniquet tightly in place on the donor's arm, a sterile needle is inserted into a vein. As the tourniquet is released, blood flows through plastic tubing into a plastic blood bag. The donor may be asked to open and close a fist to encourage blood to flow. Usually only one unit of blood is collected. Pressure is applied to the site of the venipuncture until the blood flow has been stopped. Donors are then escorted to an observation area, given light refreshments that include liquid, and allowed to rest. Positive identification of the donor and the blood bag from that donor are essential. The same unique identification number is assigned to the bag, all samples from the bag used for testing, and on all donor and testing records.

Plasma, the liquid portion of whole, anticoagulated blood in which blood cells, coagulation factors, and other blood constituents are suspended, is also collected. This is often done by commercial enterprises that sell it to companies manufacturing clotting factors and specific plasma protein products, or to companies and institutions engaged in medical research.

Plasma is collected using a process known as apheresis, in which whole blood is collected, the desired blood component is removed, and the remainder is returned to the donor. Collecting plasma generally takes one to two hours. Apheresis may also be used to collect other blood components, such as platelets and granulocytes.

Different blood components vary in how long they can be stored. Red blood cells can be refrigerated for up to 42 days or coated with a protective agent and frozen at extremely low temperatures in liquid nitrogen, a process that preserves them for up to 10 years. Platelets must be used soon after they are prepared; they are stored at room temperature for no more than five days. Fresh frozen plasma and cryoprecipitated AHF can be kept for as long as one year.

To ensure the safety of the blood supply, a multi-tiered process of donor screening and deferral is employed. This involves donor education, taking a detailed **health history** of each prospective donor, and giving potential donors a simple **physical examination**, which includes measuring blood pressure and pulse rate, taking a few drops of blood to test for hemoglobin, the iron-bearing protein in blood, and also measuring blood cell volume. These tests will indicate general health and help ensure that donation will not contribute to anemia in the donor. At any point in the process, a potential donor may be "deferred," or determined to be ineligible to donate blood. This deferral may be temporary or permanent, depending on the reason. Potential donors are also encouraged to "self-defer," or voluntarily decline to donate, rather than put future blood recipients at risk.

In general, blood donors must be at least 17 years old (some states allow younger people to donate blood with their parents' consent), must weigh at least 110 lb (50 kg), and must be in good health. Donors with a history of heart, lung, or liver disease or who are pregnant are usually deferred. Donors can be disqualified if they are known to have engaged in behavior that put them at risk of infection (such as having had a tattoo, having had sex with people in high-risk groups, having used illegal intravenous drugs, having had certain diseases, or having been raped) or have spent time in specific parts of the world, such as areas where malaria may be prevalent.

Preparation

All donated blood is extensively tested before being distributed for use by transfusion services. The first step is determining the blood type, which is the primary indication of who can receive the blood. Blood is also screened for any irregular antibodies that could cause complications for the recipients. In addition, donor blood is screened for infectious diseases, such as hepatitis, AIDS, and syphilis, by testing for specific markers of these diseases that will appear in the blood of those infected. These include: Hepatitis B surface antigen (donors with this antigen are immune and can be accepted), hepatitis B core antigen, hepatitis C virus antibody, HIV-1 and HIV-2 antibodies, HIV p24 antigen, and HTLV-I and HTLV-II antibodies. Other tests may be performed if a recipient's doctor requests them.

In order to detect the greatest possible number of infections, when present at even the lowest levels in donor blood, these screening tests are extremely sensitive. For this reason, however, donors sometimes receive false positive test results. In these cases, more specific confirmatory tests are performed to help rule out false positive results. Blood found to be not suitable for transfusion is discarded, and all items coming into direct contact with donors are used only once and then discarded. Donors of infected blood are entered into the Donor Deferral Register to prevent subsequent donation of their blood at other blood donation facilities.

There are eight major blood types comprising four ABO groups (A, B, AB, and O), and the presence or absence of the Rh factor, designated as either type Rh positive (+) or type Rh negative (-). These types and their approximate distribution in the U.S. population are as follows: O+ (38%), O- (7%), A+ (34%), A- (6%), B+ (9%), B- (2%), AB+ (3%), AB- (1%). In an emergency, when there may be no time for compatibility testing, anyone can safely receive type O red blood cells, and people with this blood type are known as "universal donors." People with type AB blood, known as "universal recipients," can receive any type of red blood cells and can give plasma to all blood types. Receiving the wrong blood type can result in the destruction of red cells in the recipients body and even **death**. For this reason, the transfusion service must conduct more pre-transfusion testing to determine the compatibility of the donor blood with the blood of the recipient. This compatibility testing, known as type and cross match, begins with matching the major blood types. Additional testing will include antibody screening of the recipient and, if specific antibodies are found, testing of other blood groups (the MN group or Kell and Lewis groups, for example) will be done to find compatible donor blood.

Risks

Thanks to the use of a multi-tiered donor screening system and advances in the effectiveness of screening tests, the risk of transmitting infectious diseases to recipients via transfusion has been significantly diminished. Nonetheless, there is still a minuscule risk that blood recipients could contract human immunodeficiency virus (HIV), hepatitis, or other diseases via transfusion. Other diseases that are of particular concern to blood-collection agencies include: babesiosis, Chagas disease, human T-lymphotropic virus (HTLV-I and -II), cytomegalovirus (CMV), Lyme disease, malaria, Creutzfeldt-Jakob disease, and new variant Creutzfeldt-Jakob disease.

There are few risks to healthy donors when AABB standards for donation are followed. People who donate blood replace the fluid they lose within 24 hours and the red cells within two months. A person can safely donate blood once in eight weeks. Donors' blood will be tested prior to donation to determine their eligibility; those ineligible will be advised of the temporary or permanent reasons for being disqualified. Their names will be placed on the national deferral registry to prevent donation at other sites and to help protect the blood supply.

Medical professionals who draw the blood of eligible donors will advise donors of any necessary precautions following donation. Most blood donors suffer no significant after effects. Occasionally donors may feel faint or dizzy, nauseous, or have tenderness, redness, or a bruise where the needle was inserted to draw their blood. More serious complications, which rarely occur, may include fainting, muscle spasms, or nerve damage.

AABB standards are designed to protect donors and recipients and especially to help ensure that compatible blood is transfused to each recipient. The accurate labeling of blood, blood components, and donor records, and the recording of all data is essential from the time blood is collected, through testing and preparation, and through pre-transfusion testing and issuance of the blood or blood component. Autologous blood donors run a tiny risk of having the wrong blood returned to them due to clerical error. There is also a faint possibility of bacterial contamination of the autologous blood. These rare occurrences apply to all other transfusions as well.

Resources

BOOKS

McClatchey, Kenneth D., M.D., ed. "Section XI: Blood Transfusion Medicine." *Clinical Laboratory Medicine.* Baltimore: Williams & Wilkins, 1994.

Starr, Douglass. *Blood: An Epic History of Medicine and Commerce.* New York: Alfred A Knopf, 1998.

PERIODICALS

McKenna, C. "Blood Minded." *Nursing Times* (April 6, 2000): 27–28.

ORGANIZATIONS

American Association of Blood Banks. 8101 Glenbrook Road, Bethesda, MD 20814-2749. (301) 907-6977. http://www.aabb.org.

American Red Cross. 430 17th Street NW, Washington, D.C. 20006. http://www.redcross.org.

National Blood Data Resource Center. (301) 215-6506. http://www.nbdrc.org.

Peter Gregutt
L. Lee Culvert

Blood phosphate level

Definition

Phosphate is a mineral that is found in abundance in the body. About 85% of the body's phosphate is in bone. Phosphate is also a major component of teeth. Phosphate is involved in producing and repairing bone, as well as in the functioning of both nerves and muscles. Phosphate is used to help produce energy for the cell, as well as in the production of DNA.

Calcium and phosphate are both present in the blood, but in inverse proportions. In other words, higher blood calcium levels result in lower blood phosphate levels; lower blood calcium levels result in higher blood phosphate levels. Excess phosphate in the blood, beyond what is needed for proper functioning, is processed by the kidneys and excreted in the urine.

Phosphate acquired through the diet, in yeast, beans, lentils, grains, peanuts, and almonds. As with calcium, vitamin D is required for the proper absorption of phosphate. Excess phosphate in the body is excreted through the urine and the stool.

Purpose

A blood phosphate level is usually drawn as part of a larger panel of electrolytes. Other measurements in the electrolyte panel include calcium, chloride, potassium, and sodium. A blood phosphate level is usually checked when there are concerns about the functioning of the patient's kidneys, to monitor patients who are on renal dialysis, in the presence of bone disease, to diagnose disorders of the parathyroid glands, to monitor intestinal disorders that affect nutrient absorption, and as part of the monitoring performed when a diabetic patient goes into ketoacidosis.

KEY TERMS

Acromegaly—A condition in which an overactive pituitary gland pumps out an excess amount of growth hormone.

Dialysis—A procedure that takes over the blood filtering capacity normally provided by the kidneys. Includes both hemodialysis (in which blood passes out of the body through a tube running from a blood vessel in the arm to a special dialysis machine) and peritoneal dialysis (in which a special catheter is implanted in the abdominal cavity, a special dialysis solution is infused into the abdomen, waste products from the body enter the solution, and the solution is then drained back out of the abdominal cavity.

Hyperphosphatemia—Elevated blood phosphate levels.

Hypophosphatemia—Low blood phosphate levels.

Ketoacidosis—A condition brought on by extremely elevated blood glucose, resulting in a life-threatening metabolic acidosis.

Parathyroid—Several small glands located behind the thyroid glands in the mid-neck. The parathyroid glands secrete parathyroid hormone, which is highly involved in the chemical equilibrium of calcium and phosphate throughout the body.

Precautions

The test results can be affected by alcohol, as well as some medications, such as steroids, androgen hormones, vitamin D supplements, and enemas containing phosphate, antacids containing aluminum, insulin, acetazolamide, epinephrine, or large quantities of glucose. Patients who are taking anticoagulant medications should inform their healthcare practitioner since this may increase their chance of bleeding or bruising after a blood test.

Description

This test requires blood to be drawn from a vein (usually one in the forearm), generally by a nurse or phlebotomist (an individual who has been trained to draw blood). A tourniquet is applied to the arm above the area where the needle stick will be performed. The site of the needle stick is cleaned with antiseptic, and the needle is inserted. The blood is collected in vacuum tubes. After collection, the needle is withdrawn, and pressure is kept on the blood draw site to stop any bleeding and decrease bruising. A bandage is then applied.

Preparation

There are no restrictions on diet or physical activity, either before or after the blood test.

Aftercare

As with any blood tests, discomfort, bruising, and/or a very small amount of bleeding is common at the puncture site. Immediately after the needle is withdrawn, it is helpful to put pressure on the puncture site until the bleeding has stopped. This decreases the chance of significant bruising. Warm packs may relieve minor discomfort. Some individuals may feel briefly woozy after a blood test, and they should be encouraged to lie down and rest until they feel better.

Risks

Basic blood tests, such as blood phosphate levels, do not carry any significant risks, other than slight bruising and the chance of brief dizziness.

Results

In adults, a normal blood phosphate level is 3.0–4.5 milligrams per deciliter (mg/dL) or 0.97–1.45 millimoles per liter (mmol/L). Children and infants normally have higher blood phosphate levels because their bodies are in a phase involving rapid bone growth. In children a normal blood phosphate level is 4.5–6.5 mg/dL or 1.45–2.10 mmol/L. In infants, a normal blood phosphate level is 4.3–9.3 mg/dL or 1.4–3.0 mmol/L.

High levels

High blood phosphate levels may be due to:

- kidney disease;
- poorly functioning parathyroid glands (hypoparathyroidism);
- acromegaly (a condition in which the pituitary is overactive, and secretes too much growth hormone;
- rhabdomyolysis (a condition in which muscle is broken down, releasing phosphate, among other substances);
- bone diseases, including recent fractured bones;
- diabetic ketoacidosis (a condition in which the blood glucose becomes extremely elevated);
- excess vitamin D;
- shortage of magnesium; or
- pregnancy.

Low levels

Low blood phosphate levels may be due to:

- overactive parthyroid glands (hyperparathyroidism);
- kidney disease;
- liver disease;
- malnutrition or outright starvation;
- burns;
- severe alcoholism;
- excess blood calcium (hypercalcemia);
- vitamin D deficiency;
- bone disorders, such as osteomalacia (an adult type of rickets in which the bones becomes softer due to a vitamin D deficiency); or
- intestinal disorders that result in poor absorption of nutrients.

Resources

BOOKS

Brenner, B. M., and F. C. Rector, eds. *Brenner & Rector's The Kidney,* 7th ed. Philadelphia: Saunders, 2004.

Goldman L., D. Ausiello, eds. *Cecil Textbook of Internal Medicine,* 23rd ed. Philadelphia: Saunders, 2007.

McPherson R. A., and M. R. Pincus, eds. *Henry's Clinical Diagnosis and Management by Laboratory Methods,* 21st ed. Philadelphia: Saunders, 2006.

OTHER

Medical Encyclopedia. Medline Plus. U.S. National Library of Medicine and the National Institutes of Health. January 2, 2008. http://www.nlm.nih.gov/medlineplus/encyclopedia.html (February 10, 2008).

ORGANIZATIONS

American Association for Clinical Chemistry, 1850 K Street, NW, Suite 625, Washington, DC, 20006, (800) 892-1400, http://www.aacc.org.

Rosalyn Carson-DeWitt, M.D.

Blood potassium level

Definition

Potassium is a mineral that is found in abundance in the body, primarily within its cells. Only about 2% of the body's total potassium is not within its cells. Potassium levels are crucial to the appropriate functioning of all cells, especially nerve and muscle cells. For the body to function normally, blood potassium levels have to be maintained at a very narrow range; when potassium levels are too high or too low, there can be serious health consequences. The body keeps its potassium levels in equilibrium by prompting the kidneys to resorb more (when the body needs potassium) or excrete more (when there is excess potassium). The hormone responsible for stimulating the processing of potassium in the kidneys is called aldosterone. Aldosterone is secreted by the adrenal glands. When blood potassium levels get too high, the condition is called hyperkalemia. When blood potassium levels get too low, the condition is called hypokalemia.

Purpose

A blood potassium level is usually drawn as part of a larger panel of electrolytes. Other measurements in the electrolyte panel include sodium, chloride, and carbon dioxide. A blood potassium level is usually checked during a regular **physical examination**, when there are concerns about the functioning of the patient's kidneys, when the patient has high blood pressure (hypertension), to monitor potassium levels during the use of medications that affect its equilibrium (such as certain **diuretics**, which cause potassium to be lost in the urine), in patients on dialysis, in patients who are on intravenous fluids or receiving parenteral nutrition, and in patients who have symptoms such as unexplained weakness or abnormal heart rhythms (cardiac arrhythmias).

Precautions

Blood potassium levels can be affected by a number of medications. Patients who are on these medications should inform their doctor, so that test results can be interpreted appropriately. Medications that increase blood potassium levels include some chemotherapy agents, aminocaproic acid, high blood pressure medications (specifically angiotensin-converting enzyme or ACE inhibitors), certain diuretics (referred to as potassium-sparing or potassium-conserving diuretics), epinephrine, heparine, histamine, isoniazid, mannitol, and succinylcholine. Medications that decrease blood potassium levels include acetazolamide, aminosalicylic acid, amphotericin B, carbenicillin, cisplatin, potassium-wasting diuretics (such as thiazide diuretics and furosemide), insulin, **laxatives**, penicillin G, phenothiazines, salicylates, and sodium polystyrene sulfonate. Other factors that may skew the results of blood potassium level include intravenous infusion of fluids containing potassium, as well as intravenous infusion of either glucose-containing solutions or insulin.

Patients who are taking anticoagulant medications should inform their healthcare practitioner since this may increase their chance of bleeding or bruising after a blood test.

Proper technique in drawing the potassium blood level and in handling the sample is crucial to an accurate result. If the patient is clenching and relaxing arm muscles in the arm from which the blood is being drawn, the potassium blood level may be falsely elevated. If the flow of blood into the vacuum tubes is not carefully regulated, and the blood flows too quickly or too slowly into the tubes, then the blood cells may be damaged due to turbulence. This will cause the blood cells to leak potassium into the sample, falsely elevating the result. Delay in testing the blood at the laboratory will also result in an artificially elevated blood potassium level being reported.

Description

This test requires blood to be drawn from a vein (usually one in the forearm), generally by a nurse or phlebotomist (an individual who has been trained to draw blood). A tourniquet is applied to the arm above the area where the needle stick will be performed. The site of the needle stick is cleaned with antiseptic, and the needle is inserted. The blood is collected in vacuum tubes. After collection, the needle is withdrawn, and pressure is kept on the blood draw site to stop any bleeding and decrease bruising. A bandage is then applied.

Preparation

There are no restrictions on diet or physical activity, either before or after the blood test.

Aftercare

As with any blood tests, discomfort, bruising, and/or a very small amount of bleeding is common at the puncture site. Immediately after the needle is withdrawn, it is helpful to put pressure on the puncture site until the bleeding has stopped. This decreases the chance of significant bruising. Warm packs may relieve minor discomfort. Some individuals may feel briefly woozy after a blood test, and they should be encouraged to lie down and rest until they feel better.

Risks

Basic blood tests, such as blood potassium levels, do not carry any significant risks other than slight bruising and the chance of brief dizziness.

Results

In adults, a normal blood potassium level is 3.5–5.0 milliequivalents perliter (mEq/L) or 3.5–5.0 millimoles per liter (mmol/L). In children a normal blood potassium level is 3.4–4.7 mEq/L or 3.4–4.7 mmol/L. In infants, a normal blood potassium level is 4.13–5.3 mEq/L or 4.1–5.3 mmol/L. In newborns, a normal blood potassium level is 3.9–5.9 mEq/L or 3.9–5.9 mmol/L.

High levels

High blood potassium levels may be due to:

- kidney disease, either acute or chronic kidney failure;
- Addison's disease (a disease in which the adrenal gland is under-functioning);
- low blood levels of the hormone aldosterone, termed hypoaldosteronism;
- tissue injury, resulting in the release of potassium into the bloodstream, including trauma, heart attack, severe burns;
- infection;
- dehydration;
- diabetes;
- excess intake of foods containing potassium (in particular, fruits and fruit juices are often high in potassium;
- excess intake of potassium supplements; or
- medications that elevate potassium, including NSAIDS (ibuprofen); beta blockers (propranlol and atenolol); ACE inhibitors (captopril, enlapril, lisinopril); and diruetics such as triamterene, amiloride, and spironolactone.

Low levels

Low blood potassium levels may be due to:

- dehydration;
- severe vomiting;
- severe diarrhea;
- insulin use;
- Cushing's syndrome;
- cystic fibrosis;
- poor nutritional status due to alcoholism, eating disorder, and other causes of malnutrition;
- Bartter's syndrome;
- too much aldosterone in the blood (hyperaldosteronism);
- diuretic use (thiazide diuretics and furosemide, in particular); or
- poor dietary intake of potassium.

Resources

BOOKS

Goldman L., D. Ausiello, eds. *Cecil Textbook of Internal Medicine,* 23rd ed. Philadelphia: Saunders, 2007.
McPherson R. A., and M. R. Pincus, eds. *Henry's Clinical Diagnosis and Management by Laboratory Methods,* 21st ed. Philadelphia: Saunders, 2006.

OTHER

Medical Encyclopedia. Medline Plus. U.S. National Library of Medicine and the National Institutes of Health. January 2, 2008. http://www.nlm.nih.gov/medlineplus/encyclopedia.html (February 10, 2008).

ORGANIZATIONS

American Association for Clinical Chemistry, 1850 K Street, NW, Suite 625, Washington, DC, 20006, (800) 892-1400, http://www.aacc.org.

Rosalyn Carson-DeWitt, M.D.

Blood pressure measurement

Definition

Blood pressure measurement is the noninvasive measurement of the pressure exerted by the circulating blood on the walls of the body's arteries.

Purpose

The purpose of non-invasive blood pressure measurement is to detect any changes from normal values, which may indicate disease. Measurement is also performed to monitor the effectiveness of medication

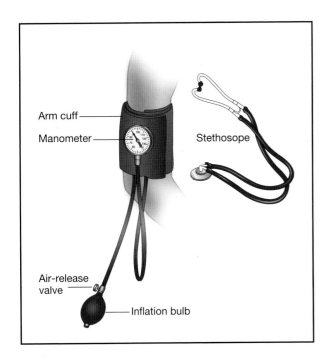

(Illustration by Electronic Illustrators Group.)

and other methods used to control elevated blood pressure.

Blood pressure should be routinely checked every one to two years and may be monitored more closely during illnesses that affect blood pressure or during medical treatments which may change blood pressure. Measurement can be taken as often as every few minutes.

Precautions

As there may be no prior knowledge of the patient's previous blood pressure for comparison, a wide range of normal values apply to patients of different ages. The inflated cuff can cause discomfort, and this should be taken into account when dealing with very ill patients. Patients with a history of sickle cell anemia should not have non-invasive blood pressure measurements made with a typical blood pressure cuff, because the sickling process can be initiated by the pressure on the arm. Blood pressure measurements should occur on a limb free of intravascular catheters and **arterial venous fistulas** (joined artery and vein) used for chronic dialysis.

Description

Blood pressure is usually recorded by measuring the force of the blood during the contraction of the ventricles (lower chambers of the heart) as blood is

pumped from the heart to the rest of the body (systolic pressure), and during the period when the heart is relaxed between beats and pressure is lowest (diastolic pressure).

The cardiac output, resistance, quality, and quantity of blood circulating through the heart, and the condition of the arterial walls are all factors that influence the blood pressure. Hypertension is an elevation in the blood pressure above normal values, with the diastolic pressure being the indicator most commonly used.

Hypotension is a reduction in the blood pressure below normal values. If a very high or very low pressure is taken, the blood pressure reading may be inaccurate and should be repeated immediately, prior to the initiation of medical treatment.

The non-invasive blood pressure is taken using a **sphygmomanometer**, a hand bulb pump, and a cuff.

The sphygmomanometer may be electronic or mercury-based. The mercury-based unit has a manually inflatable cuff attached by tubing to the unit that contains mercury and is calibrated in millimeters of mercury. The electronic unit is similar, but is mercury free and inflates and deflates automatically with the reading displayed digitally. The electronic units are also calibrated to display the measurement in millimeters of mercury. Blood pressure can be measured with either unit, although electronic units are becoming more commonplace in both **home care** and clinical use.

Children and adults with smaller or larger than average-sized limbs require special sized cuffs appropriate for their needs. The blood pressure cuff is usually placed on the arm, but can also be used on the leg.

To record blood pressure, the patient may be seated or lying down. The cuff will be positioned so that it is level with the heart. With an electronic unit the cuff is placed in accordance with manufacturer instructions on the bare upper arm, on the bare wrist, or on the bare index finger.

If the blood pressure is monitored with a manual system, a cuff is placed level with the heart and wrapped firmly but not too tightly around the bare arm 1 in (2.5 cm) above the elbow, with any creases in the cuff smoothed out. Blood pressure measurements taken on the leg require the cuff to be positioned below the groin on the bare leg.

Following the manufacturer's guidelines (electronic models), the cuff is inflated and then deflated automatically. The reading is displayed and recorded by the user. The results are charted with the systolic pressure first, then by the diastolic pressure in the following manner, xxx/xx (e.g., 120/70). A manual system requires a **stethoscope** be placed over the artery, the cuff is then inflated until the artery is occluded and no sound is heard through the stethoscope.

The cuff is then inflated a further 10 mm Hg above the last sound heard. The valve in the pump is slowly opened no faster than 5 mm Hg per second to deflate the pressure in the cuff to the point where a tapping sound is heard over the artery. This point is noted as the systolic pressure. The sounds continue as the pressure in the cuff is released and the artery is no longer occluded. At this point, the noises are no longer heard and this is noted as the diastolic pressure.

With children, the tapping noise changes to a soft muffled sound. That point is noted as the diastolic pressure, as commonly in children, sounds continue to be heard as the cuff deflates to zero.

Preparation

Medical staff should explain the procedure fully to the patient and reassure him or her that recording blood pressure is part of normal health checks and that it is necessary to ensure the patient's health is being correctly monitored. The appropriate-sized cuff should be used for the patient to give an accurate reading.

The test can be performed at any time, but is best performed when the patient has been resting for at least five minutes so that any exertion, such as climbing stairs prior to the test, will not unduly influence the outcome of the reading.

Devices should be checked and calibrated annually by a qualified technician to ensure accurate readings.

Aftercare

The health-care practitioner should make the patient comfortable. The medical staff should be notified if the blood pressure measurement is above or below normal values so that treatment can be initiated, continued, or adjusted. Repeated measurements are required for screening purposes and continuity of care.

Results

The normal values for blood pressure measurement is a systolic pressure of 120 mm Hg and a diastolic pressure of 70–80 mm Hg. Mild hypertension is a diastolic pressure above 90 mm Hg. The American Heart Association states that a systolic pressure above 130–139 mm Hg needs to be watched carefully. Significant hypertension is a systolic pressure above 200 mm Hg. The blood pressure measurement is recorded and compared with normal ranges for the patient's age and medical condition. Based on the results, a decision is made as to whether any further action is required. Hypertension increases the risk of serious diseases such as heart attack and stroke.

Hypotension is demonstrated by with a systolic blood pressure under 80 mm Hg. Treatment options depend on the patient's current health and may include blood or saline administration. Drugs to improve heart rate and function may also be administered.

Resources

BOOKS

Nagel, Rob. "Measuring Blood Pressure." In *Body by Design: From the Digestive System to the Skeleton,* edited by Betz Des Chesnes. Farmington Hills, MI: UXL, 2000.

Skeehan, Thomas, and Michael Jopling. "Monitoring the Cardiac Surgical Patient." In *The Practice of Cardiac Anesthesia,* 3rd edition. Edited by Frederick A. Hensley, Donald E. Martin, and Glenn P. Gravlee. Philadelphia: Lippincott Williams & Wilkins, 2003.

ORGANIZATIONS

American College of Nurse Practitioners. 503 Capitol Ct. NE #300, Washington, DC 20002. (202) 546-4825. acnp@nurse.org.

American Heart Association. AHA National Center, 7272 Greenville Avenue, Dallas, TX 752311. (800) AHA-USA1. http://www.americanheart.org.

OTHER

Cooper, Phyllis G. "Blood Pressure." *Clinical Reference Systems.* Annual 2000: 173.

National Library of Medicine. [cited April 2003]. http://www.nlm.nih.gov.

Margaret A Stockley, RGN
Allison J. Spiwak, MSBME

Blood pressure measurement device *see*
Sphygmomanometer

Blood removal *see* **Phlebotomy**

Blood salvage

Definition

Blood salvage is the recovery of a patient's own blood (autologous donation) from a surgical site. This blood is then readministered to the patient.

Purpose

Preoperative blood salvage can be performed prior to the surgical incision during the induction of anesthesia. This blood is collected to be administered post-operatively, because the clotting factors and platelets are protected from activation and destruction caused by the surgery. This procedure is most often used if cardiopulmonary bypass (use of a heart-lung machine) will be instituted. If the blood is not given to the patient, it will be discarded. Preoperative **blood donation** or **autologous blood donation** is a coordinated donation process planned prior to a scheduled surgical procedure, but it is not considered blood salvage.

Blood salvage is performed during surgical procedures when the risk of significant blood loss is expected. The recovered blood is collected, processed, and readministered to the patient, decreasing or preventing the need for allogeneic (from a donor) blood product administration. If the blood is not given to the patient, it will be discarded.

Postoperative blood salvage is used to collect blood from the surgical cavity as the wound heals. The blood is collected, may or may not be processed, and returned to the patient. If the blood is not given to the patient, it will be discarded.

Administration of the patient's own blood eliminates the risk of transfusion-transmitted viral disease and **transfusion** reactions. Patients with multiple red blood cell antibodies or rare blood types benefit by blood salvage during the perioperative (during surgery) and postoperative period. Shortages of rare blood types can put the patient at risk for cardiovascular

KEY TERMS

Allogeneic—Blood and blood products collected from a blood donor for administration to a recipient.

Autologous—Blood and blood products collected from an individual for readministration to self.

Catheter—A tube for transferring fluids out of the body. Patients experiencing open heart surgery will have at least one chest tube placed in the chest cavity to provide removal of blood from the chest cavity for collection and readministration.

Transfusion container—An administration bag made of polyvinyl chloride or other latex-free polymer for collection of blood products for administration to the patient.

collapse caused if hemorrhage occurs during the surgical procedure.

Some Jehovah's Witnesses patients refuse allogeneic blood donation. Blood salvage provides an opportunity for autologous blood donation for these patients. Certain modifications in collection technique make autologous blood donation an acceptable treatment for members of this faith.

Neurological, vascular, cardiac, liver transplant, and orthopedic procedures make extensive use of blood salvage techniques. Patients having surgical procedures involving amniotic fluid, malignancies, bowel contamination, or microfibrillar collagen materials are not eligible for blood salvage. In the presence of amniotic fluid or bowel contamination, thorough rinsing of the surgical site may allow for blood salvage.

Description

Preoperative blood salvage

The patient will be provided with cardiac monitoring prior to the initiation of autologous blood collection. A venous access site will be gained with a catheter. The 500–1,000 ml of whole blood is collected into a transfusion container treated with anticoagulant. The container is properly labeled for the patient and clearly marked "AUTOLOGOUS DONOR." The blood can be stored for six hours if refrigerated, and will be destroyed if not used within that time.

Blood collected in this manner is not processed further, but stored for later administration. The whole blood product provides not only red blood cells, but more importantly, plasma proteins including clotting factors and platelets. This technique is most often associated with cardiopulmonary bypass, since the heart-lung machine can damage clotting factors and platelets. The preoperative collection protects the blood components.

Perioperative blood salvage

During surgery, the surgeon suctions blood in the surgical cavity for collection. Anticoagulant is mixed with the blood at the tip of the suction apparatus. The blood is filtered as it is collected into a container. From this collection container the blood may be placed into a transfusion container for direct administration to the patient. This blood will be anticoagulated and will contain all plasma proteins, including activated clotting factors and platelets. More commonly, the blood is processed by centrifugation. The blood is centrifuged to separate the red blood cells from the plasma. The plasma is removed as saline enters the centrifuge to wash the blood. Washing the blood removes anticoagulation, plasma-free hemoglobin, and plasma proteins, including activated clotting factors and platelets. This product is called washed packed red cells. After washing is complete, the blood is collected into a transfusion container free of anticoagulant, since all clotting factors have been removed during washing. The container is properly labeled for the patient and clearly marked "AUTOLOGOUS DONOR." The blood can be stored for six hours if refrigerated, and will be destroyed if not used within that time.

Postoperative blood salvage

Postoperative blood salvage is used to remove shed blood from the surgical cavity that has been closed at the completion of the surgical procedure. At wound closure, a catheter is left in the cavity and penetrates the skin for connection to the collection reservoir. If the blood is collected from the chest cavity, no anticoagulation is required. If the blood is collected from a joint, it must receive anticoagulation during collection. The blood from the chest cavity is usually reinfused without additional processing, but may be washed. Blood collected from a joint must be washed prior to infusion. Washing involves centrifugation of the blood to separate the red blood cells from the plasma. The plasma contains anticoagulant-free hemoglobin and plasma proteins, including activated clotting factors and platelets. Once the red blood cells and plasma are separated, saline is introduced to the centrifuge to displace the plasma. The end product, called washed packed red blood cells, is collected into a transfusion container. The container is properly labeled for the patient and clearly marked "AUTOLOGOUS DONOR." The blood can be stored for six hours if refrigerated, and will be destroyed if not used within that time.

Normal results

The patient will receive autologous blood donation when the red blood cell volume, as measured by hemoglobin or **hematocrit** values, falls below the desired level, commonly 18–21% or 6–7 g/dl, respectively. These values will be dictated by the physician in the orders for patient care.

If the patient's condition is acceptable, autologous blood donation with preoperative blood collection occurs immediately following the termination of cardiopulmonary bypass. Blood collected postoperatively will be administered as need for maintenance of blood pressure or red cell volume.

The patient benefits from blood salvage by the elimination of risk of blood-transmitted virus or blood transfusion reactions. Blood transfusion reactions are experienced by about 10% of recipients for each unit transfused.

Resources

BOOKS

AABB Perioperative Standards Unit.*Standards for Perioperative Autologous Blood Collection and Administration, 3rd Edition.* Amer Assn of Blood Banks, 2007.

Spiess, Bruce D., et al. eds. *Perioperative Transfusion Medicine.* Baltimore: Williams & Wilkins, 1998.

PERIODICALS

Henry, D. A., et al. "Pre-operative Autologous Donation for Minimizing Perioperative Allogeneic Blood Transfusion." *Cochrane Review,* Issue 1 (January 20, 2003).

OTHER

"Autologous Blood Donation Basics." February 10, 2006. Bloodbook.com. http://www.bloodbook.com/autolog-1.html [Accessed April 7, 2008].

"Guidance for Autologous Blood and Blood Components." *Autologous Blood and Blood Components.* FDA, Division of Blood and Blood Products, HFB-400, Bethesda, MD 20892. March 15, 1989. http://www.fda.gov/cber/bldmem/031589.pdf [Accessed April 7, 2008].

ORGANIZATIONS

American Association of Blood Banks. 8101 Glenbrook Rd., Bethesda, MD 20814. (301) 907-6977. http://www.aabb.org/content.

American Red Cross. 431 18th St., NW, Washington, DC 20006. (202) 639-3520. http://www.redcross.org.

Allison Joan Spiwak, MSBME
Laura Jean Cataldo, RN, EdD

Blood sodium level

Definition

Sodium is a mineral that is found throughout the body and is crucial (along with other electrolytes) to the appropriate balance of fluid in the body. Sodium is primarily found in bodily fluids and blood. For the body to function normally, blood sodium levels have to be maintained at a very narrow range; when sodium levels are too high or too low, serious health consequences can result. The body keeps its sodium levels in equilibrium by prompting the kidneys to resorb more (when the body needs sodium) or excrete more (when there is excess sodium). The hormones responsible for stimulating the processing of sodium in the kidneys are called natriuretic peptides, which prompt the kidneys to excrete sodium into the urine and out of the body; aldosterone, which prompts the kidneys to hold onto or resorb sodium; and antidiruetic hormone or ADH, which prompts the retention of fluids in the bloodstream, thus increasing the amount of water in the bloodstream and diluting the blood sodium level. The mechanism of thirst is another important way that blood sodium levels are controlled; as small as a 1% increase in blood sodium level will prompt thirst, which initiates drinking behavior and serves to drop the elevated blood sodium level. When blood sodium levels get too high, the condition is called hypernatremia. When blood sodium levels get too low, the condition is called hyperkalemia.

Purpose

A blood sodium level is usually drawn as part of a larger panel of electrolytes. Other measurements in the electrolyte panel include chloride, potassium, and carbon dioxide. A blood sodium level is usually checked during a routine **physical examination**, as well as when there are concerns about the functioning of the patient's kidneys; when the patient has high blood pressure (hypertension); to monitor sodium levels during the use of intravenous fluid therapy; in patients on dialysis; in patients who have symptoms of heart failure or who are known to have heart failure; in patients with liver disease; in patients with lower leg swelling or other fluid accumulation; and in patients with symptoms that could possibly be due to electrolyte imbalance, specifically low blood sodium levels or hyponatremia. These symptoms can include confusion, severe fatigue and weakness, extreme thirst, low urine output, muscle twitching, irritability, or agitation.

Precautions

Blood sodium levels can be affected by a number of medications. Patients who are on these medications should inform their doctor, so that test results can be interpreted appropriately. Medications that increase blood sodium levels include birth control pills, some **antibiotics**, clonidine, steroid medications, anabolic steroid use, cough preparations, **laxatives**, methyldopa, and nonsteroidal anti-inflammatory agents (including ibuprofen). Medications that decrease blood sodium levels include carbamazepine, **diuretics**, sulfonylureas, triamterene, and vasopressin. Other factors that may skew the results of blood sodium level include intravenous infusion of fluids containing sodium; excess ingestion of food or beverages containing salt; excess consumption of fluids; use of the hormone aldosterone; and recent severe injury, surgery, or shock.

Patients who are taking anticoagulant medications should inform their healthcare practitioner since this may increase their chance of bleeding or bruising after a blood test.

Description

This test requires blood to be drawn from a vein (usually one in the forearm), generally by a nurse or phlebotomist (an individual who has been trained to draw blood). A tourniquet is applied to the arm above the area where the needle stick will be performed. The site of the needle stick is cleaned with antiseptic and the needle is inserted. The blood is collected in vacuum tubes. After collection, the needle is withdrawn and pressure is kept on the blood draw site to stop any bleeding and decrease bruising. A bandage is then applied.

Preparation

There are no restrictions on diet or physical activity, either before or after the blood test.

Aftercare

As with any blood tests, discomfort, bruising, and/or a very small amount of bleeding is common at the puncture site. Immediately after the needle is withdrawn, it is helpful to put pressure on the puncture site until the bleeding has stopped. This decreases the chance of significant bruising. Warm packs may relieve minor discomfort. Some individuals may feel briefly woozy after a blood test, and they should be encouraged to lie down and rest until they feel better.

KEY TERMS

Addison's disease—A condition in which the adrenal glands are not functioning properly. Addison's disease can be caused by a problem in the adrenal glands themselves, or in the pituitary gland, which secretes a hormone that affects the adrenal glands.

Aldosterone—A hormone secreted by the adrenal glands that prompts the kidneys to hold onto sodium.

Antidiuretic hormone (ADH)—Also called vasopressin. A hormone produced by the hypothalamus and stored in and excreted by the pituitary gland. ADH acts on the kidneys to reduce the flow of urine, increasing total body fluid.

Cushing's syndrome—A disorder affecting the adrenal glands and their secretion of coritsol.

Diuretic—A medication that increases the flow of urine through the kidneys and out of the body.

Hypernatremia—Elevated blood sodium levels.

Hyponatremia—Low blood sodium levels.

Natriuretic peptides—Peptides that prompt the kidneys to excrete sodium into the urine and out of the body.

Risks

Basic blood tests, such as blood sodium levels, do not carry any significant risks other than slight bruising and the chance of brief dizziness.

Results

A normal blood sodium level is 136–145 milliequivalents per liter (mEq/L), or 136–145 millimoles per liter (mmol/L).

High levels

High blood sodium levels may be due to:

- dehydration (increased loss of body water without sufficient replacement by drinking, which often occurs in febrile illnesses, with severe diarrhea and/or vomiting, or in situations involving heavy exercise in hot weather, resulting in fluid loss through sweating);
- high blood levels of the hormone aldosterone, termed hyperaldosteronism;
- Cushing's syndrome;
- diabetes insipidus (caused by a shortage of antidiuretic hormone);

- diabetic keoacidosis;
- diuretic use;
- head injury or brain surgery, particularly if the pituitary gland is affected;
- sickle cell anemia;
- kidney disease;
- medications including lithium, demeclocycline, or diuretics; or
- ingestion of an extremely high-sodium diet.

Low levels

Low blood sodium levels may be due to:

- Addison's disease;
- thyroid insufficiency;
- severe diarrhea;
- diuretic use;
- excess sweating;
- serious burns;
- kidney disease, including those resulting in the loss of protein from the body (nephrotic syndrome);
- cirrhosis of the liver;
- cystic fibrosis;
- increased retention of water in the body, due to excess consumption of water, heart failure, or cirrhosis of the liver
- poor nutritional status due to alcoholism, eating disorder, other causes of malnutrition;
- disorders involving the pituitary gland;
- medications such as chlorpropamide, carbamazepine, vincristine, clofibrate, antipsychotic medications, aspirin, ibuprofen, synthetic vasopressin, and oxytocin;
- too much antidiuretic hormone (also called vasopressin) in the blood (referred to as syndrome of inappropriate antidiuretic hormone or SIADH). This syndrome can occur due to a wide variety of conditions involving the lung and brain, including brain injury, infections such as meningitis and encephalitis, pneumonia, acute respiratory failure, brain tumors, lung cancer, and psychosis;
- a number of conditions can also stimulate release of ADH from the pituitary, such as pain, stress, exercise, dehydration, increased levels of other blood electrolytes, and low blood sugar levels; or
- poor dietary intake of sodium (this is extremely rare).

Resources

BOOKS

Goldman L., D. Ausiello, eds. *Cecil Textbook of Internal Medicine*, 23rd ed. Philadelphia: Saunders, 2007.

McPherson R. A., and M. R. Pincus, eds. *Henry's Clinical Diagnosis and Management by Laboratory Methods,* 21st ed. Philadelphia: Saunders, 2006.

OTHER

Medical Encyclopedia. Medline Plus. U.S. National Library of Medicine and the National Institutes of Health. January 2, 2008. http://www.nlm.nih.gov/medlineplus/encyclopedia.html (February 10, 2008).

ORGANIZATIONS

American Association for Clinical Chemistry, 1850 K Street, NW, Suite 625, Washington, DC, 20006, (800) 892-1400, http://www.aacc.org.

Rosalyn Carson-DeWitt, MD

Blood sugar test *see* **Glucose tests**

Blood thinners *see* **Anticoagulant and anti-platelet drugs**

Blood transfusion *see* **Transfusion**

Blood type test

Definition

A blood type test determines to which of the major blood groups an individual's blood belongs. Blood typing categorizes blood by identifying the presence or absence of particular substances on the surface of the red blood cell. The substances are called "antigens," and may be molecules of protein, carbohydrate, glycolipid, or glycoprotein.

Although there are a large number (perhaps as many as 690) of blood group systems that can identify unique attributes of antigens on red blood cells, two are commonly used and seem to be the most clinically relevant. These are the ABO blood group system and the Rhesus or Rh blood group system. These two blood group systems are the most well known, well-defined, and also the most important as regards known reactions to situations involving blood transfusions.

Blood typing is particularly important when an individual needs to receive a blood **transfusion**. If the wrong blood type is given, there is a high risk of an adverse transfusion reaction. The recipient's immune system will recognize the antigen on the donor blood as foreign, and will being to produce antibodies directed against that antigen. The antibodies will attack the donor blood, damaging and bursting the donor red blood cells. This results in high serum levels of hemoglobin spilling from the burst red blood cells

(called hemoglobinemia), disseminated intravascular coagulation or DIC (a condition in which clotting factors are used up very rapidly, resulting in the potential for severe, uncontrollable bleeding), kidney failure, and eventually complete cardiovascular collapse (a combination of heart attack, shock, and lack of blood flow to all major organs and tissues).

The Rh system identifies the presence (denoted as positive) or absence (denoted as negative) of another type of antigen termed the Rhesus antigen, because it was first identified on the red blood cell surfaces of Rhesus monkeys. The major blood type, then, is reported as a combination of the ABO and Rh blood group system; for example, A-positive, or A-negative, etc.

Knowing a pregnant woman's Rh-factor is crucial because there is always a chance during pregnancy, labor, and delivery that some of the baby's blood will get into the mother's bloodstream. If this happens in an Rh-negative mother with an Rh-positive baby, the mother's body will identify the baby's Rh-negative blood as foreign and begin producing antibodies against the Rh-factor. This is called Rh-sensitization. The first time this sensitization occurs between a mother and her baby, the baby usually doesn't suffer any ill-effects. But in subsequent pregnancies, if the mother is again carrying an Rh-positive baby, having already been exposed to the Rh-antigen previously, her body will begin to produce Rh-antibodies more quickly and in greater numbers. If these cross over into the baby's bloodstream, they can begin destroying the baby's red blood cells, resulting in severe illness. This problem is referred to as Rh disease, hemolytic disease of the newborn, or erythroblastosis fetalis. In order to avoid this problem, Rh testing is done prior to pregnancy or early in pregnancy. Rh-negative women can be given a special shot called Rh-immune globulin which can prevent Rh-sensitization.

Purpose

Blood typing is ordered prior to a blood transfusion, to make sure that the donor blood type is appropriately compatible with the recipient's blood type. It is also done on donor blood, on a donor who is giving an organ to be used for transplantation, as well as prior to surgery (so that the patient's blood type is known, should the individual needs an unexpected, emergency blood transfusion). Rh-typing is also important in pregnant women. When the mother and the baby have different Rh-types, there is a risk to the baby of illness caused by the mother's antibodies; if the mother is identified as having Rh-negative blood, a shot called Rh-immune globulin can prevent the problem from developing.

Precautions

Some situations may confuse the results of blood typing, including a recent x-ray test using contrast, use of medications such as methyldopa, levodopa, and certain **antibiotics** (including cephalexin). Other factors that may confuse test results include having received a blood transfusion in the previous three months, having had a bone marrow transplant in the past, or having a history of cancer or leukemia.

Description

This test requires blood to be drawn from a vein (usually one in the forearm), generally by a nurse or phlebotomist (an individual who has been trained to draw blood). A tourniquet is applied to the arm above the area where the needle stick will be performed. The site of the needle stick is cleaned with antiseptic, and the needle is inserted. The blood is collected in vacuum tubes. After collection, the needle is withdrawn, and pressure is kept on the blood draw site to stop any bleeding and decrease bruising. A bandage is then applied.

Preparation

There are no restrictions on diet or physical activity, either before or after the blood test.

Aftercare

As with any blood tests, discomfort, bruising, and/or a very small amount of bleeding is common at the puncture site. Immediately after the needle is withdrawn, it is helpful to put pressure on the puncture site until the bleeding has stopped. This decreases the chance of significant bruising. Warm packs may relieve minor discomfort. Some individuals may feel briefly woozy after a blood test, and they should be encouraged to lie down and rest until they feel better.

Risks

Basic blood tests, such as blood typing, do not carry any significant risks, other than slight bruising and the chance of brief dizziness.

Results

The ABO blood group system identifies a type of protein antigen on the red blood cell surface. The types of blood types within this system include type A, type B, type AB, and type O:

- People with type A blood have the A antigen on their red blood cell surface; they produce antibodies that can destroy B-type antigens. They can only safely receive either types A or O blood in transfusion.

- People with type B blood have the B antigen on their red blood cell surface; they produce antibodies that can destroy A-type antigens. They can only safely receive either types B or O blood in transfusion.

- People with type AB blood have both A and B antigens on their red blood cell surface; they do not produce any antibodies against A or B antigens. Type AB individuals have both types of major antigens present on their red blood cells, therefore they can safely receive any of the blood types (A, B, or O) in a transfusion without the risk of producing antibodies against the donor blood types. People with type AB blood are sometimes called "universal recipients."

- People with type O blood have neither A nor B antigens on their red blood cell surface, and they produce antibodies against both A and B antigens. Type O blood is sometimes called the "universal donor" type because it displays no antigens on its red blood cell surface and can be transfused into people with types A, B, or AB blood without causing adverse effects; however, people with type O blood can only safely receive type O blood in a transfusion.

The most common ABO blood type in the United States is type O; the most common Rh factor in the United States is positive. Distribution of blood types in the United States is as follows:

- 45% type O, of which 38% are O-positive and 7% are O-negative

- 40% type A, of which 34% are A-positive and 6% are A-negative

- 11% type B, of which 3% are B-positive and 1% are B-negative
- 4% type AB, of which 3% are AB-ositive and 1% are AB-negative

Resources

BOOKS

Goldman L., D. Ausiello, eds. *Cecil Textbook of Internal Medicine,* 23rd ed. Philadelphia: Saunders, 2007.

Hoffman R., et al. *Hematology: Basic Principles and Practice,* 4th ed. Philadelphia: Elsevier, 2004.

McPherson R. A., and M. R. Pincus, eds. *Henry's Clinical Diagnosis and Management by Laboratory Methods,* 21st ed. Philadelphia: Saunders, 2006.

OTHER

Medical Encyclopedia. Medline Plus. U.S. National Library of Medicine and the National Institutes of Health. January 2, 2008. http://www.nlm.nih.gov/medlineplus/encyclopedia.html (February 10, 2008).

ORGANIZATIONS

American Association for Clinical Chemistry, 1850 K Street, NW, Suite 625, Washington, DC, 20006, (800) 892-1400, http://www.aacc.org.

Rosalyn Carson-DeWitt, M.D.

Blood typing *see* **Type and screen**

Blood urea nitrogen test

Definition

Blood urea nitrogen (BUN) is a chemical waste product of protein metabolism. Proteins are broken down into amino acids within the liver; these amino acids are metabolized, giving rise to nitrogen. Nitrogen is coupled with other molecules within the liver, producing the waste product urea that circulates in the bloodstream and goes to the kidneys. Healthy kidneys filter out this waste material from the blood. It passes into the urine and out of the body. Unhealthy kidneys, however, are unable to filter urea out of the blood. The urea remains circulating in the bloodstream, and blood urea nitrogen (BUN) levels rise as the liver continues to metabolize proteins.

The blood urea nitrogen level is used to predict how the kidneys are functioning. In many cases, the blood urea nitrogen level will begin to rise before a patient is even aware of any symptoms of kidney malfunction. High BUN levels indicate the need for further investigation into the possibility that kidney failure is ensuing. If a BUN level is elevated, then other tests such as a **serum creatinine level** or a 24-hour urine creatinine will be performed. Calculations involving serum and urine creatinine levels will give the creatinine clearance, a figure which reflects the capacity of the kidneys to filter small molecules out of the bloodstream.

Purpose

A blood urea nitrogen level is usually drawn as part of a larger metabolic panel or screen. Other tests performed in this panel include electrolytes (sodium, potassium, chloride, and carbon dioxide), as well as calcium, glucose, and serum creatinine level. A blood urea nitrogen level is usually checked during a routine **physical examination**, as well as to evaluate acutely or chronically ill patients for the presence of kidney or liver disease, to monitor patients who have illnesses or who are taking medications that might affect the functioning of their kidneys, or to make sure that treatment for kidney disease (including hemodialysis or peritoneal dialysis) is effective.

Precautions

Blood urea nitrogen levels can be affected by a number of medications. Patients who are on these medications should inform their doctor, so that test results can be interpreted appropriately. Medications that may affect blood urea nitrogen levels include **diuretics**, amphotericin B, nafcillin, aminoglycosides, kanamycin, tobramycin, steroid medications, tetracycline **antibiotics**, and chloramphenicol. Additionally, if the blood urea nitrogen level is going to be used in calculations with serum or urine creatinine levels to evaluate kidney functioning, results may be skewed by the following medications: methyldopa, trimethoprim, vitamin C, cimetidine, certain diuretics, cephalosporin antibiotics, phenytoin, captopril, quinine, quinidine, and procainamide.

Patients who are taking anticoagulant medications should inform their healthcare practitioner since this may increase their chance of bleeding or bruising after a blood test.

Description

This test requires serum to be drawn from a vein (usually one in the forearm), generally by a nurse or phlebotomist (an individual who has been trained to draw serum). A tourniquet is applied to the arm above the area where the needle stick will be performed. The site of the needle stick is cleaned with antiseptic, and the needle is inserted. The serum is collected in vacuum

KEY TERMS

Creatine—Creatine is a substance produced from protein and stored in the muscles. Creatine is a source for energy, allowing muscle contraction to take place. Some creatine is converted to creatinine, and enters the bloodstream, where it is filtered out by healthy kidneys and leaves the body in the urine. When the kidneys are not functioning properly, creatinine levels in the blood become abnormally elevated.

Creatinine—Creatinine is a chemical waste product that is produced by the muscles. Creatinine enters the bloodstream and goes to the kidneys. Healthy kidneys filter out this waste material from the blood. It passes into the urine and out of the body. Unhealthy kidneys, however, are unable to filter out the creatinine from the blood. The creatinine remains circulating in the bloodstream, and levels rise as the muscles continue to produce more and more.

Urine creatinine level—A value obtained by testing a 24-hour collection of urine for the amount of creatinine present.

tubes. After collection, the needle is withdrawn, and pressure is kept on the serum draw site to stop any bleeding and decrease bruising. A bandage is then applied.

Preparation

In the 24–48 hours prior to a blood urea nitrogen level, patients should be advised to limit the amount of protein they ingest. Because urea is a waste product of protein metabolism, ingesting more than eight ounces of meat (particularly beef) or other protein sources in the 24 hours prior to the blood urea nitrogen level is performed may affect the results.

Aftercare

As with any blood tests, discomfort, bruising, and/or a very small amount of bleeding is common at the puncture site. Immediately after the needle is withdrawn, it is helpful to put pressure on the puncture site until the bleeding has stopped. This decreases the chance of significant bruising. Warm packs may relieve minor discomfort. Some individuals may feel briefly woozy after a serum test, and they should be encouraged to lie down and rest until they feel better.

Risks

Basic serum tests, such as blood urea nitrogen levels, do not carry any significant risks, other than slight bruising and the chance of brief dizziness.

Results

A normal blood urea nitrogen level is 10–20 milligrams per deciliter (mg/dL) or 3.6–7.1 millimoles per liter (mmol/L). Women and children metabolize protein slightly differently than do men, so their BUN levels may normally be lower than those of men. BUN levels also regularly rise with age, and

High levels

High blood urea nitrogen levels suggest that the kidneys are suffering from damage or disease. Kidneys can be damaged by severe infections, shock, cancer, dehydration, high blood pressure, diabetes, or conditions that limit the blood flow reaching the kidneys (such as heart attack, stress, shock, congestive heart failure, or severe burns). High blood urea nitrogen levels can also occur when the urinary tract is blocked (by a kidney stone or tumor). Other causes of increased BUN include excess Addison's disease, dietary intake of protein, bleeding in the gastrointestinal tract (resulting in the metabolism of these blood proteins generating increased urea), tissue damage that increases protein levels that reach the liver (such as may occur with very severe burns), or increases in the rate of protein metabolism in the body. BUN levels may also be elevated during a completely normal pregnancy.

Low levels

Low blood urea nitrogen levels are not diagnostic; however, they may reflect the presence of conditions such as overhydration, poor nutrition, liver disease, or pregnancy.

Resources

BOOKS

Brenner, B. M., and F. C. Rector, eds. *Brenner & Rector's The Kidney,* 7th ed. Philadelphia: Saunders, 2004.

Goldman L., D. Ausiello, eds. *Cecil Textbook of Internal Medicine,* 23rd ed. Philadelphia: Saunders, 2007.

McPherson R. A., and M. R. Pincus, eds. *Henry's Clinical Diagnosis and Management by Laboratory Methods,* 21st ed. Philadelphia: Saunders, 2006.

OTHER

Medical Encyclopedia. Medline Plus. U.S. National Library of Medicine and the National Institutes of Health. January 2, 2008. http://www.nlm.nih.gov/medlineplus/encyclopedia.html (February 10, 2008).

ORGANIZATIONS

American Association for Clinical Chemistry, 1850 K Street, NW, Suite 625, Washington, DC, 20006, (800) 892-1400, http://www.aacc.org.

Rosalyn Carson-DeWitt, M.D.

Bloodless surgery

Definition

Bloodless surgery is an approach to health care that began in the 1960s to avoid the use of transfused blood or blood-related products. The technique has grown over the last four decades, however, to include changed attitudes toward blood conservation, as well as new technologies that minimize the need for transfusions during surgery.

Purpose

The new interest in bloodless surgery has emerged from a variety of religious and social concerns, as well as medical, legal, and economic issues.

Religious and ethical considerations

One of the earliest motivations for bloodless surgery was finding ways to treat Jehovah's Witnesses who needed **emergency surgery** without offending their beliefs about blood **transfusion**. Many of the larger bloodless surgery centers in the United States serve areas with a large population of Jehovah's Witnesses. The specific Biblical passages that Witnesses cite as the basis for their objections are Genesis 9: 4–5, in which God forbids eating animal "flesh with its blood"; and Acts 15:29, in which the Apostles ask their first converts to "abstain from blood."

Respect for the religious beliefs of a specific group, however, is related to a more general ethical concern for patients' rights. While a majority of bloodless surgical procedures are still requested by Jehovah's Witnesses, the proportion of other patients requesting bloodless surgery has risen and is expected to continue to increase. The number of medical centers in the United States that offer bloodless surgery continues to expand. The increased demand for bloodless procedures reflects changing attitudes on the part of patients, who are aware that they have choices about health care and expect medical professionals to respect their decisions. Hospitals with bloodless surgery centers emphasize the importance of patients' ethical rights to privacy and self-determination, as well as their legal rights to refuse treatments that they find objectionable.

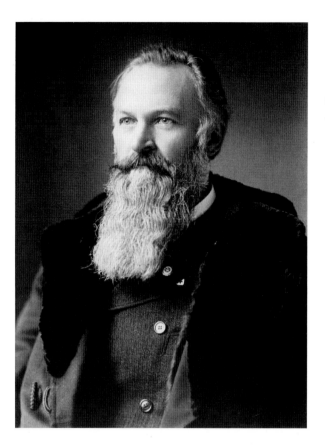

Adolf Lorenz (1854–1946), orthopedic surgeon and pioneer of bloodless surgery. (*Library of Congress / Photo Researchers, Inc.*)

Patient safety

The most important non-religious reason that patients give for requesting bloodless surgery is concern about the safety of blood transfusions. These fears are related to the quality of the American blood supply, as well as the process of blood transfusion itself, and include:

- Blood-borne diseases. Many patients are afraid of contracting such diseases as AIDS and hepatitis from allogeneic (donated) blood. The risk of contracting these specific diseases has been vastly reduced over the past several decades. The risk of contracting hepatitis from transfused blood has continued to decrease since the 1960s. The risk of contracting HIV infection has been reduced by a factor of 10,000 since the virus was first identified in 1983. However, many patients are concerned about the possibility of being infected by disease agents that have not yet been identified as blood borne.

- Transfusion reactions related to medical errors. In contrast to the reduction of risk from infection, there has been little reduction of risk since 1960 of non-infectious serious hazards of transfusion (NISHOT).

NISHOT statistics include mistransfusion and ABO/Rh-incompatibility. Although transfusion errors are only a small percentage of all medical errors reported in North American hospitals, they are the most common cause of serious mortality and morbidity associated with blood transfusions. About 25 patients die each year in the United States from transfusion errors involving ABO-Rh incompatibility. These errors are due to misidentification of type-and-crossmatch samples, laboratory errors, or misidentification of the transfusion recipient. Even patients who donate their own blood (autologous donation) in preparation for elective surgery cannot be completely certain that their blood will be correctly labeled and used during their operation.

- Immune system reactions. Allogeneic blood has been shown to disrupt the immune system and reduce longevity in cancer patients. Other studies have shown that transfused donor blood suppresses the production of B-cells and T-cells in recipients.

- Availability of blood. Many healthcare professionals are concerned about the growing shortage of blood for surgical procedures in the United States. Some blood types are less common than others; in addition, there are often seasonal shortages of blood. Additionally, there is an increasing demand for blood; three million pints of blood are used in the United States every year just for elective surgery. Also, many surgical procedures require large amounts of blood or blood products.

Economic issues

The cost of allogeneic blood transfusions is higher than most people realize. Even though the donated blood itself is free, the costs of preparing, storing, transporting, and unpackaging the blood can be very high.

Demographics

A significant problem confronting blood banks in the United States is the growing proportion of older Americans in the general population. Their numbers are not matched by any corresponding increase in the donor population; it is estimated that only 5% of American adults give blood regularly. Although a wide cross-section of the public can be found at blood drives, the statistically average donor is a college-educated married Caucasian male between the ages of 30 and 50 with an above-average income. The aging of the so-called baby boomer generation, which represents a large segment of the population, is expected to lead to a critical shortage of blood by 2030. The rise in the number of complex orthopedic procedures associated with high-volume blood loss that are performed largely in elderly patients contributes to the likelihood of a severe blood shortage over the next two decades.

Another demographic change that affects the size of the population eligible to donate blood is the increased popularity of tourism and the rising number of people stationed in other countries by their employers or the military. People who have been exposed to or have a history of certain diseases from living abroad are either indefinitely or permanently deferred from giving blood.

Description

Bloodless surgery covers a wide variety of changes in medical practice as well as new equipment and technological innovations.

Preoperative assessment of patients

A patient seeking bloodless **elective surgery** is carefully evaluated for a history of unexpected bleeding or clotting problems after medical or dental procedures. The patient will also be asked about a family history of bleeding disorders.

The patient's blood will be tested to determine hemoglobin levels. In most cases, the patient will be given medications to build up hemoglobin levels prior to surgery.

Care is taken to minimize the number and size of blood samples drawn for **presurgical testing**. The invention of microanalyzers allows hospital laboratories to run blood tests on samples of blood that are 30–60% smaller than those previously collected and to use the same blood sample for multiple tests.

New instruments and surgical techniques to reduce blood loss during surgery

The invention of several types of new **surgical instruments** has allowed surgeons to perform a variety of procedures with minimal blood loss. Miniaturized endoscopes make it possible to perform surgery on the abdomen and spine through very small incisions, often shorter than 1 in (2.5 cm) in length. The invention of argon beam coagulators, electrocautery devices, and harmonic scalpels, which use a combination of **ultrasound** vibration and friction to clot blood at the same time as cutting, also help to make transfusions unnecessary. In addition, surgeons are being trained to use extra caution during surgery and to clamp or cauterize open blood vessels as quickly as possible.

Blood transfusions can sometimes be avoided by scheduling lengthy surgical procedures in two stages. Although this approach requires additional exposure to **general anesthesia**, it can shorten the overall length of the patient's hospital stay. The patient can be discharged after the first operation relatively quickly and build up his or her hemoglobin levels before the second procedure. In addition, the second surgery can be completed without the need for allogeneic blood.

Hypotension in surgery refers to the intentional lowering of the patient's arterial blood pressure during the procedure. Lowering blood pressure has been shown to reduce blood loss and the consequent need for transfusions. It also shortens the length of time spent in the **operating room**. The limitation of hypotension is that it cannot be used in surgical procedures requiring tissue grafting or in patients with coronary artery disease.

Hemodilution is a technique in which whole blood from the patient is withdrawn before surgery for temporary storage and replaced with crystalloid or colloid solutions that restore the normal fluid volume of the blood without adding new blood cells. The patient thus loses fewer red blood cells during surgery. At the close of the operation, the patient's own blood is reinfused, thus minimizing the possibility of transfusion error or a transfusion reaction.

Blood salvage, which is also called autotransfusion, involves an automated recovery system that collects the patient's blood during surgery in a cell separation device. This device separates the red blood cells from other blood components, washes them, and concentrates them for reinfusion.

Reevaluation of postoperative anemia

Another change that has affected the frequency and number of blood transfusions is the reevaluation of anemia and its effects on the body. At one time, patients were automatically given blood transfusions if their hemoglobin level fell below 10 g/dL. More recent studies have shown that patients can tolerate hemoglobin levels of 5 g/dL or even lower. At present, the so-called transfusion trigger is a hemoglobin level of 7 g/dL, evaluated in the context of the patient's overall clinical condition.

Red cell substitutes

Researchers are presently investigating the possibility of manufacturing substitutes for red blood cells that would reduce the cost of transfusions while improving patient safety. Two approaches that have been explored are cell-free hemoglobin solutions and perfluorocarbon solutions. Neither approach has yielded satisfactory results so far: the hemoglobin solutions have a short half-life, and the perfluorocarbon solutions would be difficult to administer intravenously. Further research is underway.

Diagnosis/Preparation

Administrative

Preparation for nonemergency bloodless surgery includes a registration process as well as medical preparation. The patient is given an advance directive and enrollment form to sign. The documents are kept on file with the patient's preadmission chart. After the patient is admitted, he or she is given a red (or other distinctive color) wristband with the words "Do Not Administer Blood Products." Signs and stickers with the same warning are attached to the patient's bed and chart.

Medical

One of the basic components of bloodless surgery programs is presurgical treatment intended to boost the oxygen-carrying capacity of the patient's blood. Patients are given erythropoietin (EPO) several weeks before surgery. EPO is a hormone that stimulates the bone marrow to produce more red blood cells, as many as seven times the normal amount. The greater number of red cells increases the blood's ability to carry oxygen. In addition to the EPO, patients are given iron supplements, most commonly ferrous sulfate, iron dextran, or vitamin B.

Normal results

Patients who have been treated in bloodless surgery centers are generally satisfied with the care they receive. Hospitals have found that patients recover faster with fewer complications; it has been reported that patients requiring inpatient procedures leave the hospital on average a full day earlier than patients who have had conventional transfusions.

Resources

BOOKS

Khatri, V. P., and J. A Asensio. *Operative Surgery Manual.* 1st ed. Philadelphia: Saunders, 2003.

Townsend, C. M., et al. *Sabiston Textbook of Surgery.* 17th ed. Philadelphia: Saunders, 2004.

PERIODICALS

Cogliano, J., and D. Kisner. "Bloodless Medicine and Surgery in the OR and Beyond." *AORN Journal* 76 (November 2002): 830–837, 839, 841.

Martyn, V., S. L. Farmer, M. N. Wren, et al. "The Theory and Practice of Bloodless Surgery." *Transfusion and Apheresis Science* 27 (August 2002): 29–43.

Nuttall, Gregory A., MD. "Keeping a Finger on the Pulse of Transfusion Practices." *American Society of Anesthesiologists Newsletter* 66 December 2002 [cited May 20, 2003]. http://www.asahq.org/Newsletters/2002/12_02/nuttall.html (accessed March 7, 2008).

Ozawa, S., A. Shander, and T. D. Ochani. "A Practical Approach to Achieving Bloodless Surgery." *AORN Journal* 74 (July 2001): 34–40, 42–47, 50–54.

Yowler, Charles, MD. "Transfusion and Autotransfusion." *eMedicine* March 29, 2002 [cited May 21, 2003]. http://www.emedicine.com/med/topic3215.htm (accessed March 7, 2008).

ORGANIZATIONS

American Association of Blood Banks (AABB). 8101 Glenbrook Road, Bethesda, MD 20814-2749. (301) 907-6977. http://www.aabb.org (accessed March 7, 2008).

American Red Cross (ARC) National Headquarters. 431 18th Street, NW. Washington, DC 20006. (202) 303-4498. http://www.redcross.org (accessed March 7, 2008).

Associated Jehovah's Witnesses for Reform on Blood (AJWRB). P. O. Box 190089, Boise, ID 83719-0089. http://www.ajwrb/org (accessed March 7, 2008).

Division of Blood Diseases and Resources. The National Heart, Lung and Blood Institute (NHLBI). Two Rockledge Center, Suite 10138, 6701 Rockledge Drive, MSC 7950, Bethesda, MD 20892-7950. http://www.nhlbi.nih.gov/about/dbdr (accessed March 7, 2008).

National Blood Data Resource Center (NBDRC). 8101 Glenbrook Road, Bethesda, MD 20814-2749. (301) 215-6506. http://www.nbdrc.org (accessed March 7, 2008).

Physicians and Nurses for Blood Conservation (PNBC). P. O. Box 217, 6-2400 Dundas Street West, Mississauga, ON L5K 2R8. (905) 608-1647. http://www.pnbc.ca (accessed March 7, 2008).

Society for the Advancement of Blood Management (SABM). 350 Engle Street, Englewood, NJ 07631. (866) 894-3916. http://www.sabm.org (accessed March 7, 2008).

OTHER

American Association of Blood Banks (AABB). *All About Blood.* Bethesda, MD: AABB, 2002.

Rebecca Frey, PhD
Rosalyn Carson-DeWitt, MD

Body temperature

Definition

Temperature is a measure of an organism's ability to generate and get rid of heat. The human body has mechanisms to maintain its internal temperature within a relatively narrow, safe range despite relatively large variations in temperatures in which the body exists.

Purpose

The purpose of maintaining body temperature within a relatively narrow range is to promote and sustain life.

Demographics

Thermometers are used to measure body temperature. They are calibrated in either degrees Fahrenheit (°F) or degrees Celsius (°C). Temperatures in the United States are typically measured in degrees Fahrenheit. The standard in most countries of the world is degrees Celsius.

Description

When humans become too warm, blood vessels in the skin increase in diameter (dilate). The purpose is to carry the excess heat to the surface of the skin. In turn, this causes the body to begin to perspire. As the perspiration evaporates, it helps to cool the body. When the body becomes too cold, the blood vessels decrease in diameter (contract) so that blood flow to the skin is reduced in an attempt to conserve body heat. This often causes people to start shivering. This involves rapid, involuntary contractions of muscles. Shivering helps to generate additional heat through muscle activity. Under normal conditions, these activities maintain human body temperature within a narrow range that is healthy for the organism.

Body temperature can be measured in many locations. The mouth, ear, armpit, and rectum are the most commonly used places. Temperature can also be measured on the forehead.

Body temperature is checked for several reasons.

- To detect fever.
- To document an abnormally low body temperature (hypothermia) in people who have been exposed to cold.
- To document an abnormally high body temperature (hyperthermia) in people who have been exposed to heat.
- To monitor the effectiveness of a fever-reducing medicine (antipyretic).
- To determine when a female is ovulating, thereby increasing the probability of becoming pregnant.

Preparation

Preparation for taking a body temperature consists of ensuring that the **thermometer** is clean and disinfected.

Aftercare

Aftercare consists of ensuring that a thermometer is clean and disinfected. Electronic thermometers must be turned off to conserve their batteries.

Risks

Taking a body temperature involves little risk. Inserting a thermometer into the rectum can occasionally be painful. Breaking a thermometer that contains mercury causes exposure to a toxic substance (mercury).

Normal results

Most people consider a normal body temperature to be an oral temperature of 98.6 degrees Fahrenheit. This is more correctly an average of body temperatures. A person's body temperature varies during each 24 hour period. A normal range encompasses temperatures that are 1°F (0.6°C) above or below 98.6 degrees F. Some variation is due to fluctuations in physiology nd cellular metabolism. Bodily activities (or lack) can temporarily increase (or decrease) body temperature. Body temperature is very sensitive to hormone levels and may be higher or lower when a female is ovulating during her menstrual cycle.

A rectal or ear (tympanic membrane) temperature reading is 0.5 to 1 degree F (0.3 to 0.6 degrees C) higher than an oral temperature reading. A temperature taken in the armpit is 0.5 to 1 degree F (0.3 to 0.6 degrees C) lower than an oral temperature reading.

In adults, an oral temperature above 100 degrees F or a rectal or ear temperature above 101 degrees F is considered to be a fever. Children are considered to have a fever when their rectal temperature is 100.4 degrees F or higher.

Abnormally low body temperature is called hypothermia. It is always serious and can be life-threatening. Hypothermia can occur after exposure to cold, when a person is in shock, or after alcohol or drug usage. Metabolic disorders, such as hypothyroidism or diabetes can trigger hypothermia. An infection involving the entire body (sepsis) can cause hypothermia. Infections in older adults, newborn infants or other frail persons may be accompanied by hypothermia.

Morbidity and mortality rates

Perforations of the colon due to inserting a rectal thermometer too far have been reported. These are uncommon. The number of deaths associated with taking a temperature is essentially zero.

Alternatives

There are no alternatives to obtaining a body temperature.

Resources

BOOKS

Bickley, L. S., and P. G. Szilagyi. *Bates' Guide to Physical Examination and History Taking.* 9th ed. Philadelphia: Lippincott Williams and Wilkins, 2007.

Jarvis, C. *Physical Examination and Health Assessment.* 5th ed. Philadelphia: Saunders, 2007.

Seidel. H. M., J. Ball, J. Dains, and W. Bennedict. *Mosby's Physical Examination Handbook.* 6th ed. St. Louis: MOsby, 2006.

Swartz, M. H. *Textbook of Physical Diagnosis: History and Examination.* 5th ed. Philadelphia: Saunders, 2005.

PERIODICALS

Bruel, C., J. J. Parienti, W. Marie et al. "Mild hypothermia during advanced life support: a preliminary study in out-of-hospital cardiac arrest." *Critical Care* 12, no. 1 (2008): R31–R41.

Gunn, A. J., T. Hoehn, G. Hansmann et al. "Hypothermia: an evolving treatment for neonatal hypoxic ischemic encephalopathy." *Pediatrics* 121, no. 3 (2008): 648–650.

Mance, M. J. "Keeping Infants Warm: Challenges of Hypothermia." *Advances in Neonatal Care* 8, no. 1 (2008): 6–12.

Salerian, A. J., and N. G. Saleri. "Cooling core body temperature may slow down neurodegeneration." *CNS Spectrums* 13, no. 3 (2008): 227–229.

ORGANIZATIONS

American Academy of Family Physicians. 11400 Tomahawk Creek Parkway, Leawood, KS 66211-2672. (913) 906-6000. E-mail: fp@aafp.org. http://www.aafp.org.

American Academy of Pediatrics. 141 Northwest Point Boulevard, Elk Grove Village, IL 60007-1098. (847) 434-4000, Fax: (847) 434-8000. E-mail: kidsdoc@aap.org. http://www.aap.org/default.htm.

American College of Physicians. 190 N. Independence Mall West, Philadelphia, PA 19106-1572. (800) 523-1546, x2600, or (215) 351-2600. http://www.acponline.org.

American Medical Association. 515 N. State Street, Chicago, IL 60610. (312) 464-5000. http://www.ama-assn.org.

OTHER

HyperTextbook. "Information about body temperature." 2008 [cited February 24, 2008]. http://hypertextbook.com/facts/LenaWong.shtml.

Kid's Health. "Information about adolescent body temperature." 2008 [cited February 24, 2008]. http://www.kidshealth.org/parent/general/body/fever.html.

Mayo Clinic. "Information about low body temperature." 2008 [cited February 25, 2008]. http://www.mayoclinic.com/health/body-temperature/AN01513.

National Library of Medicine. "Information about body temperature." 2008 [cited February 22, 2008]. http://www.nlm.nih.gov/medlineplus/ency/article/001982.htm.

L. Fleming Fallon, Jr, MD, DrPH

Bone grafting

Definition

Bone grafting is a surgical procedure that places new bone or a replacement material into spaces between or around broken bone (fractures) or in holes in bone (defects) to aid in healing.

Purpose

Bone grafting is used to repair bone fractures that are extremely complex, pose a significant risk to the patient, or fail to heal properly. Bone grafting is also used to help fusion between vertebrae, correct deformities, or provide structural support for fractures of the spine. In addition to **fracture repair**, bone grafting is used to repair defects in bone caused by congenital disorders, traumatic injury, or surgery for bone cancer. Bone grafts are also used for facial or cranial reconstruction.

Demographics

Degenerative diseases of the spine increase with age. People over age 50 are more likely to need a bone graft if their condition requires surgery. Traumatic injuries occur most often in people 18–44 years.

Description

Bone tissue is a matrix-like structure primarily composed of a protein called collagen. It is strengthened by hydroxyapatite, deposits of calcium and phosphate salts. Four types of bone cells are located within and around this matrix. Together, these four types of cells are responsible for building the bone matrix, maintaining it, and remodeling the bone as needed. The four types of bone cells are:

Bone grafting

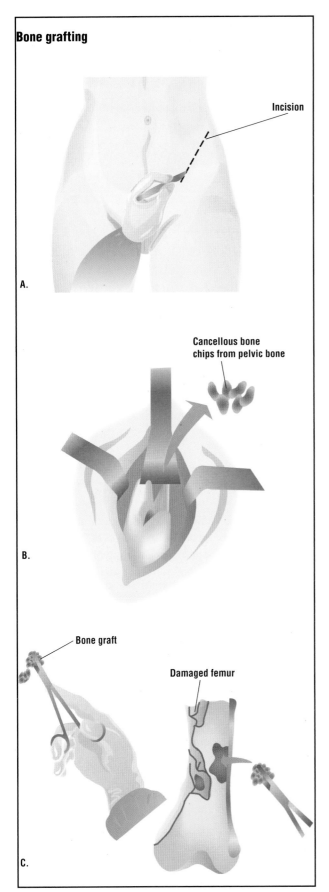

A.

Incision

Cancellous bone chips from pelvic bone

B.

Bone graft

Damaged femur

C.

- osteoblasts, which produce the bone matrix;
- osteocytes, mature osteoblasts that maintain the bone;
- osteoclasts, which break down and remove bone tissue; and
- bone lining cells, which cover bone surfaces.

There are three ways that a bone graft can help repair a defect:

- osteogenesis, the formation of new bone by the cells contained within the graft;
- osteoinduction, a chemical process in which molecules contained within the graft (bone morphogenetic proteins, abbreviated as BMP) convert the patient's cells into cells capable of forming bone; and
- osteoconduction, a physical effect whereby the graft matrix configures a scaffold on which cells in the recipient form new bone.

The term "graft" commonly refers to an autograft or allograft. A graft made of bone from the patient's own body (e.g., hip bones or ribs) is an autograft. To obtain a piece of bone for an autograft, the patient undergoes surgery under **general anesthesia**. An incision is made over the crest of the hip bone, a piece of bone is removed, and the incision is stitched closed.

An allograft uses bone from a cadaver, which has been frozen and stored in a tissue bank. Allografts are used because of the inadequate amount of available autograft material, and the limited size and shape of a person's own bone. Bones for allografts are usually available from organs and tissues donated by healthy people who die unexpectedly. Occasionally, allograft bone may be provided by a living donor. Allograft bone is commonly used in **reconstructive surgery** of the hip, knee, and long bones, as well as cases of bone loss due to trauma or tumors. Using allograft tissue eliminates the need for a second operation to remove autograft bone or tendon. It also reduces the risk of infection, and safeguards against temporary pain and loss of function at or near the secondary site.

To place an autograft or allograft, the surgeon makes an incision in the skin over the bone defect, and shapes the bone graft or replacement material to fit into it. After the graft is placed into the defect, it is held in place with pins, plates, or screws. The incision is stitched closed, and a splint or cast is often used to prevent movement of the bones while healing.

For bone grafting, an incision is made in the donor's hip (A). Pieces of bone are chipped off and removed (B). The bone materials are then transferred to the recipient area, in this case a femur that has been badly broken, to strengthen the bone (C). *(Illustration by GGS Information Services. Cengage Learning, Gale.)*

KEY TERMS

Allograft—Tissue for transplantation that is taken from another person.

Arthrodesis—Surgery that joins (or fuses) two bones so that the joint can no longer move; it may be done on joints such as the fingers, knees, ankles, or spine.

Autograft—Tissue for transplantation that is taken from the patient.

Bone morphogenetic proteins—A family of substances in human bones and blood that encourage the process of osteoinduction.

Computed tomography scan (CT)—A special type of X-ray that can produce detailed pictures of structures inside the body.

Fusion—A union, joining together; e.g., bone fusion.

Hydroxyapatite—A calcium phosphate complex that is the primary mineral component of bone.

Magnetic resonance imaging (MRI)—A test that provides images of organs and structures inside the body using a magnetic field and pulses of radio-wave energy. This form of imaging detects tumors, infection, and other types of tissue disease or damage, and helps diagnose conditions that affect blood flow. The

area of the body being studied is positioned inside a strong magnetic field.

Morbidity—A statistic that provides the rate at which an illness or abnormality occurs.

Mortality—The death rate, which reflects the number of deaths per unit of population in any specific region, age group, disease, or other classification, usually expressed as deaths per 1,000, 10,000, or 1,000,000.

Osteoblasts—Bone cells that build new bone tissue.

Osteoclasts—Bone cells that break down and remove bone tissue.

Osteoconduction—Provision of a scaffold for the growth of new bone.

Osteocytes—Bone cells that maintain bone tissue.

Osteogenesis—Growth of new bone.

Osteoinduction—Acceleration of new bone formation by chemical means. Also refers to the process of building, healing, and remodeling bone in humans.

Vertebra—The bones that make up the back bone (spine).

After the bone graft has been accepted by the body, the transplanted bone is slowly converted into new living bone or soft tissue, and incorporated into the body as a functional unit.

Bone grafts for spinal fusion

In surgery of the spine, especially **spinal fusion**, (also called arthrodesis), surgeons may decide to use bone grafts to assist in the healing and remodeling of the spine after surgery. Normally, small pieces of bone are placed into the space between the vertebrae to be fused, and sometimes larger solid pieces of bone provide immediate structural support. Spinal fusion involves the surgical treatment of abnormalities in the vertebrae, such as curvatures, scoliosis or kyphosis, or injuries (fractures). Bone grafts may be used in spinal fusion surgery involving the lower (lumbar) or upper (cervical) spine. Cervical spinal fusion joins selected bones in the neck. This surgery may also be performed by other means, such as metal rods, which would not require bone grafts.

Diagnosis/Preparation

The surgeon does a clinical examination and conducts tests to determine the necessity of a bone graft.

Diagnostic tests determine the precise location of damage. These tests include x rays, **magnetic resonance imaging** (MRI), and computed tomography **(CT) scan**. They provide an image of the affected area and indicate the exact amount of damage that has occurred due to the fracture or defect.

Orthopedic surgeries pose varying degrees of difficulty. The patient is instructed on what will take place during the procedure, as well as risks involved. A consent form is obtained before surgery.

The following activities will help the patient prepare for surgery:

- thorough physician consult before surgery;
- banking some of his or her own blood in case a transfusion is needed;
- eating well to achieve good nutritional status before and after surgery;
- following a recommended exercise program before and after surgery;
- maintaining a positive attitude; and
- smoking cessation.

Aftercare

Pain is normal for a few days following surgery and medication is given regularly to alleviate this problem. The patient will likely have a urinary catheter.

The time required for convalescence after bone grafts due to fractures or spinal fusion varies from one to 10 days. Vigorous **exercise** may be limited for up to three months. Children heal faster than adults.

If a spinal fusion was performed, the patient may be discharged from the hospital with a back brace or cast. The family will be taught how to provide **home care** for the patient. A splint or cast prevents injury or movement while healing.

Risks

The risks for any surgical procedure requiring anesthesia include reactions to the medications and breathing problems. Bleeding and infection are also risks of surgery.

There is little risk of graft rejection for autografts, but there are drawbacks:

- additional surgical and anesthesia time (typically 30 minutes per procedure) to obtain or harvest the bone for grafting;
- added costs for the additional surgery;
- pain and infection at the site from which the graft is taken;
- the relatively small amount of bone available for grafting; and
- surgical complications, such as infection and pain that sometimes last a longer period of time than the primary surgery (up to two years).

Allografts also have drawbacks:

- bone variability because it is harvested from a variety of donors;
- grafted bone may take longer to incorporate with the host bone (than in an autograft);
- graft may be less effective than an autograft;
- possibility of transferring diseases to the patient; and
- potential immune response complications (patient's immune system fighting against the grafted bone tissue). This problem is lessened through the use of anti-rejection drugs.

Normal results

Most bone grafts are successful in helping the bone defect to heal. The extent of recovery depends on the size of the defect and the condition of the bone

surrounding the graft at the time of surgery. Severe defects take some time to heal, and may require further attention after the initial graft. Less severe bone defects should heal completely without serious complications. Repeat surgery is sometimes required if the condition recurs or complications develop.

If the bone graft is done on the face or head, the surgeries usually result in a more normal appearance.

Morbidity and mortality rates

Although bone harvested from the patient is ideal, postoperative morbidity is sometimes associated with hip bone or fibula (part of the knee) autografts. Morbidity of allografts is usually related to the graft incorporating more slowly and less completely into the body.

In one study of over 1,000 patients who received very large allografts after bone cancer surgery, researchers found that approximately 85% were able to return to work or normal physical activities without crutches; however, approximately 25% required a second operation because the first graft did not heal properly.

Infections associated with bacterial contamination of allografts are rare, but can result in serious illness and **death**.

Alternatives

Despite the increase in the number of procedures requiring bone grafts, there is no ideal bone graft substitute; however, there are a variety of natural and synthetic replacement materials used instead of bone, including collagen (the protein substance of the white fibers of the skin, bone, and connective tissue); polymers, such as silicone and some acrylics; hydroxyapatite; calcium sulfate; and ceramics. Several new products are available or in development. They function as bone graft substitutes or extenders. Demineralized bone matrix (bone that has had its calcium removed) possesses some of the properties that the body uses to induce bone formation. Calcium hydroxyapatite products or coral have structures similar to bone, and act as scaffolding for new bone.

New bone morphogenetic protein (BMP) products are expected to be strong inducers of bone growth (osteoinductive). These new products will be relatively expensive, but will grow bone better than the patient's own bone, eliminating the need for bone graft harvesting. BMPs have been extracted from natural tissues and produced in the laboratory to stimulate bone production in animals and humans. Because they do not have the same drawbacks as grafts, surgeons are hopeful that they will soon be able to use BMP and laboratory-produced BMP to aid in the generation and repair of bone.

The INFUSE Bone Graft (rhBMP-2) has received U.S. Food and Drug Administration approval, and has demonstrated better patient outcomes than hip autografts with regard to length of surgery, blood loss, hospital stay, re-operation rate, median time to return to work, and fusion rates at 6, 12, and 24 months following surgery.

Advances in tissue engineering have provided polymer-based graft substitutes with degradable, porous, three-dimensional structure. New bone may be grown on these products; the grafts then slowly dissolve, leaving only the new bone behind.

Resources

BOOKS

Branemark, Per-Ingvar, Philip Worthington, Kerstin Grondahl, and Christina Darlee, eds. *Osseointegration and Autogenous Onlay Bone Grafts: Reconstruction of the Edentulous Atrophic Maxilla.* Chicago: Quintessence Publishing, 2001.

Laurencin, Cato T., ed. *Bone Graft Substitutes.* West Conshohocken, PA: American Society for Testing and Materials, 2003.

Lawrence, Peter F., Richard M. Bell, and Mohammed I. Ahmed, eds. *Essentials of General Surgery,* 2nd ed. Philadelphia, PA: Lippincott, Williams & Wilkins, 2005.

Lindholm, T. Sam, ed. *Advances in Skeletal Reconstruction Using Bone Morphogenetic Proteins.* River Edge, NJ: World Scientific Publishing, 2002.

Townsend, Courtney M., Daniel R. Beauchamp, Mark B. Evers, Kenneth L. Mattox, and David C. Sabiston, eds. *Sabiston Textbook of Surgery: The Biological Basis of Modern Surgical Practice,* 16th ed. London: W. B. Saunders Co., 2001.

PERIODICALS

Berg-Johnsen, J., and B. Magnaes. "Rib Bone Graft for Posterior Spinal Fusion in Children." *Acta Orthopaedica Scandinavica* 73, no. 6 (December 2002): 709–711.

Cowan, N., J. Young, D. Murphy, and C. Bladen. "Double-blind, Randomized, Controlled Trial of Local Anesthetic Use for Iliac Crest Donor Site Pain." *Journal of Neuroscience Nursing* 34, no. 4 (August 2002): 205–210.

Kakibuchi, M., K. Fukuda, N. Yamada, K. Matsuda, K. Kawai, T. Kubo, M. Sakagami. "A Simple Method of Harvesting a Thin Iliac Bone Graft for Reconstruction of the Orbital Wall." *Plastic and Reconstruction Surgery* 111, no. 2 (February 2003): 961–962.

Nelson C. L., J. H. Lonner, J. A. Rand, and P. A. Lotke. "Strategies of Stem Fixation and the Role of Supplemental Bone Graft in Revision Total Knee Arthroplasty." *Journal of Bone and Joint Surgery,* American volume. 85-A Suppl 1 (2003): S52–S57.

OTHER

American Academy of Orthopaedic Surgeons (AAOS) and American Association of Tissue Banks (AATB). *Bone and Tissue Transplantation.* 2007 http://orthoinfo.aaos.org/topic.cfm?topic = A00115&return_link = 0 [cited February 2008].

U.S. National Library of Medicine and the National Institutes of Health. *MEDLINE Plus Health Information.* 2003 [cited February 2008]. www.nlm.nih.gov/medlineplus.

ORGANIZATIONS

American Association of Tissue Banks, 1320 Old Chain Bridge Road, Suite 450, McLean, VA, 22101, (703) 827-9582, (703) 356-2198, aatb@aatb.org, http://www.aatb.org.

National Institutes of Health, 9000 Rockville Pike, Bethesda, MD, 20892, (301) 496-4000, NIHinfo@od.nih.gov, http://www.nih.gov/.

North American Spine Society, 22 Calendar Court, 2nd Floor, LaGrange, IL, 60525, (877) 774-6337, info@spine.org, http://www.spine.org.

Lisa Christenson, Ph.D.

Crystal H. Kaczkowski, M.Sc.

Laura Jean Cataldo, R.N., Ed.D.

Bone lengthening/shortening *see* **Leg lengthening/shortening**

Bone marrow aspiration and biopsy

Definition

Bone marrow aspiration, also called bone marrow sampling, is the removal by suction of the soft, spongy semisolid tissue (marrow) that fills the inside of the body's long and flat bones. Bone marrow biopsy, or needle core biopsy, is the removal of a small piece (about 0.75 x 0.06 in, 2 x 0.16 cm) of intact bone marrow. The bone marrow is where blood cells are made.

Purpose

Examination of the bone marrow may be the next step that follows an irregular clinical finding, such as an abnormal **complete blood count** (CBC), and/or an abnormal peripheral blood smear. It may also be performed following an abnormal bone image, such as the finding of a lesion on x rays.

A biopsy of bone marrow shows the intact tissue, so that the structure of the fat cells, lymphocytes, plasma cells, fibrous connective tissue cells, and other cells—and their relationships to each other—can be seen. A bone marrow biopsy is used for all the following:

- diagnose and manage any form of leukemia or other myeloproliferative condition such as multiple myeloma
- rule out or confirm bone marrow infiltration by malignancies such as Hodgkin's disease, non-Hodgkin's lymphoma, and metastatic carcinoma
- monitor the effects of chemotherapy and the response or lack of response to treatment of blood disease
- evaluate the success of bone marrow transplantation
- diagnose certain genetic diseases (e.g., lipid storage disease)
- investigate pancytopenia (a decrease of all blood cells in peripheral blood), neutropenia (decreased phagocytic white blood cells), or thrombocytopenia (decreased platelets)
- diagnose an infection of unknown origin
- investigate rare anemias for which a cause cannot be found or which does not respond to treatment as anticipated
- obtain intact bone marrow for laboratory analysis
- diagnose some types of cancer, or anemia and other blood disorders
- identify the source of an unexplained fever (e.g., granulomatous lesions)
- diagnose fibrosis of bone marrow and myeloma when bone marrow aspiration has failed to provide an appropriate specimen

The combination of aspiration and biopsy procedures are commonly used to ensure the availability of the best possible bone marrow specimen. The aspirate is collected at the same time as the bone core biopsy by attaching a syringe to the bone marrow needle and withdrawing the sample before the cutting blades are inserted and the bone core is removed. The aspirate is the sample of choice for studying and classifying the nucleated blood cells of the bone marrow (e.g., determining the ratio of immature white blood cells to red blood cells, which is the M:E ratio). The biopsy is the only sample that shows the blood-forming cells in relation to the structural and connective tissue elements (i.e., the microarchitecture) of the bone marrow. It provides the best sample for evaluating the cellularity of the bone marrow (the percentage of blood-forming tissue versus fat).

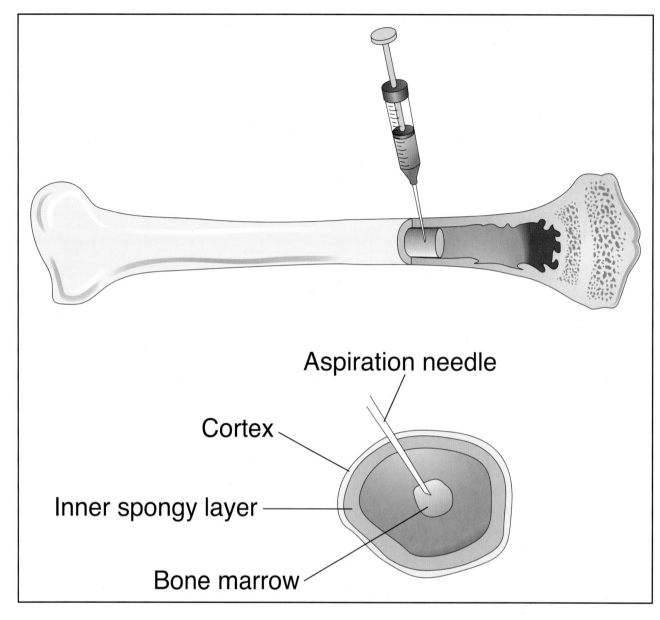

In a bone marrow aspiration, a needle is inserted beneath the skin and rotated until it penetrates the cortex, or outer covering of the bone. A small amount of marrow is suctioned out of the bone by a syringe attached to the needle. *(Illustration by Electronic Illustrators Group. Cengage Learning, Gale.)*

Description

Bone marrow aspiration and biopsy are performed by a pathologist, hematologist, or oncologist with special training in this procedure. The procedure may be performed on an outpatient basis. In adults, the specimen is usually taken from the posterior superior iliac crest (top rear part of the hip). The sternum (breastbone) may be used for aspiration, but is less desirable because it carries the risk of cardiac puncture. Other sites that are rarely used are the anterior superior iliac crest or a spinal column bone. When the

patient is a child, the biopsy site is generally the anterior tibia, the larger of the two bones in the lower leg. A vertebra may also be used.

The skin covering the biopsy site is cleansed with an antiseptic, and the patient may be given a mild sedative. A local anesthetic such as lidocaine is administered first under the skin with a fine needle and then around the bone at the intended puncture site with a somewhat larger-gauge needle. When the area is numb, a small incision is made in the skin and the biopsy needle is inserted. Pressure is applied to force

Antibodies—Proteins that are produced normally by specialized white blood cells after stimulation by a foreign substance (antigen) and that act specifically against the antigen in an immune response.

Aspiration—A procedure to withdraw fluid and cells from the body.

Connective tissue—Cells such as fibroblasts, and material such as collagen and reticulin, that unite one part of the body with another.

Fibrosis—A condition characterized by the presence of scar tissue, or reticulin and collagen proliferation in tissues to the extent that it replaces normal tissues.

Hematologist—A specialist who treats diseases and disorders of the blood and blood-forming organs.

Hematoma—Blood that collects under the skin, forms a blood clot, and causes swelling.

Hemorrhage—Heavy bleeding.

Immune system—Mechanism that protects the body from foreign substances, foreign cells, and pathogens. The thymus, spleen, lymph nodes, white

blood cells, including the B cells and T cells, and antibodies are involved in the immune response, which aims to destroy these foreign bodies.

Lymphocytes—Type of white blood cells that are part of the immune system. The lymphocytes are composed of three main cell lines: B lymphocytes, T lymphocytes, and natural killer (NK) cells.

Myeloma (multiple myeloma)—A tumor of plasma cells that originates in bone marrow and usually spreads to more than one bone.

Needle biopsy—The procedure of using a large hollow needle to obtain a sample of intact tissue.

Pathologist—A medical doctor that specializes in identifying diseases by studying cells and tissues under a microscope.

Plasma cells—Cells in the blood and bone marrow that are formed from B lymphocytes, and that produce antibodies.

White blood cells (leukocytes)—Cells of the blood that are responsible for fighting infection.

the needle through the outer bone, and a decrease in resistance signals entry into the marrow cavity. The needle most often used for bone marrow biopsy is a Jamshidi trephine needle or a Westerman-Jensen trephine needle. A syringe is placed on the top of the needle and 1–2 ml of the bone marrow is aspirated into the syringe. In some instances, the marrow cannot be aspirated because it is fibrosed, or packed with neoplastic cells. The syringe is removed and the medical technologist uses this sample to prepare several smears containing small pieces of bone (spicules). Another syringe is fitted onto the needle hub and another sample of 3 ml is removed and transferred to a tube containing EDTA for analysis by flow cytometry, cytogenetic testing, or other special laboratory procedures. Following aspiration, the cutting blades are inserted into the hollow of the needle until they protrude into the marrow. The needle is then forced over the tips of the cutting blades and the needle is rotated as it is withdrawn from the bone. This process captures the core sample inside the needle. A wire probe is inserted at the cutting end, and the bone marrow sample is pushed through the hub of the needle onto sterile gauze. The specimen is used to make several preparations on glass slides or cover glasses and is transferred to a fixative solution.

In the laboratory, the aspirate slides are stained with Wright stain or Wright-Giemsa stain. The biopsy material is sectioned onto glass slides and stained with hematoxylin-eosin, Giemsa, and Prussian blue stains. Prussian blue stain is used to evaluate the amount of bone marrow iron, and the other stains are used to contrast cell structures under the microscope. In addition, special stains may be used that aid in the classification of malignant white blood cells.

Diagnosis/Preparation

The physician should be informed of any medication the patient is using and of any heart surgery that the patient may have undergone.

Adults require no special preparation for this test. As for infants and children, they need physical and psychological preparation, depending on their age, previous medical experiences, and level of trust.

Infant preparation

Before the test, parents should know that their child will most probably cry, and that restraints might be used. To provide comfort and to help their child through this procedure, parents are commonly asked to be present during the procedure. Crying is a normal infant response to an unfamiliar environment, strangers, restraints, and separation from the parent. Infants cry more for these reasons than because they hurt. An infant will be restrained by hand or with devices because they have not yet developed the physical control, coordination, and ability to follow commands as adults have. The restraints used thus aim to ensure the infant's safety.

Toddler preparation

Parents should prepare a toddler for bone marrow aspiration directly before the procedure, because toddlers have a very short attention span. Some general guidelines for parents include the following:

- Explain the procedure in a simple language, using concrete terms and avoiding abstract terminology.
- Make sure that the child understands where on the body the procedure will be performed and that it will be limited to that area.
- Allow the child to yell, cry, or express anything, especially pain, verbally.
- Describe how the test will feel.
- Stress the benefits of the procedure and anything that the child may find enjoyable afterwards, such as feeling better or going home.

Preschooler preparation

Parents should prepare a preschooler for bone marrow aspiration directly before the procedure, so that the child does not worry about it for days in advance. Parents should ensure that the child understands that the procedure is not a punishment. Some general guidelines for parents include the following:

- Explain the procedure in a simple language, using concrete terms and avoiding abstract terminology.
- Make sure that the child understands where on the body the procedure will be performed and that it will be limited to that area.
- Allow the child to yell, cry, or express anything, especially pain, verbally.
- Describe how the test will feel and be honest about any pain that may be felt.
- Allow the child to practice different positions or movements that will be required for the procedure.
- Stress the benefits of the procedure and anything that the child may find enjoyable afterwards, such as feeling better or going for a treat on the way home.
- Practice deep breathing and other relaxation exercises. Practice also to have the child hold your hand and tell him or her to squeeze it when he or she feels pain during the procedure.

School-age child preparation

Explanations should be limited to 20 minutes, and repeated if required. The older the child, the earlier a parent can start preparation. Guidelines for parents include the ones provided for preschoolers, as well as the following:

- Suggest ways for maintaining control during the procedure; for example, counting, deep breathing, and relaxation (thinking pleasant thoughts).
- Include the child in the decision-making process; for example, the time of day or the body site where the procedure will be performed. These of course depend on the scheduling constraints of the physician and the type of procedure being performed.
- Encourage the child to participate in the procedure; for example, by holding an instrument, if allowed by the attending hospital staff.
- Encourage the child to hold your hand or the hand of a nurse. Physical contact does help reduce pain and anxiety.

Adolescent preparation

An adolescent is best prepared by being provided with detailed information and reasons for the procedure. Adolescents should be encouraged to make as many decisions as possible. An adolescent may or may not wish a parent to be present during the procedure, and such wishes should be respected, since privacy is important during adolescence. Other guidelines include the following:

- Explain the procedure in correct medical terminology, and provide the reason for it.
- As clearly as possible, describe the equipment that will be involved in concrete terms.
- Discuss potential risks honestly and openly.

Aftercare

After the needle is removed, the biopsy site is covered with a clean, dry pressure bandage. The patient must remain lying down and is observed for bleeding for one hour. The patient's pulse, breathing, blood pressure, and temperature are monitored until they return to normal. The biopsy site should be kept covered and dry for several hours.

The patient should be able to leave the clinic and resume most normal activities immediately. Patients who have received a sedative often feel sleepy for the rest of the day; so driving, cooking, and other activities that require clear thinking and quick reactions should be avoided. Walking or prescribed pain medications

WHO PERFORMS THE PROCEDURE AND WHERE IS IT PERFORMED?

A physician requests or orders the procedure. The aspirate and biopsy are most often performed in a hospital or clinic by a hematologist or pathologist that has been trained in the procedure. The analysis of the bone marrow is done by a pathologist, and a written report is added to the patient's medical record. A histologic technician performs special stains for bone marrow. Clinical laboratory scientists/medical technologists perform smear reviews and analysis of bone marrow cells by flow cytometry. Cytogenetic technologists may perform chromosomal analysis of bone marrow white blood cells.

QUESTIONS TO ASK THE DOCTOR

- What are the possible risks involved in this procedure?
- How many times will the procedure be required?
- How do I prepare for the procedure?
- Must I do anything special after the procedure?
- How long does it take to know the results?
- How many bone marrow aspirations/biopsies do you perform each year?

usually ease any discomfort felt at the biopsy site, and ice can be used to reduce swelling.

A doctor should be notified if the patient:

- feels severe pain for more than 24 hours after the procedure.
- experiences persistent bleeding or notices more than a few drops of blood on the wound dressing.
- has a temperature above 101°F (38.3°C).
- has inflammation and pus at the biopsy site and other signs of infection.

Risks

A small amount of bleeding and moderate discomfort often occur at the biopsy site. Rarely, reactions to anesthetic agents, infection, and hematoma (blood clot) or hemorrhage (excessive bleeding) may also develop. In rare instances, the heart or a major blood vessel is pierced when marrow is extracted from the sternum during bone marrow biopsy. This can lead to severe hemorrhage.

Normal results

Healthy adult bone marrow contains yellow fat cells, connective tissue, and red marrow that produces blood. Bone marrow is evaluated for cellularity, megakaryocyte production, M:E ratio, differential (classification of blood-forming cells), iron content, lymphoid, bone, and connective tissue cells, and bone and blood vessel abnormalities. The bone marrow of a healthy infant is primarily red (75–100% cellularity), but the distribution of blood-forming cells is very different than adult marrow. Consequently, age-related normal values must be used.

Microscopic examination of bone marrow can reveal leukemia, granulomas, myelofibrosis, myeloma, lymphoma, or metastatic cancers, bone marrow infection, and bone disease. Bone marrow evaluation is usually not needed to diagnose anemia, but may be useful in cases that cannot be classified by other means.

Resources

BOOKS

Abeloff, M. D., et al. *Clinical Oncology.* 3rd ed. Philadelphia: Elsevier, 2004.

Khatri, V. P., and J. A. Asensio. *Operative Surgery Manual.* 1st ed. Philadelphia: Saunders, 2003.

Townsend, C. M., et al. *Sabiston Textbook of Surgery.* 17th ed. Philadelphia: Saunders, 2004.

PERIODICALS

Azar, D., C. Donaldson, and L. Dalla-Pozza. "Questioning the Need for Routine Bone Marrow Aspiration and Lumbar Puncture in Patients with Retinoblastoma." *Clinical and Experimental Ophthalmology* 31 (February 2003): 57–60.

Jubelirer, S. J., and R. Harpold. "The Role of the Bone Marrow Examination in the Diagnosis of Immune Thrombocytopenic Purpura: Case Series and Literature Review." *Clinical and Applied Thrombosis/Homeostasis* 8 (January 2002): 73–76.

ORGANIZATIONS

The Leukemia & Lymphoma Society. 1311 Mamaroneck Avenue, White Plains, NY 10605. (914) 949-5213. http://www.leukemia.org (accessed March 7, 2008).

National Cancer Institute Cancer Information Service. 31 Center Drive, Bethesda, MD 20892-2580. (800) 422-6237. http://www.nci.nih.gov (accessed March 7, 2008).

National Marrow Donor Program. Suite 500, 3001 Broadway Street NE, Minneapolis, MN 55413-1753. (800) 627-7692. http://www.marrow.org (accessed March 7, 2008).

OTHER

"Diagnostic Tests: Bone Marrow Biopsy." *Harvard Family Health Guide.* [cited April 2003]. http://www.health.harvard.edu/fhg/diagnostics/marrow/marrow.shtml (accessed March 7, 2008).

Mark A. Best
Monique Laberge, Ph.D.
Rosalyn Carson-DeWitt, MD

Bone marrow transplantation

Definition

The bone marrow—the sponge-like tissue found in the center of certain bones—contains stem cells that are the precursors of white blood cells, red blood cells, and platelets. These blood cells are vital for normal body functions, such as oxygen transport, defense against infection and disease, and clotting. Blood cells have a limited life span and are constantly being replaced; therefore, the production of healthy stem cells is vital.

In association with certain diseases, stem cells may produce too many, too few, or abnormal blood cells. Also, medical treatments may destroy stem cells or alter blood cell production. Blood cell abnormalities can be life threatening.

Bone marrow transplantation involves extracting bone marrow containing normal stem cells or peripheral stem cells from a healthy donor, and transferring it to a recipient whose body cannot manufacture proper quantities of normal blood cells. The goal of the transplant is to rebuild the recipient's blood cells and immune system and hopefully cure the underlying disease.

Purpose

A person's red blood cells, white blood cells, and platelets may be destroyed or may be abnormal due to disease. Also, certain medical therapies, particularly chemotherapy or radiation therapy, may destroy a person's stem cells. The consequence to a person's health is severe. Under normal circumstances, red blood cells carry oxygen throughout the body and remove carbon dioxide from the body's tissues. White blood cells form the cornerstone of the body's immune system and defend it against infection. Platelets limit bleeding by enabling the blood to clot if a blood vessel is damaged.

A bone marrow transplant is used to rebuild the body's capacity to produce these blood cells and bring their numbers to normal levels. Illnesses that may be treated with a bone marrow transplant include both cancerous and non-cancerous diseases.

Cancerous diseases may or may not specifically involve blood cells; but, cancer treatment can destroy the body's ability to manufacture new blood cells. Bone marrow transplantation may be used in conjunction with additional treatments, such as chemotherapy, for various types of leukemia, Hodgkin's disease, lymphoma, breast and ovarian cancer, renal cell carcinoma, myelodysplasia, myelofibrosis, germ cell cancer, and other cancers. Non-cancerous diseases for which bone marrow transplantation can be a treatment option include aplastic anemia, sickle cell disease, thalassemia, and severe immunodeficiency.

Demographics

The decision to prescribe a bone marrow transplant is based on the patient's age, general physical condition, diagnosis and stage of the disease. A person's age or state of health may prohibit use of a bone marrow transplant. The typical cut-off age for a transplant ranges from 40 to 55 years; however, a person's general health is usually the more important factor. Before undergoing a bone marrow transplant, the bone marrow transplant team will ensure that the patient understands the potential benefits and risks of the procedure.

The first successful bone marrow transplant took place in 1968 at the University of Minnesota. The recipient was a child with severe combined immunodeficiency disease and the donor was a sibling. In 1973, the first unrelated bone marrow transplant was performed at Memorial Sloan-Kettering Cancer Center in New York City on a five-year-old patient with severe combined immunodeficiency disease. In 1984, Congress passed the National Organ Transplant Act, which included language to evaluate unrelated marrow transplantation and determine if a national donor registry was feasible. The National Bone Marrow Donor Registry (NBMDR), now called the National Marrow Donor Program (NMDP), was established in 1986.

The NMDP Network has more than 10 million volunteer donors (6 million domestically, and another 4 million through its relationships worldwide) and has 43 donor centers and transplant centers in 16 countries.

Bone marrow transplant

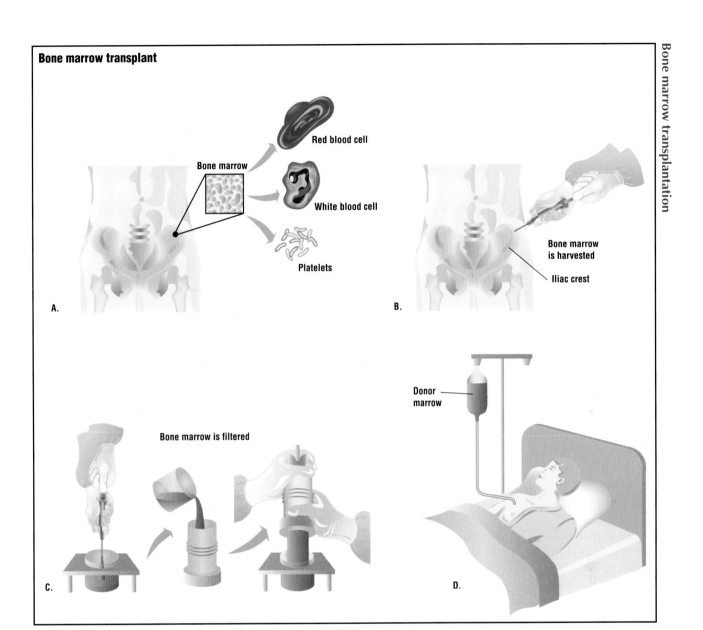

In a bone marrow transplant, bone marrow is harvested from the donor's pelvic bone at the iliac crest (B). The marrow is filtered (C) before being introduced into a large vein in the recipient's chest via a catheter (D). *(Illustration by GGS Information Services. Cengage Learning, Gale.)*

Description

Types of bone marrow transplants

AUTOLOGOUS AND ALLOGENEIC TRANSPLANTS. Two important requirements for a bone marrow transplant are the donor and the recipient. Sometimes, the donor and the recipient may be the same person. This type of transplant is called an autologous transplant. It is typically used in cases in which a person's bone marrow is generally healthy but will be destroyed due to medical treatment for diseases such as breast cancer and Hodgkin's disease. Autologous transplants are also possible if the disease affecting the bone marrow is in remission. If a person's bone marrow is unsuitable for an autologous transplant, the bone marrow must be derived from another person in an allogeneic transplant.

An allogeneic bone marrow donor may be a family member or an unrelated donor. The donated bone marrow/peripheral stem cells must perfectly match the patient's bone marrow. The matching process is called human leukocyte antigens (HLA). Antigens are markers

ABO antigen—Protein molecules located on the surfaces of red blood cells that determine a person's blood type: A, B, or O.

Acute myelogenous leukemia (AML)—Also called acute myelocytic leukemia, a malignant disorder where myeloid blast cells accumulate in the marrow and bloodstream.

Allogeneic—Referring to bone marrow transplants between two different, genetically dissimilar people.

Anemia—Decreased red cell production that results in a deficiency in oxygen-carrying capacity of the blood.

Antigen—A molecule that is capable of provoking an immune response.

Aplastic anemia—A disorder in which the body produces inadequate amounts of red blood cells and hemoglobin due to underdeveloped or missing bone marrow.

Autologous—Referring to bone marrow transplants in which recipients serve as their own donors.

Blank—If an individual has inherited the same HLA antigen from both parents, the HLA typing is designated by the shared HLA antigen followed by a "blank"(-).

Blast cells—Blood cells in early stage of cellular development.

Blast crisis—Stage of chronic myelogenous leukemia where large quantities of immature cells are produced by the marrow, and it is not responsive to treatment.

Bone marrow—A spongy tissue located within flat bones, including the hip and breast bones and the skull. This tissue contains stem cells, the precursors of platelets, red blood cells, and white blood cells.

Bone marrow biopsy—A test involving the insertion of a thin needle into the breastbone or, more commonly, the hip, in order to aspirate (remove) a sample of the marrow. A small piece of cortical bone may also be obtained for biopsy.

Bone marrow transplant—Healthy marrow is infused into people who have had high-dose chemotherapy for one of the many forms of leukemias, immunodeficiencies, lymphomas, anemias, metabolic disorders, and sometimes solid tumors.

Chemotherapy—Medical treatment of a disease, particularly cancer, with drugs or other chemicals.

Chest x ray—A diagnostic procedure in which a very small amount of radiation is used to produce an image of the structures of the chest (heart, lungs, and bones) on film.

Chronic myelogenous leukemia (CML)—Also called chronic myelocytic leukemia, a malignant disorder that involves abnormal accumulation of white cells in the marrow and bloodstream.

Cytomegalovirus (CMV)—Virus that can cause pneumonia in post bone marrow transplant patients.

Computed tomography scan (CT or CAT)—Computed axial tomography uses x rays and computers to produce an image of a cross-section of the body.

Conditioning—Process of preparing a patient to receive marrow donation, often through the use of chemotherapy and radiation therapy.

Confirmatory typing—Repeat tissue typing to confirm the compatibility of the donor and patient before transplant.

Donor—A healthy person who contributes bone marrow for transplantation.

Echocardiogram—An imaging procedure used to create a picture of the heart's movement, valves and chambers. The test uses high-frequency sound waves that come from a hand wand placed on the chest. Echocardiogram may be used in combination with Doppler ultrasound to evaluate the blood flow across the heart's valves.

Electrocardiogram (ECG, EKG)—A test that records the electrical activity of the heart using small electrode patches attached to the skin on the chest.

Graft versus host disease—A life-threatening complication of bone marrow transplants in which the donated marrow causes an immune reaction against the recipient's body.

Histocompatibility—The major histocompatibility determinants are the human leukocyte antigens (HLA), and characterize how well the patient and donor are matched.

Human leukocyte antigen (HLA)—A group of protein molecules located on bone marrow cells that can provoke an immune response. A donor's and a recipient's HLA types should match as closely as possible to prevent the recipient's immune system from attacking the donor's marrow as a foreign material that does not belong in the body.

Hodgkin's disease—A type of cancer involving the lymph nodes and potentially affecting non-lymphatic organs in the later stage.

Immunodeficiency—A disorder in which the immune system is ineffective or disabled due either to acquired or inherited disease.

Leukemia—A type of cancer that affects leukocytes, a particular type of white blood cell. A characteristic symptom is excessive production of immature or otherwise abnormal leukocytes.

Lymphoma—A type of cancer that affects lymph cells and tissues, including certain white blood cells (T cells and B cells), lymph nodes, bone marrow, and the spleen. Abnormal cells (lymphocyte/leukocyte) multiply uncontrollably.

Match—How similar the HLA typing, out of a possible six antigens, is between the donor and the recipient.

Mixed lymphocyte culture (MLC)—Test that measures level of reactivity between donor and recipient lymphocytes.

Myelodysplasia—Also called myelodysplastic syndrome, it is a condition in which the bone marrow does not function normally and can affect the various types of blood cells produced in the bone marrow. Often referred to as a preleukemia and may progress and become acute leukemia.

Myelofibrosis—An anemic condition in which bone marrow cells are abnormal or defective and become fibrotic.

Neuroblastoma—Solid tumor in children, may be treated by BMT.

Non-myeloablative allogeneic bone marrow transplant—Also called "mini" bone marrow transplants. This type of bone marrow transplant involves receiving low-doses of chemotherapy and radiation therapy, followed by the infusion of a donor's bone marrow or peripheral stem cells. The goal is to suppress the patient's own bone marrow with low-dose chemotherapy and radiation therapy to allow the donor's cells to engraft.

Peripheral stem cells—Stem cells that are taken directly from the circulating blood and used for transplantation. Stem cells are more concentrated in the bone marrow, but they can also be extracted from the bloodstream.

Peripheral stem cell transplant—The process of transplanting peripheral stem cells instead of using bone marrow. The stem cells in the circulating blood that are similar to those in the bone marrow are given to the patient after treatment to help the bone marrow recover and continue producing healthy blood cells. A peripheral stem cell transplant may also be used to supplement a bone marrow transplant.

Platelets—Fragments of a large precursor cell, a megakaryocyte found in the bone marrow. These fragments adhere to areas of blood vessel damage and release chemical signals that direct the formation of a blood clot.

Pulmonary function test—A test that measures the capacity and function of the lungs, as well as the blood's ability to carry oxygen.

Radiation therapy—The use of high-energy radiation from x rays, cobalt, radium, and other sources to kill cancer cells and shrink tumors. Radiation may come from a machine outside the body (external beam radiation therapy) or from materials called radioisotopes. Radioisotopes produce radiation and are placed in or near the tumor or in the area near the cancer cells. This type of radiation treatment is called internal radiation therapy, implant radiation, interstitial radiation, or brachytherapy. Systemic radiation therapy uses a radioactive substance, such as a radio-labeled monoclonal antibody that circulates throughout the body.

Recipient—The person who receives the donated blood marrow.

Red blood cells—Cells that carry hemoglobin (the molecule that transports oxygen) and help remove wastes from tissues throughout the body.

Remission—Disappearance of the signs and symptoms of cancer. When this happens, the disease is said to be "in remission." A remission can be temporary or permanent.

Sickle cell disease—An inherited disorder characterized by a genetic flaw in hemoglobin production. (Hemoglobin is the substance within red blood cells that enables them to transport oxygen.) The hemoglobin that is produced has a kink in its structure that forces the red blood cells to take on a sickle shape, inhibiting their circulation and causing pain. This disorder primarily affects people of African descent.

Stem cells—Unspecialized cells, or "immature" blood cells, that serve as the precursors of white blood cells, red blood cells, and platelets.

Syngeneic—Referring to a bone marrow transplant from one identical twin to the other.

Thalassemia—A group of inherited disorders that affects hemoglobin production. Because hemoglobin production is impaired, a person with this disorder may suffer mild to severe anemia. Certain types of thalassemia can be fatal.

Umbilical cord blood transplant—A procedure in which the blood from a newborn's umbilical cord, which is rich in stem cells, is used as the donor source for bone marrow transplants. Currently, umbilical cord blood transplants are mainly used for sibling bone marrow transplants or to store blood for an anonymous donation. In most cases, umbilical cord blood does not contain enough stem cells to safely use for adult bone marrow transplants.

White blood cells—A group of several cell types that occur in the bloodstream and are essential for a properly functioning immune system.

in cells that stimulate antibody production. HLA antigens are proteins on the surface of bone marrow cells. HLA testing is a series of blood tests that evaluate the closeness of tissue between the donor and recipient. If the donor and the recipient have very dissimilar antigens, the recipient's immune system regards the donor's bone marrow cells as invaders and launches a destructive attack against them. Such an attack negates any benefits offered by the transplant.

NON-MYELOABLATIVE ("MINI") ALLOGENEIC TRANSPLANTS. A "mini" transplant involves receiving low-doses of chemotherapy and radiation therapy, followed by the infusion of a donor's bone marrow or peripheral stem cells. The goal is to suppress the patient's own bone marrow with low-dose chemotherapy and radiation therapy to allow the donor's cells to engraft. If there are cancer cells remaining in the patient's body, the donated cells are able to identify the cancer cells as foreign and trigger an immune response, killing the cancer cells. This is called the graft-versus-tumor effect. Mini transplants are still under investigation, but are promising for the future.

PERIPHERAL BLOOD STEM CELL TRANSPLANTS. A relatively recent development in stem cell transplantation is the use of peripheral blood stem cells instead of cells from the bone marrow. Peripheral blood stem cells (PBSCs) are obtained from circulating blood rather than from bone marrow, but the amount of stem cells found in the peripheral blood is much smaller than the amount of stem cells found in the bone marrow. Peripheral blood stem cells can be used in either autologous or allogeneic transplants. The majority of PBSC transplants are autologous. However, clinical studies indicate that PBSCs are being used more frequently than bone marrow for allogeneic bone marrow transplantation.

The advantages of PBSC transplants when compared to bone marrow transplants are that, in allogeneic transplantation, hematopoietic and immune recovery are faster with PBSCs. In autologous transplantation, the use of PBSCs can result in faster blood count recovery. Also, some medical conditions exist in which the recipient cannot accept bone marrow transplants, but can accept PBSC transplants. A possible disadvantage to PBSC transplant versus bone marrow transplantation is that so much more fluid volume is necessary to collect enough PBSCs that, at the time that the new stem cells are infused into the recipient, the fluid can collect in the lungs. Also, the time commitment for the donor for a PBSC transplant is considerable. When the PBSCs are being collected, several outpatient sessions are needed and each session lasts approximately between two and four hours.

UMBILICAL CORD BLOOD TRANSPLANT. Umbilical cord blood transplant is a relatively new procedure in which umbilical cord blood from a newborn is used as the donor source. Umbilical cord blood is rich in stem cells, the cells that are needed for transplantation, and these cells are theoretically "immunologically naïve," reducing chances of rejection and making it a good source for donation. The matching criteria are the same as for bone marrow. Most programs to date use this procedure for a sibling or store cord blood for anonymous donation. Umbilical cord blood can be an excellent source for children. One potential problem with umbilical cord blood transplantation is the low volume of stem cells contained in the umbilical cord. In many instances, there is inadequate volume to safely use for a transplant in an adult recipient.

The transplant procedure

HLA MATCHING. There are only five major HLA classes or types—designated HLA-A, -B, -C, -D, and class III—but much variation within the groupings. For example, HLA-A from one individual may be similar to, but not the same as, HLA-A in another individual; such a situation can render a transplant from one to the other impossible.

HLA matching is more likely if the donor and recipient are related, particularly if they are siblings; however, an unrelated donor may be a potential match. The only case in which matching HLA types between two people is not an issue is if the recipient has an identical twin. Identical twins carry the same genes, therefore, the same antigens. A bone marrow transplant between identical twins is called a syngeneic transplant.

BONE MARROW TRANSPLANTATION. The bone marrow extraction, or harvest, is the same for autologous and allogeneic transplants. Harvesting is done under **general anesthesia**, and discomfort is usually minimal afterwards. Bone marrow is drawn from the iliac crest (the part of the hip bone on either side of the lower back) with a special needle and a syringe. Several punctures are usually necessary to collect the needed amount of bone marrow, approximately 1–2 quarts. (This amount is only a small percentage of the total bone marrow and is typically replaced within four weeks.) The donor remains at the hospital for 24–48 hours and can resume normal activities within a few days.

If the bone marrow is meant for an autologous transplant, it is stored at -112--320°F (-80--196°C) until it is needed. If a patient's own bone marrow can be used for transplantation or if a donor is not found, peripheral stem cells may be harvested from the patient's circulating blood. Bone marrow for an allogeneic transplant is sometimes treated to remove the donor's T cells (a type of white blood cell) or to remove ABO (blood type) antigens; otherwise, it is transplanted without modification.

The bone marrow or peripheral stem cells are administered to the recipient via a catheter (a narrow, flexible tube) inserted into a large vein in the chest. The donor cells look like a bag of blood and are infused for about 20–30 minutes. During the infusion, the patient's blood pressure, pulse, and breathing are monitored. From the bloodstream, the marrow migrates to the cavities within the bones where bone marrow is normally stored. If the transplant is successful, the bone marrow begins to produce normal blood cells once it is in place, or engrafted.

PERIPHERAL BLOOD STEM CELL TRANSPLANTATION. Before collection for a PBSC transplant, donors receive four injections daily of the drug G-CSF, or filgrastim. (Patients can give it to themselves at home, if necessary.) These pretreatments stimulate the body to release stem cells into the blood. After these pretreatments, the donors' experience is similar to that of a whole blood donor's experience—PBSC donors' blood is collected at a clinic or hospital as an outpatient procedure. The differences are that several sessions will be needed over days or weeks, and the blood is collected in a process called apheresis. The blood travels from one arm into a blood cell separator that removes only the stem cells, and the rest of the blood is returned back to the donor in the other arm. The cells are then frozen for later use.

The PBSCs are administered to the recipient using the same methods as those used in bone marrow transplantation. As stated, the amount of fluid with PBSCs infused into the recipient's body can be an issue.

Costs

Bone marrow transplantation is an expensive procedure. (Bone marrow donors are volunteers and do not pay for any part of the procedure.) Insurance companies and health maintenance organizations (HMOs) may not cover the costs. Many insurance companies require precertification letters of medical necessity. As soon as bone marrow transplantation is discussed as a treatment option, it is important for the patient to contact his or her insurance provider to determine what costs will be covered.

Diagnosis/Preparation

Several tests are performed before the bone marrow transplant to identify any potential problems ahead of time. Tests include:

- tissue typing and a variety of blood tests
- chest x ray
- pulmonary function tests
- computed tomography scan (CT or CAT)
- heart function tests, including an electrocardiogram and echocardiogram
- bone marrow biopsy
- skeletal survey

In addition, a complete dental exam is needed before the bone marrow transplant to reduce the risk of infection. Other precautions will be taken before the transplant to reduce the patient's risk of infection.

A triple lumen, central venous catheter (a slender, hollow flexible tube) is surgically inserted into a large vein in the chest during a simple outpatient procedure. The catheter is used to draw blood and infuse chemotherapy and other medications, as well as donor cells, blood product, fluids, and sometimes nutritional solutions. The central venous catheter usually stays in place for about six months after the bone marrow transplant.

Hormone-like medications called colony-stimulating factors may be given before the transplant to stimulate the patient's white blood cells. These medications stimulate the white blood cells to multiply, mature, and function. These medications also help the patient's white blood cells recover from chemotherapy and reduce the risk of infection.

A bone marrow transplant recipient can expect to spend three to four weeks in the hospital, depending on the rate of recovery. In preparation for receiving the transplant, the recipient undergoes "conditioning," a preparative regimen (also called marrow ablation) in which the bone marrow and abnormal cells are destroyed. Conditioning rids the body of diseased cells and makes room for the marrow or peripheral stem cells to be transplanted. It typically involves chemotherapy and/or radiation treatment, depending on the disease being treated. Unfortunately, this treatment also destroys healthy cells and has many side effects such as extreme weakness, nausea, vomiting, and diarrhea. These side effects may continue for several weeks.

Aftercare

A two- to four-week waiting period follows the marrow transplant before its success can begin to be evaluated. The marrow recipient is kept in isolation during this time to minimize potential infections. The recipient also receives intravenous antibiotic, antiviral, and antifungal medications, as well as blood and platelet transfusions to help fight off infection and prevent excessive bleeding. Blood tests are performed daily to monitor the patient's kidney and liver function, as well as nutritional status. Other tests are performed as necessary. Further side effects, such as nausea and vomiting, can be treated with other medications. Once blood counts are normal and the side effects of the transplant abate, the recipient is taken off **antibiotics** and usually no longer needs blood and platelet transfusions.

Following **discharge from the hospital**, the recipient is monitored through home visits by nurses or outpatient visits for up to a year. For the first several months out of the hospital, the recipient needs to be careful in avoiding potential infections. For example, contact with other people who may be ill should be avoided or kept to a minimum. Further blood transfusions and medications may be necessary, but barring complications, the recipient can return to normal activities about six to eight months after the transplant.

Risks

The procedure has a lower success rate the greater the recipient's age. Complications are exacerbated for people whose health is already seriously impaired, as in late-stage cancers.

Bone marrow transplants are accompanied by serious and life-threatening risks. Furthermore, they are not always an absolute assurance of a cure for the underlying ailment; a disease may recur in the future.

Even in the absence of complications, the transplant and associated treatments are hard on the recipient. Bone marrow transplants are debilitating. A person's ability to withstand the rigors of the transplant is a key consideration in deciding to use this treatment.

In the short term, there is the danger of pneumonia or other infectious disease, excessive bleeding, or liver disorder caused by blocked blood vessels. The transplant may be rejected by the recipient's immune system, or the donor bone marrow may launch an immune-mediated attack against the recipient's tissues. This complication is called acute graft-versus-host disease, and it can be a life-threatening condition. Characteristic signs of the disease include fever, rash, diarrhea, liver problems, and a compromised immune system.

Approximately 25–50% of bone marrow transplant recipients develop long-term complications. Chronic graft-versus-host disease symptoms include skin changes, such as dryness, altered pigmentation, and thickening, abnormal **liver function tests**, dry mouth and eyes, infections, and weight loss. Other long-term complications include cataracts (due to radiation treatment), abnormal lung function, hormonal abnormalities resulting in reduced growth or hypothyroidism, secondary cancers, and infertility.

Normal results

In a successful bone marrow transplant, the donor's marrow migrates to the cavities in the recipient's bones and produces normal numbers of healthy blood cells. Bone marrow transplants can extend a person's life, improve quality of life, and may aid in curing the underlying ailment.

Morbidity and mortality rates

Approximately 30% of people receiving allogeneic transplants do not survive. Autologous transplants have a much better survival rate—nearly 90%—but are not appropriate for all types of ailments requiring a bone marrow transplant. Furthermore, autologous transplants have a higher failure rate with certain diseases, specifically leukemia. At two years, the survival rate for patients with chronic myelogenous leukemia is 52% if they received a transplant in a chronic phase of their disease, 30% for patients in an accelerated phase and 15% for patients in the blast phase.

Alternatives

Complementary therapies are used along with standard cancer treatments. These treatments are aimed at bringing about some overall improvement in general health and well being. Complementary therapies can be helpful in managing symptoms and improving quality of life. They can be used to help alleviate pain; reduce nausea; strengthen muscles; and decrease depression, anxiety, and stress. It is

WHO PERFORMS THIS PROCEDURE AND WHERE IS IT PERFORMED?

Transplant physicians specially trained in bone marrow transplantation should perform this procedure. Bone marrow transplant physicians have extensive experience in hematology/oncology and bone marrow transplant.

Selecting a transplant center that has a multidisciplinary team of specialists is important. The bone marrow transplant team should include transplant physicians, infectious disease specialists, pharmacologists, registered nurses, and transplant coordinators. Other transplant team members may include registered dietitians, social workers, and financial counselors.

When selecting a transplant center, the patient should find out where the center is accredited. Some examples of accrediting organizations include The Foundation for the Accreditation of Cellular Therapy, the American Association of Blood Banking, the National Marrow Donor Program, and other state-level accreditation organizations.

Choosing a transplant center with experience is important. Here are some questions to consider when choosing a transplant center:

- How many bone marrow transplants are performed annually, and what are the outcomes/survival rates of those transplants?
- Does the transplant center perform transplants for the patient's type of disease? How many has it performed to date?
- Does the transplant center have experience treating patients the same age as the patient considering transplant?
- What is the required patient and unrelated donor HLA matching level at this center?
- How much does a typical bone marrow transplant cost at this facility?
- Is financial help available?
- If the transplant center is far from the patient's home, will accommodations be provided for caregivers?

important to distinguish between alternative therapies (unproven methods promoted for use instead of mainstream treatment) and complementary therapies, which are used with standard treatment. Complementary therapies are noninvasive and soothing. However, before trying them, patients should check with their oncologist to make sure the complementary therapy will not interfere with standard cancer therapy or cause harm. Examples of complementary therapies are massage therapy, aromatherapy, meditation, yoga, **biofeedback**, music, art and dance therapies, and group and individual therapy or counseling.

Hormone therapy is the treatment of cancer by removing, blocking, or adding hormones. Hormones are chemical substances produced by glands in the body that enter the bloodstream and cause effects in other tissues. Hormone therapies may be used to treat breast and prostate cancers. Hormone therapy may also be used in some situations for other cancers.

Immunotherapy, also called biological therapy, is a type of treatment that uses the body's immune system to fight cancer. The therapy mainly consists of stimulating the immune system with highly purified proteins that help it do its job more effectively.

Radiation therapy is the use of high-energy x rays, electron beams, or radioactive isotopes to attack cancer. Radiation therapy causes cancer cell death by ionization or by damaging the chromosomes in the cancer cells so they cannot multiply. Radiation therapy is a local treatment aimed directly at the cancer. Even though the radiation is aimed only at the cancer, it must often pass through skin and other organs to reach the tumor. Thus, some healthy cells may become damaged, too. The body however is able to repair the healthy cells that have been damaged and restore them to their proper function. Aside from its use as a single treatment, radiation therapy has been shown to enhance the effects of chemotherapy. It can be used in combination with chemotherapy to shrink a tumor. Successful radiation therapy depends on delivering the proper amount of radiation to the cancer in the best, and most effective way.

Resources

BOOKS

Abeloff, M. D., et al.*Clinical Oncology*. 3rd ed. Philadelphia: Elsevier, 2004.

Khatri, V. P., and J. A. Asensio. *Operative Surgery Manual*. 1st ed. Philadelphia: Saunders, 2003.

Townsend, C. M., et al. *Sabiston Textbook of Surgery*. 17th ed. Philadelphia: Saunders, 2004.

ORGANIZATIONS

American Cancer Society. 1599 Clifton Road, NE, Atlanta, GA 30329. (800) 227-2345, (404) 320-3333. http://www.cancer.org (accessed March 7, 2008).

QUESTIONS TO ASK THE DOCTOR

- What type of transplant is recommended for my condition?
- What are the potential benefits of bone marrow transplantation?
- Where does transplanted bone marrow come from?
- What types of tests are required to screen me for the bone marrow transplant?
- What is HLA/histocompatibility matching?
- What types of tests are used to screen potential bone marrow or peripheral stem donors?
- Are bone marrow or peripheral stem cell donors compensated?
- After my bone marrow transplant, can I contact an unrelated donor? How can I do this?
- Will my insurance provider cover the expenses of my bone marrow transplant?
- What types of questions should I ask my insurance provider to determine if the medical expenses of my bone marrow transplant will be covered?
- Whose insurance covers the medical expenses of the donor?
- How long does the insurance clearance process take?
- After bone marrow transplantation is approved as a treatment option for me, how long will I have to wait before I can receive the bone marrow transplant?
- What type of preparative regimen will I have before the bone marrow transplant?
- What are the side effects of the preparative regimen?

- What types of precautions must I follow before and after my bone marrow transplant?
- Will I have to have blood transfusions during the transplantation process?
- What are the risks and potential complications of bone marrow transplantation?
- What is Graft-versus-Host disease (GVHD) and can it be prevented?
- What are the signs of GVHD, rejection, and infection?
- How and when will I know if the bone marrow transplant was successful?
- How long will I have to stay in the hospital?
- What types of resources are available to me during my hospital stay and during my recovery at home?
- What types of medications will I have to take after my bone marrow transplant? How long will I have to take them?
- After I go home, when can I resume my normal activities?
- What type of follow-up care is recommended? How often will I need to go to follow-up appointments?
- Can I receive follow-up care from my primary physician, or do I need to go back to the center where I had my bone marrow transplant?
- If I live far away from my transplant center, do I have to stay near the transplant center during my recovery after discharge? If yes, for how long? Will I receive help in making accommodations?

American Society for Blood and Marrow Transplantation (ASBMT). 85 W. Algonquin Road, Suite 550 Arlington Heights, IL 60005. (847) 427-0224. mail@asbmt.org.

BMT Infonet (Blood and Marrow Transplant Information Network). 2900 Skokie Valley Road, Suite B, Highland Park, IL 60035. (847) 433-3313, (888) 597-7674. help@bmtinfonet.org. http://www.bmtinfonet.org (accessed March 7, 2008).

Cancercare. Health Resources and Services Administration. 5600 Fishers Lane, Rm. 14-45, Rockville, MD 20857. (301) 443-3376. (800) 813-HOPE (4673). http://www.cancercare.org (accessed March 7, 2008).

International Bone Marrow Transplant Registry/Autologous Blood and Marrow Transplant Registry N.

America. Health Policy Institute, Medical College of Wisconsin, 8701 Watertown Plank Road, P.O. Box 26509, Milwaukee, WI 53226. (414) 456-8325. ibmtr@mcw.edu.

Leukemia & Lymphoma Society, Inc. 1311 Mamaroneck Avenue White Plains, NY 10605. (914) 949-5213. http://www.leukemia-lymphoma.org (accessed March 7, 2008).

Lymphoma Research Foundation of America. 8800 Venice Boulevard, Suite 207, Los Angeles, CA 90034. (800) 500-9976. (310) 204-7040. helpline@lymphoma.org. http://www.lymphoma.org (accessed March 7, 2008).

National Bone Marrow Transplant Link. 20411 W. 12 Mile Road, Suite 108, Southfield, MI 48076. (800) LINK-BMT (800-546-5268).

National Foundation for Transplants. 1102 Brookfield, Suite 200, Memphis, TN, 38110. (800) 489-3863 or (901) 684-1697.http://www.transplants.org (accessed March 7, 2008).

National Marrow Donor Program. Suite 500, 3001 Broadway Street Northeast, Minneapolis, MN 55413-1753. (800) MARROW-2. http://www.marrow.org (accessed March 7, 2008).

National Organ and Tissue Donation Initiative. http://www.organdonor.gov (accessed March 7, 2008).

Julia Barrett
Laura Ruth, PhD
Angela M. Costello
Rosalyn Carson-DeWitt, MD

Bone repair *see* **Orthopedic surgery**

Bone x rays

Definition

Bone X rays are a diagnostic imaging test in which ionizing radiation passing through the bones enables an image to be produced on film. An x ray (radiograph) can produce an image of a bone from various and multiple angles. A physician may view an x-ray film to help diagnose fractures in patients and then consider treatment options based on the findings. An x ray may be taken of many bones in the body including the hand, foot, wrist, spine, rib cage, spine, and ankle.

Purpose

Bone x rays are ordered to detect bone disease or injury, such as in the case of broken bones, tumors, and other problems. They can determine bone density, texture, erosion, and changes in bone relationships. Bone x rays also evaluate the joints for such diseases as arthritis. In addition, x rays may be taken to see if a joint has been dislocated, to guide a surgeon during an orthopedic surgical procedure such as a total joint replacement operation, to visualize foreign objects, or to check bone alignment before and after cast application or repair via screw and plate orthopedic procedures.

Description

X rays are the result of the collision between electrons and a protons. German physicist Wilhelm

Conrad Röntgen (1845–1923), discovered what he called X-radiation, in 1895. This form of radiation was noted to have properties allowing transparency and fluorescence that absorbed visible light and contrasting shadows. Experiments with this new form of radiation revealed the distinction between bone and soft tissues in the body, such as in the hand. Röntgen's first x ray was of his wife's hand, which showed bones, soft tissue, and metal from the ring she was wearing. His discovery of x rays heralded a significant and valuable diagnostic tool used in the field of medicine. Röntgen was awarded the Nobel Prize for Physics in 1901 for his discovery. He was the first recipient to be honored in this category. This Nobel Laureate was honored "in recognition of the extraordinary services he has rendered by the discovery of the remarkable rays subsequently named after him."

X rays are a common diagnostic test in which a form of energy called x ray radiation penetrates the patient's body. In bone x rays, electrical current passes through an x-ray tube and produces a beam of ionizing radiation that passes through the bone(s) being examined. This produces a picture of the inside of the body on film. The doctor reads the developed x ray on a wall-mounted light box or on a computer monitor.

Digital x rays are a new type of exam in which conventional equipment is used to take the x-ray picture, but the image is produced via computer. In a digital x ray, the image is created on a reusable plate. After being read by a laser reader, the information is sent in digital form to a storage unit that is connected to a computer network. The radiologist reads the x ray from there. An electronic report can then be sent to the patient's doctor. Electronic reports can also be generated with non-digital x-ray exams.

X rays can detect problems with bones that result from injury or disease caused by malfunction in the patient's bone chemistry. Bone injuries, especially broken bones (fractures), are common and can be accurately diagnosed by evaluation of bone x rays. X rays are especially helpful in diagnosing simple and incomplete fractures, which cannot be detected during a **physical examination**. X rays can also be used to check for bone position and alignment in a fracture. Some bone diseases can be definitively diagnosed with bone x rays, while others require additional, more sophisticated imaging tests.

Osteoporosis, a common bone disease, can be detected in bone x rays, but other tests, such as bone densitometry, may need to be ordered to determine the extent of the disease. In some cases, a bone biopsy (microscopic analysis of a small amount of tissue) is also done. For arthritis, a common ailment, x rays of the bone are occasionally used in conjunction with blood tests. In bone tumors, bone x rays can be helpful, but they may not be definitive when used alone.

Bone x rays are taken by a technologist or radiologist and interpreted by a radiologist. They are taken in a doctor's office, in a hospital, or in an outpatient clinic. Bone x rays generally take less than 10 minutes to complete. There is no pain or discomfort associated with the test, but some people find it difficult to remain still throughout the procedure.

During the test, the patient lies on a table. The technician taking the x ray checks the patient's position and places the x-ray machine over the part of the body being scanned. After asking the patient to remain still, the technician steps out of the area and presses a button to take the picture.

Preparation

The patient is asked to remove clothing, jewelry, and any other metal objects from the part of the body being x rayed. If appropriate, a lead shield is placed over another part of the body to minimize exposure to the radiation that is being used.

Aftercare

The patient can immediately resume normal activities once the technician has checked that the x rays have processed well and that none need to be repeated. This takes just a few minutes.

Risks

The human body contains some natural radiation and is also exposed to radiation in the environment. There is a slight risk from exposure to radiation during bone x rays; however, the amount of radiation is small and the risk of harm is very low. If reproductive organs are to be exposed to large amounts of radiation, genetic alterations could occur in a developing fetus. Excessive or repeated doses of radiation can cause changes in other types of body tissue. No radiation remains in the body after the x ray.

Normal results

Normal bones show no fractures, dislocations, or other abnormalities.

Results that indicate the presence of bone injury or disease differ in appearance, according to the nature of the injury or disease. For example, fractures show up as clear breaks in the bones, while osteoporotic bone has the same shape as normal bone on an x ray, but is less dense.

Resources

BOOKS

Dutton, Mark. *Orthopaedic Examination, Evaluation, and Intervention*. New York: McGraw-Hill, 2004.

Fishback, Francis Talaska, ed. *A Manual of Laboratory and Diagnostic Tests*. 5th ed. Philadelphia: Lippincott, 2003.

Perry, Clayton R., and John Elstrom. *The Handbook of Fractures*, 2nd ed. New York: McGraw-Hill, 1999.

Skinner, Harry. *Current Diagnosis & Treatment in Orthopedics*. New York: McGraw-Hill, 2006.

Tierney, Lawrence M., Jr., Stephen J. McPhee, Maxine A. Papadakis. "Tumors and Tumor-Like Lesions of the Bone: Current Medical Diagnosis and Treatment." In *Current Medical Diagnosis & Treatment*, 36th ed. Stamford, CT: Appleton & Lange, 1996.

OTHER

RadiologyInfo. http://www.radiologyinfo.org.

ORGANIZATIONS

Radiological Society of North America, 820 Jorie Blvd., Oak Brook, IL, 60523-2251, (630) 571-2670, http://www.rsna.org.

Lori De Milto
Lee A. Shratter, M.D.
Laura Jean Cataldo, R.N., Ed.D.

Bowel preparation

Definition

A bowel preparation (bowel prep) involves dietary changes and the use of cathartics, laxatives, and/or enemas to clean out the colon prior to tests or procedures involving the abdomen and gastrointestinal tract. It may also include the administration of **antibiotics** to lessen the chance of infection during surgery.

Purpose

Completing a bowel prep is important prior to a radiological examination because stool in the intestine may interfere with viewing other structures/organs within the abdomen. Prior to abdominal surgery, a careful bowel prep is crucial, since the risk of severe, life-threatening infection is increased if stool remains in the colon. Because stool contains a high bacteria count, even a microscopic nick of the intestine during the course of surgery could result in contamination of the surgical field, and the development of a severe infection.

Description

Although a number of different regimens can be followed, the basic methodology is as follows. A patient who is going to undergo a test (such as **barium enema** or endoscopy) or abdominal surgery is asked to stop eating solid foods some hours prior to their surgery. Depending on the type of surgery and the timing of the surgery, they may be allowed to continue with a full liquid or clear liquid diet. At some point just prior to the surgery, they will be asked not to take anything at all by mouth.

During the twelve or so hours prior to the test or procedure, a series of preparations (in pill or liquid form) will be used in order to make sure that all stool is evacuated from the intestine. Enemas may also be used to make sure that the bowel is completely cleared of stool. Further protection from infection may involve the administration of either oral antibiotics over the twelve hours prior to surgery, or intravenous antibiotics in the several hours just prior to surgery.

Aftercare

Some people, especially those who are already in a debilitated state, may become weak or faint during the course of a bowel preparation. People at risk for this outcome should have someone stay with them as they perform the bowel prep, or should talk to their healthcare providers about having the bowel prep while an inpatient.

KEY TERMS

Cathartic—An agent which stimulates defecation.

Enema—A liquid which is injected through the anus into the lower intestine in order to stimulate defecation.

Laxative—An agent which stimulates defecation.

Risks

Most healthy patients can follow a bowel prep regimen in their own home. However, some patients may require hospitalization to complete their bowel prep if they are very weak or ill with a condition (such as kidney disease or congestive heart failure) that may require close monitoring of their hydration and electrolyte status during the course of the bowel prep.

Normal results

Normal results occur when the bowel is completely cleared of stool prior to a procedure or operation.

Resources

BOOKS

Feldman, M,, et al. *Sleisenger & Fordtran's Gastrointestinal and Liver Disease*. 8th ed. St. Louis: Mosby, 2005.

McPherson, R. A., et al. *Henry's Clinical Diagnosis and Management By Laboratory Methods*. 21st ed. Philadelphia: Saunders, 2007.

OTHER

Jensen, J. E. "Liver Function Tests." http://www.gastromd.com/lft.html [accessed May 5, 2008].

National Institutes of Health. http://www.nlm.nih.gov/medlineplus/encyclopedia.html [accessed May 5, 2008].

Rosalyn Carson-DeWitt, MD

Bowel resection

Definition

Bowel resection is a surgical procedure in which a diseased part of the large intestine is removed. The procedure is also known as colectomy, colon removal,

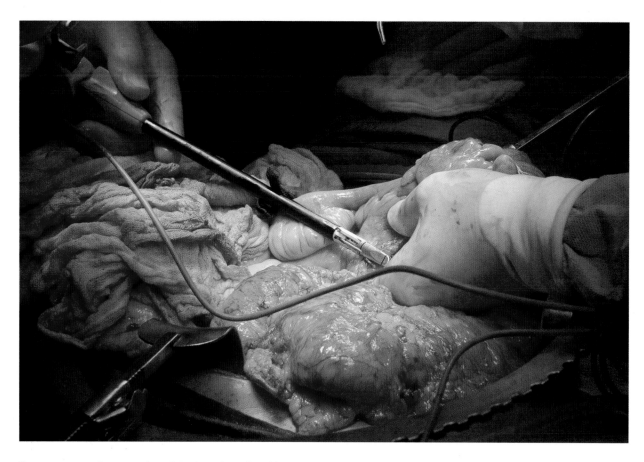

Surgeons removing a portion of the large intestine. *(Copyright Barry Slaven, MD, PhD / Phototake. Reproduced by permission.)*

colon resection, or resection of part of the large intestine.

Purpose

The large bowel, also called the large intestine, is a part of the digestive system. It runs from the small bowel (small intestine) to the rectum, which receives waste material from the small bowel. The large bowel's major function is to store waste and to absorb water from waste material. It consists of the following sections, any of which may become diseased:

- Colon. The colon averages some 60 in (150 cm) in length. It is divided into four segments: the ascending colon, transverse colon, descending colon, and sigmoid colon. There are two bends (flexures) in the colon. The hepatic flexure is where the ascending colon joins the transverse colon. The splenic flexure is where the transverse colon merges into the descending colon.

- Cecum. This is the first portion of the large bowel that is joined to the small bowel. The appendix lies at the lowest portion of the cecum.

- Ascending colon. This segment is about 8 in (20 cm) in length, and it extends upwards from the cecum to the hepatic flexure near the liver.

- Transverse colon. This segment is usually more than 18 in (46 cm) in length and extends across the upper abdomen to the splenic flexure.

- Descending colon. This segment is usually less than 12 in (30 cm) long and extends from the splenic flexure downwards to the start of the pelvis.

- Sigmoid colon. An S-shaped segment that measures about 18 in (46 cm); it extends from the descending colon to the rectum.

The wall of the colon is composed of four layers:

- Mucosa. This single layer of cell lining is flat and regenerates itself every three to eight days. Small glands lie beneath the surface.

- Submucosa. The area between the mucosa and circular muscle layer that is separated from the mucosa by a thin layer of muscle, the muscularis mucosa.

- Muscularis propria. The inner circular and outer longitudinal muscle layers.

Bowel resection (Colectomy)

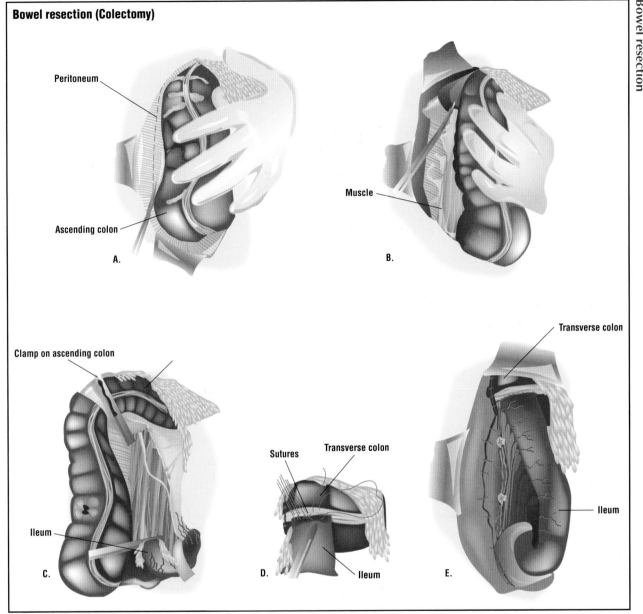

To remove a portion of the colon, or large intestine, and incision is made in the abdomen to expose the area **(A)**. Tissues and muscles connecting the colon to surrounding organs are severed **(B)**. The area to be removed is clamped and severed **(C)**. The remaining portions of the bowel, the ileum (small intestine) and transverse colon, are connected with sutures **(D)**. Muscles and tissues are repaired **(E)**. *(Illustration by GGS Information Services. Cengage Learning, Gale.)*

• Serosa. The thick outer layer that covers the bowel and is single celled. It is similar to the peritoneum, the layer of cells that lines the abdomen.

The large intestine is also responsible for bacterial production and absorption of vitamins. Resection of a portion of the large intestine (or of the entire organ) may become necessary when it becomes diseased. The exact reasons for large bowel resection in

any given patient may be complex and are always carefully evaluated by the treating physician or team. The procedure is usually performed to treat the following disorders or diseases of the large intestine:

• Cancer. Colon cancer is the second most common type of cancer diagnosed in the United States. Colon and rectum cancers, which are usually referred to as colorectal cancer, develop on the lining of the large intestine. Bowel resection may be indicated to remove the cancer.

- Diverticulitis. This condition is characterized by the inflammation of a diverticulum, especially of diverticula occurring in the colon, which may undergo perforation with abscess formation. The condition may be relieved by resecting the affected bowel section.

- Intestinal obstruction. This condition involves a partial or complete blockage of the bowel that results in the failure of the intestinal contents to pass through. It is usually treated by decompressing the intestine with suction, using a nasogastric tube inserted into the stomach or intestine. In cases where decompression does not relieve the symptoms, or if tissue death is suspected, bowel resection may be considered.

- Ulcerative colitis. This condition is characterized by chronic inflammation of the large intestine and rectum resulting in bloody diarrhea. Surgery may be indicated when medical therapy does not improve the condition. Removal of the colon is curative and also removes the risk of colon cancer. About 25–40% of ulcerative colitis patients must eventually have their colons removed because of massive bleeding, severe illness, rupture of the colon, or risk of cancer.

- Traumatic injuries. Accidents may result in bowel injuries that require resection.

- Pre-cancerous polyps. A colorectal polyp is a growth that projects from the lining of the colon. Polyps of the colon are usually benign and produce no symptoms, but they may cause rectal bleeding and develop into malignancies over time. When polyps have a high chance of becoming cancerous, bowel resection may be indicated.

- Familial adenomatous polyposis (FAP). This is a hereditary condition caused by a faulty gene. Most people discover that they have it at a young age. People with FAP grow many polyps in the bowel. These are mostly benign, but because there are so many, it is really only a question of time before one becomes cancerous. Since people with FAP have a very high risk of developing bowel cancer, bowel resection is thus often indicated.

- Hirschsprung's disease (HD). This condition usually occurs in children. It causes constipation, meaning that bowel movements are difficult. Some children with HD cannot have bowel movements at all; the stool creates a blockage in the intestine. If HD is not treated, stool can fill up the large intestine and cause

serious problems such as infection, bursting of the colon, and even death.

Description

Bowel resection can be performed using an open surgical approach (colectomy) or laparoscopically.

Colectomy

Following adequate bowel preparation, the patient is placed under **general anesthesia**, which ensures that the patient is deep asleep and pain free during surgery. Because the effects of gravity to displace tissues and organs away from the site of operation are important, patients are carefully positioned, padded, and strapped to the operating table to prevent movement as the patient is tilted to an extreme degree. The surgeon starts the procedure by making a lower midline incision in the abdomen or, alternatively, it may be preferable to perform a lateral lower transverse incision instead. The operation proceeds with the removal of the diseased portion of the large intestine, and then the two healthy ends are sutured or stapled back together before closing the incision. The amount of bowel removed can vary considerably, depending on the reasons for the operation. When possible, the procedure is performed to maintain the continuity of the bowel so as to preserve normal passage of stool.

If the bowel has to be relieved of its normal digestive work while it heals, a temporary opening of the colon onto the skin of abdominal wall, called a **colostomy**, may be created. In this procedure, the end of the colon is passed through the abdominal wall and the edges are sutured to the skin. A removable bag is attached around the colostomy site so that stool may pass into the bag, which can be emptied several times during the day. Most colostomies are temporary and can be closed with another operation at a later date. However, if a large portion of the intestine is removed, or if the distal end of the colon is too diseased to reconnect to the proximal intestine, the colostomy is permanent.

Laparoscopic bowel resection

The benefits of laparoscopic bowel resection when compared to open colectomies include reduced post-operative pain, shorter hospitalization periods, and a faster return to normal activities. The procedure is also minimally invasive. When performing a laparoscopic procedure, the surgeon makes three or four small incisions in the abdomen or in the umbilicus (belly button). He inserts specialized **surgical instruments**, including a thin, telescope-like instrument called a laparoscope, in an incision. The abdomen is then filled with gas, usually carbon dioxide, to help the surgeon view the abdominal cavity. A camera is inserted through one of the tubes and displays images on a monitor located near the operating table to guide the surgeon during the procedure. Once an adequate view of the operative field is obtained, the actual dissection of the colon can start. Following the procedure, the small incisions are closed with sutures or surgical tape.

All colon surgery involves only three maneuvers that may vary in complexity depending on the region of the bowel and the nature of the disease. The three maneuvers are retraction of the colon, division of the attachments to the colon, and dissection of the mesentery.

In a typical procedure, after retracting the colon, the surgeon proceeds to divide the attachments to the liver and the small bowel. Once the mesenteric vessels have been dissected and divided, the colon is divided with special stapling devices that close off the bowel while at the same time cutting between the staple lines. Alternatively, a laparoscopically assisted procedure may be selected, in which a small abdominal wall incision is made at this point to bring the bowel outside of the abdomen, allowing open bowel resection and reconnection using standard instruments. This technique is popular with many surgeons because an incision must be made to remove the bowel specimen from the abdomen, which allows the most time-consuming and risky parts of the procedure (from an infection point of view) to be done outside the body with better control of the colon.

Diagnosis/Preparation

Key elements of the **physical examination** before surgery focus on a thorough examination of the abdomen, groin, and rectum. Other common diagnostic tools used to evaluate medical conditions that may require bowel resection include imaging tests such as gastrointestinal barium series, **angiography**, computerized tomography (CT), **magnetic resonance imaging** (MRI), and endoscopy.

As with any surgery, the patient is required to sign a consent form. Details of the procedure are discussed with the patient, including goals, technique, and risks. Blood and urine tests, along with various imaging tests and an **electrocardiogram** (EKG), may be ordered. To prepare for the procedure, the patient is asked to completely clean out the bowel. This is a crucial step if the bowel is to be opened safely within the peritoneal cavity, or even manipulated safely through small incisions. To empty and cleanse the bowel, the patient is usually placed on a low-residue diet for several days prior to surgery. A liquid diet may be ordered for at least the day before surgery, with nothing taken by mouth after midnight. A series of enemas and/or oral preparations (Golytely or Colyte) may be ordered to empty the bowel of stool. Preoperative bowel preparation involving mechanical cleansing and administration of intravenous **antibiotics** immediately before surgery is the standard practice.

The patient may also be given a prescription for oral antibiotics (neomycin, erythromycin, or kanamycin sulfate) the day before surgery to decrease bacteria in the intestine and to help prevent postoperative infection. A nasogastric tube is inserted through the nose into the stomach during surgery and may be left in place for 24–48 hours after surgery. This removes the gastric secretions and prevents nausea and vomiting. A urinary catheter (a thin tube) may be inserted to keep the bladder empty during surgery, giving more space in the surgical field and decreasing chances of accidental injury.

Aftercare

Postoperative care for the patient involves monitoring blood pressure, pulse, respiration, and temperature. Breathing tends to be shallow because of the effect of anesthesia and the patient's reluctance to breathe deeply and experience pain that is caused by the abdominal incision. The patient is instructed how to support the operative site during deep breathing and coughing, and is given pain medication as necessary. Fluid intake and output is measured, and the operative site is observed for color and amount of wound drainage. The nasogastric tube will remain in place, attached to low intermittent suction until bowel activity resumes. Fluids and electrolytes are infused intravenously until the patient's diet can gradually be resumed, beginning with liquids and advancing to a regular diet as tolerated. The patient is generally out of bed approximately eight to 24 hours after surgery. Most patients will stay in the hospital for five to seven days, although laparoscopic surgery can reduce that stay to two to three days. Postoperative weight loss follows almost all bowel resections. Weight and strength are slowly regained over the next few months. Complete recovery from surgery may take two months. Laparoscopic surgery can reduce this time to one to two weeks.

The treating physician should be informed of any of the following problems after surgery:

• increased pain, swelling, redness, drainage, or bleeding in the surgical area

• headache, muscle aches, dizziness, or fever

• increased abdominal pain or swelling; constipation; nausea or vomiting; rectal bleeding; or black, tarry stools

Risks

Potential complications of bowel resection surgery include:

• excessive bleeding

• surgical wound infection

• incisional hernia (an organ projecting through the surrounding muscle wall; it occurs through the surgical scar)

• thrombophlebitis (inflammation and blood clot to veins in the legs)

• narrowing of the opening (stoma)

• pneumonia

• pulmonary embolism (blood clot or air bubble in the lung blood supply)

• reaction to medication

• breathing problems

• obstruction of the intestine from scar tissue

Normal results

Complete healing is expected without complications after bowel resection, but the period of time required for recovery from the surgery varies

QUESTIONS TO ASK THE DOCTOR

- What alternatives to bowel resection might be indicated in my case?
- Am I a candidate for bowel resection?
- How many patients with my specific condition have you treated?
- How long will it take to recover from surgery?
- What do I need to do before surgery?
- What happens on the day of surgery?
- What type of anesthesia will be used?
- What happens during surgery, and how is the surgery performed?

depending on the initial condition that required the procedure, the patient's overall health status prior to surgery, and the length of bowel removed.

Morbidity and mortality rates

Prognosis for bowel resection depends on the seriousness of the disease. For example, primary treatment for colorectal cancer consists of wide surgical resection of the colon cancer and lymphatic drainage after the bowel is prepared. The choice of operation for rectal cancer depends on the tumor's distance from the anus and gross extent; overall surgical cure is possible in 70% of these patients. In the case of ulcerative colitis patients, the colitis is cured by bowel resection and most people go on to live normal, active lives. As for Hirschsprung's disease patients, approximately 70–85% eventually achieve excellent results after surgery, with normal bowel habits and infrequent constipation.

Alternatives

Alternatives to bowel resection depend on the specific medical condition being treated. For most conditions where bowel resection is advised, the only alternative is medical treatment with drugs. In cases of cancer of the bowel, drug treatment alone will not cure the disease. Occasionally, it is possible to remove a rectal cancer from within the back passage without major surgery, but this only applies to very special cases. As for other conditions such as mild or moderate ulcerative colitis, drug therapy may represent an alternative to surgery; a combination of the drugs sulfonamide, sulfapyridine, and salicylate may help control inflammation. Similarly, most acute cases of

diverticulitis are first treated with antibiotics and a liquid diet.

Resources

BOOKS

Abeloff, M. D., et al. *Clinical Oncology.* 3rd ed. Philadelphia: Elsevier, 2004.

Feldman, M., et al. *Sleisenger & Fordtran's Gastrointestinal and Liver Disease.* 8th ed. St. Louis: Mosby, 2005.

Khatri, V. P., and J. A. Asensio. *Operative Surgery Manual.* 1st ed. Philadelphia: Saunders, 2003.

Townsend, C. M., et al. *Sabiston Textbook of Surgery.* 17th ed. Philadelphia: Saunders, 2004.

PERIODICALS

Alves, A., Y. Panis, D. Trancart, J. Regimbeau, M. Pocard, and P. Valleur. "Factors Associated with Clinically Significant Anastomotic Leakage after Large Bowel Resection: Multivariate Analysis of 707 Patients." *World Journal of Surgery* 26 (April 2002): 499–502.

Miller, J., and A. Proietto. "The Place of Bowel Resection in Initial Debulking Surgery for Advanced Ovarian Cancer." *Australian and New Zealand Journal of Obstetrics and Gynaecology* 42 (November 2002): 535–537.

Sukhotnik, I., A. S. Gork, M. Chen, R. Drongowski, A. G. Coran, and C. M. Harmon. "Effect of Low Fat Diet on Lipid Absorption and Fatty-acid Transport following Bowel Resection." *Pediatric Surgery International* 17 (May 2001): 259–264.

Tabet, J., D. Hong, C. W. Kim, J. Wong, R. Goodacre, and M. Anvari. "Laparoscopic versus Open Bowel Resection for Crohn's Disease." *Canadian Journal of Gastroenterology* 15 (April 2001): 237–242.

ORGANIZATIONS

American Board of Colorectal Surgeons (ABCRS). 20600 Eureka Rd., Ste. 600, Taylor, MI 48180. (734) 282-9400. http://www.abcrs.org (accessed March 7, 2008).

American Society of Colorectal Surgeons ASCRS). 85 West Algonquin, Suite 550, Arlington Heights, IL 60005. (847) 290 9184. http://www.fascrs.org (accessed March 7, 2008).

United Ostomy Association, Inc. (UOA). 19772 MacArthur Blvd., Suite 200, Irvine, CA 92612-2405. (800) 826-0826. http://www.uoa.org (accessed March 7, 2008).

OTHER

"Bowel Resection." *Patient & Family Education/NYU Medical Center.*http://www.nmh.org/nmh/pdf/pated/bowelresec-discharge07.pdf (accessed March 7, 2008).

*Health Care Corporation of St. John's.*http://www.hccsj.nf.ca (accessed March 7, 2008).

Kathleen D. Wright, RN
Monique Laberge, PhD
Rosalyn Carson-DeWitt, MD

Bowel resection, small intestine

Definition

A small **bowel resection** is the surgical removal of one or more segments of the small intestine.

Purpose

The small intestine is the part of the digestive system that absorbs much of the liquid and nutrients from food. It consists of three segments: the duodenum, jejunum, and ileum. It is followed by the large intestine (colon). A small bowel resection may be performed to treat the following conditions:

- Crohn's disease. This condition is characterized by a chronic inflammatory condition that affects the digestive tract. If other treatment does not effectively control symptoms, the physician may recommend surgery to close fistulas or remove part of the intestine where the inflammation is worst.
- Cancer. Cancer of the small intestine is a rare cancer in which malignant cells are found in the tissues of the small intestine. Adenocarcinoma, lymphoma, sarcoma, and carcinoid tumors account for the majority of small intestine cancers. Surgery to remove the cancer is the most common treatment. When the tumor is large, removal of the small intestine segment containing the cancer is usually indicated.
- Ulcers. Ulcers are crater-like lesions on the mucous membrane of the small bowel caused by an inflammatory, infectious, or malignant condition that often requires surgery and in some cases, bowel resection.
- Intestinal obstruction. This condition involves a partial or complete blockage of the bowel that results in the failure of the intestinal contents to pass through. Intestinal obstruction is usually treated by decompressing the intestine with suction, using a nasogastric tube inserted into the stomach or intestine. In cases where decompression does not relieve the symptoms, or if tissue death is suspected, bowel resection may be considered.
- Injuries. Accidents may result in bowel injuries that require resection.
- Precancerous polyps. A polyp is a growth that projects from the lining of the intestine. Polyps are usually benign and produce no symptoms, but they may cause rectal bleeding and develop into malignancies over time. When polyps have a high chance of becoming cancerous, bowel resection is usually indicated.

Demographics

According to the National Cancer Institute, adenocarcinoma, lymphoma, sarcoma, and carcinoid tumors account for the majority of small intestine cancers which, as a whole, account for only 1–2% of all gastrointestinal cancers diagnosed in the United States. About 6,110 new cases of small intestine cancer are diagnosed yearly; about 1,110 deaths occur from small intestine cancer annually.

Crohn's disease occurs worldwide with a prevalence of 10–100 cases per 100,000 people. The disorder occurs most frequently among people of European origin, is three to eight times more common among Jews than among non-Jews, and is more common among whites than nonwhites. Although the disorder can start at any age, it is most often diagnosed between 15 and 30 years of age. Some 20–30% of patients with Crohn's disease have a family history of inflammatory bowel disease.

The occurrence of polyps increases with age. The risk of cancer developing in an unremoved polyp is 2.5% at five years, 8% at 10 years, and 24% at 20 years after the diagnosis. The risk of developing bowel cancer after removal of polyps is 2.3%, compared to 8.0% for patients who do not have them removed.

Description

The resection procedure can be performed using an open surgical approach or laparoscopically. There are three types of surgical small bowel resection procedures:

- Duodenectomy. Excision of all or part of the duodenum.
- Ileectomy. Excision of all or part of the ileum.
- Jejunectomy. Excision of all or a part of the jejunum.

Open resection

Following adequate **bowel preparation**, the patient is placed under general anesthesia and positioned for the operation. The surgeon starts the procedure by making a midline incision in the abdomen. The diseased part of the small intestine (ileum or duodenum or jejunum) is removed. The two healthy ends are either stapled or sewn back together, and the incision is closed. If it is necessary to spare the intestine from its normal digestive work while it heals, a temporary opening (stoma) of the intestine into the abdomen (ileostomy, duodenostomy, or jejunostomy) is made. The ostomy can be closed and repaired at a later time.

Small bowel resection

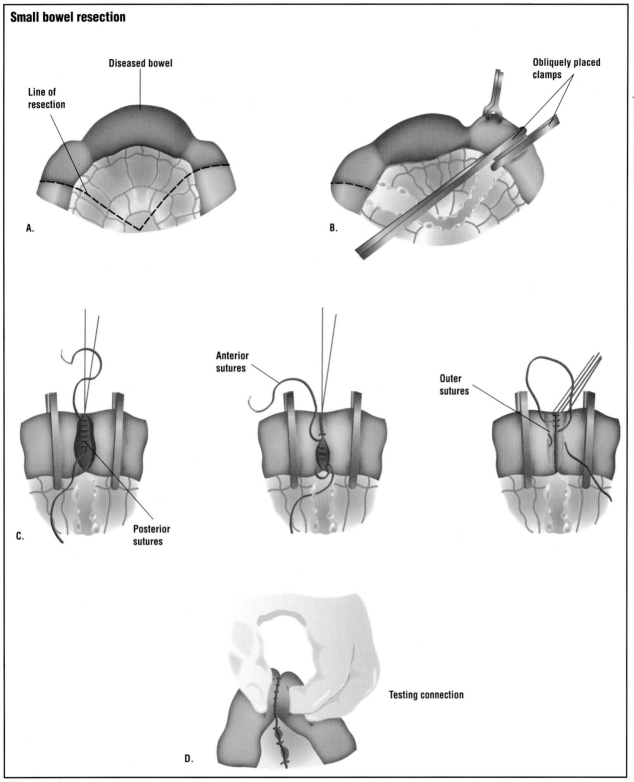

A.

Line of resection

Diseased bowel

Obliquely placed clamps

B.

C.

Posterior sutures

Anterior sutures

Outer sutures

D.

Testing connection

To remove a diseased portion of the small intestine, an incision is made into the abdomen, and the area to be treated is pulled out (A). Clamps are placed around the area to be removed and the section is cut (B). Three layers of sutures repair the remaining bowel (C). *(Illustration by GGS Information Services. Cengage Learning, Gale.)*

KEY TERMS

Adenocarcinoma—Adenocarcinoma starts in the lining of the small intestine and is the most common type of cancer of the small intestine. These tumors occur most often in the part of the small intestine nearest the stomach and often grow and block the bowel.

Anesthesia—A combination of drugs administered by a variety of techniques by trained professionals that provide sedation, amnesia, analgesia, and immobility adequate for the accomplishment of the surgical procedure with minimal discomfort and without injury to the patient.

Cancer—The uncontrolled growth of abnormal cells which have mutated from normal tissues.

Colon—Also called the large intestine, the colon has six major segments: caecum, ascending colon, transverse colon, descending colon, sigmoid colon, and rectum. Its length is approximately 5 ft (1.5 m) in the adult and it is responsible for forming, storing, and expelling waste matter.

Crohn's disease—Chronic inflammatory process, primarily involving the intestinal tract, that most commonly affects the last part of the small intestine (ileum) and/or the large intestine (colon and rectum).

Duodenectomy—Excision of the duodenum.

Ileectomy—Excision of the ileum.

Jejunectomy—Excision of all or a part of the jejunum.

Leiomyosarcoma—Leiomyosarcomas are cancers that start growing in the smooth muscle lining of the small intestine.

Lymphoma—A lymphoma starts from lymph tissue in the small intestine. Lymph tissue is part of the body's immune system, which helps the body fight infections. Most of these tumors are a type of lymphoma called non-Hodgkin's lymphomas.

Ostomy—An operation to create an opening from an area inside the body to the outside.

Polyp—Growth, usually benign, protruding from a mucous membrane, such as that lining the walls of the intestines.

Resection—Removal of a portion or all of an organ or other structure.

Small intestine—The small intestine consists of three sections: duodenum, jejunum and ileum, all of which are involved in the absorption of nutrients. The total length of the small intestine is approximately 22 ft (6.5 m).

Laparoscopic bowel resection

Laparoscopic small bowel resection features insertion of a thin, telescope-like instrument called a laparoscope through a small incision made at the umbilicus (belly button). The laparoscope is connected to a small video camera unit that shows the operative site on video monitors located in the operating room. The abdomen is inflated with carbon dioxide gas to allow the surgeon a clear view of the operative area. Four to five additional small incisions are made in the abdomen for insertion of specialized surgical instruments that the surgeon uses to perform the surgery. The small bowel is clamped above and below the diseased section and this section is removed. The small bowel ends are reattached using staples or sutures. Following the procedure, the small incisions are closed with sutures or surgical tape.

Diagnosis/Preparation

As with any surgery, the patient is required to sign a consent form. Details of the procedure are discussed with the patient, including goals, technique, and risks. Blood and urine tests, along with various imaging tests and an electrocardiogram (EKG), may be ordered as required. To prepare for the procedure, the patient is asked to completely clean the bowel and is placed on a low residue diet for several days prior to surgery. A liquid diet may be ordered for at least the day before surgery, with nothing taken by mouth after midnight. Preoperative bowel preparation involving mechanical cleansing and administration of antibiotics before surgery is the standard practice. This involves the prescription of oral antibiotics (neomycin, erythromycin, or kanamycin sulfate) to decrease bacteria in the intestine and help prevent postoperative infection. A nasogastric tube is inserted through the nose into the stomach on the day of surgery or during surgery. This removes the gastric secretions and prevents nausea and vomiting. A urinary catheter (thin tube inserted into the bladder) may also be inserted to keep the bladder empty during surgery, giving more space in the surgical field and decreasing chances of accidental injury.

Aftercare

Once the surgery is completed, the patient is taken to a postoperative or recovery unit where a nurse monitors recovery and ensures that bandages are kept clean and dry. Mild pain at the incision site is commonly experienced and the treating physician usually prescribes pain medication. Postoperative care also involves monitoring of blood pressure, pulse, respiration, and temperature. Breathing tends to be shallow because of the effect of anesthesia and the patient's reluctance to breathe deeply and experience pain that is caused by the abdominal incision. The patient is given instruction on the way to support the operative site during deep breathing and coughing. Fluid intake and output is measured, and the operative site is observed for color and amount of wound drainage. The nasogastric tube remains in place, attached to low intermittent suction until bowel activity resumes. Fluids and electrolytes are infused intravenously until the patient's diet can gradually be resumed, beginning with liquids and progressing to a regular diet as tolerated. The patient is generally out of bed approximately eight to 24 hours after surgery. Patients are usually scheduled for a follow-up examination within two weeks after surgery. During the first few days after surgery, physical activity is restricted.

Risks

Risks include all the risks associated with general anesthesia, namely, adverse reactions to medications and breathing problems. They also include the risks

associated with any surgery, such as bleeding or infection. Additional risks associated specifically with bowel resection include:

- bulging through the incision (incisional hernia)
- narrowing (stricture) of the opening (stoma)
- blockage (obstruction) of the intestine from scar tissue

Normal results

Complete healing is expected without complications after bowel resection, but the period of time required for recovery from the surgery varies depending on the condition requiring the procedure, the patient's overall health status prior to surgery, and the length of bowel removed.

Morbidity and mortality rates

According to the National Cancer Institute, the predominant treatment for small intestine cancers is surgery when bowel resection is possible, and cure depends on the ability to completely remove the cancer. The overall five-year survival rate for resectable adenocarcinoma is 20%. The five-year survival rate for resectable leiomyosarcoma, the most common primary sarcoma of the small intestine, is approximately 50%.

Crohn's disease is a chronic incurable disease characterized by periods of progression and remission with 99% of patients suffering at least one relapse. Physicians are presently unable to predict the extent and severity of the disease over time; thus, while morbidity is very high for Crohn's disease, mortality is essentially zero.

Alternatives

Alternatives to bowel resection depend on the specific medical condition being treated. For most conditions where bowel resection is advised, the only alternative is treatment with drugs.

Resources

BOOKS

Ratnaike, R. N., ed. *Small Bowel Disorders*. London: Edward Arnold, 2000.

PERIODICALS

Bines, J. E., R. G. Taylor, F. Justice, et al. "Influence of Diet Complexity on Intestinal Adaptation Following Massive Small Bowel Resection in a Preclinical Model." *Journal of Gastroenterology and Hepatology* 17 (November 2002): 1170–1179.

Dahly, E. M., M. B. Gillingham, Z. Guo, et al. "Role of Luminal Nutrients and Endogenous GLP-2 in Intestinal Adaptation to Mid-Small Bowel Resection." *American Journal of Physiology and Gastrointestinal Liver Physiology* 284 (March 2003): G670–G682.

Libsch, K. D., N. J. Zyromski, T. Tanaka, et al. "Role of Extrinsic Innervation in Jejunal Absorptive Adaptation to Subtotal Small Bowel Resection: A Model of Segmental Small Bowel Transplantation." *Journal of Gastrointestinal Surgery* 6 (March-April 2002): 240–247.

O'Brien, D. P., L. A. Nelson, J. L. Williams, et al. "Selective Inhibition of the Epidermal Growth Factor Receptor Impairs Intestinal Adaptation After Small Bowel Resection." *Journal of Surgical Research* 105 (June 2002): 25–30.

ORGANIZATIONS

American Board of Colorectal Surgeons (ABCRS). 20600 Eureka Rd., Ste. 600, Taylor, MI 48180. (734) 282-9400. www.abcrs.org.

American Society of Colorectal Surgeons (ASCRS). 85 West Algonquin, Suite 550, Arlington Heights, IL 60005. (847) 290 9184. www.fascrs.org.

United Ostomy Association, Inc. (UOA). 19772 MacArthur Blvd., Suite 200, Irvine, CA 92612-2405. (800) 826-0826. www.uoa.org.

OTHER

"Bowel Resection." Northwest Memorial Hospital. November 19, 2002. http://www.nmh.org/nmh/adam/adamencyclopedia/HIEArticles/002941.htm [accessed May 1, 2008].

Monique Laberge, Ph.D.
Rosalyn Carson-DeWitt, M.D.

Bowel surgery with ostomy *see* **Colostomy**

Brain surgery *see* **Craniotomy**

Breast augmentation *see* **Breast implants**

Breast biopsy

Definition

A breast biopsy is the removal of breast tissue for examination by a pathologist. This can be accomplished surgically or by extracting tissue through a needle.

Purpose

Breast biopsies are done to diagnose breast abnormalities. A biopsy is recommended when a significant abnormality is found by **physical examination** or an imaging test. Examples of an abnormality can include a breast lump felt during breast self-examination or tissue changes noticed from a mammogram.

Before a biopsy is performed, other simpler, less invasive tests may be done to rule out cancer. For example, a lump may be revealed simply as a fluid-filled cyst when examined by **ultrasound** imaging. If less invasive tests are not conclusive, the presence of a malignant (cancerous) or benign (noncancerous) breast condition can be definitively determined by a biopsy.

Demographics

The American Cancer Society estimated that in 2007, 78,480 new cases of invasive breast cancer and 62,030 new cases of breast carcinoma in situ (CIS) were diagnosed in the United States. CIS is the earliest, noninvasive form of breast cancer. Approximately one of every eight women will develop breast cancer at some point in her life. Since 1990, breast cancer rates have decreased among women under age 50; however, breast cancer still causes the **death** of one of every 35 women.

In 2007, the incidence of breast cancer was highest among Caucasian women, but African American women had more aggressive tumors and were more likely to die from the disease. Hispanic, Native American, and Asian women have lower breast cancer and breast cancer death rates than Caucasians or African Americans.

Description

In a biopsy, cells are removed from the breast and examined under the microscope to determine if they are malignant or benign. The type of biopsy recommended depends on whether the abnormality is large enough to be felt, how well it can be seen on mammogram or ultrasound, and how suspicious it feels or appears. Specialized equipment is needed for different types of biopsy, and its availability may vary.

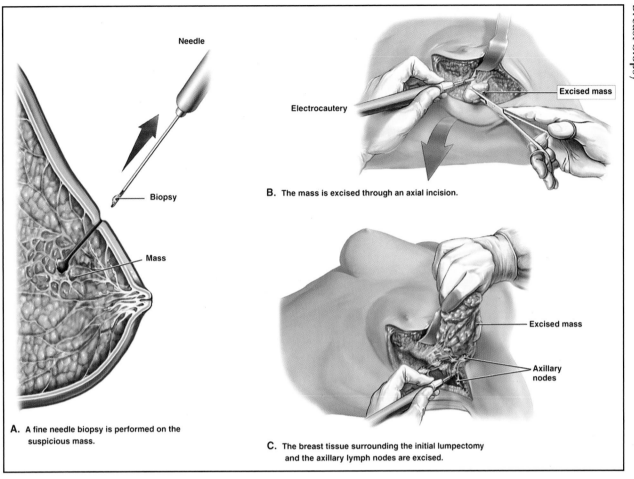

A. A fine needle biopsy is performed on the suspicious mass.

B. The mass is excised through an axial incision.

C. The breast tissue surrounding the initial lumpectomy and the axillary lymph nodes are excised.

(Nucleus Medical Art / Alamy)

Surgical biopsy

There are two types of surgical breast biopsy: excisional and incisional. An excisional biopsy is a surgical procedure that removes the entire area of concern and some surrounding tissue. It is usually done as an outpatient procedure in a hospital or free-standing surgery center. The patient may be awake, but is usually given medication to make her drowsy. The area to be operated on is numbed with a local anesthetic. Infrequently, **general anesthesia** is used. An excisional biopsy usually takes under one hour to perform. Nevertheless, the total amount of time spent at the facility depends on the type of anesthesia used, whether a needle localization was done, and the extent of the surgery.

If a mass is very large, an incisional biopsy may be performed. In this case, only a portion of the area of concern is removed and sent for analysis. The procedure is the same as an excisional biopsy in other respects.

Needle biopsies

A needle biopsy removes a sample of fluid and cells from suspicious area for examination. There are two main types or needle biopsies: aspiration biopsy, using a fine-gauge needle, and large-core needle biopsy. Either of these may be called a percutaneous needle biopsy. Percutaneous refers to a procedure done through the skin.

A fine-needle aspiration biopsy (FNAB) uses a very thin needle to withdraw (aspirate) fluid and cells that are then examined under the microscope for abnormalities. A FNAB can be done in a doctor's office, clinic, or hospital. Local anesthetic may be used, but is sometimes not needed as its administration may be more painful than the insertion of the very thin biopsy needle. Sometimes, the area to place the needle may be located by touch without using specialized equipment. However, ultrasound guidance enables the physician to feel and see the lesion at the same

Core needle biopsy (CNB)—A procedure using a larger diameter needle to remove a core of tissue from the breast.

Ductogram—A test used for imaging the breast ducts and diagnosing the cause of abnormal nipple discharges.

Fine-needle aspiration biopsy (FNAB)—A procedure using a thin needle to remove fluid and cells from a lump in the breast.

Mammogram—A set of x rays taken of the front and side of the breast used to help diagnose various breast abnormalities.

time. This helps ensure that the specimen is taken from the area of concern. The patient lies on her back or side. After the area is numbed, sterile gel is applied. The physician places a transducer, an instrument about the size of an electric shaver, over the skin. This produces an image from the reflection of sound waves. A special needle, usually in a spring-loaded device, is used to obtain the tissue. The actual withdrawal of fluid and cells can be visualized as it occurs.

A core needle biopsy (CNB) uses a larger diameter needle to remove small pieces of tissue. These are usually about the size of a grain of rice, although the needle diameter may vary based on the size and location of the suspicious mass. CNBs can be done in a clinic or hospital. Local anesthetic is routinely used. Ultrasound or x ray is used to guide the placement of the needle in a core needle biopsy. When larger cores are removed, a vacuum pump may be used to help withdraw the tissue.

If the suspicious area is seen best with x ray, a stereotactic device is used to guide the biopsy. X rays are taken from several angles. The information is fed into a computer that analyzes the data and guides the needle to the correct place. The patient may be sitting up, or she may be lying on her stomach, with her breast positioned through an opening in the table. The breast is held firmly but comfortably between a plastic paddle and a metal plate, similar to those used for mammograms. X rays may be taken before, during, and after the tissue is drawn into the needle to confirm that the correct spot is biopsied. This procedure is called a stereotactic core biopsy, or a mammotomy.

A pathologist examines the sample tissue for malignant cells, indicating the presence of cancer. If a fine-needle aspiration biopsy is performed, the pathologist looks at individual cells under the microscope to see if they appear abnormal. CNBs and surgical biopsy often provide more information than FNABs and are able to give more information on the type of cancer, whether it has invaded surrounding tissue, and how likely it is to spread quickly. The biopsy can also reveal some conditions that are not malignant but indicate high risk for future development of breast cancer. If these are identified, more frequent breast monitoring is recommended.

Diagnosis/Preparation

Sometimes an abnormality can be felt during a breast self-examination or an examination by a health-care professional. If an abnormality is not felt, there are other signs that indicate the need for medical attention. These include:

- severe breast pain
- changes in the size of a breast or nipple
- changes in the shape of both breast and nipple
- pitting, dimpling, or redness of the breast skin
- nipple redness, irritation, or inversion
- changes in the pattern of veins visible on the surface of the breast
- some types of nipple discharge

If the abnormality cannot be located easily, a wire localization may be done before the actual biopsy. After local anesthetic is administered, a fine wire is placed in the area of concern. Either x ray or ultrasound guidance is used to place the wire, and then the biopsy needle can follow the wire to the area of concern. The patient is awake and usually sitting up during this procedure.

A surgical breast biopsy may require that patient have nothing to eat or drink for some time before the operation. This will typically be from midnight the night before the procedure, if general anesthesia is planned. No food restrictions are necessary for needle biopsies, although it is advisable to eat lightly before the procedure. This is especially important if the patient will be lying on her stomach for a stereotactic biopsy.

Aftercare

After a surgical biopsy, the incision is closed with sutures and covered with a bandage. The bandage is usually removed within two days. Sutures are removed about one week later. Depending on the extent of the operation, normal activities can be resumed in one to three days. Vigorous **exercise** may be limited for one to three weeks.

The skin opening for a needle biopsy is minimal. It may be closed with thin, clear tape or covered with a small bandage. The patient can return to her usual routine immediately after the biopsy. Strenuous activity or heavy lifting should be avoided for 24 hours. Any **bandages** can be removed one or two days after the biopsy.

Risks

Infection is always a possibility when the skin is broken, although this rarely occurs in breast biopsies. Redness, swelling, or severe pain at the biopsy site indicates a possible infection and a reason for concern. Another possible consequence of a breast biopsy is a hematoma, which is a collection of blood at the biopsy site. The body usually resorbs this blood naturally without treatment. If the hematoma is very large and uncomfortable, it may need to be drained. A surgical breast biopsy may produce a visible scar on the breast. Scarring may make future mammograms harder to interpret accurately.

A false negative pathology report is another risk. In a false negative report, no cancer is found when cancer is actually present. The incidence of false negative biopsy findings varies with the biopsy technique. In general, fine-needle aspiration biopsies have the highest rate of false negative results. Different facilities also have varying rates of false negative readings, depending somewhat on the experience of their pathologist.

Normal results

A normal pathology report indicates no malignancy is present. The tissue sample may be classified

as a benign breast condition. Many women develop nonmalignant tumors of the breast (fibroadenoma) or harmless fluid-filled cysts. Some noncancerous conditions are more likely to develop into cancer. Women with these benign conditions should have more frequent breast health check-ups. Some studies have found that about 80% of all breast biopsies result in a negative (noncancer) pathology report.

Morbidity and mortality rates

The reported rate of complications for image-guided biopsies is approximately 2%. Excessive bleeding occurs after approximately 0.5% of fine needle biopsies, 3% of small needle biopsies, and 5–10% of large needle biopsies. Infection occurs in approximately 1% of biopsy sites. Organ damage such as a collapsed lung (pneumothorax) occurs in approximately 0.5% of biopsies. The rate of complications varies considerably among individual physicians and facilities.

Alternatives

While a biopsy is the only way to determine definitively if a breast abnormality is cancerous, other less invasive procedures may be done to try to rule out cancer so that a biopsy is not necessary. These include **mammography**, ultrasound imaging, and ductography (used for imaging the breast ducts and diagnosing the cause of abnormal nipple discharges).

Resources

ORGANIZATIONS

American Cancer Society. 1599 Clifton Rd., NE, Atlanta, GA 30329-4251. (800) 227-2345. http://www.cancer.org (accessed March 8, 2008).

National Cancer Institute. NCI Public Inquiries Office, 6116 Executive Boulevard Room 3036A, Bethesda, MD 20892-8322. (800) 422-6237. TTY: (800) 332-8615 http://www.nci.nih.gov (accessed march 8, 2008).

OTHER

Cardella, John F., et al. "Breast Biopsy." *MedicineNet*. April 11, 2002 [cited January 2, 2008]. http://www.medicinenet.com/breast_biopsy/article.htm.

"How is Breast Cancer Diagnosed?" *American Cancer Society*. September 13, 2007 [cited January 2, 2008]. http://www.cancer.org/docroot/CRI/content/CRI_2_4_3X_How_is_breast_cancer_diagnosed_5.asp.

"Lifetime Probability of Breast Cancer in American Women." *National Cancer Institute*. October 5, 2006 [cited January 2, 2008]. http://cis.nci.nih.gov/fact/5_6.htm.

Ellen S. Weber, MSN
Stephanie Dionne Sherk
Tish Davidson, AM

Breast implants

Definition

Breast implantation is a surgical procedure for enlarging, or augmenting, the breast. Implants are breast-shaped pouches that are saccular in shape, made of a silicone outer shell, and filled with silicone gel or saline (salt water).

Purpose

Breast implantation is usually performed to make normal breasts larger for cosmetic purposes. Sometimes a woman having **breast reconstruction** after a **mastectomy** will need the remaining breast enlarged to make the breasts more symmetrical. Breasts that are very unequal in size due to trauma or congenital deformity may also be equalized with an enlargement procedure.

Male-to-female transsexuals may use breast implantation to achieve the physical appearance of a female.

Demographics

Breast enlargement is the second-most-common cosmetic surgical procedure practiced on women in the United States. It increased by approximately 350% between 1992 and 2006. According to the American Society of Plastic and Reconstructive Surgeons, almost 150,000 breast augmentation procedures are performed each year.

Presently, more than two million, or approximately 8%, of women in the United States have breast implants. The majority of breast implant recipients are Caucasian women (95%), followed by African-American women (4%). The remaining women that have breast implants are Asian (0.5%) and other non-specified races (0.5%).

KEY TERMS

Breast augmentation—A surgery to increase the size of the breasts.

Contracture—Tissue change that is characterized by shortening of length, usually producing wrinkles or areas of thickening.

Transsexual—Person desiring to acquire the external appearance of a member of the opposite gender.

Description

Cosmetic breast enlargement or augmentation is usually performed as an outpatient procedure. It may be done under local or **general anesthesia**, depending on patient and physician preference. The incision is typically made through the armpit (axilla), along the fold line under the breast, or around the areola (the darkened area around the nipple); these techniques create the most inconspicuous scars. The implant is placed in one of two locations: between the breast tissue and underlying chest muscle, or under the chest muscle. The operation takes approximately one to two hours. The cost of a cosmetic procedure is rarely covered by insurance; however, if enlargement is part of breast reconstruction after a mastectomy, health plans may pay for some or all of it. The surgeon's fee ranges from $3,500 to $5,000, and up. The procedure may also be called breast augmentation or augmentation mammoplasty.

Diagnosis/Preparation

The diagnosis for breast reconstruction is almost always visual. The underlying medical reasons include equalizing otherwise normal breasts that are markedly different in size, replacing all or part of breast tissue that has been removed during the course of cancer treatment, or replacing breast mass that has been lost due to injury. Underlying cosmetic reasons include personal preference for larger breasts among genetic females or the creation of breasts in male-to-female transsexuals.

Before any surgery is performed, the woman should have a clear understanding of what her new breasts will look like. She and her physician should agree about the desired final result. Many surgeons find it helpful to have the patient review before and after pictures of other patients, to clarify expectations. Computer modeling is often used to assess expected results.

A person who is in poor health or has a severe or chronic disease is not a good candidate for this procedure.

Aftercare

Many normal activities such as driving may be restricted for up to one week. Sutures are usually removed in seven to 10 days. Typically, a woman can resume all routines, including vigorous **exercise**, in about three weeks. The scars will be red for approximately one month, but will fade to their final appearance within one to two years.

Risks

Risks associated with this procedure are similar to those of any surgical procedure. These risks include bleeding, infection, reaction to anesthesia, or unexpected scarring. A breast enlargement may also result in decreased sensation in the breast or interference with breast-feeding. Implants can make it more difficult to read and interpret mammograms, possibly delaying breast cancer detection. Also, the implant itself can rupture and leak, or become displaced. A thick scar that normally forms around the implant, called a capsule, can become very hard. This is called capsular contracture, and may result in pain and possible altered appearance of the breast. The chances that these problems will occur increase with the age of the implant.

There has been intermittent publicity about possible health risks associated with breast implants. Most concerns have focused on silicone gel-filled implants that leaked or ruptured. In 1992, the U.S.

Food and Drug Administration (FDA) restricted the use of this type of implant and ordered further studies. The FDA lifted the ban on silicone implants in 2007 although saline-filled implants are still more commonly used for cosmetic breast surgery. Studies have shown no evidence of long-term health risks from intact silicone implants; however, research on possible links between these implants and autoimmune or connective tissue diseases is continuing.

Normal results

Breasts of expected size and appearance are the normal results of this surgery. Normal scar formation should be expected. With any silicone prosthesis, a capsule usually forms around it. In some instances, a mild form of capsular contraction ensues. Mild ridges that can be felt under the skin categorize this condition. The capsule contracts, which occurs occasionally, and can result in a hardening of the breast. There is no way to predict who will excessively scar.

Morbidity and mortality rates

In addition to scarring, other risks include infection, excessive bleeding, problems associated with anesthesia, rupturing of the implant, and leakage. There have been approximately 120,000 reports of ruptured silicone implants. Approximately 50,000 reports of breakage have been received for saline implants.

Deaths associated with breast augmentation are extremely rare. Most postsurgical mortality has been attributed to anesthesia errors or overdoses of pain medications.

Alternatives

Alternatives to breast implant surgery include using external breast forms that fit into brassiere cups or are attached to the skin of the chest. Creams that allege to increase breast size usually produce no noticeable results. The use of creams containing hormones can lead to long-term hormonal imbalance. Reputable experts do not generally recommend these preparations for breast enlargement.

Resources

BOOKS

Bruning, N. *Breast Implants: Everything You Need to Know,* 3rd ed. Alameda, CA: Hunter House, 2002.

Freund, R. M., and A. VanDyne. *Cosmetic Breast Surgery: A Complete Guide to Making the Right Decision—From A to Double D.* New York: Marlowe & Company, 2004.

Middleton, M. S., and M. P. McNamara, Jr. *Breast Implant Imaging.* Philadelphia: Lippincott Williams & Wilkins, 2002.

Spear, S. L., S. C. Willey, G. L. Robb, D. C. Hammond, and N. Y. Nahabedian. *Surgery of the Breast: Principles And Art,* 2nd ed. Philadelphia: Lippincott Williams & Wilkins, 2005.

PERIODICALS

Crerand, C. E., A. L. Infield, and D. B. Sarwer. "Psychological considerations in cosmetic breast augmentation." *Plastic Surgical Nursing* 27, no. 3 (July/September 2007): 146–154.

Gampper, T. J., H. Khoury, W. Gottlieb, and R. F. Morgan. "Silicone gel implants in breast augmentation and reconstruction." *Annals of Plastic Surgery* 59, no. 5 (November 2007): 581–590.

Holmich, L. R., V. B. Breiting, J. P. Fryzek, B. Brandt, M. S. Wolthers, K. Kjoller, J. K. McLaughlin, and S. Friis. "Long-Term Cosmetic Outcome After Breast Implantation." *Annals of Plastic Surgery* 59, no. 6 (December 2007): 597–604.

McLaughlin, J. K., L. Lipworth, D. K. Murphy, and P. S. Walker. "The safety of silicone gel-filled breast implants: a review of the epidemiologic evidence." *Annals of Plastic Surgery* 59, no. 5 (November 2007): 569–580.

OTHER

American Society of Cosmetic Breast Surgery. *Information about Breast Surgery.* 2007 [cited December 23, 2007]. http://www.ascbs.org/.

National Library of Medicine. *Breast Implants.* 2007 [cited December 23, 2007]. http://vsearch.nlm.nih.gov/vivisimo/cgi-bin/query-meta?v%3Aproject = medlineplus&query = breast + implant.

Public Broadcasting System. *Breast Implants on Trial.* 2007 [cited December 23, 2007]. http://www.pbs.org/wgbh/pages/frontline/implants/cron.html.

U.S. Food and Drug Administration. *Breast Implants.* 2007 [cited December 23, 2007]. http://google2.fda.gov/search?output = xml_no_dtd&lr = &proxystylesheet = FDA&client = FDA&site = FDA&getfields = *&q = breast + implant.

ORGANIZATIONS

American Board of Plastic Surgery, Seven Penn Center, Suite 400, 1635 Market Street, Philadelphia, PA, 19103-2204, (215) 587-9322, http://www.abplsurg.org.

American College of Surgeons, 633 North Saint Claire Street, Chicago, IL, 60611, (312) 202-5000, http://www.facs.org.

American Society for Aesthetic Plastic Surgery, 11081 Winners Circle, Los Alamitos, CA, 90720, (888) 272-7711, http://www.surgery.org/.

American Society of Plastic Surgeons, 444 E. Algonquin Rd., Arlington Heights, IL, 60005, (847) 228-9900, http://www.plasticsurgery.org.

L. Fleming Fallon, Jr., M.D., Dr.P.H.

Breast radiography *see* **Mammography**

Breast reconstruction

Definition

Breast reconstruction consists of a series of surgical procedures performed to recreate a breast. Reconstructions are commonly begun after portions of one or both breasts are removed as a treatment for breast cancer. A breast may have to be refashioned for other reasons such as trauma or to correct abnormalities that occur during breast development.

Purpose

Many experts consider reconstruction to be an integral component of the therapy for breast cancer. A naturally appearing breast offers a sense of wholeness and normalcy, which can aid in the psychological recovery from breast cancer. It eliminates the need for an external prosthesis (false breast), which many women find to be physically uncomfortable as well as inconvenient.

Demographics

Breast surgery, including reconstruction, is the second most commonly performed cosmetic surgical procedure practiced on women in the United States. According to the American Society of Plastic and Reconstructive Surgeons, more than 200,000 breast augmentation or reconstruction procedures are performed each year.

Presently, more than 2.1 million, or approximately 8%, of women in the United States have **breast implants**. The majority of breast implant recipients are

Breast reconstruction

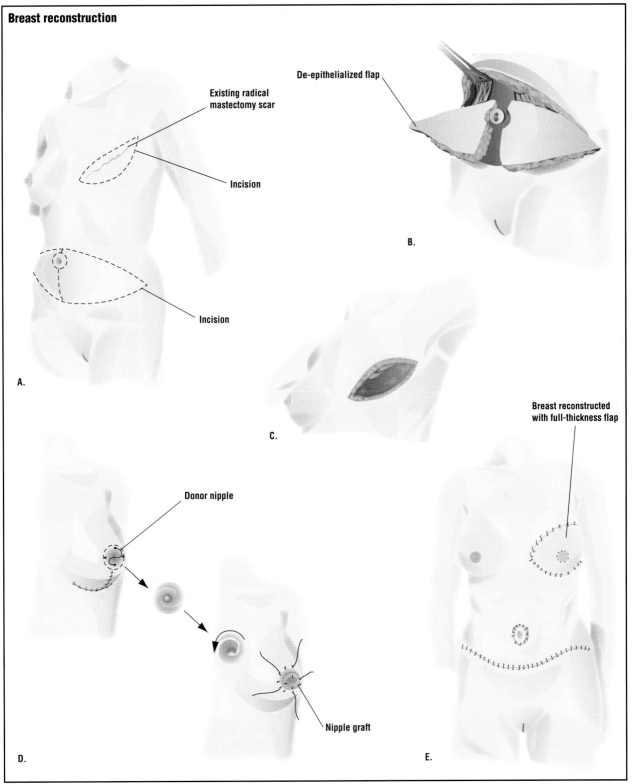

Existing radical mastectomy scar

Incision

Incision

A.

De-epithelialized flap

B.

C.

Donor nipple

Nipple graft

D.

Breast reconstructed with full-thickness flap

E.

Breast reconstruction is often performed after a mastectomy. In an autologous procedure, a section of tissue from the patient's abdomen (B) is used to create a natural-looking new breast. In a separate procedure, a layer of the patient's existing nipple can be grafted onto the new breast (D). *(Illustration by GGS Information Services. Cengage Learning, Gale.)*

KEY TERMS

Autologous—From the same person; an autologous breast reconstruction uses the woman's own tissues, while an autologous blood transfusion is blood removed then transfused back to the same person at a later time.

Capsular contracture—Thick scar tissue around a breast implant, which may tighten and cause discomfort and/or firmness.

Flap—A section of tissue moved from one area of the body to another.

Free flap—A section of tissue is detached from its blood supply, moved to another part of the body, and reattached by microsurgery to a new blood supply.

Mastectomy—Removal of all or a portion of breast tissue.

Mastopexy—Surgical procedure to lift up a breast; may be used on opposite breast to achieve symmetrical appearance with a reconstructed breast.

Pedicle flap—Also called an attached flap; a section of tissue, with its blood supply intact, which is maneuvered to another part of the body.

Caucasian women (95%), followed by African-American women (4%). The remaining women that have breast implants are Asian (0.5%) and other non-specified races (0.5%).

Description

Breast reconstruction is performed in two stages, with the ultimate goal of creating a breast that looks and feels as natural as possible. It is important to remember that while a good result may closely mimic a normal breast, there will inevitably be scars and some loss of sensation. The reconstructed breast cannot exactly match the original.

The first step is to create a structure called a breast mound. This can be accomplished using artificial materials called breast implants, or by using tissues from other parts of the woman's body. The second step involves creating a balance between the newly constructed breast and the breast on the opposite side. The nipple and areolar complex (darker area around the nipple) are recreated. This is usually done several months after the mound is created, to allow swelling to subside. Other procedures may be necessary, such as lifting the opposite breast (mastopexy) or making it larger or smaller to match the reconstructed breast.

Immediate or delayed reconstruction

While immediate reconstruction (IR) is not recommended for women with breast cancer who need to undergo other, more important treatments, breast reconstruction can be done almost anytime. It can be delayed, or it can be completed during the same procedure as the **mastectomy**. There are psychological benefits to IR. The ability to return to normal activities and routines is often enhanced when reconstruction follows immediately after mastectomy. A better final appearance may result from IR. There is less skin removal, often resulting in a shorter scar. The surgeon is better able to preserve the normal boundaries of the breast, so it is easier to more closely match the opposite breast.

The cost of IR is generally lower than the cost of delayed reconstruction (DR). There is one less operation and hospital stay. Surgeon's fees may be lower for a combined procedure than for two separate surgeries.

There are disadvantages of IR as well. The surgery itself is longer, resulting in more time under anesthesia. Postoperative pain and recovery time will be greater than for mastectomy alone.

Other authorities contend that delayed reconstruction (DR) offers different physical and psychological advantages. The initial mastectomy procedure alone takes less time, and has a shorter recovery period and less pain than mastectomy and IR. The woman has more time to adjust to her diagnosis and recover from additional therapy. She is better able to review and evaluate her options and to formulate realistic goals for reconstruction. Some **reconstructive surgery** requires blood transfusions. With DR, the patient can donate her own blood ahead of time (**autologous blood donation**), and/or arrange to have family and friends donate blood for her use (directed donation).

The psychological stress of living without a breast is a disadvantage of DR. The extra procedure needed to perform DR results in higher costs. Although initial recovery is faster, an additional recuperation period is required after the delayed operation.

Type of reconstruction

There are two basic choices for breast reconstruction. The breast tissue can be replaced with an implant, or the breast is created using some of the woman's own tissues (autologous reconstruction).

ARTIFICIAL IMPLANTS. In general, implant procedures take less time and are less expensive than autologous ones. Implants are breast-shaped pouches. They are made of silicone outer shells, which may be smooth or textured. The inside contains saline (salt water). Implants made prior to 1992 were filled with silicone gel. In 1992, the U.S. Food and Drug Association (FDA) discontinued the use of silicone as a filling material. In 2006, the FDA again allowed silicone gel for use in implants.

An implant may be a fixed-volume type, which cannot change its size. Implants that have the capacity to be filled after insertion are called tissue expanders. These may be temporary or permanent.

The initial procedure for any implant insertion uses the mastectomy incision to make a pocket of tissue, usually underneath the chest wall muscle. In DR, the mastectomy scar may be reopened and used for this purpose, or a more cosmetic incision may be made. The implant is inserted into the pocket, the skin is stretched as needed, and sutured closed.

If there is inadequate tissue to achieve the desired size, or a naturally sagging breast is desired, a tissue expander is used. It resembles a partially deflated balloon, with an attached valve or port through which saline can be injected. After the initial surgical incision is healed, the woman returns to the doctor's office on a weekly or bi-weekly basis to have small amounts of saline injected. Injections can continue for about six to eight weeks, until the preferred size is obtained. In some cases, it may initially be overfilled and later partially deflated to allow for a more pliable, natural result. A temporary tissue expander is removed after several months and replaced with a permanent implant.

IR surgery using an implant takes approximately two to three hours, and usually requires up to a three-day hospital stay. Implant insertion surgery that is accomplished as part of DR takes one to two hours and can sometimes be done as an outpatient procedure. Alternatively, it may entail overnight hospitalization.

AUTOLOGOUS RECONSTRUCTION. Attached flap and free flap are two types of surgery where a woman's own tissue is used in reconstruction. An attached flap uses skin, muscle, and fat, leaving blood vessels attached to their original source of blood. The flap is maneuvered to the reconstruction site, keeping its original blood supply for nourishment; this is also known as a pedicle flap. The second kind of surgery is called a free flap, which also uses skin, muscle, and fat, but the surgeon severs the blood vessels and reattaches them to other vessels where the new breast is to

be created. The surgeon uses a microscope to accomplish the delicate task of sewing blood vessels together (anastomosis). Sometimes, the term **microsurgery** is used to refer to free flap procedures. Either type of surgery may also be called a myocutaneous flap. This refers to the skin and muscle used.

The skin and muscle used in autologous reconstruction can come from one of several possible places on the body, including the abdomen (tummy tuck flap), the back (latissimus dorsi flap), or the buttocks (gluteus maximus free flap).

Finishing the reconstruction

Other procedures may be necessary to achieve the goal of symmetrical breasts. It may be necessary to make the opposite breast larger (augmentation), smaller (reduction), or higher (mastopexy). These, or any other refinements, should be completed before the creation of a nipple and areola. Tissue to form the new nipple may come from the reconstructed breast itself, the opposite breast, or a more distant donor site such as the inner thigh or behind the ear. The nipple and areolar construction is usually accomplished as an outpatient procedure. A final step, often done in the doctor's office, is tattooing the new nipple and areola to match the color of the opposite nipple and areola as closely as possible.

Insurance

Insurance coverage varies widely for breast reconstruction. Some policies will allow procedures on the affected breast, but refuse to pay for alterations to the opposite breast. Other plans may cover the cost of an external prosthesis or reconstructive surgery, but not both. The Women's Health and Cancer Rights Act of 1998 requires group health plans and health issuers to provide medical and surgical benefits with respect to mastectomy and to cover the cost of reconstructive breast surgery for women who have undergone a mastectomy.

Implants may pose additional insurance concerns. Some companies will withdraw coverage for women with implants, or add a disclaimer for future implant-related problems. Careful reading of insurance policies, including checking on the need for pre-approval and a **second opinion**, is strongly recommended.

Diagnosis/Preparation

The diagnosis for breast reconstruction is almost always made on a visual basis. The underlying medical reasons include replacing all or part of breast tissue that has been removed during the course of cancer treatment, replacing breast mass that has been lost due to injury, or equalizing otherwise normal breasts that are markedly different in size. Underlying cosmetic reasons include personal preference for larger breasts among genetic females or the creation of breasts in male-to-female transsexuals.

Routine preoperative preparations, such as having nothing to eat or drink the night before surgery, are needed for reconstructive procedures. Blood transfusions are often necessary for autologous reconstructive surgeries. The patient may donate her own blood and/or have family and friends donate blood for her use several weeks prior to the surgery.

Emotional preparation is also important. Breast reconstruction will not resolve a psychological problem the woman had before mastectomy, nor make an unstable relationship strong. An expectation of physical perfection is also unrealistic. A woman who cites any of these reasons for reconstruction shows that she has not been adequately informed or prepared. Complete understanding of the benefits and limitations of this surgery are necessary for a satisfactory result.

Not all women are good candidates for breast reconstruction. Overall poor physical health, or specific problems such as cigarette smoking, obesity, high blood pressure, or diabetes will increase the chance of complications. Also, a difficult or prolonged recovery period or failure of the reconstruction may be a result. A woman's physical ability to cope with major surgery and recuperation should also be considered.

Aftercare

The length of the hospital stay, recovery period, and frequency of visits to the doctor after surgery vary considerably with the different types of reconstruction. In general, autologous procedures require longer hospitalization and recovery times than implant procedures. For all surgical procedures, **bandages** and drainage tubes remain in place for at least a day. Microsurgical or free flap procedures are most closely monitored in the first day or two after surgery. The circulation to the breast may be checked as often as every hour. Complete breast reconstruction requires at least one additional surgery to create a nipple and areola. Scars may remain red and raised for a month or longer. They will fade to their final appearance within one to two years. The true, final appearance of the breasts usually will not be visible for at least one year.

Risks

Some women have reported various types of autoimmune-related connective tissue disorders,

which they attribute to their implants—usually involving silicone gel implants. Lawsuits have been filed against the manufacturers of these implants. In 1992, FDA issued guidelines to greatly curtail the use of silicone implants, restricting their use to women who had to replace an existing silicone gel-filled implant. The order required recipients to sign a consent form that details the potential risks of silicone gel-filled implants and become enrolled in a long-range study. Saline became the filling of choice for breast implants. Saline-filled implants were permitted for all uses, although manufacturers were ordered to continue to collect data on possible risks.

The FDA issued "A Status Report on Breast Implant Safety" in 1995, and revised it in March 1997. It noted that studies have not shown a serious increase in the risk of recognized autoimmune diseases in women with silicone gel-filled breast implants. It also addressed concerns about other complications and emphasized the need for further study of this issue.

In 2006, the FDA once again approved silicone gel-filled implants for breast reconstruction in women of all ages and breast augmentation in women aged 22 and older. The FDA required both approved manufacturers to study 40,000 women each for 10 years to assess potential health problems.

There are a number of risks common to any surgical procedure, such as bleeding, infection, anesthesia reaction, or unexpected scarring. Hematoma (accumulation of blood at the surgical site), or seroma (collection of fluid at the surgical site) can delay healing if they are not drained. Any breast reconstruction also poses a risk of asymmetry and the possible need for an unplanned surgical revision. Persistent pain is another potential complication of all types of breast reconstruction.

Implants have some unique problems that may develop. A thick scar, called a capsule, forms around the implant as part of the body's normal reaction to a foreign substance. Capsular contracture occurs when the scar becomes firm or hardened. This may cause

QUESTIONS TO ASK THE DOCTOR

- What will be the resulting appearance?
- Is the surgeon board certified in plastic and reconstructive surgery?
- How many procedures has the surgeon performed?
- What is the surgeon's complication rate?

pain accompanied by changes in the texture or appearance of the breast. Implants can rupture and leak, deflate, or become displaced. The chances of capsular contracture or rupture increase with the age of the implant. These complications can usually be remedied with **outpatient surgery** to loosen the capsule and remove or replace the implant as needed. There is some evidence that using implants with textured surfaces may decrease the incidence of these problems. An implant tends to remain firm indefinitely. It will not grow larger or smaller as a woman's weight changes. Asymmetry can develop if a woman gains or loses a large amount of weight.

The autologous procedures all carry a risk of flap failure, which is a loss of blood supply to the tissue forming the new breast. If a large portion of the flap develops inadequate blood supply, another reconstructive technique may be necessary. Tummy tuck flap procedures can result in decreased muscle tone and weakness in the abdomen, or lead to an abdominal hernia. Arm weakness may occur after latissimus dorsi flap surgery.

Normal results

A normal result of breast reconstruction depends on the woman's goals and expectations. It will not be the same as the breast it replaces. In general, the reconstructed breast should be similar in size and shape to the opposite breast, but will have less sensation and be less mobile than a natural breast. A reconstruction using an implant will usually be firmer and rounder than the other breast. It may feel cooler to the touch, depending on the amount of tissue over it. Scars are unavoidable, but should be as inconspicuous as possible.

Morbidity and mortality rates

Normal scar formation should be expected. With any silicone prosthesis, a capsule usually forms around it; however, in some instances, a mild form of capsular contraction may develop. Mild ridges that can be felt under the skin categorize this condition. If the capsule contracts, as occasionally occurs, it results in a hardening of the breast. There is no way to predict who will excessively scar. Other risks include infection, excessive bleeding, problems associated with anesthesia, rupturing of the implant, and leakage. There have been a total of 120,000 reports of ruptured silicone implants. Approximately 50,000 reports of breakage have been received for saline implants. Most studies have failed to link implants to serious or chronic diseases such as cancer and lupus, but questions remain over how often the implants rupture and what happens if the silicone enters the body. One of the approved manufacturers reported that its implants have a 14 percent likelihood of rupturing over a 10-year period. The other conducted a three-year study and reported that the rupture rate after three years was negligible.

Deaths associated with breast reconstruction are extremely rare. Most post-surgical mortality has been attributed to anesthesia errors or overdoses of pain medications.

Alternatives

Alternatives to breast reconstruction surgery include using external breast forms that fit into brassiere cups or are attached to the skin of the chest. Creams that allege to increase breast size usually produce no noticeable results. The use of creams containing hormones can lead to long-term hormonal imbalances. Reputable experts do not generally recommend these preparations for breast enlargement.

Resources

BOOKS

Disa, J. J., and M. C. Kuechel. *100 Questions and Answers About Breast Surgery*. Sudbury, MA: Jones and Bartlett, 2005.

Dixon, J. M. *Breast Surgery: A Companion to Specialist Surgical Practice*, 3rd ed. Philadelphia: Saunders, 2006.

Freund, R. M., and A. VanDyne. *Cosmetic Breast Surgery: A Complete Guide to Making the Right Decision—From A to Double D*. New York: Marlowe & Company, 2004.

Mang, W., K. Lang, F. Niedel, N. S. Mackowski, N. Rossman, and M. Stock. *Manual of Aesthetic Surgery 2*. New York: Springer, 2005.

Spear, S. L., S. C. Willey, G. L. Robb, D. C. Hammond, and N. Y. Nahabedian. *Surgery of the Breast: Principles And Art*, 2nd ed. Philadelphia: Lippincott Williams & Wilkins, 2005.

Steligo, K. *The Breast Reconstruction Guidebook*, 2nd ed. San Carlos, CA: Carlo Press, 2005.

PERIODICALS

Dehn, T. "The timing of breast reconstruction." *Annals of the Royal College of Surgeons of England* 89, no. 8 (November 2007): 754–759.

Guyomard, V., S. Leinster, and M. Wilkinson. "Systematic review of studies of patients' satisfaction with breast reconstruction after mastectomy." *Breast* 16, no. 6 (December 2007): 547–567.

Yano, K., K. Hosokawa, T. Masuoka, K. Matsuda, A. Takada, T. Taguchi, Y. Tamaki, and S. Noguchi. "Options for immediate breast reconstruction following skin-sparing mastectomy." *Breast Cancer* 14, no. 4 (2007): 406–413.

OTHER

"Breast Implants." U.S. Food and Drug Administration, Centers for Devices and Radiological Health. November 17, 2006. http://www.fda.gov/cdrh/breastimplants/ (December 23, 2007).

"Breast Implants on Trial." *Frontline*. Public Broadcasting System. http://www.pbs.org/wgbh/pages/frontline/implants/ (December 23, 2007).

"Breast Reconstruction." American Society of Plastic Surgeons. 2008. http://www.plasticsurgery.org/patients_consumers/procedures/BreastReconstruction.cfm?CFID=92081034&CFTOKEN=88819197 (December 23, 2007).

"Breast Reconstruction." Medline Plus. March 21, 2008. http://www.nlm.nih.gov/medlineplus/breastreconstruction.html (December 23, 2007).

"Breast Reconstruction After Mastectomy." American Cancer Society. September 6, 2007. http://www.cancer.org/docroot/CRI/content/CRI_2_6X_Breast_Reconstruction_After_Mastectomy_5.asp (December 23, 2007).

"Breast Reconstruction After Mastectomy." Mayo Clinic. August 18, 2006. http://www.mayoclinic.com/health/breast-reconstruction/WO00083 (December 23, 2007).

"Breast Reconstruction Guide for Patients." M. D. Anderson Cancer Center, University of Texas. 2008. http://www.mdanderson.org/Diseases/BreastCancer/reconstruction/ (December 23, 2007).

ORGANIZATIONS

American Board of Plastic Surgery, Seven Penn Center, Suite 4001635 Market Street, Philadelphia, PA, 19103-2204, (215) 587-9322, http://www.abplsurg.org.

American College of Surgeons, 633 North Saint Claire Street, Chicago, IL, 60611, (312) 202-5000, http://www.facs.org.

American Society for Aesthetic Plastic Surgery, 11081 Winners Circle, Los Alamitos, CA, 90720, (888) 272-7711, http://www.surgery.org/.

American Society of Plastic Surgeons, 444 E. Algonquin Rd., Arlington Heights, IL, 60005, (847) 228-9900, http://www.plasticsurgery.org.

L. Fleming Fallon, Jr., M.D., Dr.P.H.

Breast reduction

Definition

Breast reduction is a surgical procedure performed to decrease the size of the breasts.

Purpose

Women with very large breasts (macromastia, or mammary hyperplasia) seek breast reduction for relief of back, shoulder, and neck pain. They may also feel uncomfortable about their breast size and have difficulty finding clothing that will fit properly. Breast reduction may be needed after **reconstructive surgery** following the surgical removal of cancerous breast tissue (**mastectomy**), to make the breasts more symmetric.

Men who have enlarged breasts (gynecomastia) may also be candidates for breast reduction surgery. Excessive alcohol intake, marijuana use, or using anabolic steroids may cause gynecomastia. Surgery is not recommended for men who continue to use these products.

Demographics

According to the American Society of Plastic Surgeons, more than 113,000 women underwent breast reduction surgery in 2003, the most recent year for which accurate data are available. The number of breast reduction procedures is increasing each year. Women most likely to undergo breast reduction range in age from 19 to 50.

Description

Breast reduction is also called reduction mammoplasty. It is most often performed in a hospital, under general anesthetic. Studies have suggested that an outpatient procedure, using local anesthetic and mild sedation, may be appropriate for some persons. The operation requires approximately two to four hours. The most commonly made incision encircles the areola (darkened area around the nipple) and extends downward and around the underside of the breast. This produces the least conspicuous scar. Excess tissue, fat, and skin are removed, and the nipple and areola are repositioned. In certain cases, **liposuction** (fat suctioning) is used to remove extra fat from the armpit area. A hospital stay of up to three days may be needed for recovery.

Breast reduction surgery for males with gynecomastia is similar to that described for females.

If deemed medically necessary, breast reduction is covered by some insurance plans; however, a specified

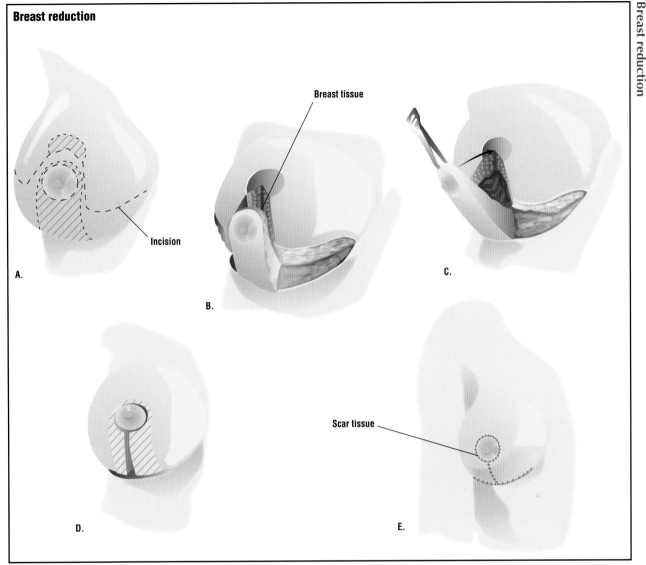

Breast tissue

Incision

A.

B.

C.

Scar tissue

D.

E.

In a breast reduction surgery, the breast tissue is cut along predetermined lines and excess tissue is removed (B). The nipple is placed higher on the breast (C), and the two sides of the incision are brought together (D), removing any excess skin. (E)
(Illustration by GGS Information Services. Cengage Learning, Gale.)

amount of breast tissue may need to be removed in order to qualify for coverage. As of 2007, surgeon's fees range from $5,400 to $6,500, or more.

Diagnosis/Preparation

Consultation between surgeon and patient is important to ensure that there is understanding and agreement with the expected final results of the procedure. Measurements and photographs may be taken. Many doctors also recommend a mammogram before the operation to ensure that there is no cancer.

Aftercare

After the surgery, an elastic bandage or special supportive bra is placed over gauze **bandages** and drainage tubes. The bandages and tubes are removed in a day or two. The bra is worn around the clock for several weeks. **Stitches** are removed one to three weeks after the operation. Normal activities, including sexual relations, may be restricted for several weeks. Scars will typically remain red and perhaps raised for up to several months, but will gradually fade and become less noticeable. It may take up to a year before the breasts achieve their final position and size.

Risks

Breast reduction surgery is not recommended for women whose breasts are not fully developed or who plan to breast-feed.

Risks common to any operation include bleeding, infection, anesthesia reactions, or unexpected scarring. Breast reduction may result in decreased feeling in the breasts or nipples and/or impaired ability to breast-feed. When healing is complete, the breasts may be slightly uneven, or the nipples may be asymmetric. This is consistent with normal breast tissue.

Normal results

Smaller breast size should be achieved and, with that, the accompanying pain and discomfort should be alleviated. Self-esteem should be improved for both females and males having breast reduction surgery.

Morbidity and mortality rates

Deaths associated with breast reduction surgery are extremely rare. Most post-surgical mortality has been attributed to anesthesia errors, overdoses of pain medications, or postoperative infections.

In very rare cases, the skin of the breast or nipple does not heal properly and additional surgery is necessary to graft skin. Approximately 10% of women experience some loss of sensation in their nipples.

Permanent scars are left after breast reduction surgery. At first, the scars usually appear red and raised but will become less obvious over time. Women who smoke often experience more prominent scars. This is because smoking interferes with the healing process.

Alternatives

There are no alternatives to surgery as a way to reduce breast tissue, although significant weight loss can decrease the size of the breast.

Resources

BOOKS

Disa, J. J., and M. C. Kuechel. *100 Questions and Answers About Breast Surgery.* Sudbury, MA: Jones and Bartlett, 2005.

Dixon, J. M. *Breast Surgery: A Companion to Specialist Surgical Practice,* 3rd ed. Philadelphia: Saunders, 2006.

Freund, R. M., and A. VanDyne. *Cosmetic Breast Surgery: A Complete Guide to Making the Right Decision—From A to Double D.* New York: Marlowe & Company, 2004.

Mang, W., K. Lang, F. Niedel, N. S. Mackowski, N. Rossman, and M. Stock. *Manual of Aesthetic Surgery 2.* New York: Springer, 2005.

Spear, S. L., S. C. Willey, G. L. Robb, D. C. Hammond, and N. Y. Nahabedian. *Surgery of the Breast: Principles And Art.* 2nd ed. Philadelphia: Lippincott Williams & Wilkins, 2005.

PERIODICALS

Bartsch, R. H., G. Weiss, T. Kastenbauer, K. Patocka, M. Deutinger, E. D. Krapohl, and H. C. Benditte-Klepetko. "Crucial aspects of smoking in wound healing after breast reduction surgery." *Journal of Plastic, Reconstructive and Aesthetic Surgery* 60, no. 9 (2007): 1045–1049.

Bikhchandani, J., S. K. Varma, and H. P. Henderson. "Is it justified to refuse breast reduction to smokers?" *Journal of Plastic, Reconstructive and Aesthetic Surgery* 60, no. 9 (2007): 1050–1054.

Hidalgo, D. A. "Y-scar vertical mammaplasty." *Plastic and Reconstructive Surgery* 120, no. 7 (2007): 1749–1754.

Spector, J. A., and N. S. Karp. "Reduction mammaplasty: a significant improvement at any size." *Plastic and Reconstructive Surgery* 120, no. 4 (2007): 845–850.

OTHER

American Society for Aesthetic Plastic Surgery. *Information about Breast Reduction Surgery.* 2007 [cited December 23, 2007]. http://www.surgery.org/public/procedures/breast_reduction.

American Society of Plastic Surgeons. *Information about Breast Reduction.* 2007 [cited December 23, 2007]. http://www.plasticsurgery.org/search-results.cfm.

- What will be the resulting appearance?
- Is the surgeon board certified in plastic and reconstructive surgery?
- How many breast reduction procedures has the surgeon performed?
- What is the surgeon's complication rate?

Mayo Clinic. *Information about Breast Reduction Surgery.* 2007 [cited December 23, 2007]. http://www.mayoclinic.com/health/breast-reduction/WO00021.

National Library of Medicine. *Reduction Mammaplasty.* [cited December 23, 2007]. http://vsearch.nlm.nih.gov/vivisimo/cgi-bin/query-meta?server = searchprod5& v%3aproject = medlineplus&v:sources = medlineplus-bundle&v:project = medlineplus&query = reduction %20mammaplasty&orig-query = reduction %20mammaroplasty&.

U.S. Food and Drug Administration. *Breast Reduction.* [cited December 23, 2007]. http://google2.fda.gov/ search?client = FDA&site = FDA&lr = &proxystyle-sheet = FDA&output = xml_no_dtd&getfields = *&q = breast + reduction.htm.

ORGANIZATIONS

American Board of Plastic Surgery, Seven Penn Center, Suite 400, 1635 Market Street, Philadelphia, PA, 19103-2204, (215) 587-9322, http://www.abplsurg.org/.

American College of Surgeons, 633 North Saint Claire Street, Chicago, IL, 60611, (312) 202-5000, http://www.facs.org/.

American Society of Plastic Surgeons, 444 E. Algonquin Rd., Arlington Heights, IL, 60005, (847) 228-9900, http://www.plasticsurgery.org.

American Society for Aesthetic Plastic Surgery, 11081 Winners Circle, Los Alamitos, CA, 90720, (888) 272-7711, http://www.surgery.org/.

L. Fleming Fallon, Jr., M.D., Dr.P.H.

Breast x ray *see* **Mammography**

Bronchoscopy

Definition

Bronchoscopy is a procedure in which a hollow, flexible tube called a bronchoscope is inserted into the airways through the nose or mouth to provide a view of the tracheobronchial tree. It can also be used to collect bronchial and/or lung secretions and to perform tissue biopsy.

Purpose

During a bronchoscopy, the physician can visually examine the lower airways, including the larynx, trachea, bronchi, and bronchioles. The procedure is used to examine the mucosal surface of the airways for abnormalities that might be associated with a variety of lung diseases. Its use may be diagnostic or therapeutic.

Bronchoscopy may be used to examine and help diagnose all of the following:

- diseases of the lung, such as cancer or tuberculosis
- congenital deformity of the lungs
- suspected tumor, obstruction, secretion, bleeding, or foreign body in the airways
- airway abnormalities, such as tracheal stenoses
- persistent cough, or hemoptysis, that includes blood in the sputum

Bronchoscopy may also be used for the following therapeutic purposes:

- remove a foreign body in the lungs
- remove excessive secretions
- remove tumors in the airway
- treat stenosis (narrowing) of the airways, by using balloon dilatation or placing a stent

Bronchoscopy can also be used to collect the following biopsy specimens:

- sputum
- tissue samples from the bronchi or bronchioles
- cells collected from washing the lining of the bronchi or bronchioles

If the purpose of the bronchoscopy is to take tissue samples, or biopsy, a forceps or bronchial brush are used to obtain cells. Alternatively, if the purpose is to identify an infectious agent, a bronchoalveolar lavage can be performed to gather fluid for culture purposes. If any foreign matter is found in the airways, it can be removed as well. Tumors can be debulked (made smaller) through the use of laser, electrocautery, or **cryotherapy** during the bronchoscopy. A balloon can be passed into a narrowed area of the airway and inflated in order to treat stenosis. A stent (tiny artificial tube) can be placed during bronchoscopy, in order to keep a portion of the airway open.

The instrument used in bronchoscopy, a bronchoscope, is a slender, flexible tube less than 0.5 in (2.5 cm)

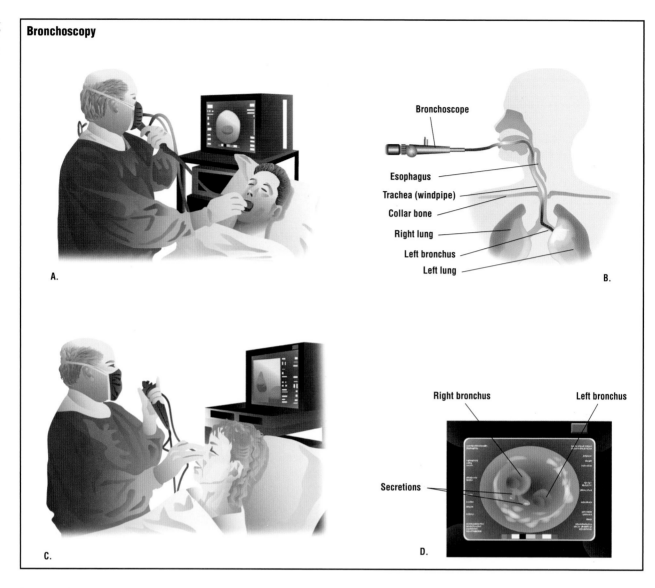

Bronchoscopy

A.

B.

Bronchoscope

Esophagus

Trachea (windpipe)

Collar bone

Right lung

Left bronchus

Left lung

C.

D.

Right bronchus

Left bronchus

Secretions

Bronchoscopy can be performed via the patient's mouth (A) or through the nose (C). During the procedure, the scope is fed down the trachea and into the bronchus leading to the lungs (B), providing the physician with a view of internal structures (D). *(Illustration by GGS Information Services. Cengage Learning, Gale.)*

wide and approximately 2 ft (0.3 m) long that uses fiber-optic technology (very fine filaments that can bend and carry light). There are two types of bronchoscopes: a standard tube that is more rigid and a fiberoptic tube that is more flexible. The rigid instrument does not bend, does not see as far down into the lungs as the flexible one, and may carry a greater risk of causing injury to nearby structures. Because a standard tube can cause more discomfort than the flexible bronchoscope, it usually requires **general anesthesia**. However, it is useful for taking large samples of tissue and for removing foreign bodies from the airways. During the procedure, the airway is not blocked since oxygen can be supplied through the bronchoscope.

Demographics

Nearly 500,000 bronchoscopies are performed annually in the United States. According to the National Cancer Institute, cancer of the lung and bronchi is the second most common cancer among both men and women and is the leading cause of cancer **death** in both sexes in the United States. Among men, lung cancer incidence rates per 100,000 people range from a low of approximately 14 among American Indians to a high of 117 among African Americans. Between these two extremes, rates fall into two groups ranging from 42 to 53 for Hispanics, Japanese, Chinese, Filipinos, and Koreans, and from

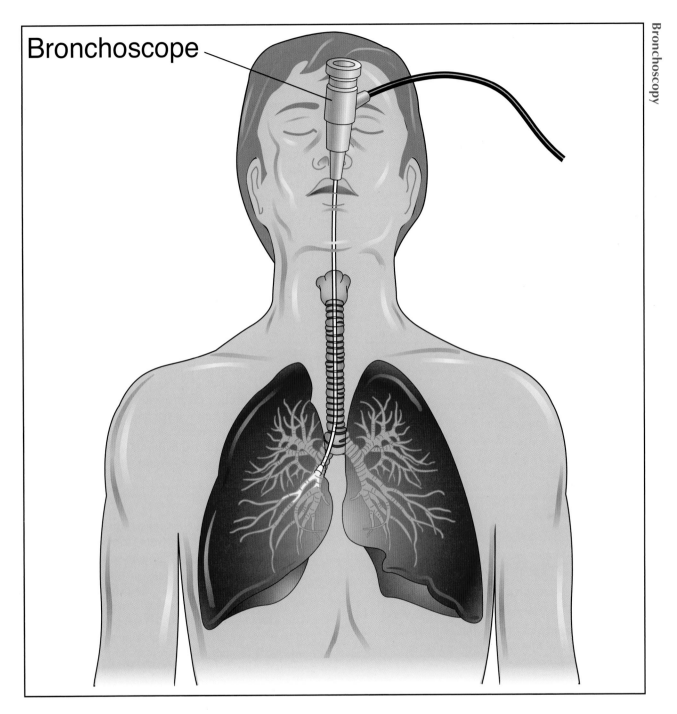

Bronchoscope

Bronchoscopy is a procedure in which a hollow, flexible tube is inserted into the airways, allowing the physician to visually examine the lower airways, including the larynx, trachea, bronchi, and bronchioles. It can also be used to collect specimens for bacteriological culture to diagnose infectious diseases such as tuberculosis. *(Illustration by Electronic Illustrators Group. Cengage Learning, Gale.)*

71 to 89 for Vietnamese, Caucasians, Alaska Natives, and Hawaiians. The range among women is much narrower, from a rate of about 15 among Japanese to nearly 51 among Alaska Natives, only a three-fold difference. Rates for the remaining female populations fall roughly into two groups with low rates of 16–25 for Korean, Filipino, Hispanic, and Chinese women, and rates of 31–44 among Vietnamese, Caucasian, Hawaiian, and African American women. The rates among men are about two to three times greater than the rates among women in each of the racial/ethnic groups.

KEY TERMS

Anesthetic—A drug that causes loss of sensation. It is used to lessen the pain of surgery and medical procedures.

Biopsy—Procedure that involves obtaining a tissue specimen for microscopic analysis to establish a precise diagnosis.

Bronchi—The network of tubular passages that carry air to the lungs and allow air to be expelled from the lungs.

Bronchioles—Small airways extending from the bronchi into the lobes of the lungs.

Bronchoalveolar lavage—Washing cells from the air sacs at the end of the bronchioles.

Computed tomography (CT)—A special radiographic imaging technique that uses a computer to acquire multiple x rays into a two-dimensional sectional image.

Emesis basin—A basin used to collect sputum or vomit.

Endoscope—A highly flexible viewing instrument.

Endoscopy—The visual inspection of any cavity of the body using an endoscope.

Hemoptysis—The expectoration of blood or of blood containing sputum.

Larynx—The voice box.

Lavage—Washing out.

Neoplasm—A new growth or tumor.

Sputum—Matter ejected from the lungs, bronchi, and trachea through the mouth.

Stenosis—Narrowing of a duct or canal.

Trachea—The windpipe.

Tracheobronchial—Pertaining both to the tracheal and bronchial tubes or to their junction.

Description

Bronchoscopy is usually performed in an endoscopy room, but may also be performed at the bedside. The patient is placed on the back or sits upright. A pulmonologist, a specialist trained to perform the procedure, sprays an anesthetic into the patient's mouth or throat. When anesthesia has taken effect and the area is numb, the bronchoscope is inserted into the mouth and passed into the throat. If the bronchoscope is passed through the nose, an anesthetic jelly is inserted into one nostril. While the bronchoscope is

WHO PERFORMS THE PROCEDURE AND WHERE IS IT PERFORMED?

The test is usually performed in a hospital or clinic by a pulmonologist, a physician specializing in diseases of the lungs. Nursing staff assist by providing education, monitoring the patient, and conducting tests, including checking blood pressure, pulse, and respiratory rate prior to the patient's discharge.

moving down the throat, additional anesthetic is put into the bronchoscope to anesthetize the lower airways. The physician observes the trachea, bronchi, and the mucosal lining of these passageways looking for any abnormalities that may be present. If samples are needed, a bronchial lavage may be performed, meaning that a saline solution is used to flush the area prior to collecting cells for laboratory analysis. Very small brushes, needles, or forceps may also be introduced through the bronchoscope to collect tissue samples from the lungs. If the procedure is therapeutic in nature, laser, electrocautery, cryotherapeutic, or balloon dilatation instruments may be passed through the bronchoscope, as well as a stent may be placed.

Preparation

The patient should fast for six to 12 hours prior to the procedure and refrain from drinking any liquids the day of the procedure. Smoking should be avoided for 24 hours prior to the procedure, and patients should also avoid taking any **aspirin** or ibuprofen-type medications. The bronchoscopy itself takes about 45–60 minutes. Prior to the bronchoscopy, several tests are usually done, including a **chest x ray** and blood work. Sometimes a bronchoscopy is done under general anesthesia, in which case the patient will have an intravenous (IV) line in the arm. More commonly, the procedure is performed under **local anesthesia**, which is sprayed into the nose or mouth. This is necessary to inhibit the gag reflex. A sedative may also be given. A signed consent form is necessary for this procedure.

Aftercare

After the bronchoscopy, the **vital signs** (heart rate, blood pressure, and breathing) are monitored. Sometimes patients have an abnormal reaction to anesthesia. Any sputum should be collected in an emesis basin so that it can be examined for the presence of blood. If a biopsy was taken, the patient should not cough or clear the throat as this might dislodge any blood clot that has formed and cause bleeding. No food or drink should be consumed for about two hours after the procedure or until the anesthesia wears off. There is a significant risk for choking if anything (including water) is ingested before the anesthetic wears off, and the gag reflex has returned. To test if the gag reflex has returned, a spoon is placed on the back of the tongue for a few seconds with light pressure. If there is no gagging, the process is repeated after 15 minutes. The gag reflex should return in one or two hours. Ice chips or clear liquids should be taken before the patient attempts to eat solid food. Patients should be informed that the throat may be irritated for several days.

Patients should notify their healthcare provider if they develop any of these symptoms:

- hemoptysis (coughing up blood)
- shortness of breath, wheezing, or any trouble breathing
- chest pain
- fever, with or without breathing problems

Risks

Use of the bronchoscope mildly irritates the lining of the airways, resulting in some swelling and inflammation, as well as hoarseness caused from abrading the vocal cords. If this abrasion is more serious, it can lead to respiratory difficulty or bleeding of the lining of the airways.

The bronchoscopy procedure is also associated with a small risk of disordered heart rhythm (arrhythmia), heart attacks, low blood oxygen (hypoxemia), and pneumothorax (a puncture of the lungs that allows air to escape into the space between the lung and the chest wall). These risks are greater with the use of a rigid bronchoscope than with a fiberoptic

bronchoscope. If a rigid tube is used, there is also a risk of chipped teeth. The risk of transmitting infectious disease from one patient to another by the bronchoscope is also present. The Centers for Disease Control (CDC) reported cases of patient-to-patient transmission of infections following bronchoscopic procedures using bronchoscopes that were inadequately reprocessed by the automated endoscope reprocessing (AER) system. Investigation of the incidents revealed inconsistencies between the reprocessing instructions provided by the manufacturer of the bronchoscope and the manufacturer of the AER; or that the bronchoscopes were inadequately reprocessed.

Normal results

If the results of the bronchoscopy are normal, the windpipe (trachea) appears as smooth muscle with C-shaped rings of cartilage at regular intervals. There are no abnormalities either in the trachea or in the bronchi of the lungs.

Bronchoscopy results may also confirm a suspected diagnosis. This may include swelling, ulceration, or deformity in the bronchial wall, such as inflammation, stenosis, or compression of the trachea, neoplasm, and foreign bodies. The bronchoscopy may also reveal the presence of atypical substances in the trachea and bronchi. If samples are taken, the results could indicate cancer, disease-causing agents, or other lung diseases. Other findings may include constriction or narrowing (stenosis), compression, dilation of vessels, or abnormal branching of the bronchi. Abnormal substances that might be found in the airways include blood, secretions, or mucous plugs.

Morbidity and mortality rates

Bronchoscopy belongs to the group of procedures associated with highest inpatient mortality with a 12.7% mortality rate.

Alternatives

Depending upon the purpose of the bronchoscopy, alternatives may include a chest x ray or a computed tomography (CT) scan. If the purpose is to obtain biopsy specimens, one option is to perform surgery, which carries greater risks. Another option is percutaneous biopsy guided by CT.

Resources

BOOKS

Abeloff, M. D., et al. *Clinical Oncology.* 3rd ed. Philadelphia: Elsevier, 2004.

Cummings, C. W., et al. *Otolayrngology: Head and Neck Surgery*. 4th ed. St. Louis: Mosby, 2005.

Khatri, V. P., and J. A. Asensio. *Operative Surgery Manual*. 1st ed. Philadelphia: Saunders, 2003.

Koppen, W., J. F. Turner, and A. C. Mehta, eds. *Flexible Bronchoscopy*. 2nd ed. Oxford: Blackwell Publishers, 2004.

Mason, R. J., et al. *Murray & Nadel's Textbook of Respiratory Medicine*. 4th ed. Philadelphia: Saunders, 2007.

Townsend, C. M., et al. *Sabiston Textbook of Surgery*. 17th ed. Philadelphia: Saunders, 2004.

PERIODICALS

Diette, G. B., N. Lechtzin, E. Haponik, A. Devrotes, and H. R. Rubin. "Distraction Therapy with Nature Sights and Sounds Reduces Pain during Flexible Bronchoscopy: A Complementary Approach to Routine Analgesia." *Chest* 123 (March 2003): 941–948.

Starobin, D., G. Fink, D. Shitrit, G. Izbicki, D. Bendayan, I. Bakal, and M. R. Kramer. "The Role of Fiberoptic Bronchoscopy Evaluating Transplant Recipients with Suspected Pulmonary Infections: Analysis of 168 Cases in a Multi-organ Transplantation Center." *Transplantation Proceedings* 35 (March 2003): 659–660.

Wu, K. H., T. T. Man, K. L. Wong, C. F. Lin, C. C. Chen, and C. R. Cheng. "Bronchoscopy and Anesthesia for Preschool-aged Patients: A Review of 228 Cases." *Internal Surgery* 87 (October–December 2002): 252–255.

Yang, C. C., and K. S. Lee. "Comparison of Direct Vision and Video Imaging during Bronchoscopy for Pediatric Airway Foreign Bodies." *Ear, Nose, and Throat Journal* 82 (February 2003): 129–133.

ORGANIZATIONS

American College of Chest Physicians. 3300 Dundee Road, Northbrook, IL 60062. (800) 343-2227.

The Association of Perioperative Registered Nurses, Inc. (AORN). 2170 South Parker Rd, Suite 300, Denver, CO 80231-5711. (800) 755-2676. http://www.aorn.org (accessed March 8, 2008).

OTHER

"Bronchoscopy." *Medline Plus*. [cited April 2003]. http://www.nlm.nih.gov/medlineplus/ency/article/003857.htm (accessed March 8, 2008).

"Public Health Advisory: Infections from Endoscopes Inadequately Reprocessed by an Automated Endoscope Reprocessing System." U. S. Food and Drug Administration, Center for Devices and Radiological Health. September 1999 [cited April 2003]. http://www.fda.gov/cdrh/safety/endoreprocess.html (accessed March 8, 2008).

Maggie Boleyn, RN, BSN
Monique Laberge, PhD
Rosalyn Carson-DeWitt, MD

BUN-creatinine ratio

Definition

Blood Urea Nitrogen (BUN) and creatinine are both waste products of normal metabolism in the human body. BUN represents the amount of nitrogen produced from the metabolism of proteins. Creatinine is a normal waste product of muscle. The ratio of BUN to creatinine is a relationship between these two end products found in blood, and paints a clinical picture for physicians describing kidney functionality.

Why BUN-creatinine is measured

The BUN-creatinine ratio provides specific clinical information about the kidney that can be used for multiple purposes. The BUN-creatinine ratio is obtained to assess normal kidney function, help identify possible kidney diseases, to monitor the progression of kidney disease, or to monitor the effectiveness of medications in treating kidney disease.

Demographics

BUN-creatinine ratio is obtained whenever medically appropriate regardless of age, gender, or race. It is commonly measured in patients before a surgical procedure to assess general function, after some types of surgical procedures, and in patients with kidney disease or failure. The BUN-creatinine ratio is also obtained to assess the degree and effectiveness of kidney filtration prior to some radiology studies.

Description

The BUN-creatinine ratio is a value measured in the blood to help assess the health of the kidney.

BUN

As a normal part of protein metabolism in the liver, protein is broken down into a compound called urea. Urea can be measured by nitrogen in the blood. Once in the blood, urea nitrogen is carried to the kidneys to be filtered out of the blood into the urine. Some of the urea nitrogen is reabsorbed back into the body for further use, but most is left in the urine. Hence, products of protein breakdown are excreted from the body. Females have lower normal BUN values than males. Women in the second or third trimester of pregnancy may present with a lower BUN value as normal. Normal BUN values in the elderly may be elevated.

Abnormal BUN Values

If the BUN value not within the normal range, it is a sign that either there is an excess of protein breakdown products in the blood, or some part of the system of BUN filtration is not functioning normally. A BUN value higher or lower than normal demonstrates a potential problem in urea removal from the blood.

The BUN filtration system relies on both kidney filtration function and on a sufficient amount of blood traveling to the kidney to be filtered. An abnormal BUN value may indicate a breakdown somewhere in this system. The kidney may not be filtering properly due to disease or injury, or blood flow may be decreased to the kidney and so not available for filtration. Either of these scenarios may cause an increased BUN value. Kidney damage can be caused by diabetes, high blood pressure, and pathologies that block the urinary tract such as kidney stones. Decreased blood flow to the kidneys may be caused by multiple disease states or physiological disorders, including congestive heart failure, dehydration, shock, or gastrointestinal bleeding.

Diets that involve consuming large amounts of protein, such as the Atkins diet, may cause an excess of protein breakdown products to be present in the blood. The more protein is ingested, the greater the amount of urea and nitrogen will be present in the blood for the kidneys to filter. Even with a healthy pair of kidneys, an excess amount of protein to be filtered can stress the kidney filtration system and result in higher than normal BUN levels. Lower than normal BUN values may occur due to a state of malnutrition where not enough protein is ingested, over hydration where the amount of BUN is diluted, or liver damage where protein breakdown is defective.

Creatinine

Creatinine is a waste product formed when the amino acid creatine in muscle tissue is metabolized. Creatinine is released into the blood, where it is carried to the kidneys for filtration into the urine. When creatinine levels are measured in the blood it is known as serum creatinine (used to help calculate the BUN-creatinine ratio). When creatinine levels are measured in the urine it is known as urine creatinine. Once creatinine is filtered by the kidney, it is not reabsorbed into the body. All the creatinine that is filtered is excreted in the urine. This is an important trait of creatinine, and makes it useful as a monitor of kidney filtration capability. Since creatinine originates from muscle breakdown, females may have lower normal serum creatinine values than males due to lower muscle mass. Pregnancy may cause low normal serum creatinine.

Abnormal Creatinine Values

Some types of kidney disease affect the ability of the kidney to filter waste products such as creatinine from the blood. The kidney diseases acute tubular necrosis, diabetic nephropathy, and glomerulonephritis may all increase serum creatinine values. Diseases that decrease the amount of blood that reaches the kidney for filtration may also increase serum creatinine values. The muscle disease rhabdomyolysis and any other disease that causes excessive breakdown of muscle tissue can cause abnormally high serum creatinine levels. Pathologies that block the urinary tract such as kidney stones will increase serum creatinine. Lower than normal serum creatinine values may be caused by decreased muscle mass due to age or diseases such as muscular dystrophy. Very low protein diets may also cause decreased serum creatinine levels.

BUN-creatinine ratio

The BUN-creatinine ratio is determined by measuring the concentrations of BUN and creatinine in the blood. A change in either component will influence the value of the ratio. A normal BUN-creatinine ratio is based on the normal values for BUN and serum creatinine. A normal BUN value is 10–20 mg/dl. A normal serum creatinine value is 0.5–1.2 mg/dl. Hence, a normal BUN-creatinine ratio lies between 10:1 and 20:1. The normal value of the BUN-creatinine ratio is different in infants less than 12 months old, where it may be as high as 30:1 and still be normal.

Abnormal BUN-creatinine ratio values

Abnormal BUN-creatinine ratios may be caused by many different types diseases, disorders, or injury to the kidney. The ratio may be abnormally high with any pathology that increases BUN or decreases creatinine. The ratio may be abnormally low with any pathology that decreases BUN or increases creatinine.

BUN-creatinine ratio and acute renal failure

Acute Renal Failure (ARF), or kidney failure, may be caused by kidney disease or injury. The cause of ARF may be due to a pathology that occurs outside of the kidney before the blood reaches the kidney filtration apparatus, or within the actual kidney. Depending on where the cause for kidney failure lies, ARF is categorized as being "prerenal" or "renal or intrinsic." The BUN-creatinine ratio is a useful tool for identifying which category of ARF is present in a patient. Prerenal causes of ARF create extremely high BUN-creatinine ratios. Renal or intrinsic causes of ARF create BUN-creatinine ratios that are higher than normal but less than those created by prerenal ARF.

How to prepare for a BUN-creatinine ratio test

BUN-creatinine ratios are measured using blood samples. Having blood drawn from a vein with a syringe, usually in the arm, is necessary. Since some medications may affect the results, it is critical that the physician take into account all prescription medications, non-prescription medications, herbal, and nutritional supplements that the patient is taking before running the BUN-creatinine ratio test. Age and gender may also affect the results in predictable patterns. To prepare for the BUN-creatinine test patients should not do any strenuous **exercise** for 2 days (48 hours) prior; not eat meat, especially beef, or other protein for 24 hours prior; drink a normal amount of fluids.

Drugs that affect BUN

- Allopurinol;
- Aminoglycosides;
- Amphotericin B;
- Bacitracin;
- Carbamazepine;
- Cephalosporins;
- Chloramphenicol;
- Cimetidine;
- Cisplatin;
- Corticosteriods;
- Furosemide;
- Gentamicin;
- Guanethidine;
- High-Dose Aspirin;
- Indomethacin;
- Methicillin;
- Methotrexate;
- Methyldopa;
- Neomycin;
- Penicillamine;
- Polymixin B;
- Probenecid;
- Propranolol;
- Rifampin;
- Spironolactone;
- Tetracyclines;
- Thiazide Diuretics;
- Triamterene; and
- Vancomycin.

Drugs that affect creatinine

- Aminoglycosides;
- Bactrim;
- Cimetidine;
- Cisplatin;
- Cephalosporins;
- Methyldopa;
- Trimethoprim; and
- Any drug toxic to kidneys.

Risks associated with testing the BUN-creatinine ratio

There is very little risk associated with having blood drawn for a BUN-creatinine ratio test. Most people have no side effects or a small bruise; however, with any blood draw there is a small chance that the area around the punctured vein may develop phlebitis, the inflammation of a vein. Phlebitis may also involve a bacterial infection if the site of the blood draw was not appropriately cleaned before the needle was inserted. Phlebitis can be locally painful but usually resolves in a short period of time. Additionally, patients with disorders involving the inability of the blood to form normal blood clots should discuss their condition and their medications with the physician before the blood draw and BUN-creatinine ratio test is done.

Risks associated with the test result include a deceptively normal value for the BUN-creatinine ratio. It is important that the physician note both the value of the BUN-creatinine ratio and the values of BUN and serum creatinine individually. Kidney damage may present with abnormal values for BUN and creatinine, but a normal value for their ratio. If the individual values are not noted, this scenario may present a seemingly normal picture of health that is not accurate. For example, in patients with chronic kidney failure, the BUN-creatinine ratio may be 10:1

Acute Renal Failure (a.k.a. Acute Kidney Failure)—The rapid loss of the kidney's ability to function due to kidney damage. Acute renal failure decreases the kidney's ability to filter waste products from the blood for excretion in the urine.

Acute Tubular Necrosis—A kidney disease involving damage to the portion of the kidney known as the tubules that causes kidney failure.

Atkins Diet—A diet that involves eating a high amount of protein and fat with a low amounts of carbohydrates.

Blood Serum—The fluid portion of the blood.

Congestive Heart Failure—A serious condition caused by disease or damage to the heart that weakens the heart's ability to pump a sufficient amount of blood to the body tissues.

Diabetic Nephropathy—A progressive kidney disease associated with diabetes that interferes with the kidney's ability to function in filtering waste products from the blood.

Gastrointestinal Tract—The path in the body from the mouth, through the stomach, intestines, rectum, and the anus.

Glomerulonephritis—A disease of the kidneys mediated by the immune system that causes inflammation of the part of the kidney known as the glomerulus.

Muscular Dystrophy—A genetic muscle disease that causes progressive muscle weakness along with the breakdown and death of muscle tissue.

Phlebitis—Inflammation of a vein.

Rhabdomyolysis—A condition causing the rapid breakdown of muscle tissue that may be caused by severe injuries or toxic chemicals. It causes the release of muscle tissue breakdown products into the blood in such excess that it may lead to acute renal failure.

with a BUN level of 60mg/dl and a **serum creatinine level** of 2mg/dl. In conclusion, a normal looking BUN-creatinine ratio does not always mean that the kidneys are functioning normally.

Resources

BOOKS

Chaudhry, H. J., et al. *Fundamentals of Clincal Medicine*, 4th ed. Philadelphia: Lippincott Williams & Wilkins, 2004.

Gennari, F. J. *Medical Management of Kidney and Electrolyte Disorders*. New York: Informa Healthcare, 2001.

Le, Tao, Vikas Bhushan, and Chirag Amin. *First Aid for the Wards*, 2nd ed. New York: McGraw-Hill, 2002.

Maxwell, R. W. *Maxwell Quick Medical Reference*, 5th ed. Tulsa, OK: Maxwell Publishing Company, 2006.

OTHER

"Blood Urea Nitrogen." WebMD. August 21, 2006. http://www.webmd.com/a-to-z-guides/blood-urea-nitrogen (April 8, 2008).

"Creatinine and Creatinine Clearance." WebMD. August 21, 2006. http://www.webmd.com/a-to-z-guides/creatinine-and-creatinine-clearance (April 8, 2008).

Maria Basile, Ph.D.

BUN test *see* **Kidney function tests**

Bunionectomy

Definition

A bunionectomy is a surgical procedure to excise, or remove, a bunion. A bunion is an enlargement of the joint at the base of the big toe and is comprised of bone and soft tissue. It is usually a result of inflammation and irritation from poorly fitting (narrow and tight) shoes in conjunction with an overly mobile first metatarsal joint and over-pronation of the foot. Over time, a painful lump appears at the side of the joint, while the big toe appears to buckle and move sideway towards the second toe. New bone growth can occur in response to the inflammatory process, and a bone spur may develop. Therefore, the development of a bunion may involve soft tissue as well as a hard bone spur. The intense pain makes walking and other activities extremely difficult. Since the involved joint is a significant structure in providing weight-bearing stability, walking on the foot while trying to avoid putting pressure on the painful area can create an unstable gait.

Purpose

A bunionectomy is performed when conservative means of addressing the problem, including properly fitting, wide-toed shoes, a padded cushion against the joint, orthotics, and anti-inflammatory medication, are unsuccessful. As the big toe moves sideways, it can push the second toe sideways as well. This can result in extreme deformity of the foot, and the patient may complain not only of significant pain, but of an inability to find shoes that fit.

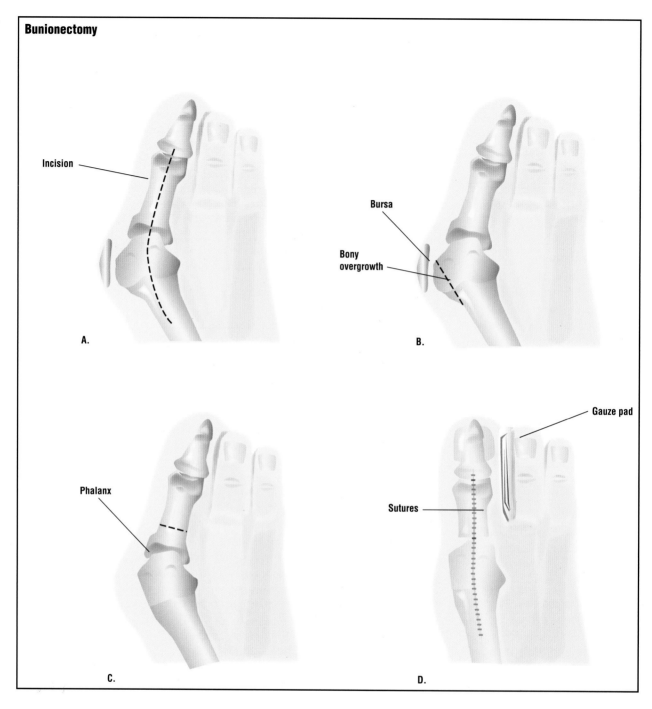

Bunionectomy

A bunion results in a bony overgrowth in the foot, causing the big toe to curve outward. To repair this, an incision is made in the top of the foot (A). The overgrowth and fluid-filled sac called a bursa are removed (B). The phalanx bone of the big toe is shortened to straighten it (C). The foot is realigned, and incision is closed (D). *(Illustration by GGS Information Services. Cengage Learning, Gale.)*

Demographics

Bunion formation can be hereditary, which means that if the individual's mother or father had the condition, he or she is at an increased risk of developing one as well. Bunions can also be a result of a congenital deformity, which means that the individual was born with an anatomical condition that made the development of a bunion more likely. Women are nine to 10 times more likely to develop bunions than men. The American Orthopaedic Foot & Ankle Society reports a study estimating that about 88% of women wear shoes that are too small and that 55% have developed bunions. The condition may begin to form in adolescence. Other conditions that contribute to bunion formation include flat-footedness, a tight Achilles tendon, and rheumatoid arthritis. The earlier the diagnosis, the better the chance that significant deformity will be avoided.

Description

Bunions become more common later in life. One reason is that with age the foot spreads and proper alignment is not maintained. In addition, the constant friction of poorly fitting shoes against the big toe joint creates a greater problem over time. Ignoring the problem in its early stages leads to a shifting gait that further aggravates the situation.

Once surgery has been decided on, the extent of the procedure will depend on the degree of deformity that has taken place. There are several different surgical techniques, mostly named after the surgeons who developed them, such as McBride, Chevron, and Keller. The degree and angle of deformity as well as the patient's age and physical condition play a significant role in the surgeon's choice of technique, which will determine how much tissue is removed and whether or not bone repositioning will occur. If bone repositioning is done, that part of the surgery is referred to as an osteotomy (*osteo* means bone). The type of anesthesia, whether ankle block (the most common, in which the foot is numb but the patient is awake), general, or spinal, will depend on the patient's condition and the anticipated extent of the surgery. For surgery done on an ambulatory basis, the patient will usually be asked to arrive one to two hours before the surgery and stay for about two to three hours after the procedure. The procedure itself may take about an hour.

The surgeon will make an incision over the swollen area at the first joint of the big toe. The enlarged lump will be removed. The surgeon may need to reposition the alignment of the bones of the big toe. This may require more than one incision. The bone itself may need to be cut. If the joint surfaces have been damaged, the surgeon may hold the bones together with screws, wires, or metal plates. In severe cases, the entire joint may need to be removed and a joint replacement inserted. If pins were used to hold the bones in place during recovery, they will be removed a few weeks later. In some mild cases, it may be sufficient to repair the tendons and ligaments that are pulling the big toe out of alignment. When finished, the surgeon will close the incision with sutures and may apply steri-strips as an added reinforcement. A compression dressing will be wrapped around the surgical wound. This helps to keep the foot in alignment as well as help reduce postoperative swelling.

Diagnosis/Preparation

Intense pain at the first joint of the big toe is what most commonly brings the patient to the doctor. Loss of toe mobility may also have occurred. Severe deformity of the foot may also make it almost impossible for the patient to fit the affected foot into a shoe. The condition may be in either foot or in both. In addition, there may be a crackling sound in the joint when it moves. Diagnosis of a bunion is based on a **physical examination**, a detailed history of the patient's symptoms and their development over time, and x rays to determine the degree of deformity. Other foot disorders such as gout must be ruled out. The patient history should include factors that increase the pain, the patient's level of physical activity, occupation, amount of time spent on his or her feet, the type of shoe most frequently worn, other health conditions such as diabetes that can affect the body's ability to heal, a thorough medication history, including home remedies, and any allergies to food, medications, or environmental aspects. The physical exam should include an assessment while standing and walking to judge the degree to which stability and gait have been affected, as well as an assessment while seated or lying down to measure range of motion and anatomical integrity. An examination of the foot itself will check for the presence of unusual calluses, which indicate abnormal patterns of friction. Circulation in the affected foot will be noted by checking the skin color and temperature. A neurological assessment will also be conducted.

Conservative measures are usually the first line of treatment and target dealing with the acute phase of the condition, as well as attempting to stop the progression of the condition to a more serious form. Measures may include:

- rest and elevation of the affected foot
- eliminating any additional pressure on the tender area, perhaps by using soft slippers instead of shoes
- soaking the foot in warm water to improve blood flow
- use of anti-inflammatory oral medication
- an injection of a steroidal medication into the area surrounding the joint
- systematic use of an orthotic, either an over-the-counter product or one specifically molded to the foot
- the use of a cushioned padding against the joint when wearing a shoe

If these measures prove unsuccessful, or if the condition has worsened to significant foot deformity and altered gait, then a bunionectomy is considered. The doctor may use the term *hallux valgus* when referring to the bunion. *Hallux* means big toe and *valgus* means bent outward. In discussing the surgical option, it is important for the patient to clearly understand the degree of improvement that is realistic following surgery.

X rays to determine the exact angle of displacement of the big toe and potential involvement of the second toe will be taken. The angles of the two toes in relation to each other will be noted to determine the severity of the condition. Studies in both a standing as well as a seated or lying down position will be considered. These will guide the surgeon at the time of the surgery as well. In addition, blood tests, an EKG, and a **chest x ray** will most likely be ordered to be sure that no other medical condition has gone undiagnosed that could affect the success of the surgery and the patient's recovery.

Aftercare

Recovery from a bunionectomy takes place both at the surgical center as well as in the patient's home. Immediate post-surgical care is provided in the surgical recovery area. The patient's foot will be monitored for bleeding and excessive swelling; some swelling is considered normal. The patient will need to stay for a few hours in the recovery area before being discharged. This allows time for the anesthesia to wear off. The patient will be monitored for nausea and vomiting, potential aftereffects of the anesthesia, and will be given something light to eat, such as crackers

WHO PERFORMS THE PROCEDURE AND WHERE IS IT PERFORMED?

Bunionectomies are performed by orthopedic surgeons, podiatric surgeons, and general surgeons. In selecting a surgeon, it is best to consider those who perform at least 20 bunionectomies each year. Most bunionectomies are performed as same-day, or ambulatory, surgery, in which the patient goes home the same day of the procedure. Sometimes a patient's condition may warrant staying overnight in the hospital.

and juice or ginger ale, to see how the food is tolerated. Hospital policy usually requires that the patient have someone drive them home, as there is a safety concern after having undergone anesthesia. In addition, the patient will most likely be on pain medication that could cause drowsiness and impaired thinking.

It is important to contact the surgeon if any of the following occur after discharge from the surgical center:

- fever
- chills
- constant or increased pain at the surgical site
- redness and a warmth to the touch in the area around the dressing
- swelling in the calf above the operated foot
- dressing that has become wet or that has fallen off
- dressing that has become bloody

While the patient can expect to return to normal activities within six to eight weeks after the surgery, the foot is at increased risk for swelling for several months. When the patient can expect to bear weight on the operated foot will depend on the extent of the surgery. The milder the deformity, the less tissue is removed and the sooner the return to normal activity level. During the six-to-eight-week recovery period, a special shoe, boot, or cast may be worn to accommodate the surgical bandage and to help provide stability to the foot.

Risks

All surgical procedures involve some degree of risk. The most likely problems to occur in a bunionectomy are infection, pain, nerve damage to the operated foot, and the possibility that the bunion will recur. Sharing all pertinent past and present medical

QUESTIONS TO ASK THE DOCTOR

- How many bunionectomies do you perform each year?
- Are there any clinical trials for new medications or new types of procedures available?
- What complications have you seen with this procedure?
- What choices do I have for anesthesia?
- What can I expect during the recovery period?
- When can I return to my work and other regular activities?
- How soon after the surgery can I drive?
- How much improvement can I expect after surgery?

history with the **surgical team** helps to lower the chance of a complication. In addition to the risk of the surgery itself, anesthesia also has risks. It is important to share with the anesthesia team the list of all the vitamins, herbs, and supplements, over-the-counter medications, and prescription medications that the patient is taking.

Normal results

The expected result will depend on the degree of deformity that has occurred prior to surgery, the patient's medical condition and age, and the adherence to the recovery regimen prescribed. Some degree of swelling in the foot is normal for up to six months after the surgery. Once wound healing has taken place, the surgeon may recommend exercises or physical therapy to improve foot strength and range of motion. It is important to be realistic about the possible results before consenting to the surgery. Since over-pronation of the foot is not corrected with the surgery, orthotics to help keep the foot/feet in alignment are usually prescribed.

Morbidity and mortality rates

According to the American Orthopaedic Foot & Ankle Society, less than 10% of patients undergoing bunionectomy experience complications, and 85–90% of patients feel the surgery was successful.

Alternatives

It may be possible to avoid surgery by preventing bunion growth from worsening. Wearing shoes that are the right size and shape is a key factor. Try on new shoes in the afternoon when the foot is more tired and perhaps has some fluid buildup. Rather than going by size alone, make sure the shoe fits well, and that there is proper arch support. Additionally, there should be enough space in the toe box for the toes to wiggle around.

If diagnosed early, an injection of a steroidal anti-inflammatory medication around the joint may be enough to decrease the irritation in the area and allow the joint to recuperate. This, along with proper shoes, may halt progression of the condition. If there is no pain accompanying the bunion, surgery is not necessary. Some people find that a cream containing the same ingredient as found in chili peppers, capsaicin, applied locally to the joint can decrease the pain. However, once deformity and its accompanying severe pain has occurred, it is unlikely that surgery can be avoided.

Resources

BOOKS

Barker, L. Randol, John R. Burton, and Phillip D. Zieve, eds. *Principles of Ambulatory Medicine.* 5th edition. Baltimore: William & Wilkins, 1999.

Skinner, Harry B. *Current Diagnosis & Treatment in Orthopedics.* Appleton & Lange, 2000.

ORGANIZATIONS

American Orthopaedic Foot & Ankle Society. 2517 Eastlake Avenue East, Seattle, WA 98102. http://www.aofas.org.

American Podiatric Medical Association. http://www.apma.com.

Esther Csapo Rastegari, RN, BSN, EdM

Burch procedure *see* **Retropubic suspension**

Bypass surgery *see* **Coronary artery bypass graft surgery**

C

C-reactive protein tests *see* **Cardiac marker tests**

C-section *see* **Cesarean section**

CABG surgery *see* **Coronary artery bypass graft surgery**

Cancer surgery *see* **Surgical oncology**

Carcinoembryonic antigen test *see* **Tumor marker tests**

Cardiac blood pool scan *see* **Multiple-gated acquisition (MUGA) scan**

Cardiac catheterization

Definition

Cardiac catheterization, also called heart catheterization, is a diagnostic and occasionally therapeutic procedure that allows a comprehensive examination of the heart and surrounding blood vessels. It enables the physician to take angiograms; record blood flow; calculate cardiac output and vascular resistance; perform an endomyocardial biopsy; and evaluate the heart's electrical activity. Cardiac catheterization is performed by inserting one or more catheters (thin flexible tubes) through a peripheral blood vessel in the arm (antecubital artery or vein) or leg (femoral artery or vein) under x-ray guidance.

Purpose

Cardiac catheterization is most commonly performed to examine the coronary arteries, because heart attacks, angina, sudden **death**, and heart failure most often originate from disease in these arteries. Cardiac catheterization may reveal the presence of other conditions, including enlargement of the left ventricle; ventricular aneurysms (abnormal dilation of a blood vessel); narrowing of the aortic valve; insufficiency of the aortic or mitral valve; and septal defects that allow an abnormal flow of blood from one side of the heart to the other.

Symptoms and diagnoses that may be associated with the above conditions and may lead to cardiac catheterization include:

- chest pain characterized by prolonged heavy pressure or a squeezing pain
- abnormal results from a treadmill stress test
- myocardial infarction (heart attack)
- congenital heart defects
- valvular disease

Cardiac catheterization with coronary **angiography** is recommended in patients with angina (especially unstable angina); suspected coronary artery disease; suspected silent ischemia and a family history of heart attack; congestive heart failure; congenital heart disease; and pericardial disease. (The pericardium is the layer of thin tissue covering the heart.) Catheterization is also recommended for patients with suspected heart valve disease, including aortic valve stenosis (narrowing) or regurgitation, and mitral valve stenosis or regurgitation.

Patients with congenital cardiac defects are also evaluated with cardiac catheterization to visualize the abnormal direction of blood flow associated with these diseases. In addition, the procedure may be performed after acute myocardial infarction (heart attack); before major noncardiac surgery in patients at high risk for cardiac problems; before cardiac surgery in patients at risk for coronary artery disease; and before such interventional technologies and procedures as stents and percutaneous transluminal coronary **angioplasty** (PTCA) or closure of small openings between the atria (upper chambers of the heart), called atrial septal defects.

Aneurysm—An abnormal dilatation of a blood vessel, usually an artery. It may be caused by a congenital defect or weakness in the vessel's wall.

Angiography—A procedure that allows x-ray examination of the heart and coronary arteries following injection of a radiopaque substance (often referred to as a dye or contrast agent).

Angioplasty—A procedure in which a balloon catheter is used to mechanically dilate the affected area of a diseased artery and enlarge the constricted or narrowed segment; it is an alternative to vascular surgery.

Aortic valve—The valve between the heart's left ventricle and ascending aorta that prevents regurgitation of blood back into the left ventricle.

Arrhythmia—A variation in the normal rhythm of the heartbeat.

Catheter—A flexible or pre-shaped curved tube, usually made of plastic, used to evacuate fluids from or inject fluids into the body.

Computed tomography (CT)—A diagnostic imaging procedure that uses x rays to produce cross-sectional images of the anatomy.

Coronary bypass surgery—A surgical procedure that places a shunt to allow blood to travel from the aorta to a branch of the coronary artery at a point below an obstruction.

Echocardiography—An ultrasound examination of the heart.

Fluoroscopy—A diagnostic imaging procedure that uses x rays and contrast agents to visualize anatomy and motion in real time.

Hematoma—An accumulation of clotted blood that may occur in the tissue around a catheter insertion site.

Ischemia—A localized deficiency in the blood supply, usually caused either by vasoconstriction or by obstacles to the arterial blood flow.

Magnetic resonance imaging (MRI)—A diagnostic imaging procedure that uses a magnetic field to produce anatomical images.

Mitral valve—The bicuspid valve that lies between the left atrium and left ventricle of the heart.

Percutaneous transluminal coronary angioplasty (PTCA)—A cardiac intervention in which an artery blocked by plaque is dilated, using a balloon catheter to flatten the plaque and open the vessel; it is also called balloon angioplasty.

Pericardial tamponade—The collection of blood in the sac surrounding the heart that causes compression.

Pseudoaneurysm—A dilation of a blood vessel that resembles an aneurysm.

Pulmonary valve—The heart valve that separates the right ventricle and the opening into the pulmonary artery.

Septum—The muscular wall that separates the two sides of the heart; an opening in the septum that allows blood to flow from one side to the other is called a septal defect.

Shunt—A passageway (or an artificially created passageway) that diverts blood flow from one main route to another.

Stent—A small tube-like device made of stainless steel or other material, used to hold open a blocked artery.

Tricuspid valve—The right atrioventricular valve of the heart; it has three flaps, whereas the mitral valve has only two.

Left- and right-side catheterization

Cardiac catheterization can be performed on either side of the heart to evaluate different functions. Testing the right side of the heart allows the physician to evaluate tricuspid and pulmonary valve function, in addition to measuring blood pressures and collecting blood samples from the right atrium, right ventricle (lower chamber), and pulmonary artery. Catheterization of the left side of the heart is performed to test the blood flow in the coronary arteries, as well as the level of function of the mitral and aortic valves and left ventricle.

Coronary angiography

Coronary angiography, also known as coronary arteriography, is an imaging technique that involves injecting a dye into the vascular system to outline the heart and coronary vessels. Angiography allows the visualization of any blockages, narrowing, or abnormalities in the coronary arteries. If these signs are visible, the cardiologist may assess the patient's readiness for coronary bypass surgery, or a less invasive approach such as dilation of a narrowed blood vessel by surgery or the use of a balloon (angioplasty). Because some interventions may be performed during cardiac catheterization, the procedure is considered therapeutic as well as diagnostic.

Demographics

Coronary artery disease is the first-ranked cause of death for both men and women in the United States. More than 1.5 million cardiac catheterizations are performed every year in the United States, primarily to diagnose or monitor heart disease. There is an expected growth to more than 3 million procedures by 2010.

Description

Cardiac anatomy

The heart consists of four chambers separated by valves. The right side of the heart, which consists of the right atrium (upper chamber, sometimes called the right auricle) and the right ventricle (lower chamber), pumps blood to the lungs. The left side of the heart, which consists of the left atrium and the left ventricle, simultaneously pumps blood to the rest of the body. The right and left coronary arteries, which are the first vessels to branch off from the aorta, supply blood to the heart. The left anterior descending coronary artery supplies the front of the heart; the left circumflex coronary artery wraps around and supplies the left side and the back of the heart; and the right coronary artery supplies the back of the heart. There is, however, a considerable amount of variation in the anatomy of the coronary arteries.

Catheterization procedure

The patient lies face up on a table during the catheterization procedure, and is connected to a **cardiac monitor**. The insertion site is numbed with a local anesthetic, and access to the vein or artery is obtained using a needle. A sheath, a rigid plastic tube that facilitates insertion of catheters and infusion of drugs, is placed in the puncture site. Under fluoroscopic guidance, a guide-wire (a thin wire that guides the catheter insertion) is threaded through a brachial or femoral artery to the heart. The catheter, a flexible or pre-shaped tube approximately 32–43 inches (80–110 cm) long, is then inserted over the wire and threaded to the arterial side of the heart. The patient may experience pressure as the catheter is threaded into the heart. The contrast agent, or dye, used for imaging is then injected so that the physician can view the heart and surrounding vessels. The patient may experience a hot, flushed feeling or slight nausea following injection of the contrast medium. Depending on the type of catheterization (left or right heart) and the area being imaged, different catheters with various shapes and ends are used.

The radiographic/fluoroscopic system has an x-ray subsystem and video system with viewing monitors that allow the physician to observe the procedure in real time using fluoroscopy as well as taking still x rays for documentation purposes. Most newer systems use a digital angiography system that allows images to be recorded, manipulated, and stored digitally on a computer.

The procedure usually lasts two or three hours. If further intervention is necessary, an angioplasty, stent implantation, or other procedure can be performed. At the end of the catheterization, the catheter and sheath are removed, and the puncture site is closed using a sealing device or manual compression to stop the bleeding. One commonly used sealing device is called Perclose, which allows the doctor to sew up the hole in the groin. Other devices use collagen seals to close the hole in the femoral artery.

Diagnosis/Preparation

Before undergoing cardiac catheterization, the patient may have had other noninvasive diagnostic tests, including an **electrocardiogram** (ECG), **echocardiography**, computed tomography (CT), **magnetic resonance imaging** (MRI), laboratory studies (e.g., blood work), and/or nuclear medicine cardiac imaging. The results of these noninvasive tests may have indicated a need for cardiac catheterization to confirm a suspected cardiac condition, further define the severity of a previously diagnosed condition, or establish the need for an interventional procedure (e.g., cardiac surgery).

Patients should give the physician or nurse a complete list of their regular medications, including **aspirin** and **nonsteroidal anti-inflammatory drugs** (NSAIDs), because they can affect blood clotting. Diabetics who are taking either metformin or insulin to control their diabetes should inform the physician, as these drugs may need to have their dosages changed before the procedure. Patients should also notify staff members of any allergies to shellfish containing iodine, iodine itself, or the dyes commonly used as contrast agents before cardiac catheterization.

Because cardiac catheterization is considered surgery, the patient will be instructed to fast for at least six hours prior to the procedure. A mild sedative may be administered about an hour before the procedure to help the patient relax. If the catheter is to be inserted through the groin, the area around the patient's groin will be shaved and cleansed with an antiseptic solution.

Aftercare

While cardiac catheterization may be performed on an outpatient basis, the patient requires close monitoring following the procedure; the patient may have to remain in the hospital for up to 24 hours. The patient will be instructed to rest in bed for at least eight hours immediately after the test. If the catheter was inserted into a vein or artery in the leg or groin area, the leg will be kept extended for four to six hours. If a vein or artery in the arm was used to insert the catheter, the arm will need to remain extended for a minimum of three hours.

Most doctors advise patients to avoid heavy lifting or vigorous **exercise** for several days after cardiac catheterization. Those whose occupation involves a high level of physical activity should ask the doctor when they could safely return to work. In most cases, a hard ridge will form over the incision site that diminishes as the site heals. A bluish discoloration under the skin often occurs at the point of insertion but usually fades within two weeks. The incision site may bleed during the first 24 hours following surgery. The patient may apply pressure to the site with a clean tissue or cloth for 10–15 minutes to stop the bleeding.

The patient should be instructed to call the doctor at once if tenderness, fever, shaking, or chills develop, which may indicate an infection. Other symptoms requiring medical attention include severe pain or discoloration in the leg, which may indicate that a blood vessel was damaged.

Risks

Cardiac catheterization is categorized as an invasive procedure that involves the heart, its valves, and coronary arteries, in addition to a large artery in the arm or leg. Cardiac catheterization is contraindicated (not advised) for patients with the following conditions:

- a bleeding disorder, or anticoagulation treatment with Coumadin (sodium warfarin), which may adversely affect bleeding and clotting during the catheterization procedure

- renal insufficiency or poor kidney functioning (especially in diabetic patients), which may worsen following angiography

- severe uncontrolled hypertension

- severe peripheral vascular disease that limits access to the arteries

- untreated active infections, severe anemia, electrolyte imbalances, or coexisting illnesses that may affect recovery or survival

- endocarditis (an inflammatory infection of the heart's lining that often affects the valves)

Radiation hazards

Cardiac catheterization involves radiation exposure for staff members as well as the patient. The patient's dose of radiation is minimized by using lead shielding in the form of blankets or pads over certain body parts and by choosing the appropriate dose during fluoroscopy. To monitor staff members' exposure to radiation, they wear radiation badges that detect exposure and lead aprons that shield the body. The radiographic/fluoroscopic system may be equipped with movable lead shields that do not interfere with access to the patient and are placed between staff members and the source of radiation during the procedure.

Morbidity and mortality rates

As with all invasive procedures, cardiac catheterization involves some risks. The most serious complications include stroke and myocardial infarction. Other complications include cardiac arrhythmias, pericardial tamponade, vessel injury, and renal failure. One study demonstrated a total risk of major complications under 2% for all patients. The risk of death from cardiac catheterization has been demonstrated at 0.11%. The most common complications resulting from cardiac catheterization are vascular related, including external bleeding at the arterial puncture site, hematomas, and pseudoaneurysms.

The patient may be given anticoagulant medications to lower the risk of developing an arterial blood clot (thrombosis) or of blood clots forming and traveling through the body (embolization).

The risk of complications from cardiac catheterization is higher in patients over the age of 60, those who have severe heart failure, or those with advanced valvular disease.

Allergic reactions related to the contrast agent (dye) and anesthetics may occur in some patients during cardiac catheterization. Allergic reactions may range from minor hives and swelling to severe shock. Patients with allergies to seafood or penicillin are at a higher risk of allergic reaction; giving antihistamines prior to the procedure may reduce the occurrence of allergic reactions to contrast agents.

Normal results

Normal findings from a cardiac catheterization will indicate no abnormalities in the size or configuration of the heart chamber, the motion or thickness of its walls, the direction of blood flow, or motion of the valves. Smooth and regular outlines indicate normal structure of the coronary arteries.

The measurement of intracardiac pressures, or the pressure in the heart's chambers and vessels, is an essential part of the catheterization procedure. Pressure readings that are higher than normal are significant for a patient's overall diagnosis. Pressure readings that are lower, other than those resulting from shock, are usually not significant.

The ejection fraction is also determined by performing a cardiac catheterization. The ejection fraction is a comparison of the quantity of blood ejected from the heart's left ventricle during its contraction phase with the quantity of blood remaining at the end of the left ventricle's relaxation phase. The cardiologist will look for a normal ejection fraction reading of 60–70%.

Abnormal results are obtained by viewing the still and live motion x rays during cardiac catheterization for evidence of coronary artery disease, poor heart function, disease of the heart valves, and septal defects.

The most prominent sign of coronary artery disease is narrowing or blockage (stenosis) in the coronary arteries, with narrowing greater than 50% considered significant. A clear indication for intervention by angioplasty or surgery is a finding of significant narrowing of the left main coronary artery and/or blockage or severe narrowing in the high left anterior descending coronary artery.

A finding of impaired wall motion is an additional indicator of coronary artery disease, an aneurysm, an enlarged heart, or a congenital heart problem. Using an ejection fraction test that measures wall motion, cardiologists regard an ejection fraction reading under 35% as increasing the risk of complications while also decreasing the possibility of a successful long- or short-term outcome from surgery.

Detecting the difference in pressure above and below the heart valve can verify the presence of valvular disease. The greater the narrowing, the higher the difference in pressure.

To confirm the presence of septal defects, measurements are taken of the oxygen content on both the left and right sides of the heart. The right heart pumps unoxygenated blood to the lungs, and the left heart pumps blood containing oxygen from the lungs to the rest of the body. Elevated oxygen levels on the right side indicate the presence of a left-to-right atrial or **ventricular shunt**. Low oxygen levels on the left side indicate the presence of a right-to-left shunt.

Alternatives

Other methods of visualization are available that limit radiation exposure, by using **ultrasound** imaging to observe the coronary arteries. Imaging of general cardiac architecture and valvular function can be visualized by noninvasive cardiac ultrasound. Cardiac ultrasound and Doppler ultrasound can be used together to observe valvular insufficiency and stenosis. Areas of poor myocardial function can also be evaluated by ultrasound.

Nuclear medicine scans of the heart can show the perfusion of blood to a region of the myocardium. If blockages of the coronary artery exist, blood flow will be reduced. By adding a radioactive marker to the blood, images are generated to show areas of poor perfusion. Combined with exercise, these tests can accurately demonstrate cardiovascular disease. However, the imaging process can take several hours, and the patient is still internally exposed to high levels of radiation.

Resources

BOOKS

Grainger R. G., et al. *Grainger & Allison's Diagnostic Radiology: A Textbook of Medical Imaging.* 4th ed. Philadelphia: Saunders, 2001.
Libby, P., et al. *Braunwald's Heart Disease.* 8th ed. Philadelphia: Saunders, 2007.
Mettler, F. A. *Essentials of Radiology.* 2nd ed. Philadelphia: Saunders, 2005.

PERIODICALS

Norris, Teresa G. "Principles of Cardiac Catheterization." *Radiologic Technology* 72, no. 2 (November–December 2000): 109–136.

ORGANIZATIONS

American College of Cardiology. Heart House, 9111 Old Georgetown Road, Bethesda, MD 20814-1699. (800) 253-4636. http://www.acc.org (accessed March 8, 2008).
American Heart Association National Center. 7272 Greenville Avenue, Dallas, TX 75231. (800) AHA-USA1. http://www.americanheart.org (accessed March 8, 2008).

OTHER

Cardiology Channel. *Cardiac Catheterization.* http://www.cardiologychannel.com/cardiaccath/ (accessed March 8, 2008).

Jennifer E. Sisk, MA
Allison J. Spiwak, MSBME
Rosalyn Carson-DeWitt, MD

Cardiac event monitor

Definition

A cardiac event monitor is an electronic device that attaches to the body and records the rhythm of the heart while the patient is experiencing pathological symptoms. The cardiac event monitor allows recording of the heart without the inconvenience of staying in the hospital or undergoing invasive procedures.

Purpose

Patients who have symptoms of heart disease such as angina (pain from a lack of oxygen flow to the heart) or arrhythmias (irregular heartbeats) use the cardiac event monitor to record the rhythm of their heart while they are experiencing the symptoms. The cardiac event monitor was designed to record pathological events in real time, allowing for continuous heart monitoring over long periods of time. The heart is thus effectively monitored without necessity for invasive procedures or staying in the hospital. The longer the cardiac event monitor is worn by the patient, the greater the chances of catching and recording the abnormal heart rhythm of a spontaneous cardiac event. Cardiac event monitors were designed as a useful tool for patients who experience symptoms that do not occur regularly, or involve fainting, and so are difficult to analyze.

Demographics

Cardiac event monitors are used to aid in the diagnosis of heart conditions that cause irregular rhythms. They are designed for a demographic of patients that do not experience symptoms on a predictable, daily basis. Cardiac event monitors can be used for patients with abnormal heart rhythms regardless of age, race, or gender.

Description

Cardiac event monitors allow the recording of heart rhythms over long periods of time. When used properly, the monitor is able to record information about heart rhythms that assists cardiologists in diagnosing different types of heart disease. There are multiple types and designs of cardiac event monitors. Each type offers unique features.

Heart Rhythm

The heart is a contracting muscle that pumps blood to the body tissues. Oxygenated blood leaves the heart and supplies tissues with the oxygen necessary for life. Deoxygenated blood carrying carbon dioxide waste travels from the tissues back to the heart. The heart sends the deoxygenated blood carrying carbon dioxide to the lungs to be oxygenated. The oxygenated blood from the lungs returns to the heart and the cycle begins again. During this cycle of pumping blood, valves in the heart create the sound of the heartbeat as they close.

The heart rhythm should be a regular pattern of heartbeats occurring at a regular rate that is considered normal. Many types of disease may cause an irregularity in this pattern. A cardiac arrhythmia is an irregular rhythm of heartbeats that does not allow the heart to pump blood properly. Cardiac arrhythmias may cause symptoms of palpitations (pounding heart), syncope (fainting), chest pain, dizziness, lightheadedness, shortness of breath, weakness, or fatigue. When a cardiac arrhythmia does not occur regularly and so is difficult to diagnose with an **electrocardiogram** (ECG) reading in a hospital setting, cardiac event monitors may be utilized to help elucidate the relationship between a patient's symptoms and the heart rhythms recorded. Cardiac event monitors may be used on patients with different types of heart conditions, including arrhythmias, myocardial infarctions (heart attacks), stroke, or during recovery from **coronary artery bypass graft surgery** (CABG).

Holter Cardiac Event Monitors

A Holter monitor is a general type of **cardiac monitor** which records heart rhythm continuously for 24 to 48 hours. Holter monitors are useful when a patient experiences symptoms on a daily basis. Holter monitors record each heartbeat, using electrodes attached to the chest. Patients using Holter monitors go through their normal daily activities (except bathing) and keep a diary of how they feel physically during the monitoring time period. When the monitoring time period is over, the Holter monitor and the accompanying diary are turned in to the diagnostic center for evaluation of the recorded results. While Holter monitors are effective, patients whose symptoms occur less frequently require the cardiac event monitor.

Looping Memory Cardiac Event Monitors

Cardiac event monitors are small black boxes attached to several wires with electrodes. The cardiac event monitor is monitoring heart rhythm as the patient goes through their daily activities. Cardiac event monitors do not record heart rhythm for more than a few minutes at a time in a cycling stream of memory. When the patient experiences symptoms it is known as a cardiac event. The patient immediately presses a button on the event monitor that records the activity of the heart while the symptom is occurring. Many cardiac events are fleeting experiences and it may take the patient a moment to press the event button, therefore, cardiac event monitors have been designed with a continuous memory "loop" that allows the recording to backtrack about 30 seconds to a minute before the event button was pressed, and obtain a complete picture of the cardiac event. If the event button is not pressed, no permanent record will be kept of the event within the basic monitor design. Some types of cardiac event monitors have been preset to record cardiac events if the heart goes into an arrhythmia and circumvent the need for the event button; however, these monitors may be less specific in the data they gather.

Cardiac event monitors are often used for 30 days. For this reason, cardiac events need to be transmitted to the diagnostic center frequently during the monitoring time frame, rather than at the end of the monitoring period. Cardiac event monitors can have their data transmitted via a telephone line to a computer system that turns the transmitted data into an ECG reading. Essentially, the cardiac event monitor provides the ability to obtain an ECG of an irregularly occurring symptom that would likely otherwise be missed in an office visit. Since transmission of data is done approximately every other time a symptom is experienced, the cardiologist is able to keep track of the patient's condition in real time over the duration of the cardiac event monitoring. Event monitors notify physicians in a timely manner if intervention is needed for a serious cardiac arrhythmia that might have otherwise have been missed.

Implantable Cardiac Event Monitors

Implantable cardiac event monitors were designed for use in patients with unexplained syncope that may have a heart-related cause. The implantable monitors are surgically placed just under the skin of the chest within a one-inch incision. The implantation procedure involves only **local anesthesia**. Implantable cardiac event monitors are set to specific heart rhythm limits in order to obtain a record of heart events during syncope episodes. The implantable design that does not require pressing an event button is critical to record events that involve a patient losing

QUESTIONS TO ASK YOUR DOCTOR

- Why do I need a cardiac event monitor?
- Which type of cardiac event monitor will I be using?
- What are the advantages and disadvantages of this type of monitor over other types?
- How should I prepare for the cardiac event monitor?
- Are there any restrictions on my daily activity with the cardiac event monitor?
- How do I use the cardiac event monitor?
- How long will I use the cardiac event monitor?
- When can I expect to go over the results of my cardiac event monitor?
- Could any of my prescription or nonprescription medications, nutritional, or herbal supplements be causing my symptoms or affect the results?

consciousness. After a period of time, the monitor is removed and its data is analyzed by a diagnostic center.

Mobile Cardiovascular Telemetry

Cardiac event monitors have been designed for use with a wireless cell phone system that transmits data from the monitor without the need of calling in a transmission to a diagnostic center. These devices act as both a monitor and an alarm system for patients with potentially life threatening cardiac arrhythmias. The remote diagnostic center and patient's physician automatically receive daily reports of the patient's heart activity. In addition to daily reports, any urgent, life-threatening data gathered by the device is immediately transmitted. In this way, the remote diagnostic center and physician are notified relatively quickly in urgent circumstances and intervention can be made in a timely manner.

Results Obtained with Cardiac Event Monitors

The recordings obtained by cardiac event monitors are sent to cardiac event monitor diagnostic centers and converted into ECG readings. Trained health care professionals interpret the ECG readings. Cardiologists are heart doctors that specialize in diagnosing heart disease, and use ECGs as tools to assist in a patient's diagnosis. Cardiac event monitors alone cannot diagnose heart conditions, but only display the heart rhythm a patient is experiencing at the time of symptom onset. Cardiologists may use ECGs to help narrow down the diagnosis whether or not the condition is caused by an arrhythmia.

Risks Associated with Cardiac Event Monitors

Cardiac event monitors are useful tools, but may not be sensitive enough to catch every cardiac event or specific enough to detail it well. Different designs have different levels of sensitivity in picking up events and give different levels of detail about the events they record. Even with designs in which event recording is automatic, some data may be missed.

Resources

BOOKS

Andreoli, Thomas E., Charles C. J. Carpenter, Robert Griggs, and Joseph Loscalzo *Cecil Essentials of Medicine,* 6th ed. Philadelphia: Saunders, 2004.

Costanzo, Linda S. *Physiology,* 3rd ed. Philadelphia: Saunders, 2006.

OTHER

Chang, Bernard S. Steven C. Schachter, and Donald L. Schomer. "Event Monitoring," in *Atlas of Ambulatory EEG.* 2005. http://books.google.com/books?id =
MOcDuNt9kqwC&pg = PA20&dq = cardiac + event + monitoring&sig = zkviXpNDvhViSqYH5La-ViTBStiE (April 9, 2008).

Committee on Congenital Cardiac Defects of the Council on Cardiovascular Disease in the Young. "What are Holter, Event, and Transtelephonic Monitors?" American Heart Association. http://www.americanheart.org/presenter.jhtml?identifier = 3005149 (April 9, 2008).

Khandpur, Raghbir Singh. *Biomedical Instrumentation: Technology and Applications.* New York: McGraw-Hill Professional, 2004.http://books.google.com/books?id = BMNLEoz8S0MC&pg = PA257&dq = cardiac + event + monitoring&sig = NCQA7Q4rsC4nuhGoGO-VDk2JvAI (April 9, 2008).

Zeevi, Bejamin. "Telecardiology," in *Telemedicine and Teledermatology,* edited by Günter Burg. Basel, Switzerland: Karger, 2002. http://books.google.com/books?id = F2gy QlDgptgC&pg = PA118&dq = cardiac + event + monitoring&sig = jDUtACUMedc0-0XftNuVMQydKwI (April 9, 2008).

Maria Basile, Ph.D.

Cardiac exercise stress testing *see* **Stress test**
Cardiac mapping *see* **Electrophysiology study of the heart**

Cardiac marker tests

Definition

Cardiac marker tests identify blood chemicals associated with myocardial infarction (MI), commonly known as a heart attack. The myocardium is the middle layer of the heart wall composed of heart muscle. Infarction is tissue **death** caused by an interruption in the blood supply to an area.

Purpose

Cardiac markers are types of blood-lab tests that help physicians assess acute coronary syndromes and identify and manage high-risk patients. Creatine kinase-MB (CK-MB), myoglobin, homocysteine, C-reactive protein (CRP), troponin T (cTnT), and troponin I (cTnI) are all types of cardiac markers used for assessment of the suspected acute myocardial infarction. CK-MB, cTnT, and cTnI may also be used to identify and manage high-risk patients.

Precautions

C-reactive protein results may be affected by the use of oral contraceptives, **nonsteroidal anti-inflammatory drugs** (NSAIDs), steroids, salicylates, and intrauterine devices (IUDs). Homocysteine levels may be affected by smoking, diabetes, and coffee.

Description

Creatine kinase (CK)

Creatine kinase is an enzyme responsible for transferring a phosphate group from ATP (adenosine triphosphate) to creatine. It is composed of M and/or B subunits that form CK-MM, CK-MB, and CK-BB isoenzymes. Total CK (the activity of the MM, MB, and BB isoenzymes) is not myocardial-specific. However, the MB isoenzyme (also called CK-2) comprises about 40% of the CK activity in cardiac muscle and 2% or less of the activity in most muscle groups and other tissues. In the proper clinical setting, MB is both a sensitive and specific marker for heart attack. MB usually becomes abnormal three to four hours after a heart attack, peaks in 10–24 hours, and returns to normal within 72 hours; however, an elevated serum MB may occur in people with severe skeletal muscle damage (such as in muscular dystrophy or a crush injury) and renal (kidney) failure. In such cases, the CK index (MB divided by total CK) is very helpful. If the index is under 4%, a nonmyocardial cause of a high MB should be suspected. CK-MB is considered the benchmark for cardiac markers of myocardial injury.

CK-MB forms can be used to determine whether **thrombolytic therapy** (such as treatment with tissue plasminogen activator to dissolve a blood clot in the coronary artery) has succeeded. MB forms are different molecular forms of MB found in the circulation. When MB is released into the blood, part of the M subunit is removed by an enzyme in the plasma. This results in a molecule called CK-2_1. This is the prevalent form of MB in the blood. CK-2_2 is the unmodified cardiac form of MB. After successful thrombolytic therapy, the unmodified form of MB is rapidly flushed into the blood, causing it to become the dominant form.

Myoblobin

Myoglobin is a protein found in both skeletal and myocardial muscle. It is released rapidly after tissue injury and may be elevated as early as one hour after myocardial injury, though it may also be elevated due to skeletal muscle trauma. However, if myoglobin values do not rise within three to four hours after a person shows acute symptoms, it is highly unlikely that he or she had a heart attack.

Troponin T and troponin I

Troponin C, I, and T are proteins that form the thin filaments of muscle fibers and regulate the

movement of contractile proteins in muscle tissue. Skeletal and cardiac forms are structurally distinct, and antibodies can be produced that react only with the cardiac forms of troponin I and troponin T.

Cardiac troponin T (cTnT) and cardiac troponin I (cTnI) are the newest additions to the list of cardiac markers. Cardiac troponins are specific to heart muscle. They have enabled the development of laboratory tests that can detect heart muscle injury with great sensitivity and specificity. While these markers have been used mainly to aid in the diagnosis of chest-pain patients with nondiagnostic electrocardiograms, they also help doctors determine a prognosis for patients who have had a heart attack. According to the American Heart Association, "… it's possible that the results of a troponin test could be used to identify people at either low risk or high risk for later, serious heart problems."

C-reactive protein (CRP)

CRP is a protein found at elevated levels in serum or plasma during inflammatory processes. CRP binds to part of the capsule of *Streptococcus pneumoniae*. It is a sensitive marker of acute and chronic inflammation and infection, and in such cases is increased several hundred-fold. Several studies have demonstrated that CRP levels are useful in predicting the risk for a thrombotic event (such as a blood clot causing heart attack). These studies suggest that a high-sensitivity assay for CRP be used that is capable of measuring the very low level normally found in serum (0.1–2.5 mg/L). Heart patients who have persistent CRP levels between 4 and 10 mg/L, with clinical evidence of low-grade inflammation, should be considered to be at increased risk for thrombosis (blood clots). People can be stratified into four groups of increased risk based on their CRP levels.

Homocysteine

Homocysteine is an amino acid. According to the American Heart Association, studies have shown that too much homocysteine in the blood is related to a higher risk of coronary heart disease, stroke, and peripheral vascular disease; and that it may also have an effect on atherosclerosis. High levels of homocysteine are the result of a lack of certain B vitamins, inheritance, or dietary excess and have been implicated in vascular-wall injury. It is believed that laboratory testing for plasma homocysteine levels can improve the assessment of risk, particularly in patients with a personal or family history of cardiovascular disease, but in whom the well-established risk factors (smoking, high blood cholesterol, high blood pressure, physical inactivity, obesity, and diabetes) do not exist.

Preparation

These tests require a sample of blood, which is typically obtained via a standard vein puncture procedure. Homocysteine tests require the patient to fast before the test.

Aftercare

Discomfort or bruising may occur at the puncture site, or the person may feel dizzy or faint. Applying pressure to the puncture site until the bleeding stops reduces bruising. Warm packs to the puncture site can relieve discomfort.

Risks

There are no complications associated with these tests.

Results

Normal results vary, based on the laboratory and method used. Unless otherwise specified, the following information is from the American College of Cardiology and the American Heart Association.

- Total CK: Reference value is 38–174 units/L for men and 96–140 units/L for women. The values begin to rise within four to six hours and peak at 24 hours. Values return to normal within three to four days.
- CK-MB: Reference value is 10–13 units/L. The values begin to rise within three to four hours and peak at 10–24 hours. Values return to normal within two to four days.
- Troponin T: Reference value is less than 0.1 ng/mL. The values begin to rise within two to four hours and peak at 10–24 hours. Values return to normal within five to 14 days.
- Troponin I: Reference value is less than 1.5 ng/mL. The values begin to rise within two to four hours and peak at 10–24 hours. Values return to normal within five to 10 days.
- CK-MB forms: Reference value is a ratio of 1.5 or greater. The values begin to rise within two to four hours and peak at six to 12 hours. Values return to normal within 12–24 hours.
- Myoglobin: Reference value is less than 110 ng/mL. The values begin to rise within one to two hours and peak at four to eight hours. Values return to normal within 12–24 hours.
- Homocysteine: The normal fasting level for plasma is 5–15 micromol/L. Moderate, intermediate, and severe hyperhomocysteinemia refer to concentrations between 16 and 30, between 31 and 100, and less than 100 micromol/L, respectively.
- C-reactive protein: According to the U.S. Food and Drug Administration, in healthy people, reference values are below 5 mg/dL; in various diseases, this threshold is often exceeded within four to eight hours after an acute inflammatory event, with CRP values reaching approximately 20–500 mg/dL.

Resources

BOOKS

McPherson, Richard A. and Matthew R. Pincus, eds. *Henry's Clinical Diagnosis and Management by Laboratory Methods,* 21st ed. Philadelphia: Saunders, 2007.

Wallach, Jacques. *Interpretation of Diagnostic Tests,* 8th ed. Philadelphia: Lippincott Williams & Wilkins, 2006.

Wu, Alan H. B., ed. *Cardiac Markers,* 2nd ed. Totowa, NJ: Humana Press, 2003.

PERIODICALS

Kucia, M., D. Buddhadeb, G. Hunt, Yiru Guo, et al. "Cells Expressing Early Cardiac Markers Reside in the Bone Marrow and Are Mobilized Into the Peripheral Blood After Myocardial Infarction," *Circulation Research* 95 (November 2004): 1191–1199.

ORGANIZATIONS

American Heart Association, 7272 Greenville Avenue, Dallas, TX, 75231, (800) 242-8721, http://www. americanheart.org.

Victoria E. DeMoranville
Mark A. Best
Robert Bockstiegel

Cardiac monitor

Definition

The cardiac monitor is a device that shows the electrical and pressure waveforms of the cardiovascular system for measurement and treatment. Parameters specific to respiratory function can also be measured. Because electrical connections are made between the cardiac monitor and the patient, it is kept at the patient's bedside.

Purpose

The cardiac monitor continuously displays the cardiac **electrocardiogram** (EKG) tracing. Additional monitoring components allow cardiovascular pressures and cardiac output to be monitored and displayed as required for patient diagnosis and treatment. Oxygen saturation of the arterial blood can also be monitored continuously. Most commonly used in emergency rooms and critical care areas, bedside monitors can be interconnected to allow for continual observation of several patients from a central display. Continuous cardiovascular and pulmonary monitoring allows for prompt identification and initiation of treatment.

Description

The monitor provides a visual display of many patient parameters. It can be set to sound an alarm if any parameter changes outside of an expected range determined by the physician. Parameters to be monitored may include, but are not limited to, electrocardiogram, noninvasive blood pressure, intravascular pressures, cardiac output, arterial blood oxygen saturation, and blood temperature.

Equipment required for continuous cardiac monitoring includes the cardiac monitor, cables, and disposable supplies such as electrode patches, pressure transducers, a pulmonary artery catheter (Swan-Ganz catheter), and an arterial blood saturation probe.

KEY TERMS

Artifact—Extra electrical activity typically caused by interference.

Cardiomyopathies—Diseases of the heart muscle; usually refers to a disease of obscure etiology.

Electrodes—Adhesive pads that are placed on the skin and attached to the leads.

Lead—Color-coded wires that connect the electrode to the monitor cable.

QRST complex—The combined waves of an electrocardiogram for monitoring the heart.

Preparation

As the cardiac monitor is most commonly used to monitor electrical activity of the heart, the patient can expect the following preparations. The sites selected for electrode placement on the skin will be shaved and cleaned causing surface abrasion for better contact between the skin and electrode. The electrode will have a layer of gel protected by a film, which is removed prior to placing the electrode to the skin. Electrode patches will be placed near or on the right arm, right leg, left arm, left leg, and the center left side of the chest. The cable will be connected to the electrode patches for the measurement of a five-lead electrocardiogram. Additional configurations are referred to as three-lead and 12-lead electrocardiograms. If noninvasive blood pressure is being measured, a blood pressure cuff will be placed around the patient's arm or leg. The blood pressure cuff will be set to inflate manually or automatically. If manual inflation is chosen, the cuff will only inflate at the prompting of the health care provider, after which a blood pressure will be displayed. During automatic operation, the blood pressure cuff will inflate at timed intervals and the display will update at the end of each measurement.

Disposable pressure transducers require a reference to atmosphere, called zeroing, which is completed before monitoring patient pressures. This measurement will occur once the patient is comfortably positioned since the transducer must be level with the measurement point. The pressure transducer will then be connected to the indwelling catheter. It may be necessary for as many as four or five pressure transducers to be connected to the patient.

The arterial blood saturation probe will be placed on the finger, toe, ear, or nasal septum of the patient, providing as little discomfort as possible, while achieving a satisfactory measurement.

Aftercare

After connecting all equipment, the health care provider will observe the monitor and evaluate the quality of the tracings, while making size and position adjustments as needed. The provider will confirm that the monitor is detecting each heartbeat by taking an apical pulse and comparing the pulse to the digital display. The upper and lower alarm limits should be set according to physician orders, and the alarm activated. A printout may be recorded for the medical record, and labeled with patient name, room number, date, time, and interpretation of the strip.

Maintenance and replacement of the disposable components may be necessary as frequently as every eight hours, or as required to maintain proper operation. The arterial saturation probe can be repositioned to suit patient comfort and to obtain a tracing. All connections will be treated in a gentle manner to avoid disruption of the signal and to avoid injury to the patient.

Normal results

The monitor will provide waveforms and/or numeric values associated with the patient status. These may include, but are not limited to, heart rate, arterial blood pressure, central venous pressure, pulmonary artery pressure, pulmonary capillary wedge pressure, left atrial pressure, cardiac output, arterial blood saturation, and blood temperature. Furthermore, these values can be used to calculate other values, or parameters, or used to diagnose and treat the patient's condition.

Patient movement may cause measurement errors; the patient will be requested to remain motionless. Depending on the mobility of the patient, assistance should be provided by the health care provider prior to changing from a laying down position to sitting or standing.

As the patient's condition improves, the amount of monitoring equipment may be decreased. The electrocardiogram and arterial blood saturation probe should be expect to remain attached until discharge is imminent.

Resources

BOOKS

Cahill, Matthew. "Providing Cardiovascular Care." In *Nursing Photobook.* Springhouse, PA: Springhouse Corporation, 1996.

Griffiths, Mark. *Management of Cardiovascular Conditions of Adults in Acute Care,* 1st ed. Malden, MA: Blackwell Publishers, 2008.

Marriott, Henry J. L. *Pearls and Pitfalls in Electrocardiography: Pithy, Practical Pointers,* 2nd ed. Baltimore: Williams & Wilkins, 1998.

Milford, Cheryl, and Gladys Purvis. "Cardiovascular Care." In *Nursing Procedures,* 3rd ed. Springhouse, PA: Springhouse Corporation, 2000.

Skeehan, Thomas, and Michael Jopling. "Monitoring the Cardiac Surgical Patient." In *A Practical Approach to Cardiac Anesthesia,* 3rd ed., edited by Frederick A. Hensley, Donald E. Martin, and Glenn P. Gravlee. Philadelphia, PA: Lippincott Williams & Wilkins, 2003.

Woods, Susan, Erika Sivarajan, Sandra Adams Motzer, and Elizabeth Bridges. *Cardiac Nursing,* 5th ed. Philadelphia: Lippincott, 2004.

PERIODICALS

Perry, A., et al."Measuring the Costs and Benefits of Heart Disease Monitoring." *Heart* 83 (June 2000): 651–656.

OTHER

Advanced Cardiac Monitoring: Ventricular Ectopy vs. Aberrancy. Videotape. RamEx Inc., 1987.

ORGANIZATIONS

American Association of Critical-Care Nurses, 101 Columbia, Aliso Viejo, CA, 92656-4109, (800) 899-2226, http://www.aacn.org/.

The American College of Cardiology, Heart House, 2400 N. Street NW, Washington, DC, 20037, (800) 253-4636, http://www.acc.org.

American Heart Association, 7272 Greenville Ave., Dallas, TX, 75231, (800) 242-8721, http://www. american heart.org.

Applied Biometrics, 501 East Highway Thirteen, Suite 108, Burnsville, MN, 55337, (952) 890-1123

Maggie Boleyn, R.N., B.S.N.
Allison Spiwak, M.S.
Laura Jean Cataldo, R.N., Ed.D.

Cardiopulmonary bypass machine *see* Heart-lung machines

Cardiopulmonary resuscitation

Definition

Cardiopulmonary resuscitation, commonly called CPR, combines rescue breathing (one person breathing into another person) and chest compression in a lifesaving procedure performed when a person has stopped breathing or a person's heart has stopped beating.

Purpose

When performed quickly enough, CPR can save lives in such emergencies as loss of consciousness, heart attacks or heart "arrests," electric shock, drowning, excessive bleeding, drug overdose, and other conditions in which there is no breathing or no pulse. The purpose of CPR is to bring oxygen to the victim's lungs and to keep blood circulating so oxygen gets to every part of the body. When a person is deprived of oxygen, permanent brain damage can begin in as little as four minutes and **death** can follow only minutes later.

Description

There are three physical symptoms that indicate a need for CPR to be performed immediately and for emergency medical support to be called: unconsciousness, not breathing, and no pulse detected.

Unconsciousness

Unconsciousness is when the victim seems to be asleep but has lost all awareness and is not able to respond to questions, touch, or gentle shaking. A sleeping person will usually respond to a loud noise, shouting, or gentle shaking. An unconscious person will not respond to noise or shaking. When unconscious, a person can not cough or clear the throat, which may allow the windpipe to become blocked, causing suffocation and death. People with a major illness or injury or who have had recent surgery are at risk for losing consciousness. If a person has fainted, which is brief unconsciousness, the cause may be dehydration (lack of body fluids), low blood pressure, or low blood sugar. This is a temporary condition. If the victim is known to have diabetes, a bit of fruit juice may revive the person once they have regained consciousness.

Just before a person loses consciousness, symptoms may include:

- lack of response to voice or touch
- disorientation or stupor
- light-headedness
- headache
- sleepiness

Not breathing

Not breathing, which is also called apnea, is the lack of spontaneous breathing. It requires immediate medical attention. The victim may become limp and lifeless, have a seizure, or turn blue. Prolonged apnea is called respiratory arrest. In children, this can lead quickly to cardiac arrest in which the heart stops beating. In adults, cardiac arrest usually happens first and

then respiratory arrest. In adults, the common causes of apnea are obstructive sleep apnea (something blocks the airway during sleep), choking, drug overdose, near-drowning, head injury, heart irregularities (arrhythmia, fibrillation) or cardiac arrest, nervous system disorders, or metabolic disorders. In children the causes may be different, such as prematurity, bronchial disturbances or pneumonia, airway blockage or choking on a foreign object, holding the breath, seizures, meningitis, regurgitating food, or asthma attacks.

No pulse detected

If the rescuer is unable to detect a pulse or has difficulty feeling a pulse, it can be an indication of the use of improper technique by the rescuer, or it may be due to shock or cardiac arrest in the victim. If a sudden, severe decrease occurs in pulse quality (such as pulse weakness) or pulse rate (how many beats in a minute) when other symptoms are also present, life-threatening shock is suspected. The rescuer may need to explain to a doctor or medical professional where on the victim's body the pulse was measured, whether or not the pulse is weak or absent, and what other symptoms are present.

Medical help and CPR are needed immediately if any of these symptoms are found. Time is critical. A local emergency number should be called immediately. If more than one person is available to help, one person can call 911 or a local emergency medical service, while the other person begins CPR. If needed, the emergency dispatcher (the person who picks up emergency 911 calls) can give step-by-step CPR instructions over the telephone. Local medical personnel, staff at hospitals and fire departments, and members of the American Heart Association teach CPR courses. If a critically ill patient or postoperative patient is being cared for at home, it is a good idea for a family member to take a CPR course to be better prepared to help in the event of an emergency.

The steps usually followed in *adult* CPR by a layperson are as follows:

1. If the victim appears to be unconscious with either no breathing or no pulse, the person should be shaken or tapped gently to check for any movement. The victim should be spoken to loudly, asking if he or she is OK. If there is no response, the rescuer should leave to call 911 immediately, send someone to call for help, or call from a cell phone. If the rescuer is alone, they should call 911 before beginning CPR. If an automated external defibrillator (AED) is found close by, the rescuer should bring the AED back with them to the victim's side.

2. The victim should be placed on his or her back on a level surface such as the ground or the floor. The rescuer should kneel next to the victim and tilt the victim's head back. The rescuer should then put their ear to the victim's open mouth and look for chest movement, listen for air flowing through the mouth or nose, and feel for air on his or her cheek. If there is no breathing, they should pinch the victim's nose, make a seal over the victim's mouth with theirs, and give the victim a breath big enough to make the chest rise. The rescuer should use a CPR mask if there is one available. The rescuer should let the chest fall, then repeat the rescue breath once more. If the chest does not rise, the victim's head should be repositioned to help ensure the tongue is kept away from the windpipe, then the rescuer should try again to give a breath.

3. If the victim is found to be breathing and has perhaps fainted, he or she can be placed in the recovery position until medical assistance arrives. This is done by straightening the victim's legs and pulling the closest arm out away from the body with the elbow at a right angle (or three o'clock position), and the other arm across the chest. The far leg should be pulled up over the victim's body with the hip and knee bent. This allows the victim's body to be rolled onto its side. The head should be tilted back slightly to keep the windpipe open. The head should not be propped up.

4. If the victim is not breathing, the rescuer should begin chest compressions. Chest compressions are needed to restore circulation (the victim has no pulse). The rescuer should push down one and a half to two inches on the chest, placing the heel of one hand in the middle of the chest, putting the other hand on top of the first, and interlacing the fingers. When performing compressions, the rescuer should keep the elbows straight, center his or her shoulders over the victim, develop an up-and-down rhythm, and keep their hands firmly on the victim's chest. Compressions should be done on the center of the chest midway between the nipples. Compressions should be hard and fast, at a rate of 100 times per minute. The rescuer should perform 30 compressions at this rate, then give 2 breaths and the again, 30 compressions (this ratio is the same whether it is performed by one or by two people at the scene). The rescuer should allow the chest to completely recoil before the next compression. The sequence of 30 compressions and two breaths should continue to be repeated until professional medical help arrives. Note: If an AED is immediately available, deliver one shock if advised by the device, then begin CPR. If an AED is not available initially, but later becomes available and the person is still unresponsive, stop doing CPR and quickly follow the directions for using the AED.

Precautions

There are certain important precautions for rescuers to remember in order to protect the victim and get the best result from CPR. These include:

- Do not leave the victim alone.
- Do not give the victim anything to eat or drink.
- Avoid moving the victim's head or neck if spinal injury is a possibility. The person should be left as found if breathing freely. To check for breathing when spinal injury is suspected, the rescuer should only listen for breath by the victim's mouth and watch the chest for movement.
- Do not slap the victim's face, or throw water on the face to try and revive the person.
- Do not place a pillow under the victim's head.

The description above is not a substitute for CPR training and is not intended to be followed as a procedure.

Normal results

Successful CPR will restore breathing and circulation in the victim. Medical attention is required immediately even if successful CPR has been performed and the victim is breathing freely.

Prevention

Loss of consciousness is an emergency that is potentially life threatening. To avoid loss of consciousness and protect themselves from emergency situations, people at risk can follow these general guidelines:

- People with such conditions as diabetes or epilepsy should wear a medical alert tag or bracelet.
- People with diabetes should avoid situations that will lower their blood sugar level.
- People who feel weak, become dizzy or light-headed, or have ever fainted, should avoid standing in one place too long without moving.
- People who feel faint can lie down or sit with their heads lowered between their knees.
- Risk factors that contribute to heart disease should be reduced or eliminated. People can reduce risks if they stop smoking, lower blood pressure and cholesterol, lose excess weight, and reduce stress.
- Illegal recreational drugs should be avoided.
- Seeing a doctor regularly and being aware of any disease conditions or risk factors can help prevent or complicate illness, as can seeking and following the doctor's advice about diet and exercise.
- Using seat belts and driving carefully can help avoid accidental injury.
- People with poor eyesight or those who have difficulty walking because of disability, injury, or recovery from illness, can use a cane or other assistive device to help them avoid falls and injury.

Resources

BOOKS

Ornato, Joseph P. and Mary Ann Peberdy. *Cardiopulmonary Resuscitation,* 1st ed. Totowa, NJ: Humana Press, 2004.

Ribes, Ramon and Sergio Mejia Viana. *Cardiovascular English,* 1st ed. New York: Springer, 2008.

OTHER

American Heart Association. *Emergency Cardiovascular Care* [cited February 2008]. http://www.americanheart.org/presenter.jhtml?identifier=3011764.

ORGANIZATIONS

American CPR Training, 444 Sante Fe Drive #127, Encinitas, CA, 92024-5134, (760) 944-1048, http://www.cpr-training-classes.com.

American Heart Association, National Center, 7272 Greenville Avenue, Dallas, TX, 75231, (800) 242-8721, http://www.americanheart.org.

L Lee Culvert, Ph.D.
Laura Jean Cataldo, R.N., Ed.D.

Cardioversion

Definition

Cardioversion refers to the process of restoring the heart's normal rhythm either by applying a controlled electric shock to the exterior of the chest or by giving certain medications. The first type is called synchronized electrical cardioversion; the second is called pharmacologic or chemical cardioversion. Abnormal heart rhythms are called arrhythmias or dysrhythmias.

Purpose

When the heart beats too fast, blood no longer circulates effectively in the body. Cardioversion is used to stop this abnormal beating so that the heart can begin its normal rhythm and pump more efficiently.

Demographics

Cardioversion is used to treat many types of fast and/or irregular heart rhythms. Most often, cardioversion is used to treat atrial fibrillation or atrial flutter. Life-saving cardioversion can be used to treat ventricular tachycardia and ventricular fibrillation; implantable cardioverter-defibrillators (ICDs) are designed to treat these two conditions.

Abnormal heart rhythms are slightly more common in men than in women and the prevalence of abnormal heart rhythms, especially atrial fibrillation, increases with age. Atrial fibrillation is relatively uncommon in people under age 20 but affects 5% of the American population over 65, and 8% of the population over 80. It is responsible for 15–25% of all strokes.

Description

Synchronized electrical cardioversion

Elective synchronized electrical cardioversion is usually scheduled ahead of time. After arriving at the hospital, the patient will have an intravenous (IV) catheter placed in the arm to deliver medications and fluids. Oxygen may be given through a face mask.

In some people, a test called a transesophageal echocardiogram (TEE) may need to be performed before the cardioversion to make sure there are no blood clots in the heart.

A short-acting general anesthetic will be given through the IV to put the patient to sleep. During the

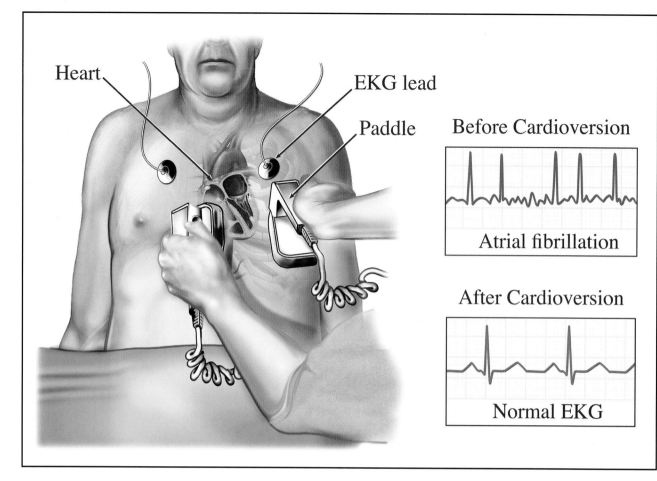

Heart   EKG lead

Paddle   Before Cardioversion

Atrial fibrillation

After Cardioversion

Normal EKG

Cardioversion. *(Nucleus Medical Art, Inc./Phototake. Reproduced by permission.)*

five or 10 minutes of anesthesia, an electric shock is delivered through paddles or patches placed on the exterior of the chest and sometimes on the back. It may be necessary for the doctor to administer the shock two or three times to stop the abnormal heartbeat and allow the heart to resume a normal rhythm. During the procedure, the patient's breathing, blood pressure, and heart rhythm are continuously monitored.

Pharmacologic cardioversion

Pharmacologic, or chemical, cardioversion is a less immediate method of restoring normal hear rhythm, and is somewhat less effective than electrical cardioversion, having a success rate between 60% and 80%. It has the advantage of being simpler and more convenient, particularly for patients who are afraid of electrical devices. The patient does not need to undergo anesthesia and can receive the drugs immediately after eating; there is no need to fast for several hours.

There are two basic groups of drugs given in pharmacologic cardioversion: those given to control

the heart rate and those given to normalize the heart rhythm. The first group includes such medications as digoxin (Lanoxin), diltiazem (Cardizem), verapamil (Calan), esmolol (Brevibloc), metoprolol (Lopressor), and propranolol (Inderal). These drugs may be given either intravenously or orally. With the exception of digoxin, which takes about 30 minutes to take effect, these drugs begin to work in 5–7 minutes.

Drugs given to normalize the heart rhythm are called antiarrhythmics. Quinidine (Quinaglute), the oldest drug in this group, is given by mouth, while procainamide, propafenone (Rythmol), flecainide (Tambocor), amiodarone (Cordarone), sotalol (Betapace), dofetilide (Tikosyn) and ibutilide (Corvert) may be given intravenously or orally. Unlike the drugs given to control the heart rate, these medications take longer to work, one hour for procainamide and ibutilide, and 3–8 hours for the others. These drugs should be administered in a hospital setting where the patient can be monitored. Dofetilide can be prescribed only by physicians who have had special training in the risks and side effects of the drug.

Diagnosis/Preparation

Diagnosis of abnormal heart rhythms

A doctor may be able to detect an irregular heart beat during a physical exam by taking the patient's pulse. In addition, the diagnosis may be based upon the presence of certain symptoms, including:

- palpitations (feeling of skipped heart beats or fluttering in the chest)
- pounding in the chest
- shortness of breath
- chest discomfort
- fainting
- dizziness or feeling light-headed
- weakness or fatigue

Not everyone with abnormal heart rhythms will experience symptoms, so the condition may be discovered upon examination for another medical condition.

DIAGNOSTIC TESTS. Tests used to diagnose an abnormal heart rhythm or determine its cause include:

- blood tests
- chest x rays
- electrocardiogram
- ambulatory monitors such as the Holter monitor, loop recorder, and transtelephonic transmitter
- stress test
- echocardiogram
- cardiac catheterization
- electrophysiology study (EPS)
- head-upright tilt table test
- nuclear medicine test, such as a MUGA scan (multiple-gated acquisition)

Preparation for synchronized electrical cardioversion

Medication to thin the blood (blood thinner or anticoagulant) is usually given for at least three weeks before elective cardioversion. The patient should take all usual medications as prescribed, unless other instructions have been given. Patients who take diabetes medications or anticoagulants should ask their doctor for specific instructions.

The patient should not eat or drink anything for six to eight hours before the procedure.

It is advisable to arrange for transportation home, because drowsiness may last several hours and driving is not permitted after the procedure. The patient is also advised not to apply any lotion or ointments to the chest or back before the procedure.

Aftercare

The patient generally wakes quickly after the procedure. Medical personnel will monitor the patient's heart rhythm for a few hours, after which the patient is usually sent home. The patient should not drive home; driving is not permitted for 24 hours after the procedure.

Medications

The doctor may prescribe anti-arrhythmic medications (such as beta-blockers, digitalis, or calcium channel blockers) to prevent the abnormal heart rhythm from returning.

Some patients may be prescribed anticoagulant medication, such as warfarin and **aspirin**, to reduce the risk of blood clots.

The medications prescribed may be adjusted over time to determine the best dosage and type of medication so the abnormal heart rhythm is adequately controlled.

Discomfort

Some chest wall discomfort may be present for a few days after the procedure. The doctor may recommend that the patient take an over-the-counter pain reliever such as ibuprofen to relieve discomfort. Skin irritation may also be present after the procedure. Skin lotion or ointment can be used to relieve irritation.

Risks

Cardioverters have been in use for many years and the risks are few. The unlikely risks that remain include those instances when the device delivers greater or lesser power than expected or when the power setting and control knobs are not set correctly. Unfortunately, in about 50% of cases, the heart prefers its abnormal rhythm and reverts to it within one year, despite cardioversion. Cardioversion can be repeated for some patients whose abnormal heart rhythm returns.

Normal results

About 90% of cardioversions are successful and, at least for a time, restore the normal heart rhythm safely and prevent further symptoms.

KEY TERMS

Ablation—The removal or destruction of tissue.

Ablation therapy—A procedure used to treat arrhythmias, especially atrial fibrillation. During the procedure, a catheter (small flexible tube) is inserted in a vein and threaded to the heart. High-frequency electrical energy is delivered through the catheter to disconnect the pathway causing the abnormal heart rhythm in the heart.

Ambulatory monitors—Small portable electrocardiograph machines that record the heart's rhythm. Ambulatory monitors include the Holter monitor, loop recorder, and transtelephonic transmitter. Each type of monitor has specific features related to the length of recording time and the ability to send the recordings over the phone.

Antiarrhythmic—Medication used to treat abnormal heart rhythms.

Anticoagulant—A medication, also called a "blood thinner," that prevents blood from clotting. This type of medication is used for people at risk of stroke or blood clots.

Arrhythmia—An irregular heart rhythm.

Atria (singular, atrium)—The right and left upper chambers of the heart.

Atrial fibrillation—A condition in which the upper chamber of the heart quivers instead of pumping in an organized way.

Atrial flutter—A rapid pulsation of the upper chambers of the heart that interferes with normal heart function. Atrial flutter is usually more organized and regular than atrial fibrillation, although it often converts to atrial fibrillation. Atrial flutter occurs most often in people with heart disease and in the first week after heart surgery.

Cardiac catheterization—An invasive procedure used to create x-ray images of the coronary arteries, heart chambers and valves. During the procedure, a catheter is inserted into an artery in the groin or arm and is guided to the heart. Contrast material (dye) is injected into the catheter to produce the x ray images.

Echocardiogram—An imaging procedure used to create a picture of the heart's movement, valves and chambers. The test uses high-frequency sound waves that come from a hand wand placed on the chest. Echocardiogram may be used in combination with Doppler ultrasound to evaluate the blood flow across the heart's valves.

Electrocardiogram (ECG, EKG)—A test that records the electrical activity of the heart using small electrode patches attached to the skin on the chest.

Electrophysiology study (EPS)—A test that evaluates the electrical activity within the heart. The test is used to help determine the cause of the abnormal heart rhythm and find the best treatment. During the test, the doctor may safely reproduce the abnormal heart rhythm and give the patient medications to determine which medication works best to control the abnormal heart rhythm.

Head-upright tilt table test—A test used to determine the cause of fainting spells. During the test, the patient is tilted at different angles on special table for a period time. During the test, the patient's heart rhythm, blood pressure and other measurements are evaluated with changes in position.

Morbidity and mortality rates

Controlling a patient's heart rate is as important as controlling the patient's heart rhythm to prevent **death** and complications from cardiovascular causes. Anticoagulant therapy is important to reduce the risk of stroke and is appropriate therapy for patients who have recurring, persistent atrial fibrillation even after they were treated with cardioversion. In patients who did not receive anticoagulant therapy after cardioversion, there was a reported 2.4% increase of embolic events (such as stroke or blood clots), even though there were no signs of these events prior to the procedure.

Alternatives

Atrial fibrillation and atrial flutter often revert to normal rhythms without the need for cardioversion. Healthcare providers usually try to correct the heart rhythm with medication or recommend lifestyle changes before recommending electrical cardioversion.

Lifestyle changes often recommended to treat abnormal heart rhythms include:

• quitting smoking

• avoiding activities that prompt the symptoms of abnormal heart rhythms

• limiting alcohol intake

Implantable cardioverter-defibrillator (ICD)—An electronic device that is surgically placed to constantly monitor the patient's heart rate and rhythm. If a very fast abnormal heart rate is detected, the device delivers electrical energy to the heart to beat in a normal rhythm again.

Maze procedure—A surgical procedure used to treat atrial fibrillation. During the procedure, precise incisions are made in the right and left atria to interrupt the conduction of abnormal impulses. When the heart heals, scar tissue forms and the abnormal electrical impulses are blocked from traveling through the heart.

Nuclear imaging—Method of producing images by detecting radiation from different parts of the body after a radioactive tracer material is administered.

Pacemaker—A small electronic device implanted under the skin. This device sends electrical impulses to the heart to maintain a suitable heart rate and prevent slow heart rates.

Pharmacologic cardioversion—The use of medications to restore normal heart rhythm. It is also called chemical cardioversion.

Pulmonary vein isolation—A surgical procedure used to treat atrial fibrillation. During the procedure, a radio frequency probe, microwave probe, or cryoprobe is inserted and, under direct vision, used to create lesion lines in the heart to interrupt the conduction of abnormal impulses.

Stress test—A test used to determine how the heart responds to stress. It usually involves walking on a treadmill or riding a stationary bike at increasing levels of difficulty, while the electrocardiogram, heart rate and blood pressure are monitored. If the patient is unable to walk on a treadmill or ride a stationary bike, medications may be used to produce similar results.

Synchronized electrical cardioversion—The term used to describe cardioversion by the application of a controlled electric shock to the patient's chest.

Transesophageal echocardiogram (TEE)—An invasive imaging procedure used to create a picture of the heart's movement, valves, and chambers. The test uses high-frequency sound waves that come from a small transducer passed down the patient's throat. TEE may be used in combination with Doppler ultrasound to evaluate the blood flow across the heart's valves.

Ventricles—The lower, pumping chambers of the heart. The heart has two ventricles: the right and the left ventricle.

Ventricular fibrillation—An erratic, disorganized firing of impulses from the ventricles, the lower chambers of the heart. The ventricles quiver instead of pumping in an organized way, preventing blood from pumping through the body. Ventricular fibrillation is a medical emergency that must be treated with cardiopulmonary resuscitation (CPR) and defibrillation as soon as possible.

Ventricular tachycardia—A rapid heart beat, usually over 100 beats per minute. Ventricular tachycardia originates from the lower chambers of the heart (ventricles). The rapid rate prevents the heart from filling adequately with blood, so less blood is able to pump through the body. Ventricular tachycardia can be a serious type of arrhythmia and may be associated with more symptoms.

- limiting or not using caffeine (caffeine products may produce more symptoms in some people with abnormal heart rhythms)

- avoiding medications containing stimulants, such as some cough and cold remedies (these medications contain ingredients that may cause abnormal heart rhythms)

If cardioversion is not successful in restoring the normal heart rhythm, other treatments for abnormal heart rhythms are considered. These include an **implantable cardioverter-defibrillator** (ICD). Since first approved by the Food and Drug Administration (FDA) in 1985, ICDs have been continually improved.

Current models are much smaller and easier to implant than the early ICDs, can be programmed to deliver low-energy or high-energy shocks, and have batteries that last as long as six years. Originally considered a treatment of last resort, ICDs are now considered first-line therapy for some abnormal heart rhythms. The chief drawback of ICDs is the anxiety some patients feel about the possibility of the device's firing (emitting a shock).

Other treatments for abnormal heart rhythms include permanent **pacemakers**, ablation therapy, and heart surgery, including the Maze procedure and the pulmonary vein isolation procedure.

WHO PERFORMS THE PROCEDURE AND WHERE IS IT PERFORMED?

Heart doctors (cardiologists) specially trained in cardioversion (called electrophysiologists) should perform this procedure. To find a heart rhythm specialist or an electrophysiologist, patients can contact the Heart Rhythm Society (formerly the North American Society of Pacing and Electrophysiology). Cardioversion usually takes place in the hospital setting in a special lab called the electrophysiology (EP) laboratory. It may also be performed in an intensive care unit, recovery room or other special procedure room.

Resources

BOOKS

Elefteriades, John A., and Lawrence S. Cohen. *Your Heart: An Owner's Guide: Answers to Your Questions about Heart Disease.* Amherst, NY: Prometheus Books, 2007.

McGoon, Michael D., ed., and Bernard J. Gersh, MD. *Mayo Clinic Heart Book: The Ultimate Guide to Heart Health, Second Edition.* New York: William Morrow and Co., Inc., 2000.

Topol, Eric J., ed. *Textbook of Cardiovascular Medicine*, 3rd ed. Philadelphia: Lippincott Williams and Wilkins, 2007.

Trout, Darrell, and Ellen Welch. *Surviving with Heart: Taking Charge of Your Heart Care.* Golden, CO: Fulcrum Publishing, 2002.

PERIODICALS

American College of Cardiology, American Heart Association, and the European Society of Cardiology. "ACC/AHA/ESC 2006 Guidelines for the Management of Patients with Atrial Fibrillation: Full Text." *Europace* 8 (September 2006): 651–745.

Bostwick, J. M., and C. L. Sola. "An Updated Review of Implantable Cardioverter/Defibrillators, Induced Anxiety, and Quality of Life." *Psychiatric Clinics of North America* 30 (December 2007): 677–688.

Cotiga, D., A. Arshad, E. Aziz, et al. "Acute Conversion of Persistent Atrial Fibrillation during Dofetilide Initiation." *Pacing and Clinical Electrophysiology* 30 (December 2007): 1527–1530.

Khan, Ijaz A. "Pharmacological Cardioversion of Recent-Onset Atrial Fibrillation." *European Heart Journal* 25, no. 15 (2004): 1274–1276.

London, B. "Amiodarone and Atrial Fibrillation." *Journal of Cardiovascular Electrophysiology* 18 (December 2007): 1321–1322.

QUESTIONS TO ASK THE DOCTOR

- Why is this procedure being performed?
- What are the potential benefits of the procedure?
- What are the risks of the procedure?
- Can I take my medications the day of the procedure?
- Can I eat or drink the day of the procedure? If not, how long before the procedure should I stop eating or drinking?
- When can I drive after the procedure?
- What should I wear the day of the procedure?
- Will I be awake during the procedure?
- What kinds of monitors are used during the procedure to evaluate my condition?
- Will I have to stay in the hospital after the procedure?
- When can I resume my normal activities?
- When will I find out the results?
- What if the procedure was not successful?
- If I have had the cardioversion procedure once, can I have it again to correct an abnormal heart rhythm, if necessary?
- Will I have any pain or discomfort after the procedure? If so, how can I relieve this pain or discomfort?
- Are there any medications, foods or activities I should avoid to prevent my symptoms from recurring?
- Is an ICD suitable for my condition?

Miller, Karl E. "Amiodarone for Cardioversion on Recent-Onset Atrial Fibrillation." *American Family Physician* 68 (July 15, 2003): 355.

ORGANIZATIONS

American College of Cardiology. Heart House, 2400 N Street, NW, Washington, DC 20037. (202) 375-6000. http://www.acc.org (accessed March 8, 2008).

American Heart Association (AHA). 7272 Greenville Ave. Dallas, TX 75231. (800) 242-8721 or (214) 373-6300. http://www.americanheart.org (accessed March 8, 2008).

Cleveland Clinic Heart and Vascular Institute, The Cleveland Clinic Foundation. 9500 Euclid Avenue, F25, Cleveland, Ohio, 44195. (216) 445-9288. http://www.clevelandclinic.org/heartcenter (accessed March 8, 2008).

HeartCenterOnline. http://www.heartcenteronline.com (accessed March 8, 2008).

Heart Rhythm Society (HRS). 1400 K Street NW, Suite 500, Washington, DC 20005. (202) 464-3400. http://www. hrsonline.org/ (accessed March 8, 2008).

National Heart, Lung and Blood Institute (NHLBI). NHLBI Health Information Center, P.O. Box 30105, Bethesda, MD 20824-0105. (301) 592-8573. http:// www.nhlbi.nih.gov (accessed March 8, 2008).

OTHER

Beyerbach, Daniel M. "Implantable Cardioverter-Defibrillators." *eMedicine*, September 6, 2006. http://www. emedicine.com/med/topic3386.htm (accessed January 8, 20080.

Chauhan, Vijai V., and Antonella Quattromani. "Synchronized Electrical Cardioversion." *eMedicine*, July 18, 2006. http://www.emedicine.com/med/top ic2968.htm (accessed January 8, 2008).

Dorothy Elinor Stonely

Angela M. Costello

Rebecca Frey, PhD

Carotid artery stenting *see* **Endovascular stent surgery**

Carotid endarterectomy

Definition

Carotid endarterectomy (CEA) is a surgical procedure that is performed to remove deposits of fat, called plaque, from the carotid arteries in the neck. These two main arteries, one on each side of the neck, deliver blood and oxygen to the brain. Plaque builds up in large- and medium-sized arteries as people get older, more in some people than others depending on lifestyle and hereditary factors. This buildup is a vascular disease called atherosclerosis, or hardening of the arteries. When this happens in either one or both of the carotid arteries, they can become narrowed, a condition called stenosis. During a carotid endarterectomy, a surgeon removes the fatty deposits to correct the narrowing and to allow blood and oxygen to flow freely to the brain.

Purpose

Carotid endarterectomy is a protective procedure intended to reduce the risk of stroke, a vascular condition also known as a cardiovascular accident (CVA). In studies conducted by the National Institute of Neurological Disorders and Stroke (NINDS), endarterectomy has proven to be especially protective for people who have already had a stroke, and for people who are at high risk for stroke or who have already been diagnosed with significant stenosis (between 50% and 70% blockage).

Demographics

The National Stroke Association reports that two-thirds of stroke victims are over age 65. Risk is shown to double with each 10 years over age 55. Men are more at risk than women, although most stroke survivors over age 65 are women, which may be partly because there are more women than men in this age group. African Americans have been shown to be at greater risk for stroke than other racial groups in the United States. Risk is also higher in people who have a family history of stroke, as well as people with diabetes because of the circulatory problems associated with diabetes. People with high blood pressure, called hypertension, have four to six times the risk of stroke.

Nearly 750,000 strokes occur in the United States each year, with about 160,000 deaths, making stroke the third leading cause of **death** behind heart disease and cancer. Stroke is also responsible for the high number of disabled adults in the United States; two million stroke survivors have some permanent disability. The annual cost to the country for treating stroke and disabilities caused by stroke is about $40 billion.

Description

The presence of fatty deposits in the carotid arteries of the neck is the most significant risk factor for ischemic stroke, which represents 80% of all strokes. A stroke can be either ischemic, which is an interruption of blood flow in a narrowed carotid artery, or hemorrhagic, which involves bleeding in the brain. Carotid endarterectomy is performed as prevention of ischemic strokes.

Some people at high risk for ischemic stroke have disturbing symptoms that can occur periodically and last from minutes to up to 24 hours, and then disappear. These episodes are called transient ischemic attacks (TIA). The symptoms are the same as actual stroke symptoms. The symptoms of TIA and ischemic stroke may include:

- numbness, muscle weakness, or paralysis of the face, arm, or leg, usually on one side of the body, and usually occurring suddenly
- speech or vision difficulties
- sudden loss of understanding, confusion
- lightheadedness or fainting spells

Carotid endarterectomy

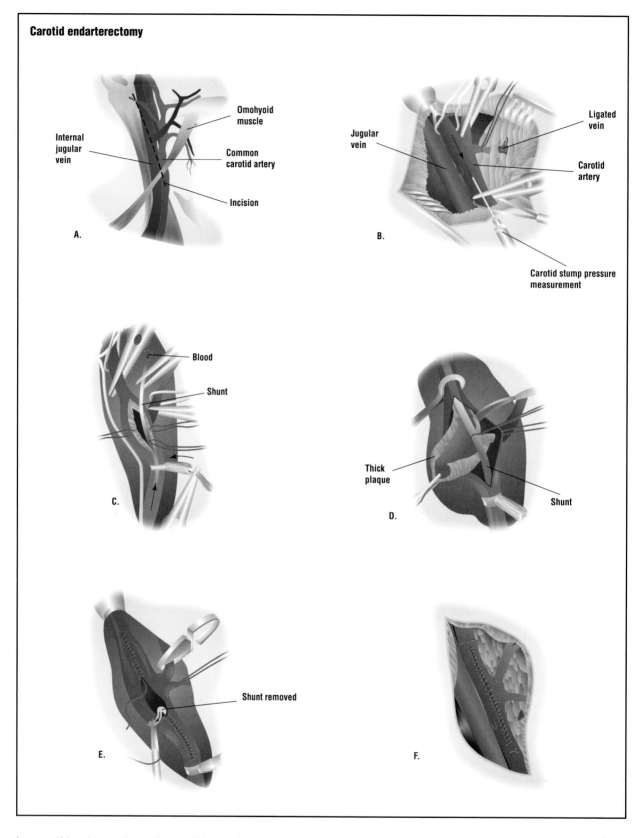

In a carotid endarterectomy, the carotid artery is access through an incision in the neck (A). A measure the pressure inside the vessel is taken to assess the degree of blockage (B). The carotid is clamped above and below the incision, and a shunt is inserted to maintain blood flow (C). Plaque lining the artery is removed (D). The shunt is taken out (E), and the incisions are repaired (F). *(Illustration by GGS Information Services. Cengage Learning, Gale.)*

KEY TERMS

Atherosclerosis—A disease characterized by the buildup of fatty deposits on the insides of artery walls, which results in thickening and hardening of the arteries and the narrowing of space for the passage of blood; also known as arteriosclerosis and hardening of the arteries, it can lead to high blood pressure, stroke, and heart attack.

Neurosurgeon—A surgeon who specializes in surgery of the nervous system, including the brain and nerves.

Plaque—A collection of wax-like fatty deposits on the insides of artery walls.

Restenosis—The repeated narrowing of blood vessels.

Stenosis—The narrowing of blood vessels in the body as a result of blockage.

Vascular—Pertaining to the veins, arteries, and organs in the body's circulatory system.

- loss of balance with difficulty walking and moving; poor coordination
- severe headache with no obvious cause, either sudden or persistent

About 35% of people who have TIAs will have a stroke within five years. The risk of stroke goes up with age and is greatest in people whose blood pressure is higher than normal. High blood pressure stresses the walls of blood vessels, particularly when the vessels are blocked with plaque and space for blood to pass is reduced.

Carotid endarterectomy has been performed since the 1950s as a stroke-prevention method. Because the surgery itself presents a high risk of complications, surgeons will look at the possible benefits and risks for each patient and compare them with medical treatment such as drug therapy to reduce plaque, cholesterol, and blood pressure. Carotid endarterectomy is typically performed on those who will benefit most from the surgery and who have the lowest risk for postoperative complications. Good candidates include:

- people who have already had one or more TIA episodes in a six-month period, with 70% narrowing of the carotid arteries supplying the part of the brain affected by the TIA.
- people who have had a mild stroke in the past six months but who are not significantly disabled and whose carotid arteries are at least 70% narrowed.

- people who have not had a stroke or TIA, but their carotid arteries are narrowed 60% or more and they have low risk of complication from having the surgery.

Carotid endarterectomy is not recommended for:

- people whose risk of complications from the surgery (such those with heart disease) is greater than the intended benefits.
- people who have had a TIA but their carotid arteries are less than 50% narrowed.
- people who have had a stroke or TIA because arteries other than the carotid arteries are blocked.
- people whose carotid arteries are blocked above a point on the neck where they can be reached easily during surgery.

The endarterectomy procedure takes about an hour to perform. **General anesthesia** is usually administered. A vascular surgeon or neurosurgeon will usually perform the surgery. During the procedure, a small incision is made in the neck below the jaw to expose the carotid artery. Blood that normally flows through the artery must be diverted in order to perform the surgery. This is accomplished by rerouting the blood through a tube (shunt) connecting the vessels below and above the surgical site. The carotid artery is opened and the waxy fat deposit is removed, sometimes in one piece. If the carotid artery is observed to be too narrow or too damaged to perform the critical job of delivering blood to the brain, a graft using a vein from the patient's leg may be created and stitched (grafted) onto the artery to enlarge or repair it. The shunt is then removed, and incisions in the blood vessels, the carotid artery, and the skin are closed.

Diagnosis/Preparation

Diagnosis

The presence and degree of stenosis in the carotid artery must be determined before a doctor decides that carotid endarterectomy is necessary. Carotid stenosis can sometimes be detected in a routine checkup, especially when a detailed history reveals that the patient has experienced symptoms of TIA or stroke. The doctor will use a **stethoscope** to listen to blood flow in the carotid artery and may hear an abnormal rushing sound called a "bruit" that will indicate narrowing in the artery. The absence of sound, however, does not mean there is no risk. More extensive testing will most likely have to be done to determine the degree of stenosis and the potential of risk for the patient. These tests may include:

- Ultrasound imaging with Doppler. A painless, non-invasive imaging test that measures sound waves directed into the body and returned to the ultrasound machine as echoes. Usually these echoes are visualized as an image on a screen; Doppler captures the sound as the echoes bounce off of moving blood in the carotid artery, giving some indication of the amount of blockage as the ultrasound probe moves up and down the arteries on each side of the neck.
- Computed tomography (CT) or computer-assisted tomography (CAT) scan. A series of cross-sectional x rays of the head and brain that can rule out other causes for the symptoms but cannot detect carotid artery stenosis.
- Oculoplethysmography (OPG). A procedure that measures the pulsing of arteries behind the eye, which can show carotid artery blockage.
- Arteriography and digital subtraction angiography (DSA). Special x-ray procedures using dye in the patient's vascular system. These tests are invasive and can actually cause a stroke, but they do indicate more exactly what degree of stenosis is present. The doctor will have to weigh the extent of risk and how much the patient will benefit from the tests.
- Magnetic resonance angiography (MRA). An imaging test that does not use dyes or x rays and relies on special computer software and powerful magnetic fields to create a highly detailed image of the inside of the brain's arteries.

Preparation

If carotid ultrasonography or arteriography procedures were not performed earlier to diagnose carotid stenosis, these tests will be performed before surgery to evaluate the amount of plaque and the extent and location of narrowing in the patient's carotid arteries. Other blood vessels in the body are also evaluated. If other arteries show significant signs of atherosclerosis or damage, the patient's risk for surgery may be too great, and the procedure will not be performed. **Aspirin** therapy or other clot-prevention medication may be prescribed before surgery. Any underlying medical condition such as high blood pressure or heart disease will be treated prior to carotid endarterectomy to help achieve the best result from the surgery. Upon **admission to the hospital**, routine blood and urine tests will be performed.

Aftercare

A person who has had carotid endarterectomy will be monitored in a hospital **recovery room** immediately after the surgery and will then go to an **intensive care**

unit at least overnight to be observed for any sign of complications. The total hospital stay may be two to three days. When the patient returns home, activities can be resumed gradually, as long as they are not strenuous. During recuperation, the patient's neck may ache slightly. The doctor may recommend against turning the head often or too quickly during recovery. The most important thing people can do after endarterectomy is to follow their doctor's guidelines for stroke prevention, which will reduce the progression of atherosclerosis and avoid repeat narrowing of the carotid artery. Repeat stenosis (restenosis) has been shown to occur frequently in people who do not make the necessary changes in lifestyle such as in diet, **exercise**, and quitting smoking, or excessive use of alcohol. The benefits of the surgery may only be temporary if underlying disease such as atherosclerosis, high blood pressure, or diabetes is not also treated.

Risks

Serious risks are associated with carotid endarterectomy. They involve complications that can arise during or following the surgery, as well as underlying conditions that led to blockage of the patient's arteries in the first place. Stroke is the most serious postoperative risk. If it occurs within 12–24 hours after surgery, the cause is usually an embolism, which is a clot or tissue from the endarterectomy site. Other major complications that can occur are:

- heart attack or other heart problems
- death
- breathing difficulties
- high blood pressure
- nerve injury, which can cause problems with vocal cords, saliva management, and tongue movement
- bleeding within the brain
- restenosis, the continuing buildup of plaque, which can occur from five months to 13 years after surgery

The risks of carotid endarterectomy surgery depend upon age, overall health, and the skill and experience levels of the surgeons treating the patient. The likelihood of complications is lower when the surgeon performing the procedure has acknowledged skills and experience. According to the Stroke Council of the American Heart Association, surgery is best performed by a surgeon who has only had complications occur in less than 3% of patients. Hospitals, too, should be able to show that fewer than 3% of their patients undergoing endarterectomy have had complications. These recommendations are based not only on skill levels, but also on the ability to accurately weigh the stroke risks for each patient against the potential risk of complication because of age, hereditary factors, and the presence of underlying conditions or diseases.

Normal results

The desired outcome of carotid endarterectomy is improved blood flow to the brain and a reduced risk of stroke. The National Stroke Association has reported that successful carotid endarterectomy surgery reduces risk of stroke by as much as 80% in people who have had either transient ischemic attacks or symptoms of stroke, or who have been diagnosed with 70% or more arterial blockage. Studies show that for people who have no symptoms but have been found to have stenosis from 60–99%, endarterectomy surgery also reduces the risk of stroke by more than 50%. These groups of people at higher risk for stroke will benefit most from having carotid endarterectomy. The benefit for people who have lesser degrees of blockage is shown to be much lower than that of high-risk stroke candidates. Surgery is not indicated for people with artery narrowing less than 50%.

Morbidity and mortality rates

Death and disabling stroke occur more often in symptomatic and asymptomatic patients at high risk for stroke who have not been treated with carotid endarterectomy surgery. A well-respected study, the North American Symptomatic Carotid Endarterectomy Trial (NASCET), along with a corresponding European study (ECST), showed that death or disabling stroke are reduced by 48% among those with severe stenosis (greater than 70%) when they undergo carotid endarterectomy surgery. In patients with less severe stenosis (50–69%), endarterectomy was shown to reduce risk by 27%. Patients with less than 50% stenosis were actually harmed by surgery, increasing the risk of death or disability by 20%. The conclusion of the study was that death and disability could be reduced overall if carotid endarterectomy was performed only on patients with the more severe stenosis

who are also surgically fit, and that that the procedure should be performed only by surgeons whose complication rates are less than 6%.

Alternatives

The carotid endarterectomy removes plaque directly from blocked arteries and there is no alternative way to mechanically remove plaque. However, there are alternative ways to prevent the buildup of plaque and thus help to prevent stroke or heart attack. Certain vitamin deficiencies in older people are known to promote high levels of homocysteine, an amino acid that contributes to atherosclerosis, putting people at greater risk for stroke or heart attack. Certain nutritional supplements have been shown to reduce homocysteine levels.

Nutritional supplements and alternative therapies that are sometimes recommended to help reduce risks and promote good vascular health include:

- Folic acid helps lower homocysteine levels and increases the oxygen-carrying capacity of red blood cells.

- Vitamins B_6 and B_{12} help lower homocysteine levels; B_6 is also a mild diuretic and helps to balance fluids in the body.

- Antioxidant vitamins C and E work together to promote healthy blood vessels and improve circulation.

- Angelica, an herb that contains Coumadin, a recognized anticoagulant, may help to prevent clot formation in the blood (blood thinner).
- Essential fatty acids help reduce blood pressure and cholesterol, and maintain elasticity of blood vessels.
- Chelation therapy can be used to break up plaque and improve circulation.

Resources

BOOKS

Khatri, V. P., and J. A. Asensio. *Operative Surgery Manual.* 1st ed. Philadelphia: Saunders, 2003.

Libby, P., et al. *Braunwald's Heart Disease.* 8th ed. Philadelphia: Saunders, 2007.

Townsend, C. M., et al. *Sabiston Textbook of Surgery.* 17th ed. Philadelphia: Saunders, 2004.

PERIODICALS

Chaturvedi S. "Carotid Endarterectomy—An Evidence-based Review: Report of the Therapeutics and Technology Assessment Subcommittee of the American Academy of Neurology." *Neurology* 65 (September 2005).

ORGANIZATIONS

National Institute of Neurological Disorders and Stroke (NINDS). National Institutes of Health, Bethesda, MD 20892. http://www.ninds.nih.gov (accessed March 8, 2008).

National Stroke Association. 9707 E. Easter Lane, Englewood, CO 80112. (800) Strokes or (303) 649-9299. http://www.stroke.org (accessed March 8, 2008).

OTHER

Carotid Endarterectomy. Harvard Medical School and Aetna. http://www.intelihealth.com (accessed March 8, 2008).

National Stroke Association, Stroke Prevention Guidelines. http://www.stroke.org (accessed March 8, 2008).

L. Lee Culvert
Rosalyn Carson-DeWitt, MD

Carpal tunnel release

Definition

A carpal tunnel release is a surgical procedure performed to relieve pressure on the nerve located inside the carpal tunnel, an area in the wrist that supplies nerve function to the fingers. The condition for which the release is performed is called carpal tunnel syndrome.

Purpose

Carpal tunnel syndrome is a relatively common problem affecting the wrist and hand. Individuals afflicted with carpal tunnel syndrome complain of numbness, tingling, and pain in the hand, with pain radiating up into the arm, shoulder, and even the neck. Some patients may experience an aching or burning sensation in the affected hand. The fingers may feel swollen, although they are no larger in size. If the condition is left unattended, symptoms may begin to awaken the individuals during sleep. If left unattended medically, muscle weakness can develop, leading to an inability to grasp objects or engage in any action requiring the opposition of the thumb and the other fingers in the affected hand. It is known as a repetitive stress injury, as it most commonly occurs in individuals who engage in motions that require the hands to repeat the same movements over and over again, especially with strong, forceful hand movements or ones that involve vibrating tools. Many individuals develop carpal tunnel syndrome in both hands. For some, the condition is worse in the dominant hand.

Demographics

Individuals who perform repetitive wrist movements, either at work or play, are at risk of developing carpal tunnel syndrome. Repetitive movements include computer work, typing, computer games; sports such as tennis; scanning items at the supermarket checkout; playing musical instruments for extended periods of time on a daily basis; assembly-line work, especially that requiring heavy gripping or the use of vibrating machinery; and the use of power tools such as for lawn care. It is more common in women, perhaps as much as three to seven times more than in men, especially during pregnancy, and also in individuals who are obese, or have diabetes or rheumatoid arthritis. It is also more common with advancing age. Carpal tunnel release is one of the most common hand surgeries performed in the United States.

Description

The carpal tunnel is a channel inside the hand, on the palm side, that surrounds and protects the main nerve and the tendons that help bend the fingers. This nerve is called the median nerve. The symptoms start gradually and continue to increase if the problem is not addressed. Numbness and tingling in the fingers are usually the first signs of the condition. It may come on while driving, sleeping, holding a telephone, or reading a book. It may also occur after a long bicycle ride, which involves gripping the handlebars. The pain

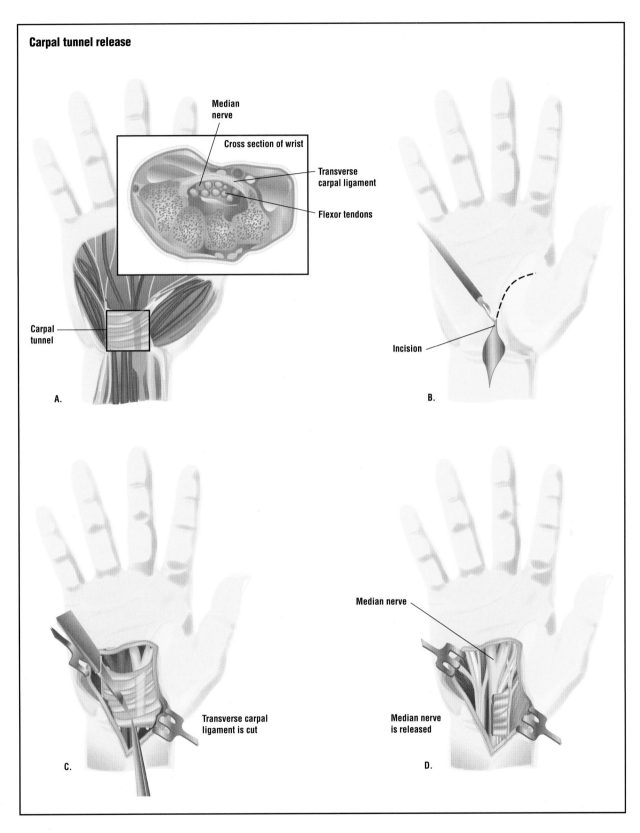

Carpal tunnel release

To perform a carpal tunnel release, the surgeon makes an incision in the palm of the hand, above the area of the carpal tunnel (B). The carpal ligament going across the hand is severed (C), releasing pressure on the median nerve (D). *(Illustration by GGS Information Services. Cengage Learning, Gale.)*

KEY TERMS

Dominant hand—The hand that the individual prefers to use for most activities, especially writing.

Edema—The abnormal accumulation of fluid in the body tissues.

Endoscopic—Surgery done making a few small incisions and inserting specialized instruments, one of which is a camera, that function as extended hands of the surgeon.

Innervate—To carry nerve impulses to a particular body part.

Neurosurgeon—A surgeon who specializes in dealing with nerve-related conditions.

or tingling might begin to travel up the arm to the shoulder. The individual may appear clumsy, drop objects, or have difficulty holding on to a glass. There may be a decrease in the ability to feel sensations in the hand. Once the problem interferes with daily activity, including sleep, or persists for longer than two weeks, it is important to seek medical advice. This is because the symptoms, even if they are not terribly disabling, can become permanent, as the damage to the tissues themselves becomes permanent.

Because of the nerve innervation routes, the one finger that is not involved in carpal tunnel syndrome is the pinkie.

Conditions associated with carpal tunnel syndrome, or that appear to put the individual at higher risk for developing the condition, include:

- obesity
- pregnancy
- certain thyroid conditions
- arthritis, especially rheumatoid
- diabetes
- menopause
- taking oral contraceptives
- conditions involving hormonal changes
- gout
- cigarette smoking

Conditions such as carpal tunnel syndrome are sometimes referred to as cumulative trauma disorders. In these disorders, the injury is not related to one major incident that causes damage, such as a fall that results in a fractured limb, but is the buildup of small microtraumas, in which the affected area is repeatedly damaged. Each small injury causes the area to become irritated or inflamed, and there is not enough time in between injuries for complete healing to occur. Treatment focuses on relieving the compression of the nerve and decreasing or eliminating the irritation and inflammation of the area. A term often associated with microtraumas or repetitive stress injuries is ergonomics, which means the way in which the body is set up to perform a certain function. If the function is typing, an ergonomic assessment would include looking at the height of the desk, the height of the chair in which one is sitting to work at the desk, the height of the hands in relation to the work area, such as the keyboard, and the angle of the wrist, elbow, hips, and knees. An ergonomically designed work station would have all components at the right height and angle for work so that there is no strain put on any joint as it performs its necessary function, and therefore no injury can take place. For those who use vibrating tools at work, special gloves exist that are padded and designed to decrease the effect of the vibration.

Diagnosis/Preparation

The diagnosis of carpal tunnel syndrome most commonly occurs because the individual seeks medical advice for numbness and tingling in the hand, especially while holding a telephone, newspaper, or holding onto the steering wheel in a car, or has experienced dropping objects. A thorough medical and medication history and a **physical examination**, especially for checking the nerve pathway functioning in the arms and hands, are essential components of a full diagnostic workup for carpal tunnel syndrome. It is important to be able to rule out other medical conditions such as a pinched nerve in the neck, which may present with similar symptoms. A complete account of symptoms, including which fingers are involved, is important because the median nerve, the nerve involved in carpal tunnel syndrome, does not innervate the little finger. The timing of the symptoms is also important because it indicates what activities set off the symptoms, such as while reading a book or having the hands placed on the steering wheel. Symptoms often occur at night because the hand gets set in a certain position for extended periods of time. Many people find that their hand is numb when they wake up in the morning, or that they wake up during the night with pain in the affected hand. To get relief, the individual may hang the hand off the bed, rub the hand, or shake it until the tingling goes away. Since, for many sufferers, the symptoms are worse at night than during the day, it may take time to associate the symptoms with the problem causing them. For some people, the symptoms come on, especially at first, only at work, because that is where the hand has to exert more than usual force in an awkward position. For others, the symptoms may come on when engaging in a hobby such as painting, gardening, knitting, woodworking, lifting weights, or playing a musical instrument. What begins as periodic symptoms may progress to constant symptoms, and mundane tasks such as unscrewing a bottle top or turning a key in a lock become extremely painful, or even impossible to perform. The doctor will want to try to elicit the symptoms by placing the hands in the same position as when the symptoms come on naturally.

Carpal tunnel syndrome is sometimes referred to as entrapment neuropathy, which means that a nerve, in this case the median nerve, is entrapped or compressed. In carpal tunnel syndrome, the median nerve is compressed, usually by swelling and inflammation, as it passes from the forearm into the hand through the carpal tunnel. The compression puts pressure on the nerve, which is what elicits the tingling and numbness felt by the patient. Compression can arise from a condition that causes the carpal tunnel to become smaller or narrower, or by something such as fluid retention, which would increase the volume inside the tunnel. In addition to trying to assess what nerve is involved in the problem, the doctor will want to see if strength in the hand has been affected. As part of the neurological exam, the doctor may tap at the base of the crease of the wrist. If this tapping brings on tingling in all the fingers except the pinkie, it is said that the Tinel's sign was positive. A positive Phalen test occurs when the two hands are placed back-to-back and held in that position for 60 seconds, bringing on symptoms. By extending the hands out of that position, symptoms are relieved. If these tests are positive, the doctor may want to order nerve conduction studies, although it is possible for conduction tests to be normal when the individual suffers from carpal tunnel syndrome.

Treatment

Once diagnosed, the first line of treatment for carpal tunnel syndrome is usually conservative in nature. This means that surgery is reserved as a last resort. Initial treatment may include taking frequent rest breaks from aggravating activity (if the activity cannot be completely avoided), anti-inflammatory medication, physical therapy, and using a splint or brace to keep the wrist in a neutral position; the splint is usually worn at night. Activities that bring on the symptoms are eliminated, avoided, or altered in some way to change the stress on the nerve. Tests to rule out conditions such as hypothyroidism may be conducted. If the problem is work related, an assessment of the

work environment from an ergonomic standpoint will be important. Work positions and tools used may need to be modified or changed completely.

If symptoms persist after conservative treatment, the injection of a corticosteroid medication may be the next line of treatment suggested. This is an anti-inflammatory medication, but because it is injected directly into the area affected, it has a greater impact than medication that is taken orally. If injections are being considered, it is important that the doctor have considerable skill and experience in administering these injections, with a thorough understanding of the anatomy of the wrist and hand. After the injection, a restriction on any wrist movement will be imposed for several days, usually followed by the wearing of a wrist splint for about one month. Finally, hand and wrist exercises to stretch the tendons as well as increase hand strength may be recommended. While the injection tends to give good short-term results, long-term results are less promising. When symptoms are not relieved by these more conservative measures, then surgery may be the next step. It is estimated that about one third of patients will not respond to conservative treatment and will require surgery.

Surgery may be performed in the more tradition fashion, or endoscopically. In traditional surgical treatment, an incision is made in the palm of the hand to openly expose the underlying structures. In endoscopic surgery, a smaller incision is made in the palm or wrist into which endoscopic instruments are inserted. In both techniques, entry into the carpal tunnel is made and the tissue called the transverse carpal ligament is cut, which stops the compression on the median nerve from continuing. Extreme caution is taken to avoid cutting additional anatomical structures or damaging the surrounding nerves.

Aftercare

Initial **postoperative care** while the individual is still in the surgical center involves making sure that circulation in the hands and fingers has not been compromised. There should be a strong radial (wrist) pulse, and the fingers should be their normal skin color and warm to the touch. The individual should be able to move all fingers equally, and there should be no edema.

Once discharged, it will be important for the patient to be aware of signs of complications, including:

- fever
- pale or bluish color to the operated hand
- if the operated hand feels significantly colder than the non-operated hand

WHO PERFORMS THE PROCEDURE AND WHERE IS IT PERFORMED?

The carpal tunnel release surgery is done by an orthopedic, plastic, or neurosurgeon. Patients considering carpal tunnel release should find a surgeon who performs this and other hand surgeries on a regular basis. The surgery is done on an outpatient or ambulatory basis.

QUESTIONS TO ASK THE DOCTOR

- Can I expect a full recovery?
- Will I be able to return to my regular work?
- Can both wrists be done at the same time?
- Is this a work-related condition?
- How soon will I be able to drive?
- When can I return to playing sports?
- How many of these surgeries have you performed?
- What complications have you seen in the surgeries you performed?
- What other complications might I encounter?

- inability or difficulty moving the fingers in the operated hand
- numbness in the operated hand
- bleeding from the bandaged hand
- swelling of the operated arm

A splint may be worn for about a month to help keep the wrist in a neutral position. This may be followed by exercises to both stretch and strengthen the hand, fingers, and wrist. Any accommodations in the work or home environment will need to be made to prevent further problems.

Risks

All surgical procedures involve some risk of infection through the operated site. Sharing all pertinent past and present medical history with the **surgical team** helps to lower the chance of a complication. In addition to the risk of the surgery itself, there are the risks associated with anesthesia. In carpal tunnel release surgery, anesthesia is more localized, which lowers the chance of complications. Nonetheless, it is important to share with the anesthesia team the list of all the vitamins, herbs, and supplements, over-the-counter medications, and prescription medications that the patient is taking. Drug interactions can be significant, especially if the anesthesia team does not have all the necessary information to make the best anesthesia choices for a particular patient. Complications such as nerve damage are linked with poor surgical technique.

Normal results

Whether or not a full recovery is achieved depends on several factors. The most important factor is if there has been permanent damage to the nerve or tissue fibers. If muscle atrophy occurred because the condition went untreated for a significant period of time, full recovery is unlikely. If no permanent damage resulted, then full recovery would be expected. Recovery is expected to take about six to eight weeks. Occupational rehabilitation may take an additional month. Those for whom the condition was work related will need to address the causative factors before returning to work.

Morbidity and mortality rates

The research literature does not indicate a significant mortality risk with carpal tunnel release. Morbidity complications are small, and it is a safe enough procedure to be done during pregnancy. Nerve block anesthesia decreases morbidity and offers pain relief from the wrist to the fingertips. According to a study, recurrent scar formation was the most common complication. Individuals considering surgery should investigate the complication rates with the surgeon, as well as the surgeon's and the facility's record.

Alternatives

Conservative treatment is the main alternative to surgery. A "wait and see" method is not a realistic form of treatment, as symptoms worsen over time, and the risk of permanent damage exists. Some acupuncturists treat carpal tunnel syndrome with success, though research studies have not been done in this area. A 2002 British study looked at the use of the homeopathic medicine, Arnica, for postoperative pain following carpal tunnel release. In the 37 patients tested, researchers found a significant decrease in pain reported by those taking the Arnica. A July 1998 study reported that about 70% of patients who undertook a specific **exercise** program for their carpal tunnel condition reported good results and were able to avoid surgery.

Resources

BOOKS

Canale, S. T., ed. *Campbell's Operative Orthopaedics.* 10th ed. St. Louis: Mosby, 2003.

DeLee, J. C., and D. Drez. *DeLee and Drez's Orthopaedic Sports Medicine.* 2nd ed. Philadelphia: Saunders, 2005.

PERIODICALS

Braun, R. M., M. Rechnic, and E. Fowler. "Complications Related to Carpal Tunnel Release." *Hand Clinics* 18, no. 2 (May 2002): 347–57.

Filippi, R., R. Reisch, D. El-Shki, and P. Grunert. "Uniportal Endoscopic Surgery of Carpal Tunnel Syndrome: Technique and Clinical Results." *Minimally Invasive Neurosurgy* 45, no. 2 (June 2002): 78–83.

Jeffrey, S. L., and H. J. Belcher. "Use of Arnica to Relieve Pain after Carpal-tunnel Release Surgery." *Alternative Therapies in Health and Medicine* 8, no. 2 (March/April 2002): 66–68.

ORGANIZATIONS

Mayo Clinic. 200 First St. S.W., Rochester, MN 55905. (507) 284-2511. http://www.mayoclinic.com (accessed March 8, 2008).

Esther Csapo Rastegari, RN, BSN, EdM
Rosalyn Carson-DeWitt, MD

Castration *see* **Orchiectomy**

CAT scan *see* **CT scans**

Cataract cryotherapy *see* **Cryotherapy for cataracts**

Catheterization, cardiac *see* **Cardiac catheterization**

Catheterization, female

Definition

Urinary catheterization is the insertion of a catheter through the urethra into the urinary bladder for withdrawal of urine. Straight catheters are used for intermittent withdrawals, while indwelling (Foley) catheters are inserted and retained in the bladder for continuous drainage of urine into a closed system.

Purpose

Intermittent catheterization is used for the following reasons:

• Obtaining a sterile urine specimen for diagnostic evaluation.

• Emptying bladder contents when an individual is unable to void (urinate) due to urinary retention, bladder distention, or obstruction.

• Measuring residual urine after urinating.

• Instilling medication for a localized therapeutic effect in the bladder.

• Instilling contrast material (dye) into the bladder for cystourethralgraphy (x-ray study of the bladder and urethra).

• Emptying the bladder for increased space in the pelvic cavity to protect the bladder during labor and delivery or during pelvic and abdominal surgery.

• Monitoring accurately the urinary output and fluid balance of critically ill patients.

Indwelling catheterization is used for the following reasons:

• Providing palliative care for incontinent persons who are terminally ill or severely impaired, and for whom bed and clothing changes are uncomfortable.

• Managing skin ulceration caused or exacerbated by incontinence.

• Maintaining a continuous outflow of urine for persons undergoing surgical procedures that cause a delay in bladder sensation, or for individuals with chronic neurological disorders that cause paralysis or loss of sensation in the perineal area.

• Keeping with standard preoperative preparation for urologic surgery and procedures for bladder outlet obstruction.

• Providing relief for persons with an initial episode of acute urinary retention, allowing the bladder to regain its normal muscle tone.

Description

The female urethral orifice is a vertical, slit-like, or irregularly ovoid (egg-shaped) opening, 0.16–0.2 in (4–5 mm) in diameter, located between the clitoris and the vagina. The urinary meatus (opening) is concealed between the labia minora, which are the small folds of tissue that need to be separated to view the opening and insert a catheter. With proper positioning, good lighting, and gloved hands, these anatomical landmarks can be identified. Perineal care or cleansing may be required to ensure a clean procedural environment.

Catheterization of the female patient is traditionally performed without the use of local anesthetic gel to facilitate catheter insertion. But since there are no lubricating glands in the female urethra (as are found in the male urethra), the risk of trauma from a simple catheter insertion is increased. Therefore, an ample

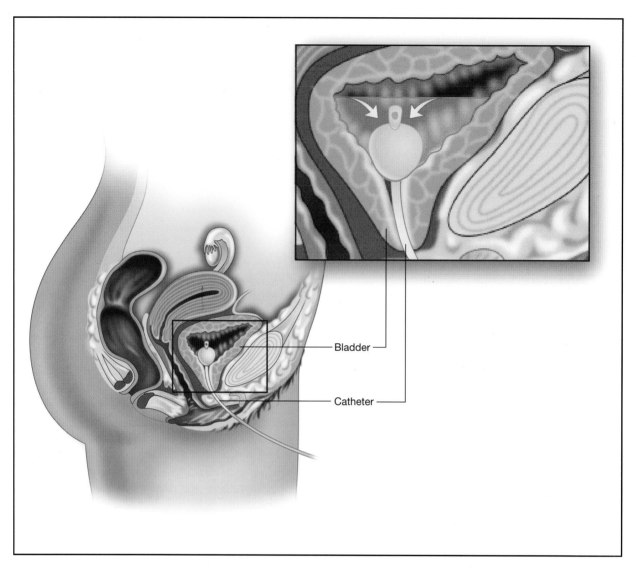

(Illustration by Electronic Illustrators Group.)

supply of an anesthetic or antibacterial lubricant should be used.

Once the catheter is inserted, it is secured as appropriate for the catheter type. A straight catheter is typically secured with adhesive tape. An indwelling catheter is secured by inflating a bulb-like device inside of the bladder.

Diagnosis/Preparation

Healthcare practitioners performing the catheterization should have a good understanding of the anatomy and physiology of the urinary system, be trained in antiseptic techniques, and have proficiency in catheter insertion and catheter care.

After determining the primary purpose for the catheterization, practitioners should give the woman

to be catheterized and her caregiver a detailed explanation. Women requiring self-catheterization should be instructed and trained in the technique by a qualified health professional.

Sterile disposable catheterization sets are available in clinical settings and for home use. These sets contain most of the items needed for the procedure, such as antiseptic agent, perineal drapes, gloves, lubricant, specimen container, label, and tape. Anesthetic or antibacterial lubricant, catheter, and a drainage system may need to be added.

Catheter choices

TYPES. Silastic catheters have been recommended for short-term catheterization after surgery because they are known to decrease incidence of urethritis (inflammation of the urethra). However, due to lower cost and acceptable outcomes, latex is the catheter of choice for long-term catheterization. Silastic catheters should be reserved for individuals who are allergic to latex products.

Additional types of catheters include:

- PTFE (plastic)-coated latex indwelling (Foley) catheters
- hydrogel-coated latex indwelling catheters
- pure silicone indwelling catheters
- silicone-coated latex indwelling catheters

SIZE. The diameter of a catheter is measured in millimeters. Authorities recommend using the narrowest and softest tube that will serve the purpose. Rarely is a catheter larger than size 18 F(rench) required, and sizes 14 or 16 F are used more often. Catheters greater than size 16 F have been associated with patient discomfort and urine bypassing. A size 12 catheter has been successfully used in children and in female patients with urinary restriction.

DRAINAGE SYSTEM. The healthcare provider should discuss the design, capacity, and emptying mechanism of several urine drainage bags with the patient. For women with normal bladder sensation, a catheter valve for intermittent drainage may be an acceptable option.

PROCEDURE. When inserting a urinary catheter, the healthcare provider will first wash the hands and put on gloves and clean the skin of the area around the urethra. An anesthetic lubricating gel may be used. The catheter is threaded up the urethra and into the bladder until the urine starts to flow. The catheter is taped to the upper thigh and attached to a drainage system.

Aftercare

Women using intermittent catheterization to manage incontinence may require a period of adjustment as they try to establish a catheterization schedule that is adequate for their normal fluid intake.

Antibiotics should not be prescribed as a preventative measure for women at risk for urinary tract infection (UTI). Prophylactic use of antibacterial agents may lead to the development of drug-resistant bacteria. Women who practice intermittent self-catheterization can reduce their risk for UTI by using antiseptic techniques for insertion and catheter care.

The extended portion of the catheter should be washed with a mild soap and warm water to keep it free of accumulated debris.

Risks

Complications that may occur include:

- Trauma or introduction of bacteria into the urinary system, leading to infection and, rarely, septicemia.
- Trauma to the urethra or bladder from incorrect insertion or attempting to remove the catheter with the balloon inflated; repeated trauma may cause scarring or stricture (narrowing) of the urethra.
- Passage of urine around the catheter; inserting a different catheter size can minimize this problem.

Sexual activity and menopause can also compromise the sterility of the urinary tract. Irritation of the urethra during intercourse promotes the migration of perineal bacteria into the urethra and bladder, causing UTIs. Postmenopausal women may experience more UTIs than younger women. The presence of residual urine in the bladder due to incomplete voiding provides an ideal environment for bacterial growth.

Urinary catheterization should be avoided whenever possible. Clean intermittent catheterization, when practical, is preferable to long-term catheterization.

Catheters should not be routinely changed. Before the catheter is changed, each woman should be monitored for indication of obstruction, infection, or complications. Some women require weekly catheter changes, while others may need one change in several weeks. Fewer catheter changes will reduce trauma to the urethra and reduce the incidence of UTI.

Because the urinary tract is normally a sterile system, catheterization presents the risk of causing a UTI. The catheterization procedure must be sterile, and the catheter must be free from bacteria.

Frequent intermittent catheterization and long-term use of indwelling catheterization predisposes a woman to UTI. Care should be taken to avoid trauma to the urinary meatus or urothelium (urinary lining) with catheters that are too large or inserted with insufficient use of lubricant. Women with an indwelling catheter must be reassessed periodically to determine if alternative treatment will be more effective in treating the problem.

Normal results

A catheterization program that includes correctly inserted catheters and is appropriately maintained will usually control urinary incontinence.

The woman and her caregiver should be taught to use **aseptic technique** for catheter care. Nursing interventions and patient education can make a difference in the incidence of urinary tract infections in hospitals, **nursing homes**, and **home care** settings.

The sexuality of a woman with an indwelling catheter for continuous urinary drainage is seldom considered. If the patient is sexually active, the practitioner must explain that intercourse can take place with the catheter in place. The woman and her partner can be taught to remove the catheter before intercourse and replace it with a new one afterwards.

Morbidity and mortality rates

Injuries resulting from catheterization are infrequent. Deaths are extremely rare. Both complications are usually due to infections that result from improper catheter care.

Alternatives

An alternative to catheterization is to use a pad to absorb voided urine.

Resources

BOOKS

Altman, M. *Urinary Care/Catheterization*. Albany, NY: Delmar, 2003.

Brenner, B. M., et al. *Brenner & Rector's The Kidney*. 7th ed. Philadelphia: Saunders, 2004.

Gearhart, John P. *Pediatric Urology*. Totawa, NJ: Humana Press, 2003.

Wein, A. J., et al. *Campbell-Walsh Urology*. 9th ed. Philadelphia: Saunders, 2007.

PERIODICALS

Johnson, J. R. "Safety of Urinary Catheters." *Journal of the American Medical Association* 289(3) (2003): 300–301.

Munasinghe, R. L., V. Nagappan, and M. Siddique. "Urinary Catheters: A One-point Restraint?" *Annals of Internal Medicine* 138(3) (2003): 238–239.

Wilde, M. H., and B. L. Cameron. "Meanings and Practical Knowledge of People with Long-term Urinary Catheters." *Journal of Wound Ostomy Continence Nursing* 30(1) (2003): 33–43.

Winder, A. "Intermittent Self-catheterisation." *Nursing Times* 98(48) (2002): 50.

ORGANIZATIONS

American Board of Urology. 2216 Ivy Road, Suite 210, Chaarlottesviille, VA 22903. (434) 979-0059. http://www.abu.org (accessed March 10, 2008).

American Foundation for Urologic Disease. 1128 North Charles Street, Baltimore, MD 21201. (800) 242-2383. http://www.afudfoundation.org/ (accessed March 10, 2008).

American Urological Association. 1120 North Charles Street, Baltimore, MD 21201. (410) 727-1100. http://www.auanet.org/ (accessed March 10, 2008).

National Health Service of Great Britain. http://www.nhsdirect.nhs.uk/ (accessed March 10, 2008).

National Kidney and Urologic Diseases Information Clearinghouse. 3 Information Way, Bethesda, MD 20892. (800) 891-5390. http://www.niddk.nih.gov (accessed March 10, 2008).

OTHER

AdvancePCS. [cited February 28, 2003] http://www.building betterhealth.com/topic/topic100587629 (accessed March 10, 2008).

Harvard Pilgrim Health Care. [cited February 28, 2003] http://www.intelihealth.com (accessed March 10, 2008).

Wayne State University. [cited February 28, 2003] http://www.dmc.org (accessed March 10, 2008).

L. Fleming Fallon, Jr, MD, DrPH

Catheterization, male

Definition

Urinary catheterization is the insertion of a catheter through the urethra into the urinary bladder for withdrawal of urine. Straight catheters are used for intermittent withdrawals, while indwelling (Foley) catheters are inserted and retained in the bladder for continuous drainage of urine into a closed system.

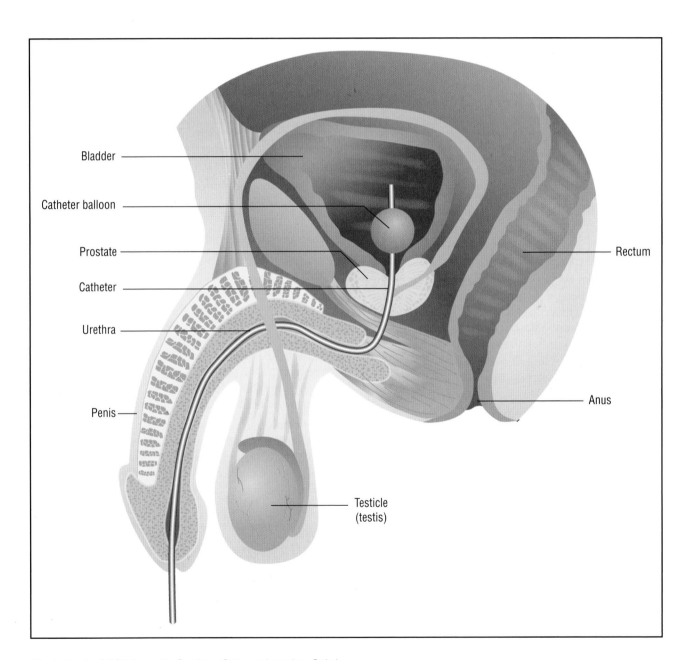

(Illustration by GGS Information Services. Cengage Learning, Gale.)

Purpose

Intermittent catheterization is used for the following reasons:

- Obtaining a sterile urine specimen for diagnostic evaluation.
- Emptying bladder contents when an individual is unable to void (urinate) due to urinary retention, bladder distention, or obstruction.
- Measuring residual urine after urinating.
- Instilling medication for a localized therapeutic effect in the bladder.
- Instilling contrast material (dye) into the bladder for cystourethralgraphy (x-ray study of the bladder and urethra).
- Emptying the bladder for increased space in the pelvic cavity to protect the bladder during labor and delivery or during pelvic and abdominal surgery.
- Monitoring accurately the urinary output and fluid balance of critically ill patients.

Indwelling catheterization is used for the following reasons:

- Providing palliative care for incontinent persons who are terminally ill or severely impaired, and for whom bed and clothing changes are uncomfortable.
- Managing skin ulceration caused or exacerbated by incontinence.
- Maintaining a continuous outflow of urine for persons undergoing surgical procedures that cause a delay in bladder sensation, or for individuals with chronic neurological disorders that cause paralysis or loss of sensation in the perineal area.
- Included in standard preoperative preparation for urologic surgery and procedures for bladder outlet obstruction.
- Providing relief for persons with an initial episode of acute urinary retention, allowing their bladder to regain its normal muscle tone.

Demographics

Men are less likely than women to use urinary catheters.

Description

The male urethral orifice (urinary meatus) is a vertical, slit-like opening, 0.15–0.2 in (4–5 mm) long, located at the tip of the penis. The foreskin of the penis may conceal the opening. This must be retracted to view the opening to be able to insert a catheter. With proper positioning, good lighting, and gloved hands,

KEY TERMS

Catheter—A tube for evacuating or injecting fluid.

Contaminate—To make an item unsterile or unclean by direct contact.

Foley catheter—A double-channel retention catheter. One channel provides for the inflow and outflow of bladder fluid, the second (smaller) channel is used to fill a balloon that holds the catheter in the bladder.

Incontinence—The inability to retain urine or control one's urine flow.

Intermittent catheterization—Periodic catheterization to facilitate urine flow. The catheter is removed when the bladder is sufficiently empty.

Urethra—The tube that allows passage of urine out of the urinary bladder.

Urethritis—Inflammation of the urinary bladder.

Urinary retention—The inability to void (urinate) or discharge urine.

Septicemia—An infection in the blood.

these anatomical landmarks can be identified. Perineal care or cleansing may be required to ensure a clean procedural environment.

The male urethra is longer than the female urethra and has two curves in it as it passes through the penis to the bladder. Catheterization of the male patient is traditionally performed without the use of local anesthetic gel to facilitate catheter insertion. Glands along the urethra provide some natural lubrication. Older men may require lubrication; in such an instance, an anesthetic or antibacterial lubricant should be used.

Once the catheter is inserted, it is secured as appropriate for the catheter type. A straight catheter is typically secured with adhesive tape. An indwelling catheter is secured by inflating a bulb-like device inside of the bladder.

Diagnosis/Preparation

Healthcare practitioners performing the catheterization should have a good understanding of the anatomy and physiology of the urinary system, be trained in antiseptic techniques, and have proficiency in catheter insertion and catheter care.

After determining the primary purpose for the catheterization, practitioners should give the male patient and his caregiver a detailed explanation. Men requiring self-catheterization should be instructed and trained in the technique by a qualified health professional.

Sterile disposable catheterization sets are available in clinical settings and for home use. These sets contain most of the items needed for the procedure, including antiseptic agent, gloves, lubricant, specimen container, label, and tape. Anesthetic or antibacterial lubricant, catheter, and a drainage system may need to be added.

Catheter choices

TYPES. Silastic catheters have been recommended for short-term catheterization after surgery because they are known to decrease incidence of urethritis (inflammation of the urethra). However, due to lower cost and acceptable outcomes, latex is the catheter of choice for long-term catheterization. Silastic catheters should be reserved for individuals who are allergic to latex products.

There are additional types of catheters:
- PTFE (plastic)-coated latex indwelling (Foley) catheters
- hydrogel-coated latex indwelling catheters
- pure silicone indwelling catheters
- silicone-coated latex indwelling catheters

SIZE. The diameter of a catheter is measured in millimeters. Authorities recommend using the narrowest and softest tube that will serve the purpose. Rarely is a catheter larger than size 18 F(rench) required, and sizes 14 or 16 F are used more often. Catheters greater than size 16 F have been associated with patient discomfort and urine bypassing. A size 12 F catheter has been successfully used in children and in male patients with urinary restriction.

DRAINAGE SYSTEM. The healthcare provider should discuss the design, capacity, and emptying mechanism of several urine drainage bags with the patient. For men with normal bladder sensation, a catheter valve for intermittent drainage may be an acceptable option.

PROCEDURE. When inserting a urinary catheter, the healthcare provider will first wash the hands and put on gloves and clean the tip of the penis. An anesthetic lubricating gel may be used. The catheter is threaded up the urethra and into the bladder until the urine starts to flow. The catheter is taped to the upper thigh and attached to a drainage system.

Aftercare

Men using intermittent catheterization to manage incontinence may require a period of adjustment as

they try to establish a catheterization schedule that is adequate for their normal fluid intake.

Antibiotics should not be prescribed as a preventative measure for men at risk for urinary tract infection (UTI). Prophylactic use of antibacterial agents may lead to the development of drug-resistant bacteria. Men who practice intermittent self-catheterization can reduce their risk for UTI by using antiseptic techniques for insertion and catheter care.

The extended portion of the catheter should be washed with a mild soap and warm water to keep it free of accumulated debris.

Risks

Phimosis is constriction of the prepuce (foreskin) so that it cannot be drawn back over the glans penis. This may make it difficult to identify the external urethral meatus. Care should be taken when catheterizing men with phimosis to avoid trauma from forced retraction of the prepuce or by incorrect positioning of the catheter.

Complications that may occur from a catheterization procedure include:
- Trauma or introduction of bacteria into the urinary system, leading to infection and, rarely, septicemia.
- Trauma to the urethra or bladder from incorrect insertion or attempting to remove the catheter with the balloon inflated; repeated trauma may cause scarring or stricture (narrowing) of the urethra.
- Passage of urine around the catheter; inserting a different catheter size can minimize this problem.

The presence of residual urine in the bladder due to incomplete voiding provides an ideal environment for bacterial growth.

Urinary catheterization should be avoided whenever possible. Clean intermittent catheterization, when practical, is preferable to long-term catheterization.

Catheters should not be routinely changed. Before the catheter is changed, each man should be monitored

QUESTIONS TO ASK THE DOCTOR

- Will the catheterization be intermittent or indwelling?
- Who will change the catheter and how long will it remain in place?
- Who will teach me or my caregiver how to insert and remove the catheter, monitor it, and perform routine care?

for indication of obstruction, infection, or complications. Some men require daily or weekly catheter changes, while others may need one change in several weeks. Fewer catheter changes will reduce trauma to the urethra and reduce the incidence of UTI.

Because the urinary tract is normally a sterile system, catheterization presents the risk of causing a UTI. The catheterization procedure must be sterile and the catheter must be free from bacteria.

Frequent intermittent catheterization and long-term use of indwelling catheterization predisposes a man to UTI. Care should be taken to avoid trauma to the urinary meatus or urothelium (urinary lining) with catheters that are too large or inserted with insufficient use of lubricant. Men with an indwelling catheter must be reassessed periodically to determine if alternative treatment will be more effective in treating the problem.

Normal results

A catheterization program that includes correctly inserted catheters and is appropriately maintained will usually control urinary incontinence.

The man and his caregiver should be taught to use **aseptic technique** for catheter care. Nursing interventions and patient education can make a difference in the incidence of urinary tract infections in hospitals, **nursing homes**, and **home care** settings.

The sexuality of a man with an indwelling catheter for continuous urinary drainage is seldom considered. If the patient is sexually active, the man and his partner can be taught to remove the catheter before intercourse and replace it with a new one afterwards.

Morbidity and mortality rates

Injuries resulting from catheterization are infrequent. Deaths are extremely rare. Both complications are usually due to infections that result from improper catheter care.

Alternatives

An alternative to catheterization is to use a pad to absorb voided urine.

Resources

BOOKS

Altman, M. *Urinary Care/Catheterization*. Albany, NY: Delmar, 2003.

Brenner, B. M., et al. *Brenner & Rector's The Kidney*. 7th ed. Philadelphia: Saunders, 2004.

Gearhart, John P. *Pediatric Urology*. Totawa, NJ: Humana Press, 2003.

Wein, A. J., et al. *Campbell-Walsh Urology*. 9th ed. Philadelphia: Saunders, 2007.

PERIODICALS

Johnson, J. R. "Safety of Urinary Catheters." *Journal of the American Medical Association* 289(3) (2003): 300–301.

Munasinghe, R. L., V. Nagappan, and M. Siddique. "Urinary Catheters: A One-point Restraint?" *Annals of Internal Medicine* 138(3) (2003): 238–239.

Wilde, M. H., and B. L. Cameron. "Meanings and Practical Knowledge of People with Long-term Urinary Catheters." *Journal of Wound Ostomy Continence Nursing* 30(1) (2003): 33–43.

Winder, A. "Intermittent Self-catheterisation." *Nursing Times* 98 (48) (2002): 50.

ORGANIZATIONS

American Board of Urology. 2216 Ivy Road, Suite 210, Chaarlottesviille, VA 22903. (434) 979-0059. http://www.abu.org (accessed March 10, 2008).

American Foundation for Urologic Disease. 1128 North Charles Street, Baltimore, MD 21201. (800) 242-2383. http://www.afudfoundation.org/ (accessed March 10, 2008).

American Urological Association. 1120 North Charles Street, Baltimore, MD 21201. (410) 727-1100. http://www.auanet.org/ (accessed March 10, 2008).

National Health Service of Great Britain. http://www.nhsdirect.nhs.uk/ (accessed March 10, 2008).

National Kidney and Urologic Diseases Information Clearinghouse. 3 Information Way, Bethesda, MD 20892. (800) 891-5390. http://www.niddk.nih.gov (accessed March 10, 2008).

OTHER

AdvancePCS. [cited February 28, 2003] http://www.buildingbetterhealth.com/topic/topic100587629 (accessed March 10, 2008).

Harvard Pilgrim Health Care. [cited February 28, 2003] http://www.intelihealth.com (accessed March 10, 2008).

Wayne State University. [cited February 28, 2003] http://www.dmc.org (accessed March 10, 2008).

L. Fleming Fallon, Jr, MD, DrPH
Rosalyn Carson-DeWitt, MD

CBC *see* Complete blood count

Cephalosporins

Definition

Cephalosporins are a type of antibiotic, or medicine that kills bacteria or prevents their growth.

Purpose

Cephalosporins are used to treat infections in different parts of the body—the ears, nose, throat, lungs, sinuses, and skin, for example. Physicians may prescribe these drugs to treat pneumonia, strep throat, staph infections, tonsillitis, bronchitis, and gonorrhea. These drugs will *not* work for colds, flu, and other infections caused by viruses.

Cephalosporins are also commonly used for surgical prophylaxis—prevention of bacterial infection during or immediately after surgery. For this purpose, a single injection may be given during the surgical procedure. In some cases, the cephalosporin may be continued for 24 to 48 hours after surgery. If, in spite of all precautions, an infection develops, the **antibiotics** may be continued until the infection has resolved.

Description

Examples of cephalosporins are cefaclor (Ceclor), cefadroxil (Duricef), cefazolin (Ancef, Kefzol, Zolicef), cefixime, (Suprax), cefoxitin (Mefoxin), cefprozil (Cefzil), ceftazidime (Ceptaz, Fortaz, Tazicef, Tazideme), cefuroxime (Ceftin), and cephalexin (Keflex). These medicines are available only with a physician's prescription. They are sold in tablet, capsule, liquid, and injectable forms.

Cephalosporins are sometimes referred to as first, second, and third generation. Each "generation" is effective against more types of bacteria than the one before it. In addition, each subsequent generation is better at getting into the central nervous system (the brain and spinal cord).

Cephalosporins are chemically similar to penicillins, and to other types of antibiotics called cephamycins.

Recommended dosage

The recommended dosage depends on the type of cephalosporin. The physician who prescribed the drug or the pharmacist who filled the prescription should be consulted for the correct dosage.

The following recommendations do not apply when cephalosporins are given as a single intravenous dose prior to or during surgery. The recommendations

---

KEY TERMS

Bronchitis—Inflammation of the air passages of the lungs.

Colitis—Inflammation of the colon (large bowel).

Gonorrhea—A sexually transmitted disease (STD) that causes infection in the genital organs and may cause disease in other parts of the body.

Inflammation—Pain, redness, swelling, and heat that usually develop in response to injury or illness.

Phenylketonuria—(PKU) A genetic disorder in which the body lacks an important enzyme. If untreated, the disorder can lead to brain damage and mental retardation.

Pneumonia—A disease in which the lungs become inflamed. Pneumonia may be caused by bacteria, viruses, or other organisms, or by physical or chemical irritants.

Sexually transmitted disease—A disease that is passed from one person to another through sexual intercourse or other intimate sexual contact. Also called STD.

Staph infection—Infection with *Staphylococcus* bacteria. These bacteria can infect any part of the body.

Strep throat—A sore throat caused by infection with *Streptococcus* bacteria. Symptoms include sore throat, chills, fever, and swollen lymph nodes in the neck.

Tonsillitis—Inflammation of a tonsil, a small mass of tissue in the throat.

---

should be considered if the drugs are used afterwards to treat a surgical infection, particularly if the cephalosporins are given by mouth.

Cephalosporins should be taken exactly as directed by the physician. The patient should never take larger, smaller, more frequent, or less frequent doses than prescribed. The drug should be taken for exactly as long as directed. No doses of the drug should be saved to take for future infections, because the medicine may not be right for other kinds of infections, even if the symptoms are the same. In addition, all of the medicine should be taken to treat the infection for which it was prescribed. The infection may not clear up completely if too little medicine is taken. Taking this medicine for too long, on the other hand, may open the door to new infections that do not respond to the drug.

Some cephalosporins work best when taken on an empty stomach. Others should be taken after meals. The physician who prescribed the medicine or the pharmacist who filled the prescription should give instructions as to how to take the medicine.

When given for surgical prophylaxis, it used to be common practice to give a dose of a cephalosporin as soon as the patient has been called to the **operating room**. More recently, the practice has been to give a single dose during the surgical procedure. This works just as well as the "on call" dose, and lowers the amount of antibiotic that the patient must take.

Precautions

The following recommendations do not apply when cephalosporins are given as a single intravenous dose prior to or during surgery. They should be considered if the drugs are used afterwards to treat a surgical infection, particularly if the cephalosporins are given by mouth.

Certain cephalosporins should not be combined with alcohol or with medicines that contain alcohol. Abdominal or stomach cramps, nausea, vomiting, facial flushing, and other symptoms may result within 15–30 minutes and may last for several hours. Alcoholic beverages as well as other medicines that contain alcohol should be avoided while being treated with cephalosporins and for several days after treatment ends.

Special conditions

People with certain medical conditions or who are taking certain other medicines can have problems if they take cephalosporins. Before taking these drugs, be sure to let the physician know about any of these conditions:

ALLERGIES. Severe allergic reactions to this medicine may occur. Anyone who is allergic to cephalosporins of any kind should not take other cephalosporins. Anyone who is allergic to penicillin should check with a physician before taking any cephalosporin. The physician should also be told about any allergies to foods, dyes, preservatives, or other substances. The type of allergic reaction should be discussed in detail, since some people have reactions to a drug that are not truly allergies. These people may be able to take cephalosporins safely.

DIABETES. Some cephalosporins may cause false positive results on urine sugar tests for diabetes. People with diabetes should check with their physicians to see if they need to adjust their medication or their diets.

PHENYLKETONURIA. Oral suspensions of cefprozil contain phenylalanine. People with phenylketonuria (PKU) should consult a physician before taking this medicine.

PREGNANCY. Women who are pregnant or who may become pregnant should check with their physicians before using cephalosporins.

BREAST-FEEDING. Cephalosporins may pass into breast milk and may affect nursing babies. Women who are breast-feeding and who need to take this medicine should check with their physicians. They may need to stop breast-feeding until treatment is finished.

OTHER MEDICAL CONDITIONS. Before using cephalosporins, people with any of these medical problems should make sure their physicians are aware of their conditions:

- History of stomach or intestinal problems, especially colitis. Cephalosporins may cause colitis in some people.
- Kidney problems. The dose of cephalosporin may need to be lower.
- Bleeding problems. Cephalosporins may increase the chance of bleeding in people with a history of bleeding problems.
- Liver disease. The dose of cephalosporin may need to be lower.

USE OF CERTAIN MEDICINES. Taking cephalosporins with certain other drugs may affect the way the drugs work or may increase the chance of side effects.

Side effects

The patient should get medical attention immediately if any of these symptoms develop while taking cephalosporins:

- shortness of breath;
- pounding heartbeat;
- skin rash or hives;
- severe cramps or pain in the stomach or abdomen;
- fever;
- severe watery or bloody diarrhea (may occur up to several weeks after stopping the drug); or
- unusual bleeding or bruising.

Other rare side effects may occur. Anyone who has unusual symptoms during or after treatment with cephalosporins should contact his or her physician.

Interactions

Some cephalosporins cause diarrhea. Certain diarrhea medicines, such as diphenoxylate-atropine

(Lomotil), may make the problem worse. Check with a physician before taking any medicine for diarrhea caused by taking cephalosporins.

Birth control pills may not work properly when taken at the same time as cephalosporins. To prevent pregnancy, other methods of birth control in addition to the pills are advised while taking cephalosporins.

Taking cephalosporins with certain other drugs may increase the risk of excess bleeding. Among the drugs that may have this effect when taken with cephalosporins are:

- blood-thinning drugs (anticoagulants) such as warfarin (Coumadin)
- blood viscosity-reducing medicines such as pentoxifylline (Trental)
- the antiseizure medicines divalproex (Depakote) and valproic acid (Depakene)

Cephalosporins may also interact with other medicines. When this happens, the effects of one or both of the drugs may change or the risk of side effects may be greater. Anyone who takes cephalosporins should let the physician know all other medicines he or she is taking.

Resources

BOOKS

AHFS: Drug Information. Washington, DC: American Society of Healthsystems Pharmaceuticals, 2003.
Weston, Debbie. *Infection Prevention and Control: Theory and Practice for Healthcare Professionals.* West Sussex, England: Wiley & Sons, 2008.

PERIODICALS

Barie, P. S. "Modern surgical antibiotic prophylaxis and therapy—less is more." *Surgical Infections* 1, no. 1 (2000): 23–29.
Cosgrove, S. E., K. S. Kaye, G. M. Eliopoulous, and Y. Carmeli. "Health and economic outcomes of the emergence of third-generation cephalosporin resistance in Enterobacter species." *Archives of Internal Medicine* 162, no. 2 (January 28, 2002): 185–190.

OTHER

Blondel-Hill, Edith, Susan Fryters, et al. "Recommended Drug Regimes for Surgical Prophylaxis." *Bugs and Drugs Antimicrobial Pocket Reference 2001.* Capital Health, 2000. http://www.dobugsneeddrugs.org/healthcare/antimicrobial/RecommendedDrugRegimensforSurgicalProphylaxis.pdf [Accessed April 11, 2008].

Nancy Ross-Flanigan
Sam Uretsky, Pharm.D.
Laura Jean Cataldo, R.N., Ed.D.

Cerclage, cervical *see* **Cervical cerclage**

Cerebral aneurysm repair

Definition

Cerebral aneurysm repair involves corrective treatment of an abnormal blood-filled sac formed by localized expansion of an artery or vein within the brain. These sacs tend to form at the juncture between a primary vessel and a branch. If the vessel involved is an artery, the lesion is also known as a berry aneurysm because of its round, berry-like appearance.

Purpose

The purpose of the surgical treatment of cerebral aneurysms is to isolate the weakened vessel area from the blood supply. This is commonly done through the strategic placement of small, surgical clips to the neck of the lesion. Thus, the aneurysm becomes isolated from the normal circulation without damaging adjacent vessels or their branches and shrinks in size until it is undetectable, a process known as aneurysm obliteration.

Demographics

Cerebral, or brain, aneurysms occur in about 2% of the American population. An estimated 15–33% of these patients have more than one aneurysm present. Occurrence of certain other medical conditions appears to increase the chances of developing aneurysms. These conditions include polycystic kidneys, systemic lupus erythematosus (SLE or lupus), and Ehlers-Danlos syndrome (EDS), a genetic disease that affects collagen, which is a primary component of connective tissue. Aneurysms in children are very rare, strongly suggesting that the condition develops, enlarges, and becomes symptomatic over a person's lifetime.

Other less frequent causes of aneurysms are infectious material from the heart, trauma, brain tumor, and brain arteriovenous malformation (AVM), which is a defect of the brain's circulatory system that results in the abnormal direct movement of blood from the arteries to the veins of the brain. The average age of cerebral aneurysm rupture is in the fifth decade of life and occurs more often in women than men by a slight margin. Environmental factors known to increase the chances of aneurysm development and rupture are cigarette smoking, excess alcohol consumption, and atherosclerotic heart disease. Some families have a definite genetic predisposition; in such families, aneurysms may run as high as 10%.

Cerebral aneurysm repair

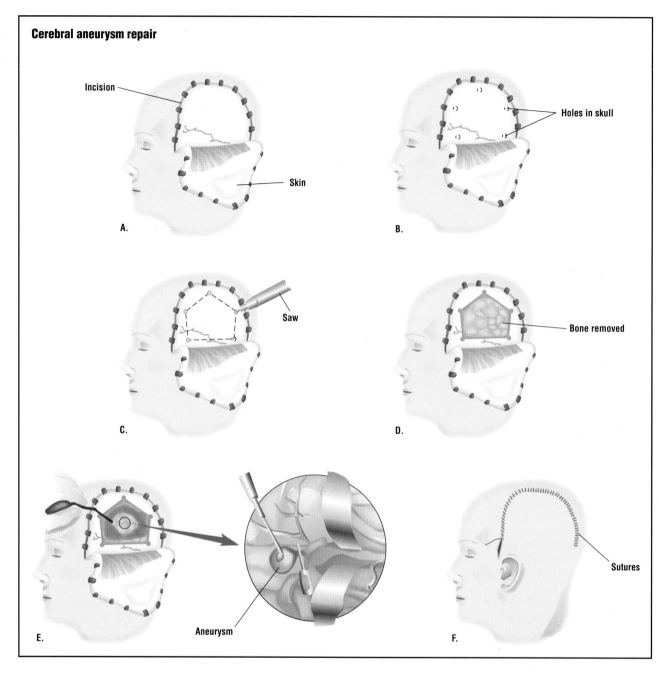

Incision

Skin

A.

Holes in skull

B.

Saw

C.

Bone removed

D.

Aneurysm

E.

Sutures

F.

To repair a cerebral aneurysm by craniotomy, an incision is made in the skin on the side of the head (A). Small holes are drilled in the skull (B), and a special saw is used to cut the bone between the holes (C). The bone is removed (D), and the aneurysm is treated (E). The bone is replaced, and the skin is sutured closed (F). *(Illustration by GGS Information Services. Cengage Learning, Gale.)*

Diagnosis/Preparation

Cerebral aneurysms become apparent in two general ways: from rupture followed by bleeding within the brain, or from enlargement and compression on surrounding critical brain structures, which leads to symptoms. The most life-threatening presentation is bleeding and is often described clinically as subarachnoid hemorrhage (SAH), a term derived from the anatomic area of the brain that becomes contaminated with blood when an aneurysm ruptures. The surface of the brain is covered by three thin membranous layers, or meninges, called the dura mater, the pia mater, and the arachnoid. The dura mater adheres to the skull, while the pia mater adheres to the brain. The arachnoid lies between the other two meninges. The space between the pia mater and the

KEY TERMS

Computerized tomography (CT)—A method of visualizing bleeding that has occurred in the brain.

Fluoroscopic angiogram—A method of precisely visualizing the brain cardiovascular system and its defects, including aneurysms.

Gugliemlimi detachable coils—A new method of treating aneurysms that is minimally invasive.

Magnetic resonance imaging (MRI)—A method of visualizing the vessels in the brain that is particularly effective at locating unruptured aneurysms.

Subarachnoid hemorrhage—Bleeding from a ruptured blood vessel in the brain that contaminates the cerebrospinal fluid.

Stroke—A brain attack that can be caused by bleeding in the brain.

Vasospasm—A deadly side effect of aneurysm rupture where the vessels in the brain spontaneously constrict; can cause brain damage or death.

arachnoid is known as the subarachnoid space and is normally filled with cerebrospinal fluid. SAH occurs when blood leaks into this space, contaminating the cerebrospinal fluid. About half of all SAH result from a ruptured cerebral aneurysm.

Clinically, the rupture causes the sudden explosive onset of a very severe headache that patients describe as the worst headache of their life. Other symptoms can include short-term loss of consciousness, neck stiffness, back pain, nausea or vomiting, and an inability to tolerate bright light. Sometimes a seizure can occur. About 40% of patients have symptoms and signs prior to the actual rupture, including minor headaches or dizziness, which are thought to result from swelling of the aneurysm or minor bleeding that occurs prior to the full rupture. Unfortunately, many of these events go undetected.

Rupture of a cerebral aneurysm is an emergency situation. About 10% of people with SAH die within the first day, and without treatment, 25% succumb within the next three months. More than half of those who survive have significant neurological damage. Partial paralysis, weakness, or numbness may linger or be permanent, as may vision and speech problems.

When SAH is suspected, a computerized tomography (CT) scan is performed to confirm the diagnosis by visualizing the bleeding. The aneurysm itself is only rarely seen using this test. CT scanning is positive

(detects the bleeding) in more than 90% of patients within the first 24 hours after the event, and for more than 50% within the first week. As time goes on, however, the bleeding becomes harder and harder to detect using this imaging method. If no bleeding is detected, a second test that could be performed is a lumbar puncture (LP), which involves drawing cerebrospinal fluid through a needle from the lower back of the patient. If SAH has occurred, the collected cerebrospinal fluid will contain blood and could be discolored yellow, caused by the presence of breakdown products of the blood cells. Other more sophisticated tests can also be performed to confirm the presence of blood and its breakdown products in the sample.

The definitive test for a cerebral aneurysm is a fluoroscopic angiogram, as it can often directly document the aneurysm, particularly its location and size. This procedure involves the placement of fluorescent material into the vein or artery of concern that increases the contrast between vessels and surrounding tissue so that their path can be clearly seen. The vessel is accessed through the insertion of a catheter in the femoral (leg) artery and threading it through the heart and into the blood vessels of the brain. A microcatheter is threaded through the larger one and used to deliver the contrast material to the precise location of the suspected aneurysm. Digital subtraction removes the bony structures from the image and leaves only the vessels. Generally, when SAH is suspected, a full cerebral angiogram that studies all four of the major cerebral arteries is performed. Modern angiograms are able to identify 85% of all cerebral aneurysms, with another 10% visible upon a second test seven to 10 days later. If this test is negative, magnetic resonance imagining (MRI), which is in some ways a more sensitive test, is often recommended.

If an aneurysm presents without rupture, some symptoms include seizures, double vision, progressive blindness in one eye, numbness on one side of the face, difficulty speaking, or, occasionally, hydrocephalus (accumulation of cerebrospinal fluid in the brain). Because of the sensitivity of available scanning techniques (particularly MRI), many aneurysms are discovered even before symptoms develop. This raises the issue of whether non-ruptured, asymptomatic aneurysms should be surgically treated.

Many health professionals view an unruptured aneurysm as a potential time bomb. In general, there is a 3% per year cumulative risk of rupture once an aneurysm is identified, or stated another way, about 0.5–0.75% of all aneurysms rupture each year. Each rupture brings with it the very high probability of serious neurological damage or even **death**. Furthermore, there are certain aneurysms that rupture more commonly than others, and environmental factors such as smoking and high blood pressure contribute to these events. However, all other things being equal, research indicates that by 10 years after diagnosis, there is an approximately 30% chance the aneurysm will rupture. Yet, the surgery itself carries significant risk. Whether or not to treat an unruptured aneurysm is a difficult decision and should be made only after careful consideration of the many influencing factors.

After diagnosis with a cerebral aneurysm, a patient will be put on strict bed rest and receive medication to avoid complications, keep blood pressure under control, and for pain relief.

Description

The exact timing for surgical treatment of cerebral aneurysms is historically a controversial subject in **neurosurgery** and is dependent on many factors including patient age, aneurysm size, aneurysm location, density of SAH, and whether the patient is comatose. Research indicates that early treatment, within the first 48 hours after hemorrhage, is generally associated with better outcomes, particularly because of the reduction of two serious complications of rupture: re-bleeding and vasospasm.

Re-bleeding is the most important cause of death if a patient survives the initial bleed and will happen in approximately 50% of all patients with a ruptured aneurysm who do not undergo surgical treatment. The peak occurrence of re-bleeding is within the first few days after rupture. About 60% of patients who re-bleed die.

The second major cause of death after rupture is vasospasm, a condition where the arteries at the base of the brain become irritated and constrict so tightly that blood cannot flow to critical brain regions. This spasm may result in further brain damage or induce re-bleeding, and much of the medical treatment after the aneurysm ruptures and prior to surgical treatment is designed to prevent this complication.

The procedure itself begins with **general anesthesia** of the patient and shaving of the area of the skull where the **craniotomy**, or opening of the skull bone, will occur. The exact position of the opening depends on the approach that the neurosurgeon will use to reach the aneurysm. The approach varies with the exact location of the aneurysm within the brain's cardiovascular system.

Once the bone flap is removed, the various layers of tissue are cut away to expose the brain. Blocking brain tissue is gently retracted back to expose the area containing the abnormal vessel formation. Surgical techniques performed through a microscope are then utilized to dissect the aneurysm away from the feeding vessels and expose the neck to receive the clip. Clips are manufactured in various types, sizes, shapes, and lengths to accommodate the needs for the various positions, shapes, and sizes of aneurysms. Clips are made of different kinds of materials, with titanium being popular because the material will not interfere with later **magnetic resonance imaging** (MRI) testing.

The clip is placed on the neck of the aneurysm in order to isolate it from the normal circulation. Careful clip placement will stop the flow of blood into the aneurysm, causing it to deflate or obliterate. Proper placement causes aneurysm obliteration and avoids damage to the adjacent vessels or their branches. Once the clip is in place, the brain tissue is carefully lowered back into place, the various layers sutured closed, and the bone flap is reseated for healing. The skin and other outer layers are also sutured closed. **Bandages** protect the area during healing.

Aftercare

Many times a postoperative angiogram is performed to confirm good clip placement, total obliteration of the aneurysm, and continued blood flow through the neighboring vessels. Because of the unpredictable nature of vessel behavior and the individual structure of each aneurysm, unexpected findings are seen in approximately 19% of postoperative angiograms. Patients stay in the hospital an average of 9.3 days after this procedure.

Risks

A major risk during surgery is a second rupture of the aneurysm during the procedure. Intraoperative rupture is very serious and associated with an approximately 30–35% morbidity and mortality of the patient. It is particularly dangerous if it occurs during the administration of the anesthesia or before the opening of the dura mater, because the surgeon is not able to reach the area immediately and control the bleeding.

Although much rarer than without surgical treatment, re-bleeding can occur even after surgery, particularly with improper placement of the clip. If too close to the parent vessel, the clip can block blood flow and promote brain damage in that area. If it is too far away from the parent vessel, a condition known as an aneurysmal rest can develop, and the area will swell and rupture later. This re-bleeding can also be described as a stroke, and occurs in between 1% and 10% of surgical patients.

Again rarer than without treatment, patients having their aneurysm clipped can also develop vasospasm after the procedure. The presence of vasospasm increases the occurrence of re-bleeding as well, making it a particularly dangerous complication. Treatments for vasospasm include giving medications that relax the smooth muscles in vessel walls, administering intravenous fluids to increase blood volume, or using drugs to increase blood pressure. In some cases, it may be necessary to open the vessel with a balloon catheter, a procedure called **angioplasty**. Angioplasty carries with it its own significant risks, including the formation of blood clots and rupture of the artery, and is effective only in some cases.

Other risks of the surgical treatment of cerebral aneurysms include neurological damage over and above what had occurred with the rupture. Special surgical procedures such as the use of temporary clips on the parent vessel, reduction of the patient's blood pressure, and administration of drugs that increase the brain tissue's ability to survive without oxygen are some techniques that minimize the amount of damage. Hypothermia (reduction of the patient's temperature during surgery) is sometimes also utilized to reduce the chance of this risk.

As this surgery involves opening of the cranium (skull), the procedure carries an increased risk of infection of brain and spinal tissues. This surgery also has all the risks of any other invasive procedure, such as infection at the incision site, and risks associated with anesthesia.

Normal results

If the postoperative angiogram indicates the clip has been properly placed, the aneurysm has been totally obliterated, and vasospasm is avoided, most patients do extremely well. However, the results of the surgery are always limited by the amount of neurological damage that occurred with the rupture itself, as much of the damage is nonreversible with current treatment methods. This issue is not a consideration with elective repair of a pre-rupture aneurysm.

Morbidity and mortality rates

Despite advances in **microsurgery**, anesthetic techniques, and critical care, the morbidity and mortality rates of SAH remains high at 25–35% and 40–50%, respectively. Age and neurologic status on hospital admission continue to be the best predictors of outcome.

In contrast, the operative mortality rate for elective clipping is close to 0, with morbidity ranging between 0% and 10%, especially if the surgeon is experienced in the procedure and utilizes the latest microsurgical techniques. In this situation, morbidity is most closely related to aneurysm size and location. Generally, elective clipping of an unruptured aneurysm is associated with better outcomes than ruptured aneurysms because the brain has not been damaged by the SAH prior to the procedure.

Alternatives

A promising new alternative to open surgery is the use of inventional neuroradiology to treat aneurysms. The greatest advantages to this technique are that it is less invasive and requires less recovery time in most patients. This technique is also more effective than craniotomy for certain positions of aneurysms or for patients that have complicating conditions that would make them unable to tolerate the stress of the more traditional surgery. The decision of whether an aneurysm should be treated surgically with a clip or through inventional neuroradiological techniques should be made as a team by the neurosurgeon and the endovascular radiologist.

Inventional neuroradiology, also known as endovascular neuroradiology, utilizes fluoroscopic **angiography**, described as a diagnostic imaging technique. Besides delivering the contrast material, the catheter can be used to place small coils, known as Gugliemlimi detachable coils, within the neck of the aneurysm using a delivery wire. Once the coil has been maneuvered into place, an electrical charge is sent through the delivery wire. This charge disintegrates the stainless steel of the coil, separating it from the delivery wire, which is removed from the body, leaving the coil. Anywhere from one to 30 coils may be necessary to block the neck of the aneurysm from the normal circulation and obliterate it, as occurs with the clip procedure. Although more research is needed to compare the two procedures, recent results indicate that intervention surgery for ruptured aneurysms may be safer than the traditionally more invasive procedure and may increase the chances of survival without disability after SAH.

Resources

BOOKS

Aldrich, E. Francois, et al. "Neurosurgery." In *Textbook of Surgery,* edited by Courtney m. Townsend. Philadelphia: W.B. Saunders Company, 2001.

Hoff, Julian T., and Michael F. Boland. "Neurosurgery." In *Principles of Surgery, Vol. 2,* edited by Seymour I. Schwartz. New York: McGraw-Hill, 1999.

PERIODICALS

"International Subarachnoid Aneurysm Trial (ISAT) of Neurosurgical Clipping versus Endovascular Coiling in 2143 Patients with Ruptured Intracranial Aneurysms: A Randomised Trial." *The Lancet* 360, no. 9342 (October 2002): 1267.

Pope, Wendi L. "Cerebral Vessel Repair with Coils & Glue." *Nursing* (July 2002): 47–49.

ORGANIZATIONS

American Association of Neurological Surgeons. http://www.aans.org.

American Society of Interventional and Therapeutic Neuroradiology. http://www.asitn.org.

OTHER

Greenberg, Mark S. *Handbook of Neurosurgery,* 1997 [cited March 1, 2003]. http://www.grgraphics.com/site/HBNS/chapters/SAH/SAH_001.html.

Michelle Johnson, MS, JD

Cerebrospinal fluid (CSF) analysis

Definition

Cerebrospinal fluid (CSF) analysis is a set of laboratory tests that examine a sample of the fluid surrounding the brain and spinal cord. This fluid is an ultrafiltrate of plasma. It is clear and colorless. It contains glucose, electrolytes, amino acids, and other small molecules found in plasma, but has very little protein and few cells. CSF protects the central nervous system from injury, cushions it from the surrounding bone structure, provides it with nutrients, and removes waste products by returning them to the blood. CSF is withdrawn from the subarachnoid space through a needle by a procedure called a lumbar puncture or spinal tap. CSF analysis includes tests in clinical chemistry, hematology, immunology, and microbiology. Usually three or four tubes are collected. The first tube is used for chemical and/or serological analysis, and the last two tubes are used for hematology and microbiology tests. This reduces the chances of a falsely elevated white cell count caused by a traumatic tap (bleeding into the subarachnoid space at the puncture site), and contamination of the bacterial culture by skin germs or flora.

Purpose

The purpose of a CSF analysis is to diagnose medical disorders that affect the central nervous system. Some of these conditions are:

- meningitis and encephalitis, which may be viral, bacterial, fungal, or parasitic infections

Normal cerebrospinal fluid values in adults	
Measurement	**Value**
Value	90–150 ml; child 60–100 ml
Clarity	Crystal clear, colorless
Pressure	50–180 mm H$_2$O
Total cell count	0–5 white blood cells/µl
Glucose	40–70 mg/dl
Protein	15–45 mg/dl (lumbar)
	15–25 mg/dl (cisternal)
	5–15 mg/dl (ventricular)
pH	7.30–7.40
CO$_2$ content	25–30 mEq/L

SOURCE: Fischbach, F.T. *A Manual of Laboratory Diagnostic Tests.* 4th ed. Philadelphia: J.B. Lippincott, 1992.

(Cengage Learning, Gale.)

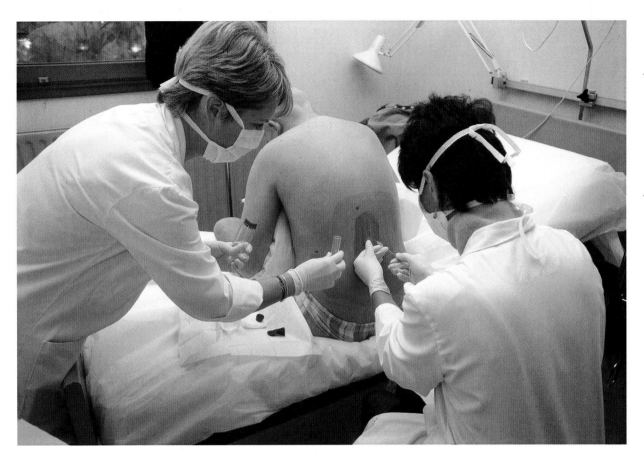

Administering a lumbar puncture for CSF analysis. *(BSIP / Phototake. Reproduced by permission.)*

- metastatic tumors (e.g., leukemia) and central nervous system tumors that shed cells into the CSF

- syphilis, a sexually transmitted bacterial disease

- bleeding (hemorrhaging) in the brain and spinal cord

- multiple sclerosis, a degenerative nerve disease that results in the loss of the myelin coating of the nerve fibers of the brain and spinal cord

- Guillain-Barré syndrome, a demyelinating disease involving peripheral sensory and motor nerves

Routine examination of CSF includes visual observation of color and clarity and tests for glucose, protein, lactate, lactate dehydrogenase, red blood cell count, **white blood cell count** with differential, syphilis serology (testing for antibodies indicative of syphilis), Gram stain, and bacterial culture. Further tests may need to be performed depending upon the results of initial tests and the presumptive diagnosis. For example, an abnormally high total protein seen in a patient suspected of having a demyelinating disease such as multiple sclerosis dictates CSF protein electrophoresis and measurement of immunoglobulin levels and myelin basic protein.

GROSS EXAMINATION. Color and clarity are important diagnostic characteristics of CSF. Straw, pink, yellow, or amber pigments (xanthochromia) are abnormal and indicate the presence of bilirubin, hemoglobin, red blood cells, or increased protein. Turbidity (suspended particles) indicates an increased number of cells. Gross examination is an important aid to differentiating a subarachnoid hemorrhage from a traumatic tap. The latter is often associated with sequential clearing of CSF as it is collected; streaks of blood in an otherwise clear fluid; or a sample that clots.

GLUCOSE. CSF glucose is normally approximately two-thirds of the fasting plasma glucose. A glucose level below 40 mg/dL is significant and occurs in bacterial and fungal meningitis and in malignancy.

PROTEIN. Total protein levels in CSF are normally very low, and albumin makes up approximately two-thirds of the total. High levels are seen in many conditions including bacterial and fungal meningitis, multiple sclerosis, tumors, subarachnoid hemorrhage, and traumatic tap.

LACTATE. The CSF lactate is used mainly to help differentiate bacterial and fungal meningitis, which

KEY TERMS

Demyelination—The loss of myelin with preservation of the axons or fiber tracts. Central demyelination occurs within the central nervous system, and peripheral demyelination affects the peripheral nervous system as with Guillain-Barré syndrome.

Encephalitis—An inflammation or infection of the brain and spinal cord caused by a virus or as a complication of another infection.

Guillain-Barré syndrome—A demyelinating disease involving nerves that affect the extremities and causing weakness and motor and sensory dysfunction.

Meningitis—An infection of the membranes that cover the brain and spinal cord.

Multiple sclerosis—A disease that destroys the covering (myelin sheath) of nerve fibers of the brain and spinal cord.

Spinal canal—The cavity or hollow space within the spine that contains the spinal cord and the cerebrospinal fluid.

Subarachnoid—The space underneath the anachnoid membrane, a thin membrane enclosing the brain and spinal cord.

Treponeme—A term used to refer to any member of the genus *Treponema,* which is an anaerobic bacteria consisting of cells, 3–8 μm in length, with acute, regular, or irregular spirals and no obvious protoplasmic structure.

Vertebrae—The bones of the spinal column. There are 33 along the spine, with five (called L1-L5) making up the lower lumbar region.

cause increased lactate, from viral meningitis, which does not.

LACTATE DEHYDROGENASE. This enzyme is elevated in bacterial and fungal meningitis, malignancy, and subarachnoid hemorrhage.

WHITE BLOOD CELL (WBC) COUNT. The number of white blood cells in CSF is very low, usually necessitating a manual WBC count. An increase in WBCs may occur in many conditions including infection (viral, bacterial, fungal, and parasitic), allergy, leukemia, multiple sclerosis, hemorrhage, traumatic tap, encephalitis, and Guillain-Barré syndrome. The WBC differential helps to distinguish many of these causes. For example, viral infection is usually associated with an increase in lymphocytes, while bacterial and fungal infections are associated with an increase in

polymorphonuclear leukocytes (neutrophils). The differential may also reveal eosinophils associated with allergy and ventricular shunts; macrophages with ingested bacteria (indicating meningitis), RBCs (indicating hemorrhage), or lipids (indicating possible cerebral infarction); blasts (immature cells) that indicate leukemia; and malignant cells characteristic of the tissue of origin. About 50% of metastatic cancers that infiltrate the central nervous system and about 10% of central nervous system tumors will shed cells into the CSF.

RED BLOOD CELL (RBC) COUNT. While not normally found in CSF, RBCs will appear whenever bleeding has occurred. Red cells in CSF signal subarachnoid hemorrhage, stroke, or traumatic tap. Since white cells may enter the CSF in response to local infection, inflammation, or bleeding, the RBC count is used to correct the WBC count so that it reflects conditions other than hemorrhage or a traumatic tap. This is accomplished by counting RBCs and WBCs in both blood and CSF. The ratio of RBCs in CSF to blood is multiplied by the blood WBC count. This value is subtracted from the CSF WBC count to eliminate WBCs derived from hemorrhage or traumatic tap.

GRAM STAIN. The Gram stain is performed on a sediment of the CSF and is positive in at least 60% of cases of bacterial meningitis. Culture is performed for both aerobic and anaerobic bacteria. In addition, other stains (e.g. the acid-fast stain for *Mycobacterium tuberculosis,* fungal culture, and rapid identification tests [tests for bacterial and fungal antigens]) may be performed routinely.

SYPHILIS SEROLOGY. This serology involves testing for antibodies that indicate neurosyphilis. The fluorescent treponemal antibody-absorption (FTA-ABS) test is often used and is positive in persons with active and treated syphilis. The test is used in conjunction with the VDRL test for nontreponemal antibodies, which is positive in most persons with active syphilis, but negative in treated cases.

Precautions

In some circumstances, a lumbar puncture to withdraw a small amount of CSF for analysis may lead to serious complications. Lumbar punctures should be performed only with extreme caution, and only if the benefits are thought to outweigh the risks. In people who have bleeding disorders, lumbar puncture can cause hemorrhage that can compress the spinal cord. If there is increased spinal column pressure, as may occur with a brain tumor and other conditions, removal of CSF can cause the brain to herniate, compressing the brain stem and other vital structures and leading to irreversible brain damage or **death**. Bacteria introduced during the puncture may cause meningitis. For this reason, **aseptic technique** must be followed strictly, and a lumbar puncture should never be performed at the site of a localized skin lesion.

Specimens should be handled with caution to avoid contamination with skin flora. They should be refrigerated if analysis cannot be performed immediately.

Description

Lumbar puncture is performed by inserting the needle between the fourth and fifth lumbar vertabrae (L4-L5). This location is used because the spinal cord stops near L2, and a needle introduced below this level will miss the cord. In rare instances, such as a spinal fluid blockage in the middle of the back, a physician may perform a spinal tap in the cervical spine.

Aftercare

After the procedure, the site of the puncture is covered with a sterile bandage. The patient should remain lying down for four to six hours after the lumbar puncture. **Vital signs** should be monitored every 15 minutes for four hours, then every 30 minutes for another four hours. The puncture site should be observed for signs of weeping or swelling for 24 hours. The neurological status of the patient should also be evaluated for such symptoms as numbness and/or tingling in the lower extremities.

Risks

The most common side effect after the removal of CSF is a headache. This occurs in 10–30% of adult patients and in up to 40% of children. It is caused by a decreased CSF pressure related to a small leak of CSF through the puncture site. These headaches usually are a dull pain, although some people report a throbbing sensation. A stiff neck and nausea may accompany the headache. Lumbar puncture headaches typically begin within two days after the procedure and persist from a few days to several weeks or months.

Normal results

- Gross appearance: Normal CSF is clear and colorless.
- CSF opening pressure: 50–175 mm H_2O.
- Specific gravity: 1.006–1.009.
- Glucose: 40–80 mg/dL.
- Total protein: 15–45 mg/dL.

- LD: 1/10 of serum level.
- Lactate: less than 35 mg/dL.
- Leukocytes (white blood cells): 0–5/microL (adults and children); up to 30/microL (newborns).
- Differential: 60–80% lymphocytes; up to 30% monocytes and macrophages; other cells 2% or less. Monocytes and macrophages are somewhat higher in neonates.
- Gram stain: negative.
- Culture: sterile.
- Syphilis serology: negative.
- Red blood cell count: Normally, there are no red blood cells in the CSF unless the needle passes through a blood vessel on route to the CSF.

Resources

BOOKS

Braunwald, Eugene, et al., eds., "Approach to the Patient with Neurologic Disease." In *Harrison's Principles of Internal Medicine*. 15th ed. New York: McGraw-Hill, 2001.

Henry, J. B. *Clinical Diagnosis and Management by Laboratory Methods*. 20th ed. Philadelphia, PA: W. B. Saunders, 2001.

Kee, Joyce LeFever. *Handbook of Laboratory and Diagnostic Tests*. 4th ed. Upper Saddle River, NJ: Prentice Hall, 2001.

Smith, Gregory P., and Carl R. Kieldsberg. *Cerebrospinal, Synovial, and Serous Body Fluids*. Philadelphia, PA: W. B. Saunders, 2001.

Wallach, Jacques. *Interpretation of Diagnostic Tests*. 7th ed. Philadelphia, PA: Lippincott Williams & Wilkins, 2000.

OTHER

National Institutes of Health. March 14, 2003 [cited April 5, 2003]. http://www.nlm.nih.gov/medlineplus/encyclopedia.html.

Victoria E. DeMoranville
Mark A. Best

Cerebrospinal fluid shunt *see* **Ventricular shunt**

Cervical biopsy *see* **Cone biopsy**

Cervical cerclage

Definition

A cervical cerclage is a minor surgical procedure in which the opening to the uterus (the cervix) is stitched closed in order to prevent a miscarriage or premature birth.

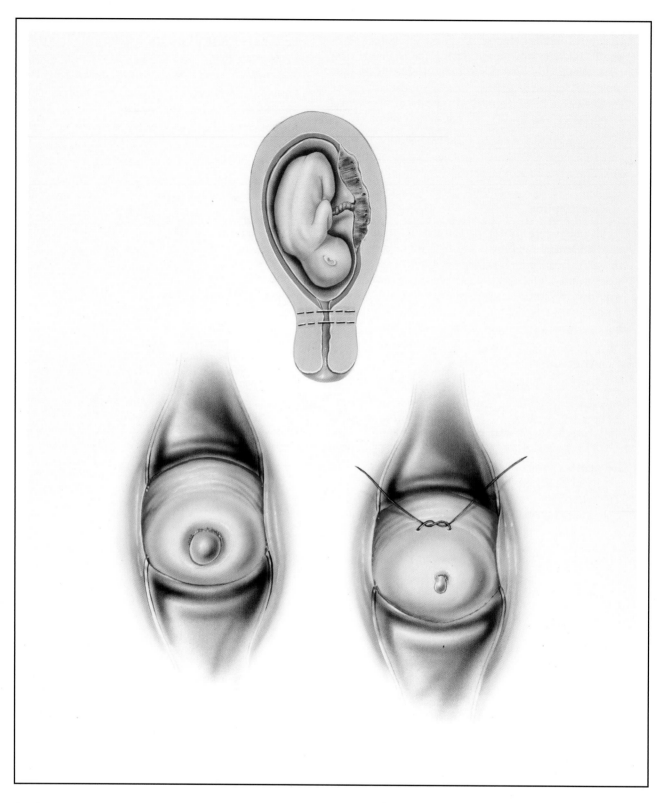

Cervical cerclage. *(Judith Glick/Phototake. Reproduced by permission.)*

Purpose

Approximately 10% of pregnancies end in preterm delivery, defined as a delivery that occurs before week 37 of pregnancy (the average pregnancy lasts 40 weeks). Premature birth is a major cause of serious health problems in neonates (newborn babies), including respiratory distress, difficulty regulating **body temperature**, and infection. More than 85% of long-term disabilities in otherwise healthy babies and 75% of deaths among newborns occur as a result of preterm delivery.

A woman with an incompetent cervix is 3.3 times more likely to deliver prematurely. The cervix is the neck-shaped opening at the lower part of the uterus and is normally closed tight during pregnancy until the baby is ready to be delivered, at which point it expands (dilates) to roughly 4 in (10 cm) in diameter. An incompetent cervix is prone to dilating and/or effacing (shortening) prematurely during the second trimester. The growing fetus subsequently places too great a strain on the cervix, leading to miscarriage (loss before week 20 of pregnancy) or premature delivery (loss after week 20). Approximately 1% of women will be diagnosed with an incompetent cervix (one in 500–2,000 pregnancies). It is the cause of 25% of losses during the second trimester.

A doctor might recommend a cerclage be performed if a woman has one or more of the following risk factors:

- a previous preterm delivery
- previous trauma or surgery to the cervix
- early rupture of membranes ("breaking water")
- hormonal influences
- abnormalities of the uterus or cervix
- exposure as a fetus to diethylstilbestrol (DES), a synthetic hormone that was used in the mid-twentieth century to treat recurrent miscarriages

Demographics

Racial and socioeconomic factors influence a woman's risk of delivering prematurely: African-American women are at more risk (16–18%) than white women (7–9%); women under 18 and over 35 are also at greater risk. Less educated women are more likely to deliver prematurely. Smoking during pregnancy is associated with a 20–30% greater risk of delivering prematurely. Male fetuses are more likely to be born prematurely and have a higher rate of fetal **death** than female fetuses (a difference of 2.8–9.8%).

KEY TERMS

Cervix—The neck-shaped opening at the lower part of the uterus.

Chorioamnionitis—Infection of the amniotic sac.

Diethylstilbestrol (DES)—A synthetic hormone that was used in the mid-twentieth century to treat recurrent miscarriages; exposure to DES as a fetus is a risk factor for premature labor.

Epidural anesthesia—Similar to the procedure for spinal anesthesia except that a catheter is inserted so that numbing medications may be administered when needed.

Neonate—A newborn baby.

Tocolytics—Drugs that are used to stop or delay labor.

Spinal anesthesia—Involves inserting a needle into a region between the vertebrae of the lower back and injecting numbing medications.

Description

Elective cervical cerclage is a minor surgical procedure that is generally performed between 12 and 14 weeks of pregnancy (at the beginning of the second trimester) before symptoms of premature labor begin. Emergent cerclages are those placed later in pregnancy when cervical changes have already begun.

The patient will usually receive regional (epidural or spinal) anesthesia during the procedure, although **general anesthesia** is sometimes used. Spinal anesthesia involves inserting a needle into a region between the vertebrae of the lower back and injecting numbing medications. An epidural is similar to a spinal except that a catheter is inserted so that numbing medications may be administered as needed. Some women experience a drop in blood pressure when a regional anesthetic is administered; this effect can be countered with fluids and/or medications.

While there are numerous techniques for performing cerclage, the McDonald and Shirodkar techniques are the most common. The McDonald cerclage involves stitching the cervix with a 0.2 in (5 mm) band of suture. The cerclage is placed high on the cervix when the lower part has already started to efface. The stitch is usually removed around week 37 of pregnancy. The classic Shirodkar procedure involves a permanent "purse-string" stitch around the cervix; because it will not be removed, a **cesarean section** will be necessary to deliver the baby. Most Shirodkar cerclages are now performed with a modified technique that allows the sutures to be later removed.

Some less common methods of cerclage include:

- Hefner (or Wurm) cerclage (usually reserved for later in pregnancy when there is little cervix to work with)
- abdominal cerclage (a permanent stitch performed through an abdominal incision instead of the vagina; reserved for when a vaginal cerclage has failed or is not possible)
- Lash cerclage (a permanent stitch performed before pregnancy because of trauma to the cervix or an anatomical abnormality)

Diagnosis/Preparation

Diagnosis of an incompetent cervix is usually done by medical history and/or by examination (manually during a pelvic exam or using **ultrasound** technology). Some symptoms of an incompetent cervix used to decide if a cerclage is necessary are:

- cervical dilation
- shortening of the cervix
- funneling of 25% or more (when the internal opening of the cervix has begun to dilate but the external opening remains closed)

Women who are more than 1.5 in (4 cm) dilated, who have already experienced rupture of membranes, or whose fetus has died are ineligible for cerclage.

Before the procedure may be performed, there are a number of preparatory steps that must be taken. A complete medical history will be taken. A cervical exam will be necessary to assess the state of the cervix; usually a transvaginal (through the vagina) ultrasound will be performed. No food or drink will be allowed after midnight before the day of surgery to avoid nausea and vomiting during and after the procedure. The patient will also be instructed to avoid sexual intercourse, tampons, and douches for 24 hours before the procedure. Before the procedure is performed, an intravenous (IV) catheter will be placed in order to administrate fluids and medications.

Aftercare

After the cerclage has been placed, the patient will be observed for at least several hours (sometimes overnight) to ensure that she does not go into premature labor. The patient will then be allowed to return home, but will be instructed to remain in bed or avoid physical activity for two to three days. Follow-up appointments will usually take place so that her doctor can

WHO PERFORMS THE PROCEDURE AND WHERE IS IT PERFORMED?

A cervical cerclage is generally performed in a hospital operating room by an obstetrician/gynecologist who specializes in the areas of women's general health, pregnancy, labor and childbirth, prenatal testing, and genetics. Anesthesia will be administered by an anesthesiologist.

monitor the cervix and stitch and watch for signs of premature labor.

Risks

While cerclage is generally a safe procedure, there are a number of potential complications that may arise during or after surgery. These include:

- risks associated with regional or general anesthesia
- premature labor
- premature rupture of membranes
- infection of the cervix
- infection of the amniotic sac (chorioamnionitis)
- cervical rupture (may occur if the stitch is not removed before onset of labor)
- injury to the cervix or bladder
- bleeding

Normal results

The success rate for cervical cerclage is approximately 80–90% for elective cerclages, and 40–60% for emergent cerclages. A cerclage is considered successful if labor and delivery is delayed to at least 37 weeks (full term).

Morbidity and mortality rates

Approximately 1–9% of women will experience premature labor after cerclage. The risk of chorioamnionitis is 1–7%, but increases to 30% if the cervix is dilated greater than 1.2 in (3 cm). The risks associated with premature delivery, however, are far greater. Babies born between 22 and 25 weeks of pregnancy are at significant risk of moderate to severe disabilities (46–56%) or death (approximately 10–30% survive at 22 weeks, increasing to 50% at 24 weeks, and 95% by 26 weeks).

Alternatives

Depending on her specific condition, a woman may have some alternative therapies available to her to avoid or delay premature labor. These include:

- Bed rest. At least 20% of pregnant women in the United States have at least one week of bed rest prescribed to them at some point of their pregnancy. The idea of bed rest is to avoid putting unnecessary pressure on the cervix.

- Tocolytics. These are drugs that are designed to stop or delay labor. Ritrodrine, terbutaline, and magnesium sulfate are some common tocolytics.

- Antibiotics. Some infections are associated with a high risk of preterm labor (e.g., upper genital tract infection). Antibiotics may be successful in preventing preterm labor from occurring by treating the infection.

Resources

BOOKS

Enkin, Murray, et al. *A Guide to Effective Care in Pregnancy and Childbirth,* 3rd ed. Oxford: Oxford University Press, 2000.

PERIODICALS

Goldenberg, Robert L. "The Management of Preterm Labor." *Obstetrics & Gynecology* 100, no. 5 (November 2002): 1020–37.

MacDonald, Hugh. "Perinatal Care at the Threshold of Viability." *American Academy of Pediatrics* 110, no. 5 (November 2002): 1024–7.

Matijevic, Ratko, Branka Olujic, Jasua Tumbri, and Asim Kurjak. "Cervical Incompetence: The Use of Selective and Emergency Cerclage." *Journal of Perinatal Medicine* 29 (2001): 31–5.

Weismiller, David G. "Preterm Labor." *American Family Physician* February 1, 1999: 593–604.

ORGANIZATIONS

American Academy of Family Physicians. 8880 Ward Parkway, Kansas City, MO 64114. (816) 333-9700. http://www.aafp.org.

American Board of Obstetrics and Gynecology. 2915 Vine Street, Dallas, TX 75204. (214) 871-1619. http://www.abog.org.

American College of Obstetricians and Gynecologists. 409 12th St., SW, PO Box 96920, Washington, DC 20090-6920. http://www.acog.org.

OTHER

Bernstein, Peter S. "Controversies in Obstetrics: Cervical Cerclage." *Third World Congress on Controversies in Obstetrics, Gynecology, and Infertility.* 2002 [cited March 1, 2003]. http://www.medscape.com/viewprogram/1964.

Pincock, Stephen. "Cervical Cerclage Associated with Good Pregnancy Outcome." *Reuters Health.* February 13, 2003 [cited March 1, 2003]. http://www.medscape.com/viewarticle/449414.

"Shortened Cervix in Second Trimester Possible Warning Sign for Premature Birth." *National Institute of Child Health and Development.* September 18, 2001 [cited March 1, 2003]. http://www.nichd.nih.gov/new/releases/cervix.cfm.

Starzyk, Kathryn A. and Carolyn M. Salafia. "A Perinatal Pathology View of Preterm Labor." *Medscape Women's Health eJournal.* 2000 [cited March 1, 2003]. http://www.medscape.com/viewarticle/408936_1.

Weiss, Robin Elise. "The Incompetent Cervix." [cited March 1, 2003.] <http://pregnancy.about.com/library/weekly/aa011298.htm>.

Stephanie Dionne Sherk

Cervical cryotherapy

Definition

Cervical **cryotherapy** is a procedure which involves freezing an area of abnormal tissue on the cervix. This tissue gradually disappears and the cervix heals. One cervical cryotherapy is usually sufficient to destroy the abnormal tissue.

Purpose

Cervical cryotherapy is a standard method used to treat cervical dysplasia, meaning the removal of abnormal cell tissue on the cervix.

Description

Cervical cryotherapy, or freezing, usually lasts about five minutes and causes a slight amount of

KEY TERMS

Biopsy—Procedure that involves obtaining a tissue specimen for microscopic analysis to establish a precise diagnosis.

Cervix—Opening of the uterus (womb) that leads into the vagina.

Colposcopy—Examination of the cervix through a magnifying device to detect abnormal cells.

Cryotherapy—The therapeutic use of cold to reduce discomfort, or remove abnormal tissue.

Dysplasia—Abnormality of development, or change in size, shape, and organization of adult cells.

Electrocautery—The cauterization of tissue using an electric current that generates heat.

Loop electrocautery excision procedure (LEEP)—Electrocautery performed to excise abnormal cervical tissue.

Pap smear—A test performed using a special stain applied on a smear taken from the cervix.

Squamous cells—Scaly or plate-like cells.

discomfort. The procedure is usually performed in an outpatient setting.

Cervical cryotherapy is done by placing a small freeze-probe (cryoprobe) against the cervix that cools the cervix to sub-zero temperatures. The cells destroyed by freezing are shed afterwards in a heavy watery discharge. The main advantage of cryotherapy is that it is a simple procedure that requires inexpensive equipment.

The cryogenic device consists of a gas tank containing a refrigerant and non-explosive, non-toxic gas (usually nitrous oxide). The gas is delivered using flexible tubing through a gun-type attachment to the cryoprobe.

Diagnosis/Preparation

Women who undergo cervical cryotherapy typically have had an abnormal Pap smear which has led to a diagnosis of cervical squamous dysplasia and usually confirmed by biopsy after an adequate colposcopic exam.

Preparation for cervical cryotherapy involves scheduling the procedure when the patient is not experiencing heavy menstrual flow. Ibuprofen, ketoprofen, or naproxen sodium may be given before cryotherapy

WHO PERFORMS THE PROCEDURE AND WHERE IS IT PERFORMED?

Cervical cryotherapy can be done in the treating physician's office. The physician is usually a gynecologist.

to decrease cramping. If there is any doubt about the pregnancy status, a pregnancy test is performed.

Aftercare

Cervical cryotherapy is often followed by a heavy and often odorous discharge during the first month after the procedure. The discharge is due to the dead tissue cells leaving the treatment site, and Aminocerv cream may be prescribed. The patient should abstain from sexual intercourse and not use tampons for a period of three weeks after the procedure. Excessive **exercise** should also be avoided to lessen the occurrence of post-therapy bleeding.

Risks

The following risks have been associated with cervical cryotherapy:

- Uterine cramping. Often occurs during the cryotherapy but rapidly subsides after treatment.
- Bleeding and infection. Rare, but incidences have been reported.
- More difficult Pap smears. Future Pap smears and colposcopy may be more difficult after cryotherapy.

Normal results

A normal result is no recurrence of the abnormal cervix cells. The first follow-up Pap smear is done within three to six months. If normal, Pap smears are repeated every six months for two years. If any, recurrences usually occur within two years of treatment. Another option is to replace the initial and each yearly Pap smear with a colposcopic examination.

If a follow-up Pap smear is abnormal, a **colposcopy** with biopsy is usually performed. Other treatment methods, usually the loop electrocautery excision procedure (LEEP) are then used if persistent disease is discovered.

Following the procedure, it is considered normal to experience the following:

- slight cramping for two to three days
- watery discharge requiring several pad changes daily
- bloody discharge, especially 12–16 days after the procedure

Alternatives

Alternatives to cryotherapy include:

- Laser treatment. A carbon dioxide laser focuses a beam of light to vaporize the abnormal cells. This technique can be used in the physician's office with very little discomfort.
- Loop electrocautery excision procedure (LEEP). This procedure uses a fine wire loop with an electric current flowing through it to remove the desired area of the cervix. Loop excision is usually done under local anesthesia and causes very little discomfort.

Resources

BOOKS

Handley, J. *What Your Doctor May Not Tell You about HPV and Abnormal Pap Smears.* New York: Warner Books, 2002.

Platzer, W., et al. *Vaginal Operations: Surgical Anatomy and Technique.* Philadelphia: Lippincott, Williams and Wilikins, 1996.

Rushing, L., and N. Joste. *Abnormal Pap Smears: What Every Woman Needs to Know.* Amherst, NY: Prometheus Books, 2001.

PERIODICALS

Sparks, R. A., D. Scheid, V. Loemker, E. Stader, K. Reilly, R. Hamm, and L. McCarthy. "Association of Cervical Cryotherapy with Inadequate Follow-up Colposcopy." *Journal of Family Practice* 51 (June 2002): 526–529.

Tate, D. R. and R. J. Anderson. "Recrudescence of Cervical Dysplasia among Women Who are Infected with the Human Immunodeficiency Virus: A Case-control Analysis." *American Journal of Obstetrics and Gynecology* 186 (May 2002): 880–882.

ORGANIZATIONS

American Society for Colposcopy and Cervical Pathology. 20 West Washington St., Suite 1, Hagerstown, MD 21740. (301) 733-3640. http://www.asccp.org/index.html

National Association for Women's Health. 300 W. Adams Street, Suite 328, Chicago, IL 60606-5101. (312) 786-1468. http://www.nawh.org

OTHER

"Cervical Cancer Prevention." *JHPIEG.* September 2002 [cited April 2003]. http://www.jhpiego.jhu.edu/cecap.

"Cytopathology." *The Internet Pathology Laboratory for Medical Education.* [cited April 2003]. <http//www-medlib.med.utah.edu/WebPath/TUTORIAL/CYTOPATH/CYTOPATH.html>.

Mayeaux Jr., E. J., M.D. "Cervical Cryotherapy Atlas." *LSUHSC-S Family Medicine Server.* [cited April 2003]. <http://lib-sh.lsumc.edu/fammed/atlases/cryo.html>.

National Women's Health Information Center. [cited April 2003]. http://www.4woman.org.

"What is cervical dysplasia?" *AMA Medical Library.* [cited April 2003]. http://www.medem.com.

Monique Laberge, PhD

Cesarean section

Definition

A cesarean section is a surgical procedure in which incisions are made through a woman's abdomen and uterus to deliver her baby.

Purpose

Cesarean sections, also called c-sections or cesarean deliveries, are performed whenever abnormal conditions complicate labor and vaginal delivery, threatening the life or health of the mother or the baby. Dystocia, or difficult labor, is the other common cause of c-sections. The procedure is performed in the United States on nearly one of every four babies delivered—more than 900,000 babies each year. The procedure is often used in cases where the mother has had a previous c-section.

The most common reason that a cesarean section is performed (in 35% of all cases, according to the United States Public Health Service) is the woman has had a previous c-section. The "once a cesarean, always a cesarean" rule originated when the uterine incision was made vertically (termed a "classical incision"); the resulting scar was weak and had a risk of rupturing in subsequent deliveries. Today, the incision

Cesarean section

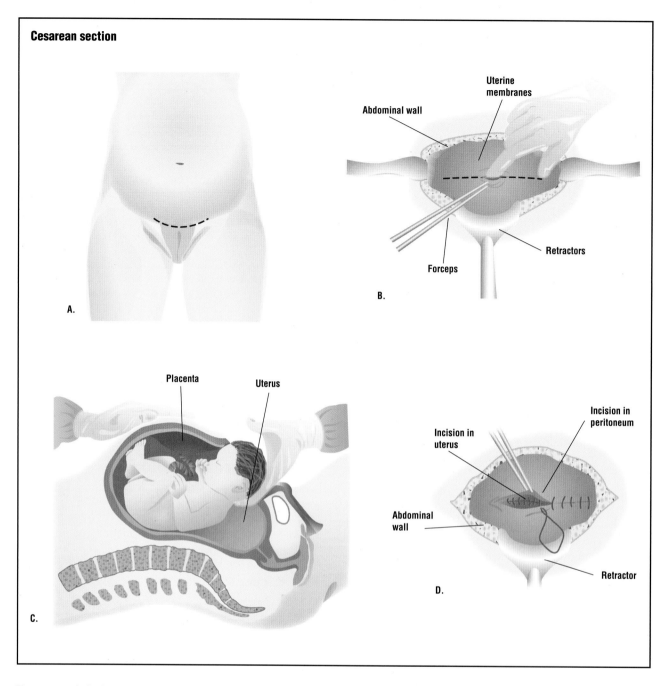

A.

B.

C.

D.

Uterine membranes

Abdominal wall

Retractors

Forceps

Placenta

Uterus

Incision in peritoneum

Incision in uterus

Abdominal wall

Retractor

To remove a baby by cesarean section, an incision is made into the abdomen, usually just above the pubic hairline (A). The uterus is located and divided (B), allowing for delivery of the baby (C). After all the contents of the uterus are removed, the uterus is repaired, and rest of the layers of the abdominal wall are closed (D). *(Illustration by GGS Information Services. Cengage Learning, Gale.)*

is almost always made horizontally across the lower end of the uterus (called a low transverse incision), resulting in reduced blood loss and a decreased chance of rupture. This kind of incision allows many women to have a vaginal birth after a cesarean (VBAC).

The second most common reason that a c-section is performed (in 30% of all cases) is difficult childbirth due to non-progressive labor (dystocia). Difficult labor is commonly caused by one of the three following conditions: abnormalities in the mother's birth canal; abnormalities in the position of the fetus; or abnormalities in the labor, including weak or infrequent contractions. The mother's pelvic structure may not allow adequate passage for birth. When the baby's head is too large to fit through the pelvis, the condition is called cephalopelvic disproportion (CPD).

KEY TERMS

Breech presentation—The condition in which the baby enters the birth canal with its buttocks or feet first.

Cephalopelvic disproportion (CPD)—The condition in which the baby's head is too large to fit through the mother's pelvis.

Classic incision—In a cesarean section, an incision made vertically along the uterus.

Dystocia—Failure to progress in labor, either because the cervix will not dilate (expand) further or (after full dilation) the head does not descend through the mother's pelvis.

Hematoma—A collection of blood localized to an organ, tissue, or space of the body.

Low transverse incision—Incision made horizontally across the lower end of the uterus.

Placenta previa—The placenta totally or partially covers the cervix, preventing vaginal delivery.

Placental abruption—Separation of the placenta from the uterine wall before the baby is born, cutting off blood flow to the baby.

Preeclampsia—A pregnancy-related condition that causes high blood pressure and swelling.

Prolapsed cord—The umbilical cord is pushed into the vagina ahead of the baby and becomes compressed, cutting off blood flow to the baby.

Respiratory distress syndrome (RDS)—Difficulty breathing; found in infants with immature lungs.

Transverse presentation—The baby is laying sideways across the cervix instead of head first.

VBAC—Vaginal birth after cesarean.

Another 12% of c-sections are performed to deliver a baby in a breech presentation (buttocks or feet first). Breech presentation is found in about 3% of all births.

In 9% of all cases, c-sections are performed in response to fetal distress, which refers to any situation that threatens the baby such as the umbilical cord wrapped around the baby's neck. This may appear on the fetal heart monitor as an abnormal heart rate or rhythm. Fetal brain damage can result from oxygen deprivation. Fetal distress is often related to abnormalities in the position of the fetus or abnormalities in the birth canal, causing reduced blood flow through the placenta.

The remaining 14% of c-sections are indicated by other serious factors. One is prolapse of the umbilical cord: the cord is pushed into the vagina ahead of the baby and becomes compressed, cutting off blood flow to the baby. Another is "placental abruption," whereby the placenta separates from the uterine wall before the baby is born, cutting off blood flow to the baby. The risk of this is especially high in multiple births (twins, triplets, or more). A third factor is "placenta previa," in which the placenta covers the cervix partially or completely, making vaginal delivery impossible. In some cases requiring c-section, the baby is in a transverse position, lying horizontally across the pelvis, perhaps with a shoulder in the birth canal.

The mother's health may make delivery by c-section the safer choice, especially in cases of maternal diabetes, hypertension, genital herpes, malignancies of the genital tract, and preeclampsia (high blood pressure related to pregnancy).

Choosing cesarean section

A 1997 survey of female obstetricians found that 31% would choose to have a c-section without trial of labor if they had an uncomplicated pregnancy. This finding mirrors a growing movement to allow women the right to choose c-section over vaginal delivery, even when no indications for c-section exist.

There are a number of reasons why a woman might choose a c-section in the absence of the usual indications. These include:

- Convenience. A scheduled c-section would allow a woman to choose the time and date of delivery to avoid conflicting with work or family obligations.

- Fear of childbirth. A woman might fear the pain of labor and delivery and feel that a scheduled c-section would allow her to circumvent it.

- Avoiding risks of vaginal delivery. Certain risks inherent to vaginal delivery (urinary or rectal incontinence, sexual dysfunction, dystocia) are avoided in a c-section.

Demographics

Women of higher socioeconomic status are more likely to have a c-section, 22.9%, compared to 13.2% of women who live in low-income families. C-section rates are highest among non-Hispanic white women (20.6%). Asian-American women have a c-section rate of 19.2%; African-American women, a rate of 18.9%, and Hispanic women, a rate of 13.9%.

Description

Regional anesthesia, either a spinal or epidural, is the preferred method of pain relief during a c-section. The benefits of regional anesthesia include allowing the mother to be awake during the surgery, avoiding the risks of **general anesthesia**, and allowing early contact between mother and child. Spinal anesthesia involves inserting a needle into a region between the vertebrae of the lower back and injecting numbing medications. An epidural is similar to a spinal except that a catheter is inserted so that numbing medications may be administered continuously. Some women experience a drop in blood pressure when a regional anesthetic is administered; this can be countered with fluids and/or medications.

In some instances, use of general anesthesia may be indicated. General anesthesia can be more rapidly administered in the case of an emergency (e.g., severe fetal distress). If the mother has a coagulation disorder that would be complicated by a drop in blood pressure (a risk with regional anesthesia), general anesthesia is an alternative. A major drawback of general anesthesia is that the procedure carries with it certain risks such as pulmonary aspiration and failed intubation. The baby may also be affected by the anesthetics since they cross the placenta; this effect is generally mild if delivery occurs within 10 minutes after anesthesia is administered.

Once the patient has received anesthesia, the abdomen is washed with an antibacterial solution and a portion of the pubic hair may be shaved. The first incision opens the abdomen. Infrequently, it will be vertical from just below the navel to the top of the pubic bone or, more commonly, it will be a horizontal incision across and above the pubic bone (informally called a "bikini cut").

The second incision opens the uterus. In most cases, a transverse incision is made. This is the favored type because it heals well and makes it possible for a woman to attempt a vaginal delivery in the future. The classical incision is vertical. Because it provides a larger opening than a low transverse incision, it is used in the most critical situations such as placenta previa. However, the classic incision causes more bleeding, a greater risk of abdominal infection, and a weaker scar.

Once the uterus is opened, the amniotic sac is ruptured and the baby is delivered. The time from the initial incision to birth is typically five minutes. The umbilical cord is clamped and cut, and the newborn is evaluated. The placenta is removed from the mother, and her uterus and abdomen are stitched closed (surgical **staples** may be used instead in closing the outermost layer of the abdominal incision). From birth through suturing may take 30–40 minutes; the entire surgical procedure may be performed in less than one hour.

Diagnosis/Preparation

There are several ways that obstetricians and other doctors diagnose conditions that may make a c-section necessary. **Ultrasound** testing reveals the positions of the baby and the placenta and may be used to estimate the baby's size and gestational age. Fetal heart monitors, in use since the 1970s, transmit any signals of fetal distress. Oxygen deprivation may be determined by checking the amniotic fluid for meconium (feces); a lack of oxygen may cause an unborn baby to defecate. Oxygen deprivation may also be determined by testing the pH of a blood sample taken from the baby's scalp; a pH of 7.25 or higher is normal, between 7.2 and 7.25 is suspicious, and below 7.2 is a sign of trouble.

When a c-section becomes necessary, the mother is prepped for surgery. A catheter is inserted into her bladder and an intravenous (IV) line is inserted into her arm. Leads for monitoring the mother's heart rate, rhythm, and blood pressure are attached. In the **operating room**, the mother is given anesthesia, usually a regional anesthetic (epidural or spinal), making her numb from below her breasts to her toes. In some cases, a general anesthetic will be administered. Surgical drapes are placed over the body, except the head; these drapes block the direct view of the procedure.

Aftercare

A woman who undergoes a c-section requires both the care given to any new mother and the care given to any patient recovering from major surgery. She should be offered pain medication that does not interfere with breastfeeding. She should be encouraged to get out of bed and walk around eight to 24 hours after surgery to stimulate circulation (thus avoiding the formation of blood clots) and bowel movement. She should limit climbing stairs to once a day, and avoid lifting anything heavier than the baby. She should nap as often as the baby sleeps, and arrange for help with the housework, meals, and care of other children. She may resume driving after two weeks, although some doctors recommend waiting for six weeks, the typical recovery period from major surgery.

Risks

Because a c-section is a surgical procedure, it carries more risk to both the mother and the baby. The maternal **death** rate is less than 0.02%, but that is four times the maternal death rate associated with vaginal delivery. Complications occur in less than 10% of cases.

The mother is at risk for increased bleeding (a c-section may result in twice the blood loss of a vaginal delivery) from the two incisions, the placental attachment site, and possible damage to a uterine artery. The mother may develop infection of the incision, the urinary tract, or the tissue lining the uterus (endometritis); infections occur in approximately 7% of women after having a c-section. Less commonly, she may receive injury to the surrounding organs such as the bladder and bowel. When a general anesthesia is used, she may experience complications from the anesthesia. Very rarely, she may develop a wound hematoma at the site of either incision or other blood clots leading to pelvic thrombophlebitis (inflammation of the major vein running from the pelvis into the leg) or a pulmonary embolus (a blood clot lodging in the lung).

Undergoing a c-section may also inflict psychological distress on the mother, beyond hormonal mood swings and postpartum depression ("baby blues"). The woman may feel disappointment and a sense of failure for not experiencing a vaginal delivery. She may feel isolated if the father or birthing coach is not with her in the operating room, or if an unfamiliar doctor treats her rather than her own doctor or midwife. She may feel helpless from a loss of control over labor and delivery with no opportunity to actively participate. To overcome these feelings, the woman must understand why the c-section was necessary. She must accept that she could not control the unforeseen events that made the c-section the optimum means of delivery, and recognize that preserving the health and safety of both her and her child was more important than her delivering vaginally. Women who undergo a c-section should be encouraged to share their feelings with others. Hospitals can often recommend support groups for such mothers. Women should also be encouraged to seek professional help if negative emotions persist.

Normal results

The aftereffects of a c-section vary, depending on the woman's age, physical fitness, and overall health. Following this procedure, a woman commonly experiences gas pains, incision pain, and uterine contractions (also common in vaginal delivery). Her hospital stay may be two to four days. Breastfeeding the baby is encouraged, taking care that it is in a position that keeps the baby from resting on the mother's incision. As the woman heals, she may gradually increase

WHO PERFORMS THE PROCEDURE AND WHERE IS IT PERFORMED?

Cesarean sections are considered to be major surgery and are therefore usually performed under the strict conditions of a hospital operating room. The procedure is generally performed by an obstetrician who specializes in the areas of women's general health, pregnancy, labor and childbirth, prenatal testing, and genetics.

appropriate exercises to regain abdominal tone. Full recovery may be achieved in four to six weeks.

The prognosis for a successful vaginal birth after a cesarean (VBAC) may be at least 75%, especially when the c-section involved a low transverse incision in the uterus and there were no complications during or after delivery.

Morbidity and mortality rates

Surgical injuries to the ureter or bowel occur in approximately 0.1% of c-sections. The risk of infection to the incision ranges from 2.5% to 15%. Urinary tract infections occur in 2–16% of patients post-c-section. The risk for developing a deep-vein thrombosis is three to five times higher in patients undergoing c-section than vaginal delivery.

Of the hundreds of thousands of women in the United States who undergo a c-section each year, about 500 die from serious infections, hemorrhaging, or other complications. The overall maternal mortality rate is estimated to be between six and 22 deaths per 100,000 births; approximately one-third of maternal deaths that occur after c-section can be attributed to the procedure. These deaths may be related to the health conditions that made the operation necessary, and not simply to the operation itself.

Alternatives

When a c-section is being considered because labor is not progressing, the mother should first be encouraged to walk around to stimulate labor. Labor may also be stimulated with the drug oxytocin. A woman should receive regular prenatal care and be able to alert her doctor to the first signs of trouble. Once labor begins, she should be encouraged to move around and to urinate. The doctor should be conservative in diagnosing dystocia and fetal distress, taking a position of "watchful waiting" before deciding to operate.

- What is your medical training and how many c-sections have you performed?
- What percentage of women receive c-sections in your practice?
- If I have an elective c-section, what happens if I go into labor before the procedure is scheduled?
- What options are available to me for pain relief during and after the c-section?
- May a person of my choice remain with me during the procedure?
- When will I be able to hold/breastfeed my child?

Approximately 3–4% of babies present at term in the breech position. Before opting to perform an elective c-section, the doctor may first attempt to reposition the baby; this is called external cephalic version. The doctor may also try a vaginal breech delivery, depending on the size of the mother's pelvis, the size of the baby, and the type of breech position the baby is in. However, a c-section is safer than a vaginal delivery when the baby is 8 lb (3.6 kg) or larger, in a breech position with the feet crossed, or in a breech position with the head hyperextended.

A vaginal birth after cesarean (VBAC) is an option for women who have had previous c-sections and are interested in a trial of labor (TOL). TOL is a purposeful attempt to deliver vaginally. The success rate for VBAC in patients who have had a prior low transverse uterine incision is approximately 70%. The most severe risk associated with TOL is uterine rupture: 0.2–1.5% of attempted VBACs among women with a low transverse uterine scar will end in uterine rupture, compared to 12% of women with a classic uterine incision. To minimize this risk, the American College of Obstetricians and Gynecologists (ACOG) recommends that VBAC be limited to women with full-term pregnancies (37–40 weeks) who have only had one previous low transverse c-section.

Resources

BOOKS

Enkin, Murray, et al. *A Guide to Effective Care in Pregnancy and Childbirth,* 3rd ed. Oxford: Oxford University Press, 2000.

PERIODICALS

Harer, W. Benson. "Vaginal Birth After Cesarean Delivery: Current Status." *Journal of the American Medical Association* 287, no. 20 (May 2002).

Murphy, Deirdre, Rachel Liebling, Lisa Verity, Rebecca Swingler, and Roshni Patel. "Early Maternal and Neonatal Morbidity Associated with Operative Delivery in Second Stage of Labour: A Cohort Study." *The Lancet* 358 (October 13, 2001): 1203–07.

Wagner, Marsden. "Choosing Cesarean Section." *The Lancet* 356 (November 11, 2000): 1677–80.

Yokoe, Deborah, et al. "Epidemiology of and Surveillance for Postpartum Infections." *Emerging Infectious Diseases* 7, no. 5 (2001).

ORGANIZATIONS

American Academy of Family Physicians. 8880 Ward Parkway, Kansas City, MO 64114. (816) 333-9700. http://www.aafp.org.

American Board of Obstetrics and Gynecology. 2915 Vine Street, Dallas, TX 75204. (214) 871-1619. http://www.abog.org.

American College of Obstetricians and Gynecologists. 409 12th St., SW, PO Box 96920, Washington, DC 20090-6920. http://www.acog.org.

International Cesarean Awareness Network. 1304 Kingsdale Ave., Redondo Beach, CA 90278. (310) 542-6400. http://www.ican-online.org.

OTHER

"Cesarean Birth." *American College of Obstetricians and Gynecologists,* March 1999 [cited February 26, 2003]. http://www.medem.com.

Duriseti, Ram. "Cesarean Section." *eMedicine,* August 29, 2001 [cited February 26, 2003]. http://www.emedicine.com/aaem/topic99.htm.

Sehdev, Harish. "Cesarean Delivery." *eMedicine,* February 22, 2002 [cited February 26, 2003]. http://www.emedicine.com/med/topic3283.htm.

Bethany Thivierge
Stephanie Dionne Sherk

Charts *see* **Medical charts**

Cheiloplasty *see* **Cleft lip repair**

Chemical debridement *see* **Debridement**

Chemistry screen

Definition

A chemistry screen is a blood test done to check for normal levels of various blood elements. A chemistry screen measures levels of the following blood parameters: electrolytes, specific proteins, lipids, sugar, enzymes associated with specific organs, blood gases, waste products, and other blood elements.

Purpose

There are many different reasons a physician may order a blood chemistry screen. A chemistry screen may be done as part of a routine examination to assess normal body function or a routine blood laboratory workup prior to surgery. Chemistry screens are used to identify potential disease states present in a patient, to monitor the progression of a patient's disease, to monitor disease treatment or recurrence of a disease, to observe levels of certain prescription medicines, or to assess the effects of prescription medicines that may be harmful.

Demographics

Chemistry screens are performed whenever medically necessary regardless of age, gender, or race. They are routinely done on patients before surgical procedures.

Description

Chemistry screens provide information on the quantity of specific chemical parameters in the blood. The patient's blood levels are listed along with a reference range of values for each component. The reference range indicates what the normal range of values is, from low to high. The chemistry screen compares the patient's blood levels to the reference range, and flags the patient's blood values as falling outside of the normal range when necessary. If the patient's values fall within the reference range, the value is considered normal. If the patient's value is higher or lower than the reference range, the physician then evaluates the results and follows a proper course of action. Whether or not a patient's blood chemistry screen demonstrates normal results can help determine whether a patient has a condition requiring surgery, or whether they are fit enough for a particular surgical procedure to be successful.

Chemistry screens can test for many different blood parameters, and can be customized by the physician to fit a particular patient's medical needs. When chemistry screens are customized, the physician merely indicates on the prescription that parameters not usually included in a standardized screen are to be included. Standardized forms of chemistry screens often used in the hospital include the Chem-6, Chem-7, Chem-12, and Chem-20, which measure 6, 7, 12, and 20 different blood components, respectively. The type of chemistry screen chosen by the physician is determined by the reason for the chemistry screen, any diseases the patient has, and specific medical symptoms the patient is experiencing that need to be explored via the results of the screen. The Chem-20 is

the most thorough, and includes all the parameters measured in the smaller screens with some additions.

The Chem-20 Chemistry Screen

The Chem-20 chemistry screen is also known as a Sequential Multi-channel Analysis -20 (SMA-20) screen. The Chem-20 tests for 20 different chemical parameters listed below.

Blood Parameters Measured in the Chem-20 Chemistry Screen

- alanine aminotransferase (ALT);
- albumin;
- alkaline phosphatase (ALP);
- aspartate aminotransferase (AST);
- bicarbonate;
- blood urea nitrogen (BUN);
- calcium;
- carbon dioxide;
- chloride;
- conjugated bilirubin;
- creatinine;
- gamma glutamyl transpeptidase (GGT);
- glucose;
- lactate dehydrogenase (LDH);
- phosphate;
- potassium;
- sodium;
- total bilirubin;
- total cholesterol; and
- uric acid.

The blood components measured in the chemistry screen may be affected by various disease or nutritional states. A physician can learn much about the health condition of a patient by interpreting the results of a chemistry screen. The overall picture of health presented by the combined measurements in the chemistry screen are more informative than any one value alone.

General Description of Blood Parameters Measured in a Chemistry Screen

Albumin is a blood component made in the liver. Albumin binds to and carries certain substances in the blood, including some medications. It is important for keeping the proper amount of fluid within blood vessels, tissue growth, and healing. Albumin is measured to help assess liver and kidney function, as well as nutritional state.

NORMAL RESULTS REFERENCE RANGE (MAY VARY SLIGHTLY BY TESTING LABORATORY)

- alanine aminotransferase: 4–36 U/L;
- albumin: 3.5–5.5 g/dl;
- alkaline phosphatase: males 38–126 U/L, females 70–230 U/L;
- aspartate aminotransferase: 8–35 U/L;
- bicarbonate: 21–27 mEq/L;
- blood urea nitrogen: 7–18 mg/dl;
- calcium: 8.4–10.2 mg/dl;
- carbon dioxide: 35–45 mm Hg;
- chloride: 98–106 mEq/L;
- conjugated bilirubin: 0–0.2 mg/dl;
- creatinine: 0.6–1.2 mg/dl;
- gamma glutamyl transpeptidase: 7–50 U/L;
- glucose: 70–115 mg/dl;
- lactate dehydrogenase: 90–190 U/L;
- phosphate: 2.7–4.5 mg/dl; males >60 years old 2.3–3.7, females 2.8–4.1 mg/dL;
- potassium: 3.5–5.1 mEq/L;
- sodium: 135–145 mEq/L;
- total bilirubin: 0.2–1.0 mg/dl;
- total cholesterol: <200 mg/dl; and
- uric acid: males 3.5–7.2 mg/dl, females 2.6–6.0 mg/dl.

QUESTIONS TO ASK YOUR DOCTOR

- Why do I need a chemistry screen?
- Is the screen being done to look for signs of a specific disease?
- Do I need to fast before the chemistry screen?
- Will any of my prescription or non-prescription medications, herbal, or nutritional supplements affect the results of the chemistry screen?
- When will I get the results of the screen?
- Could any of the results affect my surgery if they are abnormal?

Blood urea nitrogen tests how well the kidneys are functioning to remove waste from the body for excretion in the urine. Creatinine is another parameter measured to help assess kidney function. The ratio of the amount of BUN and creatinine present in the blood provides a more detailed picture of kidney function than either measurement alone. Uric acid is an indicator of kidney function in removing waste from the blood.

ALT, ALP, AST, GGT, and LDH are all enzymes associated with the liver whose levels help assess liver function and whether the liver is damaged. In addition to the liver, ALP is associated with the kidney, bones, and placenta. LDH is also associated with many different organs including the heart, brain, and skeletal muscle and is released with tissue damage. Bilirubin is a breakdown product of red blood cells that is taken up from the blood by the liver, altered, and secreted through the bile into the digestive tract where it is partially excreted in feces. Measurements involving bilirubin assess how well the liver and associated biliary tract is functioning.

Electrolytes such as potassium, sodium, and chloride are measured in chemistry screens. Electrolytes are minerals found naturally in the body; are necessary to keep a balance in body fluids; to maintain normal body functions such as heart rhythm, muscle contraction, and brain function. Electrolyte imbalances can be caused by various disease states, including kidney disease. Calcium and phosphate levels may also be affected by kidney function, parathyroid disorders, and certain bone diseases. Both chloride and bicarbonate levels are indicative of acid base disorders and the ability of the blood to buffer acid and base to determine the pH value.

Cholesterol is measured to assess the level of fatty substances in the blood that affect the arteries and the heart. Glucose levels are potential indicators of liver function, pancreatic function, and the body's ability to utilize sugar for energy. Carbon dioxide gas levels in the blood assess the function of both the lungs and the kidneys. Each component of the chemistry screen can be affected in distinct ways by many different disease states. Interpreting the results of the chemistry screen requires much training and experience.

How the Chemistry Screen is Done

Chemistry screens are done using blood samples. Having blood drawn from a vein with a syringe, usually in the arm, is necessary. Some parameters of the chemistry screen may require a period of fasting from all food and drink (except water) before the test. Patients should also avoid high fat foods or alcohol the night before the test. Since some medications may affect the results of the chemistry screen, it is critical that the physician take into account all prescription medications, non-prescription medications, herbal, and nutritional supplements that the patient is taking before running the chemistry screen. Some people may have slightly high or low values as their normal level. Age and gender may also affect the results in predictable patterns.

Risks Associated with the Procedure

There is very little risk associated with having blood drawn for a chemistry screen. Most people have no side effects; some may get a small bruise where the syringe was inserted. With any blood draw there is a small chance that the area around the punctured vein may develop phlebitis, the inflammation of a vein. Phlebitis may also involve a bacterial infection if the site of the blood draw was not appropriately cleaned before the needle was inserted. Phlebitis can be locally painful but usually resolves in a short period of time.

Additionally, patients with disorders involving the inability of the blood to form normal blood clots should discuss their condition and their medications with the physician before the blood draw and chemistry screen is done.

Who Performs the Procedure?

A chemistry screen is prescribed by a physician. It is a routine test that is run before a surgical procedure. A nurse often draws the blood sample from the patient. The blood sample is then sent to a specific hospital laboratory that tests the blood. The results of the chemistry screen are then sent to the physician for review.

Resources

BOOKS

Chaudhry, H. J., et al. *Fundamentals of Clincal Medicine*, 4th ed. Philadelphia: Lippincott Williams & Wilkins, 2004.

Maxwell, R. W. *Maxwell Quick Medical Reference*, 5th ed. Tulsa, OK: Maxwell Publishing Company, 2006.

OTHER

"Chemistry Screen." WebMD.com. May 19, 2006. http://www.webmd.com/a-to-z-guides/chemistry-screen (April 7, 2008).

Maria Basile, Ph.D.

Chest radiography *see* **Chest x ray**

Chest surgery *see* **Thoracic surgery**

Chest tube insertion

Definition

A chest tube insertion is a procedure to place a flexible, hollow drainage tube into the chest in order to remove an abnormal collection of air or fluid from the pleural space (located between the inner and outer lining of the lung).

Purpose

Chest tube insertions are usually performed as an emergency procedure. Chest tubes are used to treat conditions that can cause the lung to collapse, which occurs because blood or air in the pleural space can hamper the ability of a patient to breath.

There are four common conditions than can require surgical chest tube insertion, including:

- pneumothorax (air leak from the lung into the chest)
- hemothorax (bleeding into the chest)
- empyema (lung abscess or pus in the chest)
- pneumothorax or hemothorax after surgery or from trauma to the chest

Demographics

There is no available data concerning the demographics of chest tube insertion since this is a common procedure performed in emergency rooms and surgical departments. However, pneumothorax seems to occur most often in males 25–40 years of age.

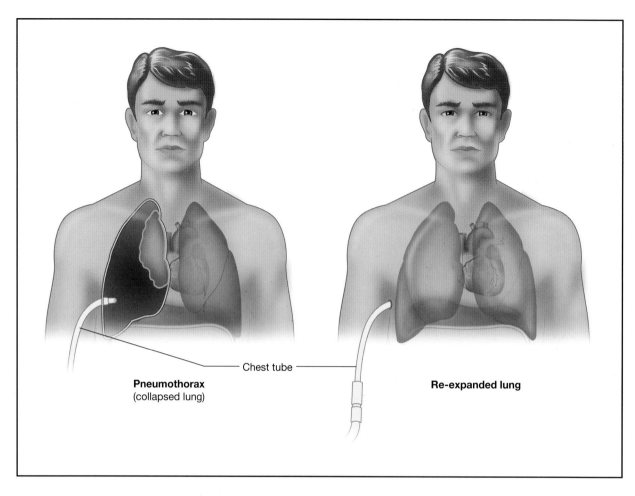

Pneumothorax
(collapsed lung)

Chest tube

Re-expanded lung

(Illustration by Electronic Illustrators Group.)

Description

The point of insertion in the chest most commonly occurs on the side (lateral thorax), at a line drawn from the armpit (anterior axillary line) to the side (lateral) of the nipple in males, or to the side (about 2 in [5 cm]) above the sternoxiphoid junction (lower junction of the sternum, or chest bone) in females. The skin is sterilized with antiseptic solution covering a wide area, and **local anesthesia** is administered to minimize discomfort. At the rib chosen for insertion, the skin over the rib is anesthetized with lidocaine (a local chemical anesthetic agent) using a 10-cc syringe and 25-gauge needle. At the rib below the rib chosen for pleural insertion, the tissues, muscles, bone, and lining covering the lung are also anesthetized using a 22-gauge needle.

All health-care providers will take precautions to keep the procedure sterile, including the usage of sterile gown, facemask, and eye protection. All equipment must be sterile as well and universal precautions are followed for blood and body fluids. Chest tube size is selected depending on the problem; an 18–20 F(rench) catheter is used for pneumothorax, a 32–26 F catheter for hemothorax, and trauma patients usually require a 38–40 F catheter size; children generally require smaller tube sizes.

The patient's arm is placed over the head with a restraint on the affected side. For an insertion line down the armpit (axillary line insertion), the patient's head is elevated from the bed 30–60°. Using the anesthetic needle and syringe, the physician will insert a needle (aspirate) into the pleural cavity to check for the presence of air or fluid. Then, an incision is made and a clamp is used to open the pleural cavity. At this stage, either air or fluid will rush out when the pleural cavity is opened. The chest tube is positioned for insertion with a clamp and attached to the suction-drain system. A silk suture is used to hold the tube firmly in place. The area is wrapped, and an x ray is taken to visualize the status of the tube placement.

Diagnosis/Preparation

The diagnosis for chest tube insertion depends on the primary cause of fluid or air in the pleural cavity.

For malignancy (cancer)-causing pleural effusion (fluid in the pleural space filled with malignant cells), the diagnosis can be established with positive cytopathology (cancer cell visualization and analysis) and a **chest x ray** that shows fluid accumulation.

The typical diagnostic signs and symptoms of empyema (lung infection) include fever, cough, and sputum discharge as well as the development of pleural effusion (causing chest pain and shortness of breath). This type of lung infection can progress to systemic disease with such signs as weakness, and loss of appetite (anorexia). Chest x rays can readily allow the clinician to view the pleural effusion and can also help to detect pneumothorax, since there is visual proof in the displacement of the tissues covering the lungs as a result of air in the pleural cavity. Additionally, during physical examinations, people with pnemothorax have diminished breath sounds, hyperesonance on percussion (a highly resonating sound when the physician taps gently on a patient's back), and diminished ability to expand the chest. Computed axial tomography (CAT) scans can be used to visualize and analyze complicated cases that may require chest tube insertion.

Aftercare

The chest tube typically remains secure and in place until imaging studies such as x rays show that air or fluid has been removed from the pleural cavity. This removal of air or fluid will allow the affected lung to fully re-expand, allowing for adequate or improved

breathing. After chest tube insertion, the patient will stay in the hospital until the tube is removed. It is common to expect complete recovery from chest tube insertion and removal. During the stay, the medical and nursing staff will carefully and periodically monitor the chest tube for air leaks or if the patient is having breathing difficulties. Deep breathing and coughing after insertion can help with drainage and lung re-expansion.

Aftercare should also include chest tube removal and follow-up care. The patient is placed in the same position in which the tube was inserted. Using precautions to maintain a sterile field, the suture holding the tube in place is loosened and the chest is prepared for tying the insertion-point wound. The chest tube is then clamped to disconnect the suction system. At this point, the patient will be asked to hold his or her breath, and the clinician will remove the tube with a swift motion. After the suture is tied, dressing (gauze with antibiotic ointment) and tape is securely applied to close the wound. A chest x ray should be repeated soon after tube removal and, within 48 hours, a routine **wound care** clinic follow-up is advised to remove the dressing and to further assess the patient's medical status and condition.

Risks

Although chest tube insertion is a commonly used as a therapeutic measure, there are several complications that can develop, including:

- bleeding from an injured intercostal artery (running from the aorta)
- accidental injury to the heart, arteries, or lung resulting from the chest tube insertion
- a local or generalized infection from the procedure
- persistent or unexplained air leaks in the tube

- the tube can be dislodged or inserted incorrectly
- insertion of chest tube can cause open or tension pneumothorax

Normal results

Chest tube insertion is a commonly used procedure, and it is typical for patients to recover fully from insertion and removal. If no complications develop, the procedure can relieve air or fluid accumulation in the pleural cavity that caused breathing impairment. Breathing is usually improved, and follow-up within the immediate 48 hours after hospital discharge is advised so that the patient can be further assessed with x rays and in the wound care clinic.

Morbidity and mortality rates

Mortality and morbidity for chest tube insertion is not strongly associated with the procedure itself. The primary cause responsible for fluid or air accumulation in the pleural cavity is related to continued illness and outcome such as pleural effusions caused by cancer (malignant pleural effusions). Cancer, and not the insertion of a chest tube, determines a patient's sickness and outcome. Chest tube insertion may be problematic in persons affected with certain connective tissue diseases.

Alternatives

The diagnosis, indications, and procedure for chest tube insertion are specific and unambiguous. There is no other alternative to rapidly remove accumulation of fluid or air within the pleural cavity.

Resources

BOOKS

Pfenninger, John. *Procedures for Primary Care Physicians,* 1st ed. St Louis: Mosby-Year Book, Inc., 1994.
Townsend, Courtney. *Sabiston Textbook of Surgery,* 16th ed. St. Louis: W. B. Saunders Company, 2001.

ORGANIZATIONS

*American Thoracic Society Homepage.*http://www.thoracic.org.

Laith Farid Gulli, MD
Nicole Mallory, MS, PA-C
Alfredo Mori, MBBS

Chest x ray

Definition

A chest x ray is a procedure used to evaluate organs and structures within the chest for symptoms of disease. Chest x rays include views of the lungs, heart, small portions of the gastrointestinal tract, thyroid gland, and the bones of the chest area. X rays are a form of radiation that can penetrate the body and produce an image on an x-ray film. Another name for the film produced by x rays is radiograph.

Purpose

Chest x rays are ordered for a wide variety of diagnostic purposes. In fact, this is probably the most frequently performed type of x ray. In some cases, chest x rays are ordered for a single check of an organ's condition, and at other times, serial x rays are ordered to compare to previous studies. Some common reasons for chest x rays include the following.

Pulmonary disorders

Chest films are frequently ordered to diagnose or rule out pneumonia. One type, tuberculosis, can be observed on chest x rays, as can cardiac disease and damage to the ribs or lungs. Other pulmonary disorders such as pneumothorax (presence of air or gas in the chest cavity outside the lungs) or emphysema may be detected or evaluated through the use of chest x ray.

Cancer

A chest x ray may be ordered by a physician to check for possible tumors of the lungs, lymphoid tissue, or bones of the thorax. These may be primary tumors, or the areas in which cancer originates in the body. X rays also check for secondary spread of cancer from another organ to the chest.

KEY TERMS

Bronchi—Plural of bronchus. The air passages in the lungs through which inhaled air passes on its way through the lungs.

Diaphragm—The large muscle that is located between the abdomen and the chest area. The diaphragm aids in breathing.

Gastrointestinal—The digestive organs and structures, including the stomach and intestines.

Interstitial lung disease—About 180 diseases fall into this category of breathing disorders. Injury or foreign substances in the lungs (such as asbestos fibers) as well as infections, cancers, or inherited disorders may cause the diseases. They can lead to breathing or heart failure.

Lymphoid—Tissues relating to the lymphatic system. A thin, yellowish fluid called lymph fluid, travels throughout the body. The lymphatic system helps control fluids in the body.

Portable chest x ray—An x ray procedure taken by equipment that can be brought to the patient. The resulting radiographs may not be as high in quality as stationary x-ray radiographs, but allow a technologist to come to the patient.

Pulmonary—Refers to the lungs and the breathing system and function.

Serial x rays—A number of x rays performed at set times in the disease progression or treatment intervals. The radiographs will be compared to one another to track changes.

Sternum—Also referred to as the breast bone, this is the long flat bone in the middle of the chest.

Thorax—The chest area, which runs between the abdomen and neck and is encased in the ribs.

X ray—A form of electromagnetic radiation with shorter wavelengths than normal light. X rays can penetrate most structures.

Cardiac disorders

While less sensitive than **echocardiography**, chest x ray can be used to check for disorders such as congestive heart failure or pulmonary edema.

Other

Chest x rays are used to see foreign bodies that may have been swallowed or inhaled, and to evaluate response to treatment for various diseases. Often the chest x ray is also used to verify correct placement of chest tubes or catheters. Chest x rays can be used to check for fluid surrounding the lungs (pleural effusion).

Description

Routine chest x rays consist of two views, the frontal view (referred to as posterioranterior or PA) and the lateral (side) view. It is preferred that the patient stand for this exam, particularly when studying collection of fluid in the lungs.

During the actual time of exposure, the technologist will ask the patient to hold his or her breath. It is very important in taking a chest x ray to ensure there is no motion that could detract from the quality and sharpness of the film image. The procedure will only take a few minutes and the time patients must hold their breath is a matter of a few seconds.

The chest x ray may be performed in a physician's office or referred to an outpatient radiology facility or hospital radiology department. In some cases, particularly for patients who cannot get out of bed, a portable chest x ray may be taken. Portable films are sometimes of poorer quality than those taken with permanent equipment, but are the best choice for some patients or situations when the patient cannot be moved or properly positioned for the chest x ray. Patients confined to bed may be placed in as upright a position as possible to get a clear picture, particularly of chest fluid.

Preparation

There is no advance preparation necessary for chest x rays. Once the patient arrives in the exam area, a hospital gown will replace all clothing on the upper body and all jewelry must be removed.

Aftercare

No aftercare is required by patients who have chest x rays.

Risks

The only risk associated with chest x ray is minimal exposure to radiation, particularly for pregnant women and children. Those patients should use protective lead aprons during the procedure. Technologists are cautioned to check carefully possible dislodging of any tubes or monitors in the chest area from the patient's placement during the exam.

Normal results

A radiologist, or physician specially trained in the technique and interpretation of x rays, will evaluate the results. A normal chest x ray will show normal structures for the age and medical history of the patient. Findings, whether normal or abnormal, will be provided to the referring physician in the form of a written report.

Abnormal findings on chest x rays are used in conjunction with a physician's physical exam findings, patient medical history, and other diagnostic tests, including laboratory tests, to reach a final diagnosis. For many diseases, chest x rays are more effective when compared to previous chest x-ray studies. The patient is asked to help the radiology facility in locating previous chest radiographs from other facilities.

Pulmonary disorders

Pneumonia shows up on radiographs as patches and irregular areas of density (from fluid in the lungs). If the bronchi (air passages in the lungs which are usually not visible) can be seen, a diagnosis of bronchial pneumonia may be made. Shifts or shadows in the hila (lung roots) may indicate enlarged lymph nodes of a malignancy. Widening of the spaces between ribs and increased lucency of the lung fields suggests emphysema. Other pulmonary diseases may also be detected or suspected through chest x ray.

Cancer

In nearly all patients with lung cancer, some sort of abnormality can be seen on a chest radiograph. Hilar masses (enlargements at that part of the lungs where vessels and nerves enter) are one of the more common symptoms as are abnormal masses and fluid buildup on the outside surface of the lungs or surrounding areas. Interstitial lung disease, which is a large category of disorders, many of which are related to exposure of substances (such as asbestos fibers), may be detected on a chest x ray as increased prominence of the interstitial pattern, often in the lower portions of the lungs.

Other

Congestive heart failure and other cardiac diseases may be indicated on the view of a heart and lung in a chest radiograph. Fractures of the sternum and ribs are sometimes detected as breaks on the chest x ray, though often dedicated bone films are needed. In some instances, the radiologist's view of the diaphragm may indicate an abdominal problem. Foreign bodies that may have been swallowed or inhaled can usually be located by the radiologist, as they will look different from any other tissue or structure in the chest. Serial chest x rays may be ordered to track changes over a period of time, usually to evaluate response to therapy of a malignancy.

Resources

ORGANIZATIONS

American Lung Association. 1740 Broadway, New York, NY 10019. (800) 586–4872. http://www.lungusa.org.

Emphysema Anonymous, Inc. P.O. Box 3224, Seminole FL 34642. (813) 391–9977.

National Heart, Lung and Blood Institute. P.O. Box 30105, Bethesda, MD 20824–0105. (301) 251–1222. http://www.nhlbi.nih.gov.

Teresa Norris, RN
Lee Shratter, MD

Children's surgery *see* **Pediatric surgery**

Chin cosmetic surgery *see* **Mentoplasty**

Chloride test *see* **Electrolyte tests**

Cholecystectomy

Definition

A cholecystectomy is the surgical removal of the gallbladder. The two basic types of this procedure are open cholecystectomy and the laparoscopic approach. It is estimated that the laparoscopic procedure is currently used for approximately 80% of cases.

Purpose

A cholecystectomy is performed to treat cholelithiasis and cholecystitis. In cholelithiasis, gallstones of varying shapes and sizes form from the solid components of bile. The presence of these stones, often referred to as gallbladder disease, may produce symptoms of excruciating right upper abdominal pain radiating to the right shoulder. The gallbladder may become the site of acute infection and inflammation, resulting in symptoms of upper right abdominal pain, nausea, and vomiting. This condition is referred to as cholecystitis. The surgical removal of the gallbladder can provide relief of these symptoms. Cholecystectomy is used to treat both acute and chronic cholecystitis when there are significant pain symptoms. The typical composition of gallstones is predominately cholesterol, or a compound called calcium bilirubinate.

Cholecystectomy (Laparoscopic)

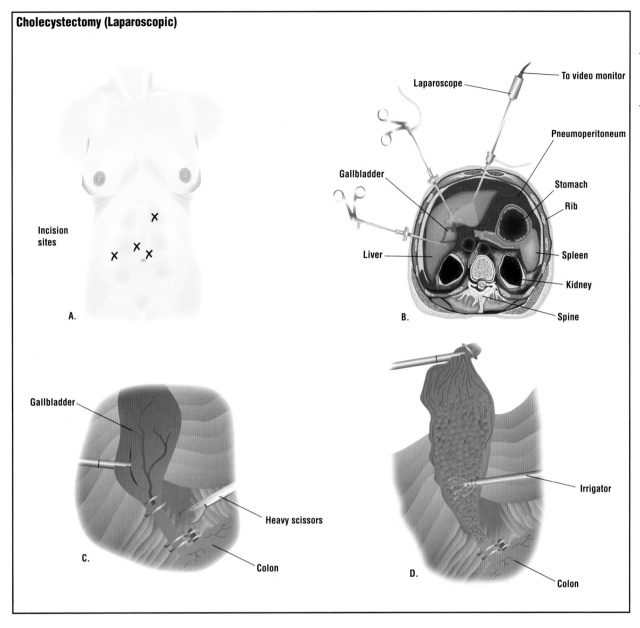

In a laparoscopic cholecystectomy, four small incisions are made in the abdomen (A). The abdomen is filled with carbon dioxide, and the surgeon views internal structures with a video monitor (B). The gallbladder is located and cut with laparoscopic scissors (C). It is then removed through an incision (D). *(Illustration by GGS Information Services. Cengage Learning, Gale.)*

Cholelithiasis

Most patients with cholelithiasis have no significant physical symptoms. Approximately 80% of gallstones do not cause significant discomfort. Patients who develop biliary colic generally do have some symptoms. When gallstones obstruct the cystic duct, intermittent, extreme, cramping pain typically develops in the right upper quadrant of the abdomen. This pain generally occurs at night and can last from a few minutes to several hours. An acute attack of cholecystitis is often associated with the consumption of a large, high-fat meal.

The medical management of gallstones depends to a great degree on the presentation of the patient. Patients with no symptoms generally do not require any medical treatment. The best treatment for patients with symptoms is usually surgery. Laparoscopic cholecystectomy is typically preferred over the open surgical

KEY TERMS

Cholecystitis—Infection and inflammation of the gallbladder, causing severe pain and rigidity in the upper right abdomen.

Cholelithiasis—Also known as gallstones, these hard masses are formed in the gallbladder or passages, and can cause severe upper right abdominal pain radiating to the right shoulder, as a result of blocked bile flow.

Gallbladder—A hollow pear-shaped sac on the under surface of the right lobe of the liver. Bile comes to it from the liver, and passes from it to the intestine to aid in digestion.

Laparoscope—A device consisting of a tube and optical system for observing the inside of the abdomen and its organs.

approach because of the decreased recovery period. Patients who are not good candidates for either type of surgery can obtain some symptom relief with drugs, especially oral bile salts.

Cholecystitis

Cholecystitis is an inflammation of the gallbladder, both acute and chronic, that results after the development of gallstones in some individuals. The most common symptoms and physical findings associated with cholecystitis include:

- pain and tenderness in the upper right quadrant of the abdomen
- nausea
- vomiting
- fever
- jaundice
- history of pain after eating large, high-fat meals

Demographics

Overall, cholelithiasis is found in about 20,000,000 Americans. An overwhelming majority of these individuals do not ever develop symptoms. Overall, about 500,000–600,000 (2–3%) are treated with cholecystectomies every year. Typically, the incidence of cholelithiasis increases with age. The greatest incidence occurs in individuals between the ages of 40 and 60 years. The following groups are at an increased risk for developing cholelithiasis:

- pregnant women
- females

- family history of gallstones
- obesity
- certain types of intestinal disease
- age greater than 40 years
- oral contraceptive use
- diabetes mellitus
- estrogen replacement therapy
- rapid weight loss

Overall, patients with cholelithiasis have about a 20% chance of developing biliary colic (the extremely painful complication that usually requires surgery) over a 20-year period.

Acute cholecystitis develops most commonly in women between the ages of 40 and 60 years. Some ethnic groups, such as Native Americans, have a dramatically higher incidence of cholecystitis.

Description

The laparoscopic cholecystectomy involves the insertion of a long, narrow cylindrical tube with a camera on the end, through an approximately 0.4 in (1 cm) incision in the abdomen, which allows visualization of the internal organs and projection of this image onto a video monitor. Three smaller incisions allow for insertion of other instruments to perform the surgical procedure. A laser may be used for the incision and cautery (burning unwanted tissue to stop bleeding), in which case the procedure may be called laser laparoscopic cholecystectomy.

In a conventional or open cholecystectomy, the gallbladder is removed through a surgical incision high in the right abdomen, just beneath the ribs. A drain may be inserted to prevent accumulation of fluid at the surgical site.

Diagnosis/Preparation

The initial diagnosis of acute cholecystitis is based on the following symptoms:

- constant, dull pain in upper right quadrant of abdomen
- fever
- chills
- nausea
- vomiting
- pain aggravated by moving or coughing

Most patients have elevated leukocyte (white blood cells) levels. Leukocyte levels are determined using laboratory analysis of blood samples. Traditional x rays are not particularly useful in diagnosing cholecystitis. Ultrasonography of the gallbladder usually provides evidence of gallstones, if they are present. Ultrasonography can also help identify inflammation of the gallbladder. Nuclear imaging may also be used. This type of imaging cannot identify gallstones, but it can provide evidence of obstruction of the cystic and common bile ducts.

Cholelithiasis is initially diagnosed based on the following signs and symptoms:

- history of biliary colic or jaundice
- nausea
- vomiting
- sudden onset of extreme pain in the upper right quadrant of the abdomen
- fever
- chills

Laboratory blood analysis often finds evidence of elevated bilirubin, alkaline phosphatase, or aminotransferase levels. Ultrasonography, computed tomography (CT) scanning, and radionuclide imaging are able to detect the impaired functioning of bile flow and of the bile ducts.

As with any surgical procedure, the patient will be required to sign a consent form after the procedure is explained thoroughly. Food and fluids will be prohibited after midnight before the procedure. Enemas may be ordered to clean out the bowel. If nausea or vomiting are present, a suction tube to empty the stomach may be used, and for laparoscopic procedures, a urinary drainage catheter will also be used to decrease the risk of accidental puncture of the stomach or bladder with insertion of the trocar (a sharp, pointed instrument).

Aftercare

Postoperative care for the patient who has had an open cholecystectomy, as with those who have had any major surgery, involves monitoring of blood pressure, pulse, respiration, and temperature. Breathing tends to be shallow because of the effect of anesthesia, and the patient's reluctance to breathe deeply due to the pain caused by the proximity of the incision to the muscles used for respiration. The patient is shown how to support the operative site when breathing deeply and coughing and is given pain medication as necessary. Fluid intake and output is measured, and the operative site is observed for color and amount of wound drainage. Fluids are given intravenously for 24–48 hours, and then the patient's diet is gradually advanced as bowel activity resumes. The patient is generally encouraged to walk eight hours after surgery and discharged from the hospital within three to five days, with return to work approximately four to six weeks after the procedure.

Care received immediately after laparoscopic cholecystectomy is similar to that of any patient undergoing surgery with **general anesthesia**. A unique postoperative pain may be experienced in the right shoulder related to pressure from carbon dioxide used in the laparoscopic tubes. This pain may be relieved by lying down on the left side with right knee and thigh drawn up to the chest. Walking will also help increase the body's reabsorption of the gas. The patient is usually discharged the day after surgery and allowed to shower on the second postoperative day. The patient is advised to gradually resume normal activities over a three-day period, while avoiding heavy lifting for about 10 days.

Risks

Potential problems associated with open cholecystectomy include respiratory problems related to location of the incision, wound infection, or abscess formation. Possible complications of laparoscopic cholecystectomy include accidental puncture of the bowel or bladder and uncontrolled bleeding. Incomplete reabsorption of the carbon dioxide gas could irritate the muscles used in respiration and cause respiratory distress. While most patients with acute cholecystitis respond well to the laparoscopic technique, about 5–30% of these patients require a conversion to the open technique because of complications. Some patients undergoing elective laparoscopic cholecystectomy will require conversion to an open procedure.

Normal results

The prognosis for cholecystitis and cholelithiasis patients who receive cholecystectomy is generally good. Overall, cholecystectomy relieves symptoms in about 95% of cases.

Morbidity and mortality rates

The complication rate is less than 0.5% with open cholecystectomy and about 1% with laparoscopic cholecystectomy. The primary complication with the open technique is infection, whereas bile leak and hemorrhage are the most common complications associated with the laparoscopic technique. The overall mortality rate associated with cholecystectomy is less than 1%. However, the rate of mortality in the elderly is higher.

In a small minority of cases, symptoms will persist in patients who receive cholecystectomy. This has been named the post-cholecystectomy syndrome, and

Cholecystectomy, including the laparoscopic approach, is usually performed by a general surgeon who has completed a five-year residency training program in all components of general surgery and, in particular, proper techniques involving the use of the laparoscope. If surgery is being considered, it is a good idea to find out how many laparoscopic cholecystectomies the surgeon performs on a yearly basis. Laparoscopic cholecystectomies are often performed in the specialized department of a general hospital, but they are also performed in specialized gastrointestinal clinics or institutes for gastrointestinal disorders.

- What are my alternatives?
- Can you recommend a surgeon who performs the laparoscopic procedure?
- If surgery is appropriate for me, what are the next steps?
- How many times have you performed open or laparoscopic cholecystectomy?
- Are you a board-certified surgeon?
- What type of outcomes have you had?
- What are the most common side effects or complications?
- What should I do to prepare for surgery?
- What should I expect following the surgery?
- Can you refer me to one of your patients who has had this procedure?
- What diagnostic procedures are performed to determine if I require surgery?
- Will I need to see another specialist for the diagnostic procedures?

usually results from functional bowel disorder, errors in diagnosis, technical errors, overlooked common bile duct stones, recurrence of common bile duct stones, or the spasm of a structure called the sphincter of Oddi.

Alternatives

Acute cholecystitis usually improves following conservative therapy in most patients. This conservative therapy involves the withholding of oral feedings, the use of intravenous feedings, and the administration of **antibiotics** and **analgesics**. This is only a short-term alternative in hospitalized patients. Most of these patients should receive cholecystectomy within a few days to prevent recurrent attacks. In the short term, patients often receive narcotic analgesics such as meperidine to relieve the intense pain associated with this condition. Patients who have evidence of gallbladder perforation or gangrene need to have an immediate cholecystectomy.

In patients with cholelithiasis who are deemed unfit for surgery, alternative treatments are sometimes effective. These individuals often have symptom improvement after lifestyle changes and medical therapy. Lifestyle changes include dietary avoidance of foods high in polyunsaturated fats and gradual weight loss in obese individuals. Medical therapy includes the administration of oral bile salts. Patients with three or fewer gallstones of cholesterol composition and with a gallstone diameter less than 0.6 in (15 mm) are more likely to receive medical therapy and have positive results. The primary requirements for receiving medical therapy include the presence of a functioning gallbladder and the absence of calcification on **CT scans**. Other non-surgical alternatives include using a solvent to dissolve the stones and using sound waves to break up small stones. A major drawback to medical therapy is the high recurrence rate of stones in those treated, as well as the possibility of successfully removing stones, but leaving an infected gallbladder behind, requiring a later operation for its removal.

Resources

BOOKS

Current Surgical Diagnosis & Treatment. New York: McGraw-Hill, 2003.

Feldman, M, et al. *Sleisenger & Fordtran's Gastrointestinal and Liver Disease*. 8th ed. St. Louis: Mosby, 2005.

Khatri, V. P., and J. A. Asensio. *Operative Surgery Manual*. 1st ed. Philadelphia: Saunders, 2003.

"Liver, Biliary Tract, & Pancreas." In *Current Medical Diagnosis & Treatment*. New York: McGraw-Hill, 2003.

Townsend, C. M., et al. *Sabiston Textbook of Surgery*. 17th ed. Philadelphia: Saunders, 2004.

Mark Mitchell
Rosalyn Carson-DeWitt, MD

Cholesterol and triglyceride tests

Definition

Cholesterol and triglyceride tests are components of a **lipid profile** that provide important data about an individual's risk for developing cardiovascular (heart) disease.

Purpose

The purpose of cholesterol and triglyceride tests is to evaluate an individual's risk of cardiovascular (heart) disease.

Description

The body uses cholesterol when building cells and producing hormones. An excess of cholesterol in the blood can build up along the inside of the artery walls, forming plaque. Large amounts of plaque increase the chances of having a heart attack or stroke.

Triglycerides are a type of fat the body uses for storing energy. Only small amounts are found in the blood. Having a high triglyceride level along with a high LDL cholesterol may increase a person's risk of having heart disease more than having only a high LDL cholesterol level.

Cholesterol and triglyceride testing is done for several reasons.

- As a component of a routine physical examination to screen for a lipid disorder.
- To evaluate an individual's risk for heart disease.
- To evaluate an individual's response to drugs used to treat lipid disorders.
- To check for a rare genetic disease that causes very high cholesterol levels in persons that have unusual symptoms such as yellow fatty deposits in the skin (xanthomas).

Cholesterol and triglyceride tests are components of a lipid profile. A lipid profile includes four blood tests: total cholesterol, HDL cholesterol, LDL cholesterol and triglycerides.

Dietary fats, including cholesterol, are absorbed from the small intestines. They are converted into triglycerides, which are then packaged into lipoproteins. All of these products are transported into the liver by chylomicrons. After a fast (not eating) lasting at least 12 hours, chylomicrons are absent from the

bloodstream. This is the reason why persons that are having an LDL test must fast overnight.

A desirable cholesterol level is less than 200 mg/dL.

- Desirable: Less than 200 mg/dL
- Borderline high: 200-239 mg/dL
- High: 240 mg/dL or more

A healthy triglyceride level is 150 mg/dL or less.

- Normal: Less than 150 mg/dL
- Borderline high: 150-199 mg/dL
- High: 200-499 mg/dL
- Very high: 500 mg/dL and higher

Pharmaceutical interventions are based, in part, on cholesterol and triglyceride test values.

Cholesterol and triglyceride levels vary according to a person's age and gender.

Ranges for cholesterol and triglyceride values vary slightly among different laboratories.

Cholesterol and triglyceride tests can be ordered at any time. Routine lipid profiles that are used to monitor the effectiveness of drugs intended to reduce serum cholesterol are usually performed every three months.

Some medical experts recommend routine cholesterol and triglyceride testing to screen for problems that affect the way cholesterol is produced, used, carried in the blood, or disposed of by the body.

Precautions

A fast (not eating) for a minimum of 12 hours before drawing blood contributes to a more accurate measurement of cholesterol and triglycerides in the blood. No other precautions are needed.

At the time of drawing blood, the only precaution needed is to clean the venipuncture site with alcohol.

Side effects

The most common side effects of cholesterol or triglyceride tests are minor bleeding (hematoma) or bruising at the site of venipuncture.

Interactions

There are no interactions for a cholesterol or triglyceride test.

Resources

BOOKS

Fischbach, F. T. and M. B. Dunning. *A Manual of Laboratory and Diagnostic Tests.* 8th ed. Philadelphia: Lippincott Williams & Wilkins, 2008.

McGhee, M. *A Guide to Laboratory Investigations.* 5th ed. Oxford, UK: Radcliffe Publishing Ltd, 2008.

Price, C. P. *Evidence-Based Laboratory Medicine: Principles, Practice, and Outcomes.* 2nd ed. Washington, DC: AACC Press, 2007.

Scott, M.G., A. M. Gronowski, and C. S. Eby. *Tietz's Applied Laboratory Medicine.* 2nd ed. New York: Wiley-Liss, 2007.

Springhouse, A. M.. *Diagnostic Tests Made Incredibly Easy!.* 2nd ed. Philadelphia: Lippincott Williams & Wilkins, 2008.

PERIODICALS

Amati, L., M. Chilorio, E. Jirillo, and V. Covelli. "Early pathogenesis of atherosclerosis: the childhood obesity." *Current Pharmaceutical Design* 13, no. 36 (2007): 3696–3700.

Leigh-Hunt, N., and M. Rudolf. "A review of local practice regarding investigations in children attending obesity clinics and a comparison of the results with other studies." *Child Care Health and Delivery* 34, no. 1 (2008): 55–58.

Shephard, M. D., B. C. Mazzachi, and A. K. Shephard. "Comparative performance of two point-of-care analysers for lipid testing." *Clinical Laboratory* 53, no. 9-12 (2007): 561–566.

Wright, J. T., S. Harris-Haywood, S. Pressel, et al. "Clinical outcomes by race in hypertensive patients with and without the metabolic syndrome: Antihypertensive and Lipid-Lowering Treatment to Prevent Heart Attack Trial." *Archives of Internal Medicine* 168, no. 2 (2008): 207–217.

ORGANIZATIONS

American Association for Clinical Chemistry. http://www.aacc.org/AACC/.

American Society for Clinical Laboratory Science. http://www.ascls.org/.

American Society of Clinical Pathologists. http://www.ascp.org/.

College of American Pathologists. http://www.cap.org/apps/cap.portal.

OTHER

American Clinical Laboratory Association. "Information about clinical chemistry." 2008 [cited February 24, 2008]. http://www.clinical-labs.org/.

Clinical Laboratory Management Association. "Information about clinical chemistry." 2008 [cited February 22, 2008]. http://www.clma.org/.

Lab Tests On Line. "Information about lab tests." 2008 [cited February 24, 2008]. http://www.labtestsonline.org/.

National Accreditation Agency for Clinical Laboratory Sciences. "Information about laboratory tests." 2008 [cited February 25, 2008]. http://www.naacls.org/.

L. Fleming Fallon, Jr, MD, DrPH

Cholesterol tests *see* **Lipid tests**

Circulation support *see* **Mechanical circulation support**

Circumcision

Definition

Circumcision is the surgical removal of the foreskin of the penis, or the prepuce of the clitoris.

Circumcision

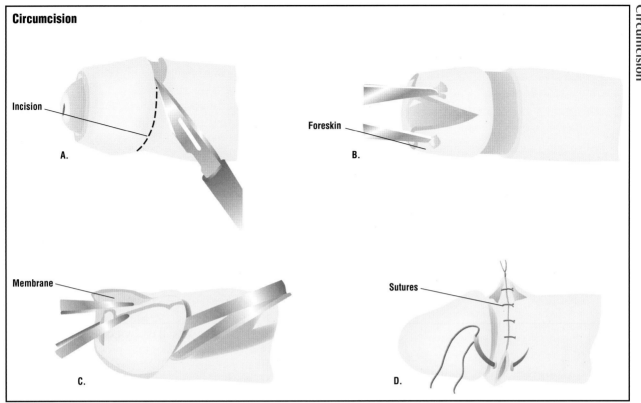

Incision

A.

Foreskin

B.

Membrane

C.

Sutures

D.

During a circumcision, the outer layer of the foreskin around the penis is cut (A). The foreskin is pulled away (B), and the remaining membrane is cut away (C). Sutures are used to stitch the area (D). *(Illustration by GGS Information Services. Cengage Learning, Gale.)*

Purpose

In the United States, circumcision in infant boys is performed for social, medical, or cultural/religious reasons. Once a routine operation urged by pediatricians and obstetricians for newborns in the middle of the twentieth century, circumcision has become an elective option that parents make for their sons on an individual basis. Families who practice Judaism or Islam may select to have their sons circumcised as a religious practice. Others choose circumcision for medical benefits.

Female circumcision (also known as female genital mutilation) is usually performed for cultural and social reasons by family members and others who are not members of the medical profession, with no anesthesia. Not only is the prepuce of the clitoris removed, but often the vaginal opening is sewn to make it smaller. This practice is supposed to ensure the virginity of a bride on her wedding day. It also prevents the woman from achieving sexual pleasure during coitus. This practice is not universally approved by the medical profession and is considered by many to be a human rights violation.

Some of the medical reasons parents of male infants choose circumcision are to protect against infections of the urinary tract and the foreskin, prevent cancer, lower the risk of getting sexually transmitted diseases, and prevent phimosis (a tightening of the foreskin that may close the opening of the penis). Though studies indicate that uncircumcised boys under the age of five are 20 times more likely than circumcised boys to have urinary tract infections (UTIs), the rate of incidence of UTIs is quite low and treatable with **antibiotics**. There are also indications that circumcised men are less likely to suffer from penile cancer, inflammation of the penis, or have many sexually transmitted diseases. Here again, there is a low rate of incidence. Good hygiene usually prevents most infections of the penis. Phimosis and penile cancer are very rare, even in men who have not been circumcised. Education and safe sex practices can prevent sexually transmitted diseases in ways that a surgical procedure cannot because these are diseases acquired through risky behaviors.

In 2002, however, research indicated that circumcised men may be less at risk for contracting HIV infections than uncircumcised men, whose foreskins have higher concentrations of cells that are targeted specifically by HIV. Genital hygiene and safe sex practices are still crucial to preventing the spread of HIV.

Another study found that circumcised men who engaged in risky sexual behaviors were less likely to contract penile human papillomavirus (HPV), which has been implicated in the incidence of cervical cancer in women. There was little difference between circumcised and uncircumcised men's incidence of the virus if the men were in a monogamous relationship.

With these factors in mind, the American Academy of Pediatrics has issued a policy statement that maintains that though there is existing scientific evidence that indicates the medical benefits of circumcision, the benefits are not strong enough to recommended circumcision as a routine practice.

Demographics

Though the incidence of male circumcision has decreased from 90% in 1979 to 60% in 1999, it is still the most common surgical operation in the United States. Circumcision rates are much lower for the rest of the industrialized world. In Britain, it is only done for religious practices or to correct a specific medical condition of the penis.

Description

The foreskin of the penis protects the sensitivity of the glans and shields it from irritation by urine, feces, and foreign materials. It also protects the urinary opening against infection and incidental injury.

In circumcision of infants, the foreskin is pulled tightly into a specially designed clamp, which forces the foreskin away from the broadened tip of the penis. The clamp applies pressure that stops bleeding from blood vessels that supply the foreskin. In older boys or adults, an incision is made around the base of the foreskin, the foreskin is pulled back, and then it is cut away from the tip of the penis. **Stitches** are usually used to close the skin edges.

Circumcision should not be performed on infants with certain deformities of the penis that may require a portion of the foreskin for repair. The most common condition for surgery using the foreskin is hypospadias, a congenital deformity of the penis where the urinary tract opening is not at the tip of the glans. Also, infants with a large hydrocele, or hernia, may suffer complications through circumcision. Premature infants and infants with serious infections are also poor candidates to be circumcised, as are infants with hemophilia, other bleeding disorders, or whose mothers had taken **anticoagulant drugs**. In older boys or men, circumcision is a minor procedure and can be performed on virtually anyone without a serious illness or unusual deformity.

Diagnosis/Preparation

Despite a long-standing belief that infants do not experience serious pain from circumcision, physicians now believe that some form of **local anesthesia** is necessary. Over 80% of pediatric residents, 80% of family practice residents, and 60% of obstetric/gynecological residents are routinely given instruction on pain control for circumcisions. Local anesthesia is often injected at the base of the penis (dorsal penile nerve block) or under the skin around the penis (subcutaneous ring block). Both anesthetics block key nerves and provide significantly lowered perceived pain. EMLA cream (lidocaine 2.5% and prilocaine 2.5%) can also be used.

Aftercare

After circumcision, the wound should be washed daily. An antibiotic ointment or petroleum jelly may be applied to the site. If there is an incision, a wound dressing will be present and should be changed each time the diaper is changed. Sometimes a plastic ring is used instead of a bandage. The ring will usually fall off in 5–8 days. The penis will heal in 7–10 days.

Infants who undergo circumcision may be fussy for some hours afterward, so parents should be prepared for crying, feeding problems, and sleep problems. Generally, these go away within a day. In older

WHO PERFORMS THE PROCEDURE AND WHERE IS IT PERFORMED?

Medical circumcisions are performed in the hospital by a pediatrician for an infant or child. For an adult, a general surgeon or urologist may perform a circumcision, especially if there are other urinary tract repairs to be made.

A Jewish religious circumcision, a *Bris Milah*, is performed when an infant male is eight days old. It is conducted by a trained *mohel*, with family and friends present, in a non-medical setting.

QUESTIONS TO ASK THE DOCTOR

- Is there a medical reason for performing a circumcision on my child?
- Is there new research about the benefits of circumcisions that I should be aware of?
- What kind of anesthesia will be used during the procedure?
- What should I be aware of when I go home with the baby?
- When should I call the doctor?

boys, the penis may be painful, but this will go away gradually. A topical anesthetic ointment or spray may be used to relieve this temporary discomfort. There may also be a bruise on the penis, which typically disappears with no particular attention.

Risks

Complications following newborn circumcision appear in between two and six of every 1,000 procedures. Most complications are minor. Bleeding occurs in half of the complications and is usually easy to control. Infections are rare and occur at the circumcision site, the opening to the bladder, or at the tip of the penis as a result of contact with urine or feces. Infections are indicated by fever and signs of inflammation, and are treatable with antibiotics.

There may be injuries to the penis itself, and these may be difficult to repair.

Normal results

When an infant or an adult is circumcised, the surgical wound should heal quickly, with normal urinary function resuming immediately. An infant or older child should have no complications. After a period of recovery, an adult male should be able to resume sexual intercourse normally.

Morbidity and mortality rates

Complications as a result of circumcision are usually minor if the physician is experienced and makes sure the Mogen or Gomco clamps that are used are in good working order. Severe penile injuries are rare, but they are serious, and include penile **amputation** (partial or total), laceration, hemorrhage, and damage to the urinary tract. Other serious complications such

as meningitis, penile necrosis, necrotizing fasciitis, and sepsis can occur. Some of these, like meningitis and sepsis, can even cause **death**.

Hidden complications also occur. Subcutaneous masses have been detected under the skin of the penis. These masses usually have no symptoms, but, left untreated, could lead to more serious outcomes. Physicians should examine the penis at every well-baby checkup during the first year. If a mass is detected, it can easily be removed under a local anesthesia and sent to a pathology lab.

Alternatives

The only alternative to this surgery is to make an informed decision not to have an infant circumcised. Some Jewish parents are even electing not to hold a *Bris Milah*, a religious circumcision, for their sons, and choosing instead to hold a *Brit Shalom*, a naming ceremony, similar to that given for their infant daughters.

Resources

BOOKS

Wein, A. J., et al. *Campbell-Walsh Urology.* 9th ed. Philadelphia: Saunders, 2007.

PERIODICALS

"Circumcision." *Harvard Men's Health Watch* 6, no. 3 (October 2001).

Imperio, Winnie Anne. "Circumcision Appears Safe, But Not Hugely Beneficial." *OB GYN News* 35, no. 7 (April 1, 2000): 9.

"Link to Uncircumcised Males Found." *Women's Health Weekly* (May 9, 2002): 10.

Schmitt, B. D. "The Circumcision Descision: Pros and Cons." *Clinical Reference Systems* (2000): 1579.

OTHER

American Academy of Pediatrics. *New AAP Circumcision Policy Released (Press Release),* March 1, 1999. http://

www.aap.org/advocacy/archives/marcircum.htm (accessed March 11, 2008).

Janie F. Franz
Rosalyn Carson-DeWitt, MD

Claw toe surgery *see* **Hammer, claw, and mallet toe surgery**

Cleft lip repair

Definition

Cleft lip repair (cheiloplasty) is a surgical procedure to correct a groove-like defect in the lip.

Purpose

A cleft lip does not join together (fuse) properly during embryonic development. Surgical repair corrects the defect, preventing future problems with breathing, speaking, and eating, and improving the person's physical appearance.

Demographics

Cleft lip is the second most common embryonic (congenital) deformity. (Club foot is the most common congenital deformity.) Cleft lip, with or without cleft palate, occurs in approximately one in 750 live births. The highest incidence exists in Native American Indians and Japanese (approximately one in 350 births). African Americans and Africans represent the lowest incidence of cleft lip deformity (approximately one in 1,500 births). There is a higher frequency of clefting in certain populations of Scandinavia and Middle European countries.

Cleft lip occurs more commonly in males, while cleft palate is more likely to occur in females. Cleft lip alone (without cleft palate) occurs in approximately 20% of cases across both genders. The majority of cases, fully 80%, have both cleft lip and cleft palate. A unilateral cleft lip, commonly occurring on the left side, is more common than a bilateral cleft lip.

Potential causes

Most cases of cleft lip have no known cause. However, there is a strong genetic correlation. Other single gene defects that are associated with cleft lip include: Van der Woude syndrome, Opitz Syndrome, Aarskog syndrome, Fryns syndrome, Waardenburg syndrome, and Coffin-Siris syndrome. Approximately 5% of cleft conditions are associated with a genetic syndrome. Most of these syndromes do not include mental retardation.

Facial cleft has been implicated with maternal exposure to environmental causes, such as rubella or medications that can harm the developing embryo. These medications include steroids, anti-seizure drugs, vitamin A, and oral anti-acne medications (such as Accutane) taken during the first three months of pregnancy. Cleft lip is also associated with fetal alcohol syndrome and maternal diabetes.

Risk of cleft lip increases with paternal age, especially over 30 years at the time of conception. Generally, the risk is higher when both parents are over 30 years of age. However, most cases seem to be isolated within the family with no obvious causation.

When the affected child has unilateral cleft lip and palate, the risk for subsequent children increases to 4.2%. Advances in high-resolution ultrasonography (prenatal **ultrasound** exam) have made it possible to detect facial abnormalities in the developing embryo (in utero).

Description

Developmental anatomy

Important structures of the embryo's mouth form at four to seven weeks of gestation. Development during this period entails migration and fusion of mesenchymal cells with facial structures. A cleft can develop along the lip if this migration and fusion is interrupted (usually by a combination of genetic and environmental factors). The type of clefting varies with the embryonic stage when its development occurred.

There are several types of cleft lip, ranging from a small groove on the border of the upper lip to a larger deformity that extends into the floor of the nostril and part of the maxilla (upper jawbone).

Unilateral cleft lip results from failure of the maxillary prominence on the affected side to fuse with medial nasal prominences. The result is called a persistent labial groove. The cells of the lip become stretched and the tissues in the persistent groove break down, resulting in a lip that is divided into medial (middle) and lateral (side) portions. In some cases, a bridge of tissue (simart band) joins together the two incomplete lip portions.

Bilateral cleft lip occurs in a fashion similar to the unilateral cleft. Patients with bilateral cleft lip may have varying degrees of deformity on each side of the defect. An anatomical structure, intermaxillary segment, projects to the front and hangs unattached. Defects associated with bilateral cleft lip are particularly problematic

Cleft lip repair

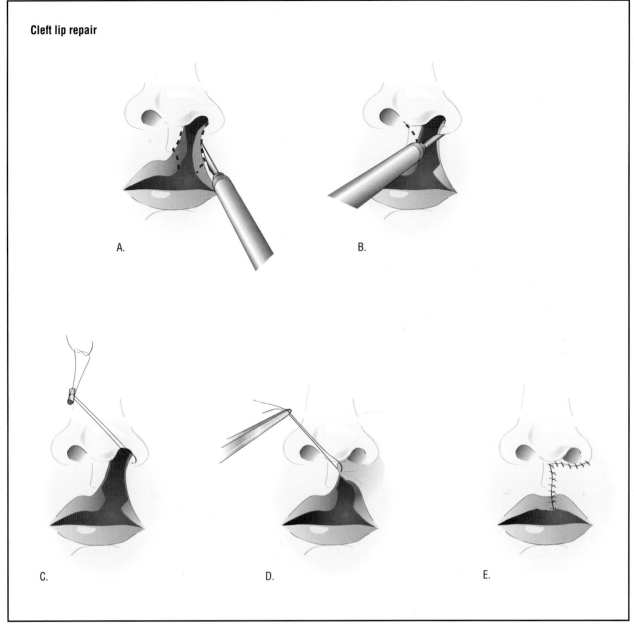

The edges of the cleft between the lip and nose are cut (A and B). The bottom of the nostril is formed with suture (C). The upper part of the lip tissue is closed (D), and the stitches are extended down to close the opening entirely (E). *(Illustration by GGS Information Services. Cengage Learning, Gale.)*

due to discontinuity of the muscle fibers of the orbicularis oris (primary muscle of the lip.) This deformity can result in closure of the mouth and pursing of the lip.

Classification

In addition to classification as unilateral or bilateral, cleft lips are further classified as complete or incomplete. A complete cleft involves the entire lip, and typically the alveolar arch. An incomplete cleft involves only part of the lip. The Iowa system (which also classifies cleft palate) classifies cleft lip in five groups, including:

- group I—clefts of the lip only
- group II—clefts of palate only
- group III—clefts of lip, alveolus, and palate
- group IV—clefts of lip and alveolus
- group V—miscellaneous

Alveolar arch—An arch formed by the ridge of the alveolar process of the mandible (jawbone) or maxilla.

Alveolar part of the maxilla—The part of the bony upper jaw that contains teeth (the upper gum).

Bilateral cleft lip—Cleft that occurs on both sides of the lip.

Buccal sulcus—Groove in the upper part of the upper jaw (where there are teeth).

Cleft—Split or opening, which can occur in the lip or palate or both.

Columella—Outer portion of the nose that divides the nostrils.

Cupid's bow—Double curve of the upper lip.

Epithelium—Protective membranous layer of tissue, usually a single layer of cells very close together, which lines the cavities outside of an organism.

Flap—Anatomical section that is surgically cut using special incisions and moved (rotated/advanced) to repair a defect.

Inferior turbinate—Bony projections on each side of the nose.

Labial—Of or pertaining to the lips.

Lateral—Of or pertaining to a side (opposite of medial).

Maxilla—Bony upper jaw.

Medial—Toward the middle or center (i.e., the chest is medial to the arm).

Medial (or lateral) nasal prominence—The medial (toward the middle) or lateral (toward the sides) are anatomical structures that form and merge the nose of the developing embryo during weeks six to nine in utero.

Mesenchymal cells—Embryonic cells that develop into many structures, including the soft tissues in the lip.

Mixed dentition—A mix of both "baby teeth" and permanent teeth.

Myringotomy—A procedure that involves making a small incision in the eardrum to release pressure caused by excess fluid accumulation.

Orbicularis oris—Concentrically shaped muscle that surrounds the upper and lower lips.

Oropharynx—The part of the throat at the back of the mouth.

Palate—The roof of the mouth composed of two anatomical structures, the hard and soft palates.

Philtral units—Consists of several anatomical landmarks: the philtral dimple (the skin or depression below the nose extending to the upper lip in the midline); philtral columns (the skin columns on the right and left side of the philtral dimple); philtral tubercle (in the midline of the upper lip); white roll (a linear tissue prominence that joins the upper lip portion of the philtral dimple and vermilion—the dark pink tissue that makes up the lip); nasal columella (the outer portion of the nose that divides the nostrils).

Philtal dimple—The skin or depression below the nose, extending to the upper lip in the midline.

Septal mucosa—The epithelium in the nasal mucosa.

Unilateral cleft lip—A cleft that occurs on either the right or left side of the lip.

Vermilion—The dark pink tissue that makes up the lip.

Another widely accepted cleft lip classification is based on recommendations of the American Cleft Palate Association. This classification divides cleft lip into unilateral or bilateral (right, left, or extent) in thirds (i.e., one-third, two-thirds, three-thirds), or median cleft lip, the extent of which is also measured in thirds.

Surgical procedure

Cleft lip repair can be initiated at any age, but optimal results occur when the first operation is performed between two and six months of age. Surgery is usually scheduled during the third month of life.

While the patient is under **general anesthesia**, the anatomical landmarks and incisions are carefully demarcated with methylene blue ink. An endotracheal tube prevents aspiration of blood. The surgical field is injected with a local anesthetic to provide further numbing and blood vessel constriction (to limit bleeding). Myringotomy (incisions in one or both eardrums) is performed, and myringotomy tubes are inserted to permit fluid drainage.

There are several operative techniques for cleft lip reconstruction. The Millard rotation advancement (R-A) technique is the most widely accepted form of repair. This method involves rotation of the entire philtral dimple (groove in the upper lip) and Cupid's bow (double curve of the upper lip). The scar falls along the new philtral column (central section of the upper lip), and is adjusted as required since the procedure allows for flexibility.

The Millard procedure begins with an incision on the edge of the cleft side of the philtrum, and the cutting continues upward, medially, and to the side. A second incision extends to the buccal sulcus (top part of the upper jaw). The length of this incision depends on the size of the gap to be closed. In this second incision, the surgeon frees soft tissue, which allows him or her to completely lift the lip from the underlying bone. This dissection should be tested to ensure free advancement toward the middle, as inadequate dissection is the root cause of poor results. Nasal deformity can be dealt with by a procedure known as the McComb nasal tip plasty, which elevates the depressed nasal dome and rim. Cartilage from the cleft side is freed from the opposite side, and is positioned and reshaped using nylon sutures.

Advantages of the Millard rotation advancement technique include:

- It is the most common procedure (i.e., surgeons are more familiar with it).
- The technique is adaptable and flexible.
- It permits construction of a normal-looking Cupid's bow.
- A minimal amount of tissue is discarded.
- The suture line is camouflaged.

The disadvantage of the Millard rotation advancement technique is the possible development of a vermilion notch (shortening of the entire lip in the vertical direction), resulting from contracture of the vertical scar. Cupid's bow is a critical part of the repair, making it very important to accurately determine the high point of Cupid's bow on the lateral lip.

Diagnosis/Preparation

Facial clefting has a wide range of clinical presentations, ranging from a simple microform cleft to the complete bilateral cleft involving the lip, palate, and nose. A comprehensive **physical examination** is performed immediately after birth, and the defect is usually evident by visual inspection and examination of the facial structures.

Care must be taken to diagnose other physical problems associated with a genetic syndrome. Weight, nutrition, growth, and development should be assessed and closely monitored.

Presurgical tests include a variety of procedures, such as hemoglobin studies. It is important for the patient's parents and physician to discuss the operation prior to surgery.

Aftercare

The postoperative focus is on ensuring proper nutrition, as well as lip care and monitoring the activity level. Breast milk or full-strength formula is encouraged immediately after surgery or shortly thereafter. Lip care for patients with sutures should include gentle cleansing of suture lines with cotton swabs and diluted hydrogen peroxide. Liberal application of topical antibiotic ointment several times a day for 10 days is recommended. There will be some scar contracture, redness, and firmness of the area for four to six weeks after surgery. Parents should gently massage the area, and avoid sunlight until the scar heals.

The patient's activities may be limited. Some surgeons use elbow immobilizers to minimize the risk of accidental injury to the lip. Immobilizers should be removed several times a day in a supervised setting, allowing the child to move the restricted limb(s).

Interaction between the orthodontist and surgeon as part of the treatment team begins in the neonatal period, and continues through the phases of mixed dentition.

Risks

There may be excessive scarring and contraction of the lips. Two types of scars, hypertrophic or keloid, may develop. Hypertrophic scars appear as raised and red areas that usually flatten, fade in color, and soften within a few months. Keloids form as a result of the accelerated growth of tissue in response to the surgery or trauma to the area. The keloid can cause itching and a burning sensation. Scratching must be avoided because it can lead to healing problems. Some patients require minimal revision surgery, but in most cases, the initial redness and contracture is part of the normal healing process.

Normal results

Ideal surgical results for cleft lip include symmetrically shaped nostrils, and lips that appear as natural as possible and have a functional muscle. Many characteristics of the natural lip can be achieved; however, the outcome ultimately depends on a number of factors, including the skill of the surgeon, accurate pre-surgery markings, alignment of bones within the affected area, uncomplicated healing of the initial repair, and the effect of normal growth on the repaired lip. Additional surgical correction to reconstruct nasal symmetry is sometimes necessary.

Morbidity and mortality rates

Generally, cleft lip repair is well-tolerated in healthy infants. No major health problems are associated with this **reconstructive surgery**. Depending on the results, it may be necessary to perform additional operations to achieve desired functional and cosmetic outcomes.

Alternatives

There are no alternatives for this surgery. Obvious deformity and impairments of speech, hearing, eating,

and breathing occur as a direct result of the malformation. These issues cannot be corrected without surgery.

Resources

BOOKS

Behrman, R. E., et al. *Nelson's Textbook of Pediatrics*. 17th ed. Philadelphia: Saunders, 2004.

Cummings, C. W., et al. *Otolayrngology: Head and Neck Surgery*. 4th ed. St. Louis: Mosby, 2005.

Bluestone, Charles. *Pediatric Otolaryngology*. Philadelphia, PA: Saunders, 2003.

ORGANIZATIONS

American Board of Plastic Surgery,Inc. Seven Penn Center, Suite 400, 1635 Market Street, Philadelphia, PA 19103-2204. (215) 587-9322. http://www.abplsurg.org (accessed March 11, 2008).

International Birth Defects Information Systems. http://ibis-birthdefects.org/start/index.htm (accessed March 11, 2008).

International Craniofacial Institute. http://www.craniofacial.net/additional_services/additional_services.asp (accessed March 11, 2008).

OTHER

Wide Smiles. http://www.communicationdisorder.net/ (accessed March 11, 2008).

Laith Farid Gulli, MD,MS
Robert Ramirez, BS
Randall J. Blazic, MD, DDS
Bilal Nasser, MD, MS
Rosalyn Carson-DeWitt, MD

Closed fracture reduction *see* **Fracture repair**

Closures: stitches, staples, and glue

Definition

Stitches, staples, surgical glue, and tapes are four methods used to close wounds. Stitches use specialized needles and thread to "sew" the wound. Staples are thin pieces of metal that are placed with a stapling device through the edges of a wound to close it. Glues and adhesive tapes are materials used to close wounds without puncturing or penetrating the skin around the edges of an incision.

Description

Wounds to the skin, fat, muscle, blood vessels, and other structures in the body may occur accidentally (as in a cut) or purposefully (as in a surgical incision). A number of different methods exist to close a wound; the method selected depends on the type of injury, the type of tissue injured, the location and depth of the injury, and the patient's general health. Stitches and staples are two commonly used wound closure methods.

Stitches

Sutures, as stitches are often called, are the way that most wounds are closed. They are the oldest method of wound closure, having been described over two millennia ago by the Indian surgeon Susruta (sixth century B.C.), sometimes called the "father of plastic surgery," and the Roman physician Claudius Galen (129–200 A.D.), who treated several Roman emperors. These ancient doctors used such natural materials as human hair, hemp, silk, and catgut (a tough thread made from the dried intestines of sheep or horses). Silk and catgut are still used for sutures in the twenty-first century. Synthetic materials were first used for sutures in the 1950s; they are preferred by some surgeons because they are less likely to cause allergic tissue reactions around the edges of the wound. On the other hand, many synthetic suture materials are more difficult to knot securely. Suture materials have various characteristics that determine their use; no single material is ideal for all purposes. The surgeon must often decide whether ease of knot tying is more important than strength or longevity in tissue. The two main components of suture materials are the needle and thread.

MATERIALS. Suture thread is often categorized by how long it retains its strength in tissue. Absorbable stitches lose their strength in a matter of days or weeks and are eventually absorbed by the tissue. This characteristic is useful for the suturing of subcutaneous tissues. Nonabsorbable stitches retain their strength for months to years and may never be absorbed by the tissue. They are generally used for skin and are removed once the wound has sufficiently healed. Suture thread is made of various natural or synthetic components and comes in different diameters for use in different types of tissues. Very fine suture threads are used to close cuts on the face, while threads with a larger diameter are required for subcutaneous tissues.

Suture thread is also categorized by its structure, as either monofilament (one strand or filament) or multifilament, which has a braided structure. Monofilament sutures are less likely to cause infection and can be pulled through tissue with less damage to the skin, but are easily damaged by **surgical instruments**.

Stainless steel wire is a specialized, nonabsorbable suturing material, used in **orthopedic surgery** or to close the sternum (breastbone) following heart surgery.

To minimize the risk of infection, all types of suture materials are sterilized before use in a chamber containing ethylene oxide, a gas that kills bacteria, mold, and fungi. A newer technique to further lower the risk of bacterial contamination is to coat the suture material with an antimicrobial substance.

In the United States, the diameter of suturing materials is defined by the United States Pharmacopoeia (USP). The largest diameter is designated as #5, for heavy multifilament sutures used in orthopedic surgery; the smallest is #11-0, extremely fine monofilament sutures used primarily in ophthalmology.

Suture needles may resemble a conventional sewing needle with an eye through which suture material is threaded, or they come with suture thread attached at one end; this connection is said to be swaged (forged). Swaged needles have the advantage of causing less damage to tissue because the swaged end is smaller than the needle body and is less likely to rip tissue than the older type of threaded needle.

Needles may be straight or curved; the most commonly used shape is the semicircle, which permits easier manipulation through tissues by the clinician. Needles vary in length from less than 0.1 in (2 mm) to 2.4 in (60 mm). The point of a needle may be cutting (for tougher tissues such as the skin), rounded (for easily penetrable tissues such as the subcutaneous layers), or blunt (for easily damaged tissues such as the liver).

TECHNIQUE. While various stitching techniques may be used depending on the location of the wound and type of tissue to be sutured, basic suturing technique remains the same. Several instruments are necessary for proper wound closure, including dissecting scissors (for cleaning the wound); suture scissors (for cutting suture thread); a needle holder (for manipulating the needle); and forceps (for manipulating tissue). Wounds resulting from an injury must be cleaned before closure; dead tissue and foreign bodies are removed and the area is cleansed with an antiseptic. Sutures may be interrupted (each stitch is separately placed, tied, and cut) or continuous (one continuous piece of thread composes all the stitches); they may be placed at different angles and depths.

Nonabsorbable stitches should be removed several days to weeks after their placement, depending on their location. For instance, sutures on the face should be removed in approximately 5 days; sutures on the legs and abdomen, in 7 to 10 days; and sutures on the back, in 10 to 14 days. Strips of adhesive tape may be placed over the wound to help support the tissue while it is healing.

Staples

Staples are a relatively new method of wound closure, having been introduced in 1908 by a Hungarian surgeon named Humer Hultl. The primary purpose of Hultl's invention was reliable closure of bowel anastomoses, that is, the joining together of two segments of intestine. Leakage of intestinal contents from anastomoses was a common cause of postoperative mortality in the early twentieth century. The early staplers were large and cumbersome. It was not until the mid-1960s that reliable and easy-to-use surgical staplers were manufactured by the United States Surgical Corporation.

A distinct advantage that modern surgical staples have over sutures is their quick placement—stapling is approximately three to four times faster than suturing. Staples are also associated with a lower risk of infection and tissue reaction than sutures. It is, however, more difficult to correctly align the edges of a wound for stapling, and staples generally cost more than sutures. Common locations of wounds that may be stapled are the arms, legs, abdomen, back, or scalp; wounds on the hands, feet, neck, or face should not be stapled. Additionally, staples are still used to connect cut ends of larger blood vessels or segments of the bowel.

A newer form of stapling uses clips that do not penetrate the skin to close the edges of a wound.

MATERIALS. Most surgical staples used inside the body are made of titanium, a lightweight silvery metal that is less likely to trigger the patient's immune system or interfere with MRI scanners. Staples used to close skin wounds or incisions are composed of stainless steel and have a crossbar that lies parallel to the skin, two legs that enter each edge of the wound, and tips that hold the staple in place. Staples are placed with the aid of a stapling device that generally holds between 5 and 25 staples. As of 2007, most skin staplers are disposable plastic instruments that contain a single cartridge of staples. Staplers used to place staples inside the body are more commonly made of stainless steel and are not disposable. Forceps are also necessary to help align the edges of the wound together and hold them in place until staples can be placed.

TECHNIQUE. The wound is first cleaned of dead tissue and foreign bodies and washed with an antiseptic. The edges of the wound are aligned and held together with forceps or the clinician's fingers. The stapling device is held against the wound at the point at which the staple is to be placed. By squeezing the trigger on the stapling device, the staple is automatically placed into the skin; the depth of placement is controlled by how firmly the stapling device is held against the skin. The staples should be removed at approximately the same time as sutures; removal is done with a specialized staple remover.

A newer type of surgical staple is bioabsorbable, meaning that it does not require removal after the wound has healed. These staples are made from polyglycolic acid (PGA), a material that is also used to make absorbable sutures and scaffolds for tissue engineering. Staples made of PGA lose about half their strength within two weeks and are completely absorbed by the body within 4 months.

Glues

Tissue glues have been used in surgery on an experimental basis since the mid-1960s; they were formally approved by the U.S. Food and Drug Administration (FDA) for surgical use in 1998. As early as 1964, Eastman Kodak submitted an application to the FDA for the use of cyanoacrylate glues in surgery; the formula was used by Dr. Harry Coover during the Vietnam War to seal chest wounds or other open wounds until the patient could be taken to a military hospital.

In addition to wound closure, surgical glues were approved by the FDA in 2001 as sealants against certain types of bacteria, including staphylococci and pseudomonads.

MATERIALS. Cyanoacrylate glues are familiar to most people in the form of such compounds as Krazy Glue or Superglue, used as household adhesives to bond nonporous materials, including metals. These glues are also used in criminal investigations to develop latent fingerprints on smooth surfaces like glass or plastics. Instructions for the use of cyanoacrylate industrial glues always contain warnings about their capacity to bond with skin; it is this characteristic that led to their use in surgery. The chemical formula of cyanoacrylate approved for medical use is 2-octyl cyanoacrylate; its trade names include Dermabond, Band-Aid Liquid Adhesive Bandage, and Soothe-N-Seal.

Dermabond has several advantages: rapid application, good cosmetic results, strength, and flexibility. It also has several drawbacks: it can only be used to close the uppermost layers of skin, as it causes inflammation to subcutaneous tissues. It cannot be used close to the eyes or mouth, on hairy parts of the body, or to close wounds with jagged or torn edges. The surgeon must use subcutaneous sutures to draw the edges of a deep wound together before applying the surgical glue to the surface of the skin. Last, a small percentage of patients are allergic to cyanoacrylate and develop a skin rash.

TECHNIQUE. Dermabond comes in an applicator that resembles a fountain pen with a thicker barrel. It contains a vial that snaps open inside the barrel when the doctor removes the cap. The adhesive itself is tinted purple and comes out through a porous tip about the size of a pencil eraser when a black button on the side of the barrel is pushed. The doctor or nurse holds the edges of the wound together while applying a layer of Dermabond to the wound with the tip of the applicator. After 15 seconds, the first layer is dry and the doctor can apply the second layer of adhesive. After about 45 seconds to a minute, the closure is complete. It reaches its full strength about three minutes after the second layer has been applied. The patient does not need to cover the Dermabond with a bandage. It is safe to get the closure wet in the course of normal bathing or showering, although patients are usually instructed not to soak the wound.

Dermabond does not have to be removed like staples or nonabsorbable stitches; it wears off the skin in 5–10 days, which is usually enough time for the upper layer of skin to heal.

Over-the-counter (OTC) forms of surgical adhesive have been available since 2004; they come in bottles that contain about 10 applications. As of 2007, these products cost between $5.50 and $7.00 in most parts of the United States.

Tapes

Surgical tapes have been used for wound closure since the Renaissance period, when the French surgeon Ambroise Paré (1510–1590) made tapes out of strips of sticking plaster for treating facial wounds. This technique allowed the wound edges to be splinted as well as joined together. In modern surgery, adhesive strips can be used to hold the edges of the wound together before suturing or by themselves without sutures.

MATERIALS. The first modern type of adhesive strip used for wound closure was introduced in the early 1960s and is commonly called Steri-Strips. Still used in the early 2000s, Steri-Strips are reinforced strips of a microporous synthetic material backed by an acrylic polymer adhesive that holds the edges of a wound together for 5–7 days. They can be removed at home by the patient after the wound has healed.

A newer type of adhesive strip was known as ClozeX when it was introduced in 2004. Its name was changed to Steri-Strip S Surgical Skin Closure in 2007. The product comes in a range of 11 different sizes to cover a variety of injuries and surgical incision. The original ClozeX was a transparent film with an adhesive backing, designed to hold the edges of a wound together. In 2005, the company introduced a second version with a center pad. According to a report published in 2006, a sample group of both surgeons and patients preferred the new method of wound closure to standard monofilament sutures for speed of application, greater comfort, lower cost, and better cosmetic effect. The limitations of the Steri-Strip S device are similar to those of surgical glues: it cannot be used on hairy portions of the body, infected wounds, wounds that are oozing tissue fluid, or wounds on parts of the body used for repetitive motion (such as knee or finger joints).

TECHNIQUE. Steri-Strips and the newer skin closure device are applied after the patient's skin has been cleansed with rubbing alcohol or sterile saline solution and dried thoroughly. If the skin closure device is to be used, the surgeon chooses the proper size for the wound and removes a series of liners inside the device, pressing the clear adhesive pad first along one side of the wound and then the other while holding the edges of the wound together. After the adhesive pad is in place, the surgeon applies a series of filament straps that hold the adhesive pad in place. The device is left in place for 7 days. It can then be removed in the doctor's office or by the patient.

Steri-Strips are commonly used with a liquid adhesive, usually either Mastisol or tincture of benzoin, to help them adhere to the wound longer. After the patient's skin has been cleansed and dried, the liquid adhesive is applied over the edges of the wound and the entire area where the Steri-Strips will be placed. After the adhesive is partly dry, the strips are placed across the wound (perpendicular to it rather than parallel) without overlapping one another.

Resources

BOOKS

Current and Emerging Wound Closure Products and Techniques in Europe and the U.S. Newport Beach, CA: Medtech Insight, 2003.

Lammers, Richard L., and Alexander T. Trott. "Methods of Wound Closure." In *Clinical Procedures in Emergency Medicine.* Philadelphia: W. B. Saunders Company, 1998.

O'Leary, J. Patrick, ed. *The Physiologic Basis of Surgery*, 4th ed. Philadelphia: Lippincott Williams & Wilkins, 2008.

PERIODICALS

Autio, L., and K. K. Olson. "The Four S's of Wound Management: Staples, Sutures, Steri-Strips, and Sticky Stuff." *Holistic Nursing Practice* 16 (January 2002): 80–88.

Barber, F. A., et al. "Sutures and Suture Anchors—Update 2006." *Arthroscopy* 22 (October 2006): 1063.

Casper, K. A. "OTC Product: Band-Aid Liquid Bandage." *Journal of the American Pharmacists Association* 46 (November-December 2006): 768.

Catena, Fausto, Michele La Donna, Stefano Gagliardi, et al. "Stapled versus Hand-Sewn Anastomoses in Emergency Intestinal Surgery: Results of a Results of a Prospective Randomized Study." *Surgery Today* 34 (February 2004): 123–126.

Groce, J. R., et al. "Endoscopic Clip Closure of a Gastric Staple-Line Dehiscence (with Video)." *Gastrointestinal Endoscopy* 65 (February 2007): 321–322.

Hancock, N. J., and A. W. Samuel. "Use of Dermabond Tissue Adhesive in Hand Surgery." *Journal of Wound Care* 16 (November 2007): 441–443.

Kuo, F., D. Lee, and G. S. Rogers. "Prospective, Randomized, Blinded Study of a New Wound Closure Film versus Cutaneous Suture for Surgical Wound Closure." *Dermatologic Surgery* 32 (May 2006): 676–681.

OTHER

Doud Galli, Suzanne K. and Minas Constantinides. "Wound Closure Technique." *eMedicine.* August 1, 2006 [cited January 3, 2008]. http://www.emedicine.com/ent/topic35.htm.

Lai, Stephen Y. and Daniel G. Becker. "Sutures and Needles." *eMedicine.* June 27, 2006 [cited January 4, 2008]. http://www.emedicine.com/ent/topic38.htm.

Terhune, Margaret. "Materials for Wound Closure." *eMedicine.* November 19, 2007 [cited January 4, 2008]. http://www.emedicine.com/derm/topic825.htm.

ORGANIZATIONS

United States Pharmacopoeia (USP), 12601 Twinbrook Parkway, Rockville, MD, 20852-1790, (800) 227-8772, http://www.usp.org/.

Stephanie Dionne Sherk
Rebecca Frey, Ph.D.

Club foot repair

Definition

Club foot repair, also known as foot tendon release or club foot release, is the surgical repair of a birth defect of the foot and ankle called club foot.

Purpose

Club foot, or *talipes equinovarus*, is the most common birth defect of the lower extremity, characterized by the foot turning both downward and inward. The defect can range from mild to severe. The purpose of club foot repair is to provide the child with a functional foot that looks as normal as possible and that is painless, plantigrade, and flexible. Plantigrade means that the child is able to stand with the sole of the foot on the ground, and not on the heels or the outside of the foot.

Demographics

In the United States, club foot is a common birth defect, and occurs at a rate of one to two cases per 1,000 live births among whites. More than 4,000 babies with club foot are born in the United States each year. Boys are affected with club foot twice as often as girls. The risk increases 30-fold in individuals who have a relative of the first degree affected by the defects.

Description

A newborn baby's club foot is first treated with applying a cast because the tendons, ligaments, and bones are quite flexible and easy to reposition. The procedure involves stretching the foot into a more normal position and using a cast to maintain the corrected position. The cast is removed every week or two, so as to stretch the foot gradually into a correct position. Serial casting goes on for approximately three months.

In 30% of cases, manipulation and casting is successful, and the foot can be placed in a brace to maintain the correction. In about 70% of cases, manipulation and castings alone do not correct the deformity completely, and the child's physicians and parents must decide whether to attempt surgery.

The type of surgery depends on how severe the club foot is. The deformity features tight and short tendons around the foot and ankle. Surgery consists of releasing all the tight tendons and ligaments in the posterior (back) and medial (inside) aspects of the foot and repairing them in a lengthened position. Metal pins may also be used to maintain the bones in place for some six weeks. Surgery usually involves an overnight stay in hospital. After surgery, the foot is put into a cast for approximately three months, followed by the use of a brace to hold the correction. The brace is worn for approximately 6–12 months after surgery.

Diagnosis/Preparation

Presurgical diagnosis requires radiography (x rays). The evaluation usually includes only the acquisition of weight-bearing images because the stress involved is reproducible. In babies, weight bearing is simulated by holding the baby upright on a flat surface.

Some surgeons prefer to wait until the child is about one year old before performing surgery, so that the foot may grow a little larger. Other surgeons operate as early as three months of age when it becomes clear that further castings will not achieve any more correction.

Aftercare

The patient usually stays in the hospital for two days after club foot repair. The foot is put into a cast and kept elevated, with application of ice packs to reduce swelling and pain. Painkillers may also be prescribed to relieve pain. During the 48 hours following surgery, the skin near the cast and the toes are examined carefully to ensure that blood circulation, movement, and feeling are maintained. After leaving the hospital, the cast is usually left on for about three months. Skin irritations due to the cast or infections may occur. A course of physical therapy may be indicated after removal of the cast to help keep the repaired foot in good position, improve its flexibility, and strengthen the muscles.

Risks

The risks involved in club foot repair are the general risks associated with anesthesia and surgery.

Risks associated with anesthesia include:
- adverse reactions to medications
- breathing problems

Risks associated with surgery include:
- excessive bleeding
- infections

QUESTIONS TO ASK THE DOCTOR

- Is there any treatment needed to prevent the club foot from coming back after surgery?
- What are the chances that my child's club foot will get corrected?
- How long will it take to recover from the surgery?
- What procedures do you follow?
- How much club foot surgery do you perform each year?

Normal results

If club foot repair is required, the foot usually becomes quite functional after surgery. In some cases, the foot and calf may remain smaller throughout the patient's life. Most children who have undergone club foot repair develop normally and participate fully in any athletic or recreational activity that they choose.

Morbidity and mortality rates

If left untreated, club foot will result in an abnormal gait, and further deformity may occur on the side of the foot due to preferential weight bearing.

Alternatives

The Ponseti non-surgical treatment

Dr. Ignacio Ponseti developed this method, which consists of a weekly series of gentle manipulations followed by the application of casts that are placed from the toes to the upper thigh. Five to seven casts are applied every week. Before applying the last cast, which is worn for three weeks, the heel cord is cut to finalize the correction of the foot. By the time the cast is removed, the heel cord has healed. After this two-month period of casting, a splint is worn full time by the patient for a few months and is then worn only at night for two to four years. Special shoes also maintain the foot in the corrected position.

The French treatment

This method consists of daily physical therapy, featuring gentle and painless stretching of the foot. The foot is then taped to maintain the corrected position until the next day's visit. At night, the taped foot is inserted into a continuous passive-motion machine at home to maximize the amount of stretching. The tape is removed for a few hours each day to wash the foot, air the skin, and perform exercises. Removable splints are also used to support the taped foot. The one-hour physical therapy sessions are conducted five days each week for approximately three months. Taping is stopped when the child starts walking.

Resources

BOOKS

Behrman, R. E., et al. *Nelson's Textbook of Pediatrics.* 17th ed. Philadelphia: Saunders, 2004.

Canale, S. T., ed. *Campbell's Operative Orthopaedics.* 10th ed. St. Louis: Mosby, 2003.

PERIODICALS

Aronson, J., and C. L. Puskarich. "Deformity and Disability from Treated Clubfoot." *Journal of Pediatrics and Orthopedics* 10 (1990): 109–112.

Cooper, D. M. and F. R. Dietz. "Treatment of Idiopathic Clubfoot. A Thirty Year Follow-up." *Journal of Bone and Joint Surgery* 77A (1995): 1477–1479.

Herzenberg, J. E., C. Radler, and N. Bor. "Ponseti Versus Traditional Methods of Casting for Idiopathic Clubfoot." *Journal of Pediatrics and Orthopedics* 22 (July–August 2002): 517–521.

Ideka, K. "Conservative Treatment of Idiopathic Clubfoot." *Journal of Pediatrics and Orthopedics* 12 (March–April 1992): 217–223.

ORGANIZATIONS

American Academy of Pediatrics. 141 Northwest Point Boulevard, Elk Grove Village, IL 60007-1098. (847) 434-4000. http://www.aap.org (accessed March 11, 2008).

Shrine and Shriner's Hospitals. 2900 Rocky Point Dr., Tampa, FL 33607-1460. (813) 281-0300. http://www.shrinershq.org/ (accessed March 11, 2008).

OTHER

The Club Foot Club. [cited April 2003]. http://home.ica.net/~maudefamily (accessed March 11, 2008).

"List of Physicians Qualified in the Ponseti Method." Virtual Children's Hospital. [cited April 2003]. http://www.uihealthcare.com/topics/medicaldepartments/orthopaedics/clubfeet/physicians.html (accessed March 11, 2008).

"Club Foot." John Hopkins Department of Orthopedic Surgery. [cited April 2003]. http://www.hopkinsortho.org/clubfoot.html (accessed March 11, 2008).

Monique Laberge, PhD
Rosalyn Carson-DeWitt, MD

Coarctation of the aorta *see* **Heart surgery for congenital defects**

Cochlear implants

Definition

A cochlear implant is a small, complex electronic device used to treat severe to profound hearing loss. It is surgically implanted underneath the skin behind the patient's ear.

Purpose

A cochlear implant delivers useful auditory signals from the environment to the patient by electronically bypassing nonfunctional parts of the ear and directly stimulating the auditory nerve. Unlike a hearing aid, it does not merely amplify sound. Instead, an implant increases the amount of nervous response to sound. Although it does not restore normal hearing, the additional input provided by the implant often improves sound detection and increases speech understanding.

Description

Normal hearing occurs because sound travels from the outer ear into the ear canal and vibrates the eardrum. The vibration is carried through the middle ear by three small bones attached to the eardrum and on to a fluid-filled part of the inner ear called the cochlea. Movement in the cochlear fluid is transferred to hair fibers within the cochlea. The movement of these hair cells stimulates nerve cells called ganglion cells, which send an electrical current to the auditory nerve. In turn, the nerve carries the current to the brain, where the electrical stimulation is recognized as sound.

A common cause of hearing loss is damage to the hair cells within the cochlea. This kind of deafness, called sensorineural deafness, can often be treated with cochlear implants. This is particularly true if damage to the hair cells is not accompanied by damage to the auditory nerve itself. It has been estimated that more than 100,000 individuals have received cochlear implants.

Cochlear implants consist of internal and external parts. The external parts include a microphone, a speech processor, and a transmitter. The internal parts include a receiver-stimulator and an electrode. Some models include a small headpiece that is worn just behind the ear and contains all the external parts, while other models also use body-worn modules that are placed in a shoulder pouch, in a pocket, or worn on a belt. The convenience of the all-in-one headpiece is balanced by shorter life for the batteries used in the smaller units, although systems using rechargeable batteries do solve some of these issues.

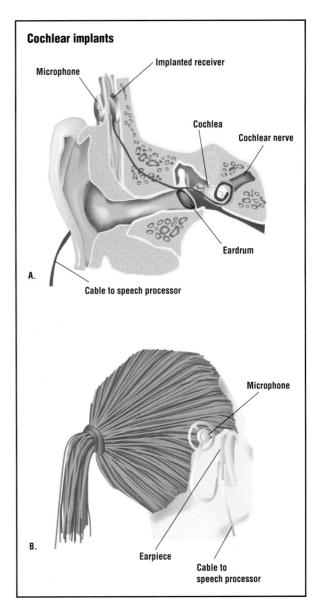

Cochlear implants

Microphone · Implanted receiver · Cochlea · Cochlear nerve · Eardrum · A. · Cable to speech processor

Microphone · B. · Earpiece · Cable to speech processor

A cochlear implant has a microphone outside the ear that transmits sounds to an implanted receiver. In turn, the receiver transmits electrical impulses to the cochlea and cochlear nerve, which is stimulated in normal hearing. *(Illustration by GGS Information Services. Cengage Learning, Gale.)*

Within the headpiece, the microphone picks up sound in the environment. The speech processor converts these sounds into a digital signal. The content of the generated digital signal is determined by the programming of the processor and is complex. It includes information about the pitch, loudness, and timing of sound signals, and attempts to filter out extraneous noise. The transmitter converts the digital signals into FM radio signals and sends them through the skin to the internal parts of the implant. The transmitter and the internal parts are kept in correct alignment by using magnets present in both the internal and external parts of the device.

The internal parts are those that are surgically implanted into the patient. The receiver-stimulator is disk-shaped and is about the size of a quarter. It receives the digital signals from the transmitter and converts them into electrical signals. A wire connects the receiver to a group of electrodes that are threaded into the cochlea when the implant is placed. As many as 24 electrodes, depending on the type of the implant, stimulate the ganglion cells in the cochlea. These cells transmit the signals to the brain through the auditory nerve. The brain then interprets the signals as sound.

The sounds heard through an implant are different from the normal hearing sounds and have been described as artificial or robot-like. This is because the implant's handful of electrodes cannot hope to match the complexity of a person's 15,000 hair cells. However, as more electrodes are added, electrode placement issues are solved, and the software for the implant speech processor takes into account more and more aspects of sound, the perceived results are moving closer to how speech and other sounds are naturally perceived.

Despite the benefits that the implant appears to offer, some hearing specialists and members of the deaf community believe that the benefits may not outweigh the risks and limitations of the device. Because the device must be surgically implanted, it carries some **surgical risk**. Manufacturers cannot promise how well a person will hear with an implant. Moreover, after getting an implant, some people say they feel alienated from the deaf community, while at the same time not feeling fully a part of the hearing world. The decision to undergo cochlear implant surgery is a complex one, and a person should take into account the risks and realistic rewards of the device.

Surgical procedure

The procedure can be preformed on an outpatient basis for adult and adolescent patients. With children, it is often performed with a one-night stay in the hospital.

The internal parts of the implant are placed under the skin behind the patient's ear. The area is shaved, although newer procedures allow for sterilization of the hair in the area so less shaving has to occur. Once the sterile field is established, the surgeon makes an 2–3 in (5–7.6 cm) incision behind the ear and opens the mastoid bone (the ridge on the skull behind the ear) leading into the middle ear. A depression is made in the bone next to the opening to allow the receiver-stimulator to sit flush with the skull surface. After seating, the receiver-stimulator is held in place with a long-lasting suture.

The surgeon then goes through the opening in the mastoid bone to create a new opening in the cochlea for the implant electrodes. The electrode is then very slowly and carefully threaded through this new opening. The electrode structure itself is designed to align the electrodes as closely as possible to the ganglion cells, as this allows the electrical signals that function to be less powerful. Once in place, the device is tested to be certain it is working. If all is well, the surgeon then closes up the incision with absorbable sutures, so the area does not need to be revisited to remove the **stitches**.

The entire operation takes between one and two hours, although the procedure is more complex for younger patients due to the smaller size of their middle ear structures and tends to take longer.

Aftercare

For a short period of time after the surgery, a special bandage is worn on the head during sleep. After about one month, the surgical wounds heal. The patient then returns to the implant clinic to be fitted with the external parts of the device and to have it turned on and mapped. Mapping involves fine tuning the speech processor and setting levels of stimulation for each electrode, from soft to loud.

The patient is then trained in how to interpret the sounds heard through the device. The length of the training varies from days to years, depending on how well the person can interpret the sounds heard through the device.

Risks

As with all operations, there are risks with this surgery, including:

- infection at the incision site
- bleeding
- complications related to anesthesia
- transient dizziness
- facial paralysis (rarely)
- temporary taste disturbances
- additional hearing loss
- device failure

However, it should be noted that serious surgical complications have been observed in only one in 10,000 procedures of this type.

Some long-term risks of the implant include the unknown effects of electrical stimulation on the nervous system. It is also possible to damage the implant's internal components by a blow to the head, which will render the device unworkable.

A further consideration is that the use of **magnetic resonance imaging** (MRI) for patients with cochlear implants is not recommended because of the magnets present in the devices. Several companies have developed implants that do not use magnets, or have altered the receiver-stimulator to make it easier to remove the magnets before testing. One fact that reduces the concern about MRI testing is that for many medical indications, MRI can be replaced with a computer assisted tomography (CAT, CT) scan, which is not a problem for persons with cochlear implants.

Additionally, in July 2002, the Food and Drug Administration (FDA) issued a warning about a possible connection between increased incidence of meningitis and the presence of a cochlear implant. This warning included special vaccine recommendations for those with implants, as well as the voluntary removal from the market of certain devices. Specifically, those implants that included a positioner to hold the electrodes in place in the cochlea appear to be associated with an increased risk of the disease.

Normal results

Most profoundly deaf patients who receive an implant are able to discern medium and loud sounds, including speech, at comfortable listening levels. Many use sound clues from the implant, together with speech reading and other facial cues, to achieve understanding. Almost all adults improve their communication skills when combining the implant with speech reading (lip reading), and some can understand spoken words without speech reading. More than half of adults who lost hearing after they learned to speak can understand some speech without speech reading. Especially with the use of accessory devices, the great majority can utilize the telephone with their implants.

Children who were born deaf or who lost their hearing before they could speak have the most difficulty in learning to use the implant. Research suggests, however, that most of these children are able to learn spoken language and understand speech using the implant. In general, the earlier the implant occurs, the greater the chance of the implant providing sufficient sound input to provide speech understanding. As with the use of the telephone in adults, accessory devices such as special microphones often help the function of the implant in classroom settings.

Resources

BOOKS

Cummings, C. W., et al. *Otolayrngology: Head and Neck Surgery.* 4th ed. St. Louis: Mosby, 2005.

Niparko, John K., ed. *Cochlear Implants: Principles and Practices.* Philadelphia: Lippincott, Williams & Wilkins, 2000.

PERIODICALS

Roland, J. T. Jr., et al. "Revision cochlear implantation." *Otolaryngol Clin North Am* 39, no. 4 (August 1, 2006): 833–839.

ORGANIZATIONS

Alexander Graham Bell Association for the Deaf. 3417 Volta Place NW, Washington, DC 20007. (202) 337-5220. http://www.agbell.org (accessed March 11, 2008).

The UCSF Cochlear Implant Center. http://cochlearim plant.ucsf.edu/page.asp?bodyid = resources (accessed March 11, 2008).

Hearing Loss Link. 2600 W. Peterson Ave., Ste. 202, Chicago, IL 60659. (312) 743-1032, (312) 743-1007 (TDD).

National Association for the Deaf. 814 Thayer Ave., Silver Spring, MD 20910. (301) 587-1788, (301) 587-1789 (TDD). http://www.nad.org (accessed March 11, 2008).

OTHER

Cochlear Implant Recipients may be at Greater Risk for Meningitis. FDA Public Health Web Notification. October 17, 2002 [cited February 23, 2003]. http://www.fda.gov/cdrh/safety/cochlear.html (accessed March 11, 2008).

Carol A. Turkington
Michelle L. Johnson
Rosalyn Carson-DeWitt, MD

Colectomy *see* **Bowel resection; Bowel resection, small intestine**

Collagen periurethral injection

Definition

Collagen periurethral injection is a procedure in which collagen is injected around the urethra and bladder neck as a treatment for stress incontinence in women.

Purpose

The bladder and urethra are supported by muscles, ligaments, and connective tissues around the base of the bladder. This support prevents the leakage of urine, along with the watertight seal provided by the urethra.

As a result of pregnancy, childbirth, and aging, or damage by scarring from surgery or radiotherapy, these structures may become damaged or weakened, thus causing stress incontinence, meaning an involuntary loss of urine that occurs during physical activity such as coughing, sneezing, laughing, or **exercise**.

The injection of bulking agents, such as collagen, around the urethra aims to improve the lost support of the bladder and urethra. The substance most commonly used for injection is collagen; other bulking agents are being developed; for example, a silicon base suspended in a viscous gel called Macroplastique. Teflon paste, introduced in the 1970s, initially gave good results, but was discontinued after reported problems with excessive scarring and with the migration of Teflon particles to other tissues in the body. The collagen used in the procedure comes from the cartilage of cattle and has been extensively sterilized to produce a viscous paste for injection. There is no risk of bovine spongiform encephalopathy (BSE) transmission because the processing of the paste destroys any bacterial or viral particles.

Description

The collagen periurethral injection procedure is quick, and usually over within 15–20 minutes. No incisions are made, meaning that it can be carried out using a local anesthetic or a regional anesthetic such as an epidural. The surgeon uses a fine fiber-optic cystoscope to examine the inside of the urethra and bladder, and then inserts a fine needle to inject the collagen. Usually three injections are made around the urethra. The exact amount of collagen used depends on how much closure the urethra requires.

Aftercare

Since the procedure is very short and there is little discomfort afterwards, it is performed on an outpatient basis, and women can go home the same day. Recovery from the operation is very quick.

Risks

Periurethral injection is not associated with major complications. Urinary tract infection is common in up to a fifth of the women having undergone the procedure, but is usually quickly and easily treated with **antibiotics**. Some women experience difficulty urinating immediately after the procedure, but this is not unexpected following an operation involving the bladder and urethra that may easily lead to swelling and bruising of the tissues. It is an uncommon problem after periurethral injection. The condition usually settles quickly, but may require catheterization. Long-term problems are very rare.

Normal results

Since periurethral injection is so quick and easy with very few complications, it would appear to be an ideal treatment for stress incontinence; however, there is a problem with the longer-term results. Within three

months after injection, good results are reported with at least 80% of women cured or improved. After two years, less than half of these women will still be cured. Longer-term studies are still being performed, but it is likely that positive results will continue to diminish. This is due to the injected collagen dispersing away from the urethra over time. Injections can be repeated and some women do require more than one injection before they are cured. Ongoing research into new injection substances may improve these results. The results in younger, physically active women are also less successful, usually lasting for a shorter time. Repeated injections are not a simple solution because collagen is very expensive and the long-term effects of repeated injections are unknown. Physicians prefer one of the alternative operations if long-term cure of stress incontinence is the aim.

Alternatives

Other treatments are available to treat incontinence. They include:

- Physiotherapy—this treatment aims to increase the strength and support provided by the pelvic floor muscles.

- Surgical procedures—operations such as colposuspension, sling procedures, needle-suspensions, and vaginal repair operations are all based on lifting and re-supporting the bladder and urethra.

Resources

BOOKS

American Medical Association. *American Medical Association Family Medical Guide,* 4th ed. Hoboken, NJ: Wiley & Sons, 2004.

Burgio, K. L., L. Pearce, A. J. Lucco, and K. F. Jeter. *Staying Dry: A Practical Guide to Bladder Control.* Baltimore: Johns Hopkins University Press, 1990.

Kaschak Newman, D. *Managing and Treating Urinary Incontinence.* Baltimore: Health Professions Press, 2002.

PERIODICALS

Block, C. A., C. S. Cooper, and C. E. Hawtrey. "Long-term Efficacy of Periurethral Collagen Injection for the Treatment of Urinary Incontinence Secondary to Myelomeningocele." *Journal of Urology* 169 (January 2003): 327–329.

Culligan, P. J., et al. "The Safety of Reusing Injectable Collagen: A Multicenter Microbiological Study." *International Urogynecological Journal of Pelvic Floor Dysfunction* 13 (2002): 232–234.

Dmochowski, R. R., and R. A. Appell. "Injectable Agents in the Treatment of Stress Urinary Incontinence in Women: Where Are We Now?" *Urology* 56 (December 2000): 32–40.

Kassouf, W., G. Capolicchio, G. Berardinucci, and J. Corcos. "Collagen Injection for Treatment of Urinary Incontinence in Children." *Journal of Urology* 165 (May 2001): 1666–1668.

OTHER

National Women's Health Information Center. http://www.womenshealth.gov/.

Rackley, Raymond. "Periurethral Injection Therapy for Incontinence." *eMedicine.* June 29, 2006. www.emedicine.com/med/topic3049.htm.

"Stress Incontinence." *Medline Encyclopedia.* May 15, 2006. www.nlm.nih.gov/medlineplus/ency/article/000891.htm.

ORGANIZATIONS

Office of Women's Health, U.S. Food and Drug Administration, 5600 Fishers Lane, Rockville, MD, 20857, (301) 827-0350, http://www.fda.gov/womens/default.htm.

Monique Laberge, Ph.D.
Laura Jean Cataldo, R.N., Ed.D.

Colon anastomosis *see* **Ileoanal anastomosis**

Colonic stent

Definition

A colonic stent is a tubular device made out of artificial materials that is positioned within the intestine in order to keep the intestine patent (open). A colonic stent is placed in order to relieve the symptoms of a bowel obstruction, which often occur when tumors are blocking the intestine. A stent is not a cure for the tumors, but it can provide relief of the unpleasant symptoms that accompany bowel obstruction, such as nausea and vomiting, intractable constipation, inability to pass gas, bloating, and abdominal pain.

Purpose

A colonic stent is used when a patient has an intestinal obstruction, meaning that there is something (often a tumor) blocking the intestine. During an intestinal obstruction, nothing can travel past the point of the obstruction. Therefore, the patient cannot pass gas or feces. If the patient continues to eat and/or drink while obstructed, he or she usually begins vomiting, since nothing he or she eats or drinks can proceed through the intestine. Other symptoms of intestinal obstruction include abdominal pain and uncomfortable bloating (abdominal swelling).

A colonic stent is often employed to relieve the symptoms of intestinal obstruction for either palliative purposes or as a bridge to surgery. "Palliative" treatments are things that are intended for symptom relief, but which do not hold the hope of cure. In the case of colon cancer, if the tumors are inoperable, a palliative procedure such as colonic stenting can allow the patient to experience a better quality of life, although it does not treat the actual underlying disease. In the case of a bridge procedure, colonic stenting can allow relief of symptoms until such time as surgery is deemed safe for the individual.

Demographics

Statistics on cancer of the large intestine (colon) are often linked with statistics on cancer of the rectum. Together, they are referred to as colorectal cancer. Colorectal cancer is the third most common cancer in the United States. Projections for 2008 suggest that 108,070 new cases of colon cancer alone will be diagnosed (about 14% of all cancer cases), with 53,760 cases striking men and 54,310 cases striking women. Colorectal cancer is an extremely serious form of cancer, and is responsible for about 14% of all cancer deaths annually. In 2008, the projection is that 49,960 people will die of colorectal cancer (24,260 men and 25,700 women). This means that colorectal cancer ranks third for causing cancer-related deaths in the United States.

About 90% of the time, colorectal cancer strikes people over the age of forty; most people receive the diagnosis while they are in their 50s or 60s. People with certain other conditions are more likely to develop colorectal cancer. This includes patients who have or have had breast, uterine, or ovarian cancer, ulcerative

KEY TERMS

Colon—The large intestine.

Colonoscope—The fiberoptic device used to view the inside of the large intestine, and through which a variety of procedures can be performed, including biopsies and colonic stent placement.

Colorectal—Pertaining to the large intestine and the rectum.

colitis, or Crohn's disease. Additionally, a family history of either intestinal polyps or colorectal cancer increases an individual's risk of colorectal cancer.

Description

Most colonic stents are placed in the intestine during the course of a **colonoscopy**. The same type of scope used for the diagnostic or screening exam is utilized. The stent is made of wire mesh, and is self-expanding.

While a regular screening colonoscopy can sometimes be performed in a clinic or doctor's office, stent placement requires that the procedure take place in a hospital, so that the position of the stent can be confirmed through x rays. The procedure is usually performed by a specialist in intestinal disease, a gastroenterologist. The procedure is performed under either extensive sedation, given through an intravenous line, or with full **general anesthesia**.

The patient is placed on his or her side, with knees pulled up towards the chest. The colonoscope is thoroughly lubricated, then introduced into the anus. As the colonoscope progresses through the colon, the gastroenterologist will be watching carefully on a monitor, to see whether there are any other problems within the intestine. Mucus, blood, or feces that block the view may be suctioned out through the colonoscope. Air may be pumped into the intestine through the colonoscope, in order to open up the field for better viewing. During the course of the procedure, samples of the intestine (biopsies) may also be taken.

When the colonoscope reaches the level of the obstruction, the colonic stent is guided through the scope into the intestine. Once inside the intestine, the stent will expand itself into a wire-mesh tube. The colonoscope is then withdrawn through the anus, and the procedure is over.

Diagnosis/Preparations

As with any procedures involving the intestine, one of the most important ways to prepare involves cleaning the colon very thoroughly of any stool. Patients whose intestine is completely obstructed may require admittance to a hospital for this to be accomplished. Patients with only partial obstruction may be able to do this at home.

Patients who are allowed to eat solid food should assume a low-residue diet three days prior to the procedure. In general, a low-fiber/low-residue diet involves avoiding whole-grain and whole-wheat foods, processed meats, heavy, deep-fried foods, and foods in thick cream sauces.

The day before the procedure, the patient must follow a careful regimen of taking oral stool softeners, and then using a colon cleansing agent. This can be in a solution that is drunk, or in the form of multiple capsules that are taken with a great deal of water. In some cases, the patient may be required to receive one or more enemas, to make sure that all stool has been evacuated from the intestine.

The patient is usually required to stop eating all solid foods for the twenty-four hours prior to the procedure. They are usually allowed to drink clear fluids until about twelve hours prior to the procedure.

Patients who are using anticoagulant (blood thinning) medications, aspirin, or **nonsteroidal anti-inflammatory drugs** should discuss with their doctor whether these should be discontinued prior to the procedure, in order to decrease the risk of bleeding.

Aftercare

Patients who have had a colonic stent placed are usually kept in the hospital for a day or two after the procedure, in order to carefully monitor them. They will be slowly progressed to clear fluids, then full fluids, then a soft diet, and then a full diet.

Normal results

Successful placement of a colonic stent allows for the passage of both gas and stool through the intestine. Pain, bloating, and nausea are relieved, and the patient can resume eating and drinking normally. In patients awaiting surgery, a normal result allows the surgery to be scheduled nonemergently, thus decreasing the risk of **colostomy** as part of the surgical outcome. Success is achieved between 93 and 95% of the time in colonic stent placement.

Morbidity and mortality rates

Complications of colonic stent placement include dislodging of the stent from its original location (has occurred in about 10-12% of patients), passage of the stent in stool, obstruction of the stent's lumen with impacted stool or expanding tumor, perforation (occurs in about 4% of patients) of the intestine, bleeding, abdominal pain, rectal spasms, embolism.

Resources

BOOKS

Abeloff, M. D., et al. *Clinical Oncology,* 3rd ed. Philadelphia: Elsevier, 2004.

Feldman, M., et al. *Sleisenger & Fordtran's Gastrointestinal and Liver Disease,* 8th ed. St. Louis: Mosby, 2005.

PERIODICALS

Fregonese, D. "Ultraflex precision colonic stent placement as a bridge to surgery in patients with malignant colon obstruction." *Gastrointestinal Endoscopy* 67 (2008): 68–73.

Repici, A. "WallFlex colonic stent placement for management of malignant colonic obstruction: a prospective study at two centers." *Gastrointestinal Endoscopy* 67 (2008): 77–84.

Rosalyn Carson-DeWitt, MD

Colonoscopy

Definition

Colonoscopy is an endoscopic medical procedure that uses a colonoscope, a long, flexible, thin, lighted tube-like instrument containing a tiny video camera, that allows a visual examination of the lining of the colon (large intestine) and rectum.

Purpose

A colonoscopy is generally recommended when the patient complains of rectal bleeding, has a change in bowel habits, and/or has other unexplained abdominal symptoms. The test is frequently used to look for colorectal cancer, especially when polyps or tumor-like growths have been detected by a **barium enema** examination and other diagnostic imaging tests. Polyps can be removed through the colonoscope, and samples of tissue (biopsies) can be taken to detect the presence of cancerous cells. In addition, colonoscopy can also be used to remove foreign bodies from the colon, control hemorrhaging, and excise tumors.

A colonoscopy allows the physician to visualize the lining of the entire colon and, therefore, it also enables physicians to check for bowel diseases such as ulcerative colitis and Crohn's disease. Colonoscopy is being used increasingly as a screening tool in asymptomatic patients. It is recommended as a screening test in all people 50 years or older and is an essential tool for monitoring patients who have a past history of polyps or colon cancer.

Description

Colonoscopy can be performed either in a physician's office or in an endoscopic procedure room of a hospital or freestanding clinic. For otherwise healthy patients, colonoscopy is usually performed by a gastroenterologist or surgeon in an office or clinic setting. When performed on patients with other medical conditions that could cause complications or that require hospitalization, it is usually performed in the endoscopy department of a hospital, where more intensive physiologic monitoring and/or **general anesthesia** can be better provided.

An intravenous line is usually inserted into a vein in the patient's arm to administer a sedative and a painkiller. During the colonoscopy, patients lie on their sides with their knees drawn up towards the abdomen. The doctor begins the procedure by inserting a lubricated, gloved finger into the anus to check for any abnormal masses or blockage. A thin, well-lubricated colonoscope is then inserted into the anus and gently advanced through the colon. The lining of the large intestine is examined through the colonoscope. The physician views images on a television monitor, and the procedure can be documented using a video recorder. Still images can be recorded and saved on a computer disk or printed. Occasionally, air may be pumped through the colonoscope to help clear the path or open the colon. If excessive secretions, stool, or blood obstructs the viewing, they are suctioned out through the scope. The doctor may press on the abdomen or ask the patient to change position in order to advance the scope through the colon.

The entire length of the large intestine can be examined in this manner. If suspicious growths are present, tiny biopsy forceps or brushes are inserted through the colon and tissue samples (biopsies) are obtained. Small polyps or inflamed tissue also can be removed using tiny instruments passed through the scope. For removing tumors or performing other types of surgery on the colon during colonoscopy, an electrosurgical device or laser system may be used in conjunction with the colonoscope. To stop bleeding in the colon, a laser, heater probe, or electrical probe is

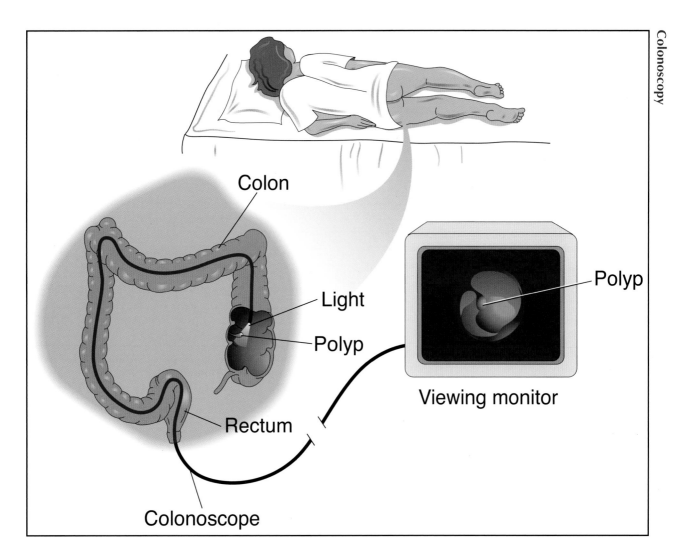

Colonoscopy is a procedure where a long and flexible tubular instrument called a colonoscope is inserted into the patient's anus in order to view the lining of the colon and rectum. It is performed to test for colorectal cancer and other bowel diseases, and enables the physician to collect tissue samples for laboratory analysis. *(Illustration by Electronic Illustrators Group. Cengage Learning, Gale.)*

used, or special medicines are injected through the scope. After the procedure, the colonoscope is slowly withdrawn and the instilled air is allowed to escape. The anal area is then cleansed with tissues. Tissue samples taken by biopsy are sent to a clinical laboratory, where they are analyzed by a pathologist.

The procedure may take anywhere from 30 minutes to two hours depending on how easy it is to advance the scope through the colon. Colonoscopy can be a long and uncomfortable procedure, and the bowel-cleansing preparation may be tiring and can produce diarrhea and cramping. During the colonoscopy, the sedative and the pain medications will keep the patient drowsy and relaxed. Some patients complain of minor discomfort and pressure from the colonoscope; however, the

sedative and pain medication usually cause most patients to dose off during the procedure.

Preparation

Patients who regularly take **aspirin, nonsteroidal anti-inflammatory drugs** (NSAIDs), blood thinners, or insulin should be sure to inform the physician at the time the colonoscopy is scheduled. The physician also should be notified if the patient has allergies to any medications or anesthetics, bleeding problems, or is pregnant. The doctor should be informed of all the medications the patient is taking and if he or she has had a barium enema x-ray examination recently. If the patient has had heart valves replaced, the doctor should be informed so that appropriate **antibiotics**

Barium enema—An X-ray test of the bowel performed after giving the patient an enema of a white chalky substance (barium) that outlines the colon and the rectum.

Biopsy—A procedure in which a sample of suspicious tissue is removed and examined by a pathologist for cancer or other disease.

Colonoscope—A thin, flexible, hollow, lighted tube that is inserted through the anus and rectum to the colon to enable the physician to view the entire lining of the colon.

Computed tomography (CT) scan—A radiologic imaging technique that uses computer processing to generate an image of the tissue density; also called computerized axial tomography (CAT) and computerized transaxial tomography (CTAT).

Crohn's disease—A chronic inflammatory disease that generally starts in the gastrointestinal tract and causes the immune system to attack one's own body.

Diverticulosis—A condition that involves the development of sacs that bulge through the large intestine's muscular walls, but are not inflamed. It may cause bleeding, stomach distress, and excess gas.

Electrosurgical device—A medical device that uses electrical current to cauterize or coagulate tissue during surgical procedures; often used in conjunction with laparoscopy.

Magnetic resonance imaging (MRI)—A test that provides pictures of organs and structures inside the body using radio waves. In many cases, an MRI provides information that cannot be obtained from X-ray tests.

Pathologist—A doctor who specializes in the diagnosis of disease by studying cells and tissues under a microscope.

Polyps—An abnormal growth that develops on the inside of a hollow organ such as the colon.

Sigmoidoscopy—A process of passing a long, hollow tubular instrument through the anus in order to permit inspection, diagnosis, treatment, and imaging, especially of the sigmoid flexure.

Ulcerative colitis—A chronic condition in which recurrent ulcers are found in the colon. It is manifested clinically by abdominal cramping and rectal bleeding.

Virtual colonoscopy—Two new techniques that provide views of the colon to screen for colon polyps and cancer. The images are produced by computerized manipulations rather than direct observation through the colonoscope; one technique uses the X-ray images from a CT scan, and the other uses magnetic images from an MRI scan.

---

can be administered to prevent infection. Patients with severe active colitis, extremely dilated colon (toxic megacolon), or severely inflamed bowel may not be candidates for colonoscopy. Patients requiring continuous ambulatory peritoneal dialysis are generally not candidates for colonoscopy due to a higher risk of developing internal bleeding. The risks associated with the procedure are explained to the patient beforehand, and the patient is asked to sign a consent form.

The colon must be thoroughly cleansed before performing colonoscopy. Consequently, for about two days before the procedure, considerable preparation is necessary to clear the colon of all stool. The patient is asked to refrain from eating any solid food for 24–48 hours before the test. Only clear liquid such as juices, broth, and gelatin are allowed. Red or purple juices should be avoided, since they can cause coloring of the colon that may be misinterpreted as blood during the colonoscopy. The patient is advised to drink plenty of water to avoid dehydration. A day before the

colonoscopy, the patient is prescribed liquid, tablet, and/or suppository **laxatives** by the physician. In addition, commercial enemas may be prescribed. The patient is given specific instructions on how and when to use the laxatives and/or enemas. This preparatory emptying of the colon assures that the colonoscope will not be obstructed and that the physician will be able to clearly see the colon lining.

On the morning of the colonoscopy, the patient is not to eat or drink anything. Unless otherwise instructed by the physician, the patient should continue to take all current medications. Vitamins with iron, iron supplements, or iron preparations should be discontinued for a few weeks before the colonoscopy because iron residue in the colon can inhibit viewing during the procedure. These preparatory procedures are extremely important to ensure a thoroughly clean colon for examination.

After the procedure, the patient is kept under observation until the medications' effects wear off.

The patient has to be driven home and can generally resume a normal diet and usual activities unless otherwise instructed. The patient is advised to drink plenty of fluids to replace those lost by laxatives and fasting.

For a few hours after the procedure, the patient may feel groggy. There may be some abdominal cramping and a considerable amount of gas may be passed. If a biopsy was performed or a polyp was removed, there may be small amounts of blood in the stool for a few days. If the patient experiences severe abdominal pain or has persistent and heavy bleeding, this information should be brought to the physician's attention immediately.

Risks

The procedure is practically free of complications and risks. Rarely, (two in 1,000 cases) a perforation (hole) may occur in the intestinal wall. Heavy bleeding due to the removal of the polyp or from the biopsy site occurs infrequently (one in 1,000 cases). Some patients may have adverse reactions to the sedatives administered during the colonoscopy, but severe reactions are very rare. Infections due to a colonoscopy are also extremely rare. Patients with artificial or abnormal heart valves are usually given antibiotics before and after the procedure to prevent an infection.

Normal results

The results are normal if the lining of the colon is a pale reddish pink and there are no abnormal masses visible. In this case, the patient probably will not have to undergo another colonoscopy for several years.

Abnormal results indicate polyps or other suspicious masses in the lining of the colon. Many polyps can be removed during the procedure, and tissue samples can be taken by biopsy. If cancerous cells are detected in the tissue samples, then a diagnosis of colon cancer is made. A pathologist analyzes the tumor cells further to estimate the tumor's aggressiveness and the extent of the disease. This is crucial before deciding on the mode of treatment for the disease. Abnormal findings could also be due to inflammatory bowel diseases such as ulcerative colitis or Crohn's disease. A condition called diverticulosis, which causes many small finger-like pouches to protrude from the colon wall, may also contribute to an abnormal result in the colonoscopy.

Morbidity and mortality rates

Colorectal cancer is the second leading cause of cancer deaths in the United States. In 2007, The American Cancer Society estimated that 52,180 people died from the disease. The World Health Organization (WHO) estimates that about 500,000 people worldwide die from colorectal cancer each year. Although colonoscopy screening can find precancerous growths (polyps), which lead to colorectal cancer, screening rates in the United States remain low. Removing polyps before they become cancerous can prevent the disease and potentially reduce deaths. Scientific evidence indicates that more than one-third of deaths from colorectal cancer could be avoided if people aged 50 years and older were screened regularly.

Alternatives

Individuals with a strong family history of colorectal cancer may wish to undergo genetic screening to detect a genetic alteration that may identify people who are more likely to develop the disease and who would benefit from earlier and more frequent screening. Only about 5% of colorectal cancers are inherited, so genetic testing provides limited benefits for most of the population.

Virtual colonoscopy is a new non-invasive technique for screening for colon polyps and cancer. The colon is cleaned out using potent laxatives just as it is for a standard colonoscopy. Instead of obtaining pictures through the insertion of a colonoscope, virtual colonoscopy uses X-ray images from a computerized tomography (CT) scan or **magnetic resonance imaging** (MRI) to create through computer manipulation two- and three-dimensional pictures of the colon.

Virtual colonoscopy offers several advantages. The procedure is non-invasive. It does not require patients to be sedated or put under anesthesia and is a good option for individuals who cannot or will not undergo standard colonoscopy. The procedure can be performed in less than one minute, compared with about 30–60 minutes plus recovery time required for standard colonoscopy. Another benefit of the **CT scan** is that it can find polyps that occasionally are missed by colonoscopy because the polyps lie behind folds within the colon.

Disadvantages of virtual colonoscopy include:

- It has difficulty finding small polyps (<0.2 in [5 mm] in size) that are easily seen in a colonoscopy.
- It is less able to find flat polyps compared to a colonoscopy.
- Small pieces of stool can look like polyps on the CT scan and lead to a diagnosis of polyp when there is none.
- It is not possible to remove suspect polyps or take a biopsy. If polyps are found by virtual colonoscopy, a standard colonoscopy must be done to remove the polyps. As a result, the individual must undergo two procedures.

Resources

BOOKS

Beers, Mark H., Robert S. Porter, and Thomas V. Jones, eds. *The Merck Manual*, 18th ed. Whitehouse Station, NJ: Merck, 2007.

Tierney, Lawrence M., Stephen J. McPhee, and Maxine A. Papadakis, eds. *Current Medical Diagnosis & Treatment 2003*. Stamford, CT: Appleton & Lange, 2002.

OTHER

"Colonoscopy." *Mayo Clinic*. June 29, 2007 [cited January 28, 2008]. http://www.mayoclinic.com/health/colonoscopy/CO00009.

"Patient Information from Your Surgeon & SAGES." *Society of American Gastrointestinal Endoscopic Surgeons*. March 2004 [cited January 28, 2008]. http://www.sages.org/sagespublication.php?doc = PI04.

"Screen for Life: National Colorectal Cancer Action Campaign." *Centers for Disease Control and Prevention*. March 10, 2008 [cited March 16, 2008]. http://www.cdc.gov/cancer/colorectal/sfl/.

"Virtual Colonoscopy." *National Digestive Diseases Information Clearinghouse*. May 2003 [cited January 28, 2008]. http://digestive.niddk.nih.gov/ddiseases/pubs/virtualcolonoscopy.

ORGANIZATIONS

American College of Gastroenterology, P.O. Box 342260, Bethesda, MD, 20827-2260, (301) 263-9000, http://www.acg.gi.org.

Colorectal Cancer Network (CCNetwork), P.O. Box 182, Kensington, MD, 20895-0182, (301) 879-1500, http://clickonium.com/colorectal-cancer.net/html/.

International Foundation for Functional Gastrointestinal Disorders (IFFGD), P.O. Box 170864, Milwaukee, WI, 53217, (414) 964-1799, (888) 964-2001, http://www.iffgd.org.

National Digestive Diseases Information Clearinghouse (NDDIC), 2 Information Way, Bethesda, MD, 20892-3570, (800) 891-5389, http://digestive.niddk.nih.gov.

Society of American Gastrointestinal Endoscopic Surgeons (SAGES), 11300 West Olympic Blvd., Suite 600, Los Angeles, CA, 90064, (310) 437-0544, http://www.sages.org.

Jennifer E. Sisk, M.A.
Crystal H. Kaczkowski, M.Sc.
Tish Davidson, A.M.

Colorectal surgery

Definition

Colorectal surgery repairs damage to the colon, rectum, and anus through a variety of procedures that may have little or great long-term consequence to the patient. It may also involve surgery to the pelvic floor to repair hernias.

Purpose

Colorectal surgery is performed to repair damage to the colon, rectum, and anus, caused by diseases of the lower digestive tract, such as cancer, **diverticulitis**, and inflammatory bowel disease (ulcerative colitis and Crohn's disease). Injury, obstruction, and ischemia (compromised blood supply) may require bowel surgery. Masses and scar tissue can grow within the rectum, causing blockages that prevent normal elimination of feces. Other diseases such as diverticulitis and ulcerative colitis can cause perforations in the rectum. Surgical removal of the damaged area or areas can return normal bowel function.

Demographics

Colorectal cancer affects 140,000 people annually, causing 60,000 deaths. Polypectomy (the removal of polyps in the colon), usually performed during a routine diagnostic test (colonscopy or flexible **sigmoidoscopy**), has been a factor in the declining incidence of this cancer. However, incidence of the disease, as reported in the Journal of the National Cancer Institute in 2001, differed among ethnic groups, with Hispanics having 10.2 cases per 100,000 people, to African Americans having 22.8 cases per 100,000. Surgery is the optimal treatment for colorectal cancer, resulting in cure in 80% of patients. Recurrence due to surgical failure is low, from 4% to 8%, when surgery is meticulously performed.

Crohn's disease and ulcerative colitis, both chronic inflammatory diseases of the colon, together affect approximately 1,000,000 young adults. Surgery is recommended when medication fails patients with ulcerative colitis. Usually, surgery is drastic, removing the colon and rectum and creating an interior or exterior pouch to collect body wastes. Nearly three-fourths of all Crohn's patients face surgery to removed a diseased section of the intestine or rectum.

Diverticulosis, the growth of pouches in the walls of the intestine, occurs in nearly half of all Americans by the time they reach age 60 and in practically everyone over 80. Sometimes these diverticuli become infected and diverticulitis occurs. Diverticulitis may also require surgery to remove part of the colon if there have been recurrent episodes with complications or perforations.

Description

Colorectal surgery is a necessary treatment option for colorectal cancer, ulcerative colitis, Crohn's disease,

KEY TERMS

Adjuvant therapy—Treatment that is added to increase the effectiveness of surgery, usually chemotherapy or radiation used to kill any cancer cells that might be remaining.

Anastomosis—The surgical connection of two sections of tubes, ducts, or vessels.

Diverticuli—Pouches in the intestinal wall usually created from a diet low in fiber.

Embolism—Blockage of a blood vessel by any small piece of material traveling in the blood; the emboli may be caused by germs, air, blood clots, or fat.

Enema—Insertion of a tube into the rectum to infuse fluid into the bowel and encourage a bowel movement. Ordinary enemas contain tap water, mixtures of soap and water, glycerine and water, or other materials.

Intestine—Commonly called the bowels, divided into the small and large intestine. They extend from the stomach to the anus.

Ischemia—A compromise in blood supply delivered to body tissues that causes tissue damage or death.

Ostomy—A surgical procedure that creates an opening from the inside of the body to the outside, usually to remove body wastes (feces or urine).

Sigmoid colon—The last third of the intestinal tract that is attached to the rectum.

and some cases of diverticulitis, often resulting in major reconstruction of the intestinal tract. Other bowel conditions that may require surgery to a lesser extent are hemorrhoids, anal fissures (tears in the lining of the anus), rectal prolapse, and bowel incontinence. Most of these surgeries repair tears, remove blockages, or tighten sphincter muscles. Patients with anal fissures, for example, experience immediate relief, with more than 90% of them never having the problem recur.

Some colorectal surgeons also treat pelvic floor disorders such as perineal hernia and rectocele (a bulging of the rectum toward the vagina).

Types of surgery

There are a variety of procedures a colorectal surgeon may use to treat intestinal disorders. Until 1990, all colorectal surgery was performed by making large incisions in the abdomen, opening up the intestinal cavity, and making the repair. Most of these repairs involved resection (cutting out the diseased or damaged portion) and anastomosis (attaching the cut ends of the intestine together). Some were tucks to tighten sphincter muscles or repair fissures, and others cut out hemorrhoids. Some colorectal surgeons perform a strictureplasty, a new procedure that widens the intestine instead of making it shorter; this is used with patients with extensive Crohn's disease.

Often colorectal surgery involves creating an ostomy, which is an opening from the inside of the body to the outside, usually to remove body wastes (feces or urine). There are several types of ostomy surgeries that colorectal surgeons do. A **colostomy** is a surgical procedure that brings a portion of the large intestine through the abdominal wall, creating an opening, or stoma, to carry feces out of the body to a pouch. An **ileostomy** removes the entire colon, the rectum, and the anus. The lower end of the small intestine (the ileum) becomes the stoma.

For all ostomies, a pouch will generally be placed around the stoma on the patient's abdomen during surgery. During the hospital stay, the patient and his or her caregivers will be educated on care of the stoma and the ostomy pouch. Determination of appropriate pouching supplies and a schedule of how often to change the pouch should be established. Regular assessment and meticulous care of the skin surrounding the stoma is important to maintain an adequate surface on which to attach the pouch. Some patients with colostomies are able to routinely irrigate the stoma, resulting in regulation of bowel function; rather than needing to wear a pouch, these patients may need only a dressing or cap over their stoma. Often, an enterostomal therapist will visit the patient in the hospital or at home after discharge to help the patient with stoma care.

Most colostomies and ileostomies are permanent. Temporary colostomies are created to divert stool from injured or diseased portions of the large intestine, allowing rest and healing. Although colorectal cancer is the most common indication for a permanent colostomy, only about 10–15% of patients with this diagnosis require a colostomy.

A new procedure called an **ileoanal anastomosis** creates an internal reservoir that is sewn to the anus and acts as an artificial rectum. It usually is not used with Crohn's disease patients because their disease often recurs.

Laparoscopic surgery is being used with many diseases of the intestinal tract, including initial cancers. For this surgery, the colon and rectal surgeon inserts a laparoscope (an instrument that has a tiny video camera attached) through a small incision in the abdomen. Other small incisions are made through which the surgeon inserts **surgical instruments**. This surgery often results in fewer complications, a shorter stay in the hospital, less postoperative pain, a quicker return to normal activities, and less scarring. It is not recommended for patients who have had extensive prior abdominal surgery, large tumors, previous cancer, or serious heart problems.

Diagnosis/Preparation

Some disease or conditions may require a minimally invasive surgery. Other diseases such as inflammatory bowel disease and colorectal cancer may require an ostomy, a more drastic procedure. Determining whether this surgery is necessary is a decision the physician makes based on a number of factors, including patient history, the amount of pain the patient is experiencing, and the results of several diagnostic tests. Due to the lifestyle impact of ostomy surgery, surgeons make that decision with careful input from the patient. Sometimes, though, an immediate decision may be necessary in emergency situations involving injuries or puncture wounds in the abdomen, or intestinal perforations related to diverticular disease, ulcers, or cancer, which can be life-threatening.

Diagnostic tests

Colonoscopy, flexible sigmoidoscopy, and a lower GI (gastrointestinal) series help determine the condition of the intestinal tract. These tests can identify masses and perforations on bowel walls.

A lower GI series is a series of x rays of the colon and rectum, which can identify ulcers, cysts, polyps, diverticuli (pouches in the intestine), and cancer. The patient is given a **barium enema**; the barium coats the intestinal tract, making any signs of disease easier to see on x rays.

Flexible sigmoidoscopy, a flexible tube with a miniature camera, is inserted into the rectum so the physician can examine the lining of the rectum and the sigmoid colon, the last third of the intestinal tract. The sigmoidoscope can also remove polyps or tissue for biopsy.

A colonoscopy is a similar procedure to the flexible sigmoidoscopy, except the flexible tube looks at the entire intestinal tract. For the patient's comfort, a sedative is given.

Magnetic resonance imaging (MRI), used both prior to and during surgery, allows physicians to determine the precise margins for resections of the colon, so that they can eliminate all of the diseased tissue. MRI can also identify patients who could most benefit from adjuvant therapy such as chemotherapy or radiation.

Preoperative preparation

The doctor will outline the procedure, possible side effects, and what the patient may experience after surgery. As with any surgical procedure, the patient will be required to sign a consent form. Blood and urine studies, along with various x rays and an electrocardiograph (EKG), may be ordered. If necessary, an enterostomal therapist will be contacted to mark an appropriate place on the abdomen for the stoma and offer preoperative education on ostomy management.

In order to empty and cleanse the bowel, the patient may be placed on a restricted diet for several days prior to surgery. A liquid diet may be ordered for at least the day before surgery, with nothing by mouth after midnight. A series of enemas and/or oral preparations (GoLytely, Colyte, or senna) may be ordered to empty the bowel of stool. Oral anti-infectives (neomycin, erythromycin, or kanamycin sulfate) may be ordered to decrease bacteria in the intestine and help prevent postoperative infection.

Aftercare

Postoperative care involves monitoring blood pressure, pulse, respiration, and temperature. Breathing tends to be shallow because of the effect of the anesthesia and the patient's reluctance to breathe deeply and experience pain that is caused by the abdominal incision. The patient is instructed how to support the operative site during deep breathing and coughing, and given pain medication as necessary. Fluid intake and output is measured, and the operative site is observed for color and amount of wound drainage.

The patient is usually helped out of bed the evening of the surgery and allowed to sit in a chair. Most patients are discharged in two to four days.

The nasogastric tube will remain in place, attached to low, intermittent suction until bowel activity resumes. For the first 24–48 hours after surgery, the ostomy will drain bloody mucus. Fluids and electrolytes are given intravenously until the patient's diet can gradually be resumed, beginning with liquids only, then adding solids. Usually within 72 hours, passage of gas and stool through the stoma begins. Initially the stool is liquid, gradually thickening as the patient begins to take solid foods. The patient is usually out of bed in eight to 24 hours after surgery and discharged in two to four days.

Risks

Potential risks of colorectal surgery are those of any major surgery and usually occur while the patient is still in the hospital. The patient's general health prior to surgery will also be an indication of the potential for risk. Of special concern are cardiac problems and stressed immune systems.

Psychological complications may result from ostomy surgery because of the fear of the social stigma attached to wearing a colostomy bag. Patients may also be depressed and have feelings of low self-worth because of the change in their lifestyle and their appearance. Some patients may feel ugly and sexually unattractive and may worry that their spouse or significant other will no longer find them appealing. Counseling and education regarding surgery and the inherent lifestyle changes are often necessary.

Normal results

Complete healing is expected without complications. The period of time required for recovery from the surgery may vary, depending on the patient's overall health prior to surgery. Dietary changes may be encouraged to prevent future disorders or to manage a current disease.

Morbidity and mortality rates

Mortality has been decreased from nearly 28% to under 6% through the use of prophylactic **antibiotics** prescribed before and after surgery. Strong indicators of survival outcome or increased complications from surgery for elderly patients are underlying medical conditions. Therefore, the underlying medical conditions of at-risk patients should be controlled prior to a colorectal surgery.

Even among higher risk patients, mortality is about 16%. This rate is greatly reduced (between 0.8% and 3.8%) when the ostomies and resections for cancer are performed by a board-certified colon and rectal surgeon.

The physician and the nursing staff monitor the patient's **vital signs** and the surgical incision, alert for:

- excessive bleeding
- wound infection
- thrombophlebitis (inflammation and blood clot in the veins in the legs)
- pneumonia
- pulmonary embolism (blood clot or air bubble in the lungs' blood supply)
- cardiac stress due to allergic reaction to the general anesthetic

---

WHO PERFORMS THE PROCEDURE AND WHERE IS IT PERFORMED?

Colorectal surgery is performed by general surgeons and board-certified colon and rectal surgeons as in-patient surgeries under general anesthesia.

Symptoms that the patient should report, especially after discharge, include:

- increased pain, swelling, redness, drainage, or bleeding in the surgical area
- flu-like symptoms such as headache, muscle aches, dizziness, or fever
- increased abdominal pain or swelling, constipation, nausea or vomiting, or black, tarry stools

Stomal complications can also occur. They include:

- Death (necrosis) of stomal tissue. Caused by inadequate blood supply, this complication is usually visible 12–24 hours after the operation and may require additional surgery.

- Retraction (stoma is flush with the abdomen surface or has moved below it). Caused by insufficient stomal length, this complication may be managed by use of special pouching supplies; elective revision of the stoma is also an option.

- Prolapse (stoma increases length above the surface of the abdomen). Most often this results from an overly large opening in the abdominal wall or inadequate fixation of the bowel to the abdominal wall; surgical correction is required when blood supply is compromised.

- Stenosis (narrowing at the opening of the stoma). Often this is associated with infection around the stoma or scarring. Mild stenosis can be removed under local anesthesia; severe stenosis may require surgery for reshaping the stoma.

- Parastomal hernia (bulge in the abdominal wall, caused by a section of bowel, next to the stoma). This occurs due to placement of the stoma where the abdominal wall is weak or an overly large opening in the abdominal wall is created. The use of an ostomy support belt and special pouching supplies may be adequate. If severe, the defect in the abdominal wall should be repaired and the stoma moved to another location.

Alternatives

When a colostomy is deemed necessary, there are usually no alternatives to the surgery, though there can be alternatives in the type of surgery involved and adjuvant therapies related to the disease.

Resources

BOOKS

Johnston, Lorraine. *Colon & Rectal Cancer: A Comprehensive Guide for Patients and Families.* Sebastopol, CA: O'Reilly, 2000.

Levin, Bernard. *American Cancer Society Colorectal Cancer.* New York: Villard, 1999.

PERIODICALS

Beets-Tan, R. G. H., et al. "Accuracy of Maganetic Resonance Imaging in Prediction of Tumour-free Resection Margin in Rectal Cancer Surgery." *The Lancet* 357 (February 17, 2001): 497.

"Laparoscopy Could Offer Long-term Survival Benefit over Conventional Surgery." *Cancer Weekly* (July 30, 2002): 14.

Schwenk, Wolfgang. "Pulmonary Function Following Laparoscopic or Conventional Colorectal Resection: A Randomized Controlled Evaluation." *Journal of the American Medical Association* 281 (April 7, 1999): 1154.

Senagore, A. J., and P. Erwin-Toth. "Care of the Laparoscopic Colectomy Patient." *Advances in Skin & Wound Care* 15 (November–December 2002): 277–284.

Walling, Anne D. "Follow-up after Resection for Colorectal Cancer Saves Lives. (Tips from Other Journals)." *American Family Physician* 66 (August 1, 2002): 485.

ORGANIZATIONS

American Board of Colon and Rectal Surgery (ABCRS). 20600 Eureka Road, Suite 713, Taylor, MI 48180. (734) 282-9400. www.fascrs.org.

Mayo Clinic. 200 First St. S.W., Rochester, MN 55905. (507) 284-2511. www.mayoclinic.org.

United Ostomy Association, Inc. (UOA). 19772 MacArthur Blvd., Suite 200, Irvine, CA 92612-2405. (800) 826-0826. http://www.uoa.org.

Wound Ostomy and Continence Nurses Society. 2755 Bristol Street, Suite 110, Costa Mesa, CA 92626. (714) 476-0268. http://www.wocn.org.

OTHER

National Digestive Diseases Information Clearinghouse. *Ileostomy, Colostomy, and Ileoanal Reservoir Surgery.* (February 1, 2000): 1.

Janie F. Franz

Colostomy

Definition

A colostomy is a surgical procedure that brings a portion of the large intestine through the abdominal wall to carry feces out of the body.

Purpose

A colostomy is a means to treat various disorders of the large intestine, including cancer, obstruction, inflammatory bowel disease, ruptured diverticulum, ischemia (compromised blood supply), or traumatic injury. Temporary colostomies are created to divert stool from injured or diseased portions of the large intestine, allowing rest and healing. Permanent colostomies are performed when the distal bowel (at the farthest distance) must be removed or is blocked and inoperable. Although colorectal cancer is the most common indication for a permanent colostomy, only about 10–15% of patients with this diagnosis require a colostomy.

Demographics

Estimates of all ostomy surgeries (those involving any opening from the abdomen for the removal of either feces or urine) range from 42,000 to 65,000 each year; about half are temporary. Emergency surgeries for bowel obstruction and/or perforation comprise 10–15% of all colorectal surgeries; a portion of these result in colostomy.

Description

Surgery will result in one of three types of colostomies:

- End colostomy. The functioning end of the intestine (the section of bowel that remains connected to the

Colostomy

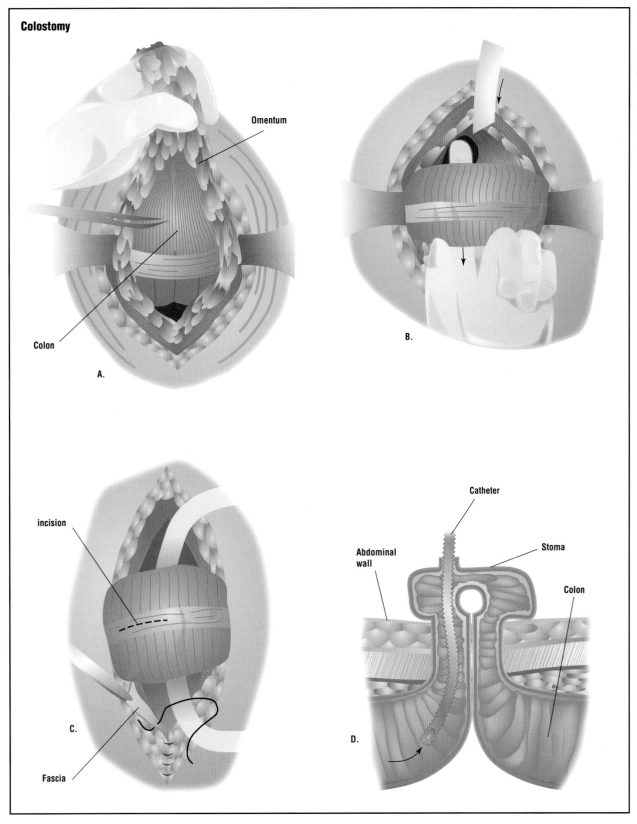

Omentum

Colon

A.

B.

incision

C.

Fascia

Catheter

Stoma

Abdominal wall

Colon

D.

To perform a colostomy, the surgeon enters the abdomen and locates the colon, or large intestine (A). A loop of the colon is pulled through the abdominal incision (B); then the colon is cut to allow the insertion of a catheter (C). The skin and tisses are closed around the new opening, called a stoma (D). *(Illustration by GGS Information Services. Cengage Learning, Gale.)*

upper gastrointestinal tract) is brought out onto the surface of the abdomen, forming the stoma (artificial opening) by cuffing the intestine back on itself and suturing the end to the skin. The surface of the stoma is actually the lining of the intestine, usually appearing moist and pink. The distal portion of bowel (now connected only to the rectum) may be removed, or sutured closed and left in the abdomen. An end colostomy is usually a permanent ostomy, resulting from trauma, cancer, or another pathological condition.

- Double-barrel colostomy. This involves the creation of two separate stomas on the abdominal wall. The proximal (nearest) stoma is the functional end that is connected to the upper gastrointestinal tract and will drain stool; the distal stoma, connected to the rectum and also called a mucous fistula, drains small amounts of mucus material. This is most often a temporary colostomy performed to rest an area of bowel, and to be later closed.

- Loop colostomy. This surgery brings a loop of bowel through an incision in the abdominal wall. The loop is held in place outside the abdomen by a plastic rod slipped beneath it. An incision is made in the bowel to allow the passage of stool through the loop colostomy. The supporting rod is removed approximately seven to 10 days after surgery, when healing has occurred that will prevent the loop of bowel from retracting into the abdomen. A loop colostomy is most often performed for creation of a temporary stoma to divert stool away from an area of intestine that has been blocked or ruptured.

Diagnosis/Preparation

A number of diseases and injuries may require a colostomy. Among the diseases are inflammatory bowel disease and colorectal cancer. Determining whether this surgery is necessary is a decision the physician makes based on a number of factors, including patient history, amount of pain, and the results of tests such as **colonoscopy** and lower G.I. (gastrointestinal) series. Due to lifestyle impact of the surgery, the decision is made after careful consultation with the patient. However, an immediate decision may be made in emergency situations involving injuries or puncture wounds in the abdomen or intestinal perforations related to diverticular disease, ulcers, or life-threatening cancer.

As with any surgical procedure, the patient will be required to sign a consent form after the procedure is explained thoroughly. Blood and urine studies, along with various x rays and an electrocardiograph (EKG), may be ordered as the doctor deems necessary. If possible, the patient should visit an enterostomal

---

KEY TERMS

Diverticulum—Pouches that project off the wall of the intestine.

Embolism—Blockage of a blood vessel by any small piece of material traveling in the blood; the emboli may be caused by germs, air, blood clots, or fat.

Enema—Insertion of a tube into the rectum to infuse fluid into the bowel and encourage a bowel movement. Ordinary enemas contain tap water, mixtures of soap and water, glycerine and water, or other materials.

Intestine—Commonly called the bowels, divided into the small and large intestine. They extend from the stomach to the anus.

Ischemia—A compromise in blood supply delivered to body tissues that causes tissue damage or death.

Ostomy—A surgical procedure that creates an opening from the inside of the body to the outside, usually to remove body wastes (feces or urine).

---

therapist, who will mark an appropriate place on the abdomen for the stoma and offer preoperative education on ostomy management.

In order to empty and cleanse the bowel, the patient may be placed on a low-residue diet for several days prior to surgery. A liquid diet may be ordered for at least the day before surgery, with nothing by mouth after midnight. A series of enemas and/or oral preparations (GoLytely or Colyte) may be ordered to empty the bowel of stool. Oral anti-infectives (neomycin, erythromycin, or kanamycin sulfate) may be ordered to decrease bacteria in the intestine and help prevent postoperative infection. A nasogastric tube is inserted from the nose to the stomach on the day of surgery or during surgery to remove gastric secretions and prevent nausea and vomiting. A urinary catheter (a thin plastic tube) may also be inserted to keep the bladder empty during surgery, giving more space in the surgical field and decreasing chances of accidental injury.

Aftercare

Postoperative care for the patient with a new colostomy, as with those who have had any major surgery, involves monitoring of blood pressure, pulse, respirations, and temperature. Breathing tends to be shallow because of the effect of anesthesia and the patient's reluctance to breathe deeply and experience pain that is caused by the abdominal incision. The patient is instructed how to support the operative site during deep breathing and coughing, and given pain medication as necessary. Fluid intake and output is measured, and the operative site is observed for color and amount of wound drainage. The nasogastric tube will remain in place, attached to low, intermittent suction until bowel activity resumes. For the first 24–48 hours after surgery, the colostomy will drain bloody mucus. Fluids and electrolytes are infused intravenously until the patient's diet can gradually be resumed, beginning with liquids. Usually within 72 hours, passage of gas and stool through the stoma begins. Initially, the stool is liquid, gradually thickening as the patient begins to take solid foods. The patient is usually out of bed in eight to 24 hours after surgery and discharged in two to four days.

A colostomy pouch will generally have been placed on the patient's abdomen around the stoma during surgery. During the hospital stay, the patient and his or her caregivers will be educated on how to care for the colostomy. Determination of appropriate pouching supplies and a schedule of how often to change the pouch should be established. Regular assessment and meticulous care of the skin surrounding the stoma is important to maintain an adequate surface on which to attach the pouch. Some patients with colostomies are able to routinely irrigate the stoma, resulting in regulation of bowel function; rather than needing to wear a pouch, these patients may only need a dressing or cap over their stoma. Often, an enterostomal therapist will visit the patient in the hospital or at home after discharge to help the patient with stoma care.

Dietary counseling will be necessary for the patient to maintain normal bowel function and to avoid constipation, impaction, and other discomforts.

Risks

Potential complications of colostomy surgery include:

- excessive bleeding
- surgical wound infection
- thrombophlebitis (inflammation and blood clot to veins in the legs)
- pneumonia
- pulmonary embolism (blood clot or air bubble in the lungs' blood supply)

Psychological complications may result from colostomy surgery because of the fear of the perceived

General surgeons and colon and rectal surgeons perform colostomies as inpatient surgeries, under general anesthesia.

social stigma attached to wearing a colostomy bag. Patients may also be depressed and have feelings of low self-worth because of the change in their lifestyle and their appearance. Some patients may feel ugly and sexually unattractive and may worry that their spouse or significant other will no longer find them appealing. Counseling and education regarding surgery and the inherent lifestyle changes are often necessary.

Normal results

Complete healing is expected without complications. The period of time required for recovery from the surgery may vary depending on the patient's overall health prior to surgery and the patient's willingness to participate in stoma care. The colostomy patient without other medical complications should be able to resume all daily activities once recovered from the surgery. Adjustments in diet and daily personal care will need to be made.

Morbidity and mortality rates

Complications after colostomy surgery can occur. The doctor should be made aware of any of the following problems after surgery:

- increased pain, swelling, redness, drainage, or bleeding in the surgical area
- headache, muscle aches, dizziness, or fever
- increased abdominal pain or swelling, constipation, nausea or vomiting, or black, tarry stools

Stomal complications can also occur. They include:

- Death (necrosis) of stomal tissue. Caused by inadequate blood supply, this complication is usually visible 12–24 hours after the operation and may require additional surgery.
- Retraction (stoma is flush with the abdomen surface or has moved below it). Caused by insufficient stomal length, this complication may be managed by use of special pouching supplies. Elective revision of the stoma is also an option.

- Prolapse (stoma increases length above the surface of the abdomen). Most often this results from an overly large opening in the abdominal wall or inadequate fixation of the bowel to the abdominal wall. Surgical correction is required when blood supply is compromised.
- Stenosis (narrowing at the opening of the stoma). Often this is associated with infection around the stoma or scarring. Mild stenosis can be removed under local anesthesia; severe stenosis may require surgery for reshaping the stoma.
- Parastomal hernia (bowel causing bulge in the abdominal wall next to the stoma). This occurs due to placement of the stoma where the abdominal wall is weak or an overly large opening in the abdominal wall was made. The use of an ostomy support belt and special pouching supplies may be adequate. If severe, the defect in the abdominal wall should be repaired and the stoma moved to another location.

Mortality rates for colostomy patients vary according to the patient's general health upon admittance to the hospital. Even among higher risk patients, mortality is about 16%. This rate is greatly reduced (between 0.8% and 3.8%) when the colostomy is performed by a board-certified colon and rectal surgeon.

Alternatives

When a colostomy is deemed necessary, there are usually no alternatives to the surgery, though there can be alternatives in the type of surgery involved and adjuvant therapies related to the disease. For example, laparoscopic surgery is being used with many diseases of the intestinal tract, including initial cancers. For this surgery, the colon and rectal surgeon inserts a laparoscope (an instrument that has a tiny video camera attached) through a small incision in the abdomen. Other small incisions are made for the surgeon to insert laparoscopic instruments to use in creating the colostomy. This surgery often results in a shorter stay in the hospital, less postoperative pain, a quicker return to normal activities, and far less scarring. It is not recommended for patients who have had extensive prior abdominal surgery, large tumors, previous cancer, or serious heart problems.

Resources

BOOKS

Doughty, Dorothy. *Urinary and Fecal Incontinence*. St. Louis: Mosby-Year Book, Inc., 1991.

Hampton, Beverly, and Ruth Bryant. *Ostomies and Continent Diversions*. St. Louis: Mosby-Year Book, Inc., 1992.

Monahan, Frances. *Medical-Surgical Nursing*. Philadelphia: W. B. Saunders Co., 1998.

ORGANIZATIONS

United Ostomy Association, Inc. (UOA). 19772 MacArthur Blvd., Suite 200, Irvine, CA 92612-2405. (800) 826-0826. http://www.uoa.org.

Wound Ostomy and Continence Nurses Society. 2755 Bristol Street, Suite 110, Costa Mesa, CA 92626. (714) 476-0268. http://www.wocn.org.

OTHER

National Digestive Diseases Information Clearinghouse. *Ileostomy, Colostomy, and Ileoanal Reservoir Surgery*. (February 1, 2000): 1.

Janie F. Franz
Kathleen D. Wright, RN

Colporrhaphy

Definition

Colporrhaphy is the surgical repair of a defect in the vaginal wall, including a cystocele (when the bladder protrudes into the vagina) and a rectocele (when the rectum protrudes into the vagina).

Purpose

A prolapse occurs when an organ falls or sinks out of its normal anatomical place. The pelvic organs normally have tissue (muscle, ligaments, etc.) holding them in place. Certain factors, however, may cause those tissues to weaken, leading to prolapse of the organs. A cystocele is defined as the protrusion or

Colporrhaphy

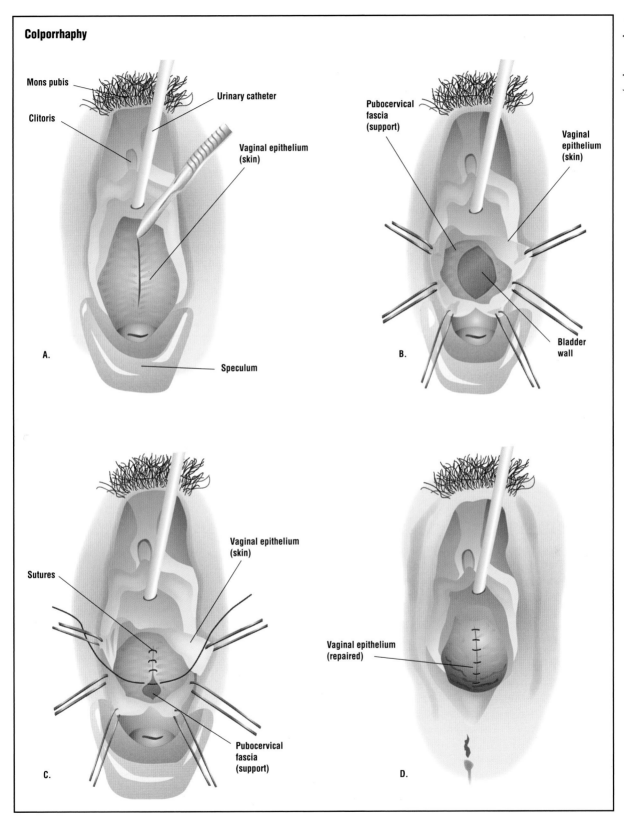

A.

- Mons pubis
- Clitoris
- Urinary catheter
- Vaginal epithelium (skin)
- Speculum

B.

- Pubocervical fascia (support)
- Vaginal epithelium (skin)
- Bladder wall

C.

- Sutures
- Vaginal epithelium (skin)
- Pubocervical fascia (support)

D.

- Vaginal epithelium (repaired)

In this anterior colporrhaphy, a speculum is used to hold open the vagina, and the cystocele is visualized (A). The wall of the vagina is cut open to reveal an opening in the supporting structures, or fascia (B). The defect is closed (C), and the vaginal skin is repaired (D). *(Illustration by GGS Information Services. Cengage Learning, Gale.)*

prolapse of the bladder into the vagina; a urethrocele is the prolapse of the urethra into the vagina. These are caused by a defect in the pubocervical fascia (fibrous tissue that separates the bladder and vagina). A rectocele occurs when the rectum prolapses into the vagina, caused by a defect in the rectovaginal fascia (fibrous tissue that separates the rectum and vagina). When a part of the small intestine prolapses into the vagina, it is called an enterocele. Uterine prolapse occurs when the uterus protrudes downward into the vagina.

Factors that are linked to pelvic organ prolapse include age, repeated childbirth, hormone deficiency, ongoing physical activity, and prior **hysterectomy**. Symptoms of pelvic organ prolapse include stress incontinence (inadvertent leakage of urine with physical activity), a vaginal bulge, painful sexual intercourse, back pain, and difficult urination or bowel movements.

Demographics

Approximately 50% of women report occasional urinary incontinence, with 10% reporting regular incontinence. This percentage increases with age; daily incontinence is experienced by 20% of women over the age of 75. According to a recent study, approximately 16% of women ages 45 to 55 experience mild pelvic organ prolapse, while only 3% experience prolapse severe enough to warrant surgical repair.

Description

Colporrhaphy may be performed on the anterior (front) and/or posterior (back) walls of the vagina. An anterior colporrhaphy treats a cystocele or urethrocele, while a posterior colporrhaphy treats a rectocele. Surgery is generally not performed unless the symptoms of the prolapse have begun to interfere with daily life.

The patient is first given general, regional, or **local anesthesia**. A speculum is inserted into the vagina to hold it open during the procedure. An incision is made into the vaginal skin and the defect in the underlying fascia is identified. The vaginal skin is separated from the fascia and the defect is folded over and sutured (stitched). Any excess vaginal skin is removed and the incision is closed with **stitches**.

Diagnosis/Preparation

Physical examination is most often used to diagnose prolapse of the pelvic organs. A speculum is inserted into the vagina, and the patient is asked to

strain or sit in an upright position. The physician then inspects the anterior, posterior, upper (apex), and side (lateral) walls of the vagina for prolapse or bulging. In some cases, a physical examination cannot sufficiently diagnose pelvic prolapse. For example, cystogram may be used to determine the extent of a cystocele; the bladder is filled by urinary catheter with contrast medium and then x-rayed.

The patient will be asked to refrain from eating or drinking after midnight on the day of the procedure. The physician may request that an enema be administered the night before the procedure if posterior colporrhaphy will be performed.

Aftercare

A Foley catheter may remain for one to two days after surgery. The patient will be given a liquid diet until normal bowel function returns. The patient will be instructed to avoid activities for several weeks that will cause strain on the surgical site, including lifting, coughing, long periods of standing, sneezing, straining with bowel movements, and sexual intercourse.

Risks

Risks of colporrhaphy include potential complications associated with anesthesia, infection, bleeding, injury to other pelvic structures, dyspareunia (painful intercourse), recurrent prolapse, and failure to correct the defect. A fistula is a rare complication of colporrhaphy in which an opening develops between the vagina and bladder or the vagina and rectum.

Normal results

A woman will usually be able to resume normal activities, including sexual intercourse, about four weeks after the procedure. After successful colporrhaphy, the symptoms associated with cystocele or rectocele will recede, although a separate procedure may be needed to treat stress incontinence. Anterior colporrhaphy is approximately 66% successful at restoring urinary continence.

Morbidity and mortality rates

There is approximately a 1% risk of serious complications associated with colporrhaphy; the procedure is generally viewed to be safe with a very low rate of overall complications.

Alternatives

Surgery is generally reserved for more severe cases of pelvic organ prolapse. Milder cases may be treated by a number of medical interventions. The physician may recommend that the patient do Kegel exercises, a series of contractions and relaxations of the muscles in the perineal area. These exercises are thought to strengthen the pelvic floor and may help prevent urinary incontinence. One study showed an decrease of 62% in the amount of urine leakage among women ages 35 to 75 who performed Kegel exercises regularly for 16 weeks.

A pessary, a device that is inserted into the vagina to help support the pelvic organs, may be recommended. Pessaries come in different shapes and sizes and must be fitted to the patient by a physician. Hormone replacement therapy may also be prescribed if the woman has gone through menopause; hormones may improve the quality of the supporting tissues in the pelvis.

Resources

PERIODICALS

Cespedes, R. Duane, Cindy A. Cross, and Edward J. McGuire. "Pelvic Prolapse: Diagnosing and Treating Cystoceles, Rectoceles, and Enteroceles." *Medscape Women's Health eJournal* 3, no. 4 (1998).

Viera, Anthony, and Margaret Larkins-Pettigrew. "Practice Use of the Pessary." *American Family Physician* 61 (May 1, 2000): 2719–26.

ORGANIZATIONS

American Academy of Family Physicians. 8880 Ward Parkway, Kansas City, MO 64114. (816) 333-9700. http://www.aafp.org.

American Board of Obstetrics and Gynecology. 2915 Vine Street, Dallas, TX 75204. (214) 871-1619. http://www.abog.org.

American Urological Association. 1120 North Charles Street, Baltimore, MD 21201. (410) 727-1100. http://www.auanet.org.

OTHER

"Cystocele (Fallen Bladder)." *National Kidney and Urologic Diseases Information Clearinghouse*, March 2002 [cited March 20, 2003]. http://www.niddk.nih.gov/health/urolog/summary/cystocel.

Jelovsek, Frederick R. "Cystocoele, Rectocoele, and Pelvic Support Surgery." *Society of Gynecologic Surgeons*, 2001 [cited March 20, 2003]. http://www.sgsonline.org/edpro002.html.

Miklos, John R., and Robert D. Moore. "Prolapse Treatment." *Atlanta Center for Laparoscopic Urogynecology*, 2002 [cited March 20, 2003]. http://www.urogynecologychannel.com/pro_treat.shtml.

Stendardo, Stef. "Urinary Incontinence: Assessment and Management in Family Practice." *American Academy of Family Physicians*, 2002 [cited March 20, 2003]. http://www.aafp.org/PreBuilt/videocme/urinary_mono.pdf.

"Surgical Treatment of Genuine Stress Incontinence." *Royal College of Obstetricians and Gynaecologists*, August 2002 [cited March 20, 2003]. http://www.rcog.org.uk/resources/worddocs/incontinencedraft.doc.

Stephanie Dionne Sherk

Colposcopy

Definition

Colposcopy is a procedure that allows a physician to examine a woman's cervix and vagina using a special microscope called a colposcope. Colposcopy is used to check for precancerous or abnormal areas.

Purpose

Colposcopy is used to identify or rule out the existence of any precancerous conditions in the cervical tissue. If a Papanicolaou (Pap) test shows abnormal cell growth, colposcopy is usually the first follow-up test performed. The physician will attempt to find the area that produced the abnormal cells and remove a sample of it for further study (biopsy) and diagnosis.

Colposcopy may also be performed if the cervix looks abnormal during a routine examination. It may be suggested for women with genital warts and for diethylstilbestrol (DES) daughters (women whose mothers took the anti-miscarriage drug DES when pregnant with them). Colposcopy is used in the emergency department to examine victims of sexual assault

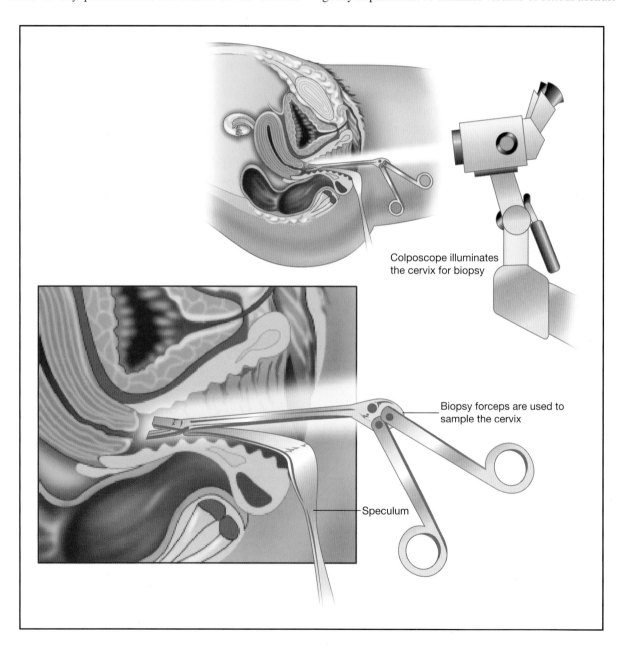

Colposcope illuminates the cervix for biopsy

Biopsy forceps are used to sample the cervix

Speculum

(Illustration by Electronic Illustrators Group.)

and abuse and document any physical evidence of vaginal injury.

Demographics

Cervical cancer affects millions of women worldwide. In the United States, the routine use of Pap tests has substantially decreased the rate of this cancer. With the introduction of a vaccine against the family of viruses associated with cervical cancer, the rate in the developed world is expected to continue to fall. Cervical cancer continues to be a major health problem for women in the developing world. Even in the United States, it is estimated that about one-third of women fail to follow up with colposcopy after an abnormal Pap test. Minority women, teenagers, and those of low socioeconomic status are the least likely to follow up.

Description

Colposcopy is usually performed in a physician's office and is similar to a regular gynecologic exam. An instrument called a speculum is inserted to hold the vagina open, and the gynecologist looks at the cervix and vagina using a colposcope, a low-power microscope designed to magnify the cervix 10–40 times its normal size. Most colposcopes are connected to a video monitor that displays the area of interest. Photographs are taken during the examination to document abnormal areas.

The cervix and vagina are swabbed with dilute acetic acid (vinegar). The solution highlights abnormal areas by turning them white (instead of a normal pink color). Abnormal areas can also be identified by looking for a characteristic pattern made by abnormal blood vessels.

If any abnormal areas are seen, the doctor takes a biopsy of the tissue, a common procedure that takes about 15 minutes. Several samples might be taken, depending on the size of the abnormal area. A biopsy may cause temporary discomfort and cramping, which usually go away within a few minutes. If the abnormal area appears to extend inside the cervical canal, a scraping of the canal may also be done. The biopsy results are usually available within a week.

If the tissue sample indicates abnormal growth (dysplasia) or is precancerous, and if the entire abnormal area can be seen, the doctor may destroy the tissue using one of several procedures, including ones that use high heat (diathermy), extreme cold (cryosurgery), or lasers. Another procedure, called loop electrosurgical excision (LEEP), uses low-voltage, high-frequency radio waves to excise tissue. If any of the abnormal tissue is within the cervical canal, a **cone biopsy**

KEY TERMS

Biopsy—Removal of a sample of abnormal tissue for more extensive examination under a microscope.

Cervix—Narrow, lower end of the uterus forming the opening to the vagina.

Cryosurgery—Freezing and destroying abnormal cells.

Diathermy—Also called electrocautery, this is a procedure that heats and destroys abnormal cells.

Diethylstilbestrol (DES)—A synthetic form of estrogen that was widely prescribed to women from 1940 to 1970 to prevent complications during pregnancy, and linked to several serious birth defects and disorders of the reproductive system in daughters of women who took DES.

Dysplasia—Abnormal cellular changes that may become cancerous.

Human papillomavirus (HPV)—A family of viruses that cause common warts of the hands and feet, as well as lesions in the genital and vaginal area. More than 50 types of HPV have been identified, some of which are linked to cancerous and precancerous conditions, including cancer of the cervix. A vaccine is now available against some of these viruses.

Loop electrosurgical excision (LEEP)—A procedure that can help diagnose and treat cervical abnormalities using a thin wire loop that emits a low-voltage high-frequency radio wave that can excise tissue.

Monsel's solution—A solution used to stop bleeding.

Pap test—The common term for the Papanicolaou test, a simple smear method of removing cervical cells to screen for abnormalities that indicate cancer or a precancerous condition.

Speculum—A retractor used to separate the walls of the vagina to make visual examination easier.

(removal of a conical section of the cervix for inspection) will be needed.

Diagnosis/Preparation

Women who are pregnant or who suspect that they are pregnant must tell their doctor before the procedure begins. Pregnant women may undergo colposcopy if they have an abnormal Pap test; special precautions, however, must be taken during biopsy of the cervix. Patients who are taking blood-thinning

Colposcopy may be performed by a gynecologist or other qualified health care provider in an outpatient setting. A gynecologist specializes in the areas of women's general health, pregnancy, labor and childbirth, prenatal testing, and genetics. In cases of sexual assault, a nurse practitioner, or registered nurse may perform the procedure. If a biopsy is performed, a pathologist examines the tissue samples under a powerful microscope in the laboratory and sends the results to the health care provider who, in turn, informs the patient of the results.

medications such as warfarin (Coumadin) should tell their doctor before the procedure.

Patients should be instructed not to douche, use tampons, or have sexual intercourse for 24 hours before colposcopy. Patients should empty their bladder and bowels before colposcopy for comfort. Colposcopy does not require any anesthetic medication because pain is minimal. If a biopsy is done, there may be mild cramps or a sharp pinching when the tissue is removed. To lessen this pain, the doctor may recommend ibuprofen (Motrin, Advil) taken the night before and the morning of the procedure (no later than 30 minutes before the appointment). Patients who are pregnant or allergic to **aspirin** or ibuprofen can instead take **acetaminophen** (Tylenol).

Aftercare

If a biopsy was done, there may be a dark vaginal discharge afterwards. After the sample is removed, the doctor applies Monsel's solution to the area to stop the bleeding. When this mixes with blood, it creates a black fluid that looks like coffee grounds. This fluid may be present for a several days after the procedure. It is also normal to have some blood spotting after colposcopy. Pain-relieving medication can be taken to lessen any post-procedural cramping.

Patients should not use tampons, douche, or have sex for at least a week after the procedure or until the doctor says it is safe because of the risk of infection.

Risks

Colposcopy is a very safe procedure. Patients may have bleeding or infection after biopsy. Bleeding is usually controlled with a topical medication prescribed

- Why is colposcopy recommended in my case?
- Will a biopsy be performed?
- How long will the procedure take?
- When will I find out the results?
- What will happen if the results are positive for cancer or another abnormality?

by the physician or health care provider. If colposcopy is performed on a pregnant patient, there is a risk of premature labor.

A patient should call her doctor right away if she notices any of the following symptoms:

- heavy vaginal bleeding (more than one sanitary pad an hour);
- fever, chills, or an unpleasant vaginal odor; or
- lower abdominal pain.

Normal results

If visual inspection shows that the surface of the cervix is smooth and pink, this is considered normal. Areas that look abnormal may actually be normal variations; a biopsy will indicate whether the tissue is normal or abnormal.

Abnormal conditions that can be detected using colposcopy and biopsy include precancerous tissue changes (cervical dysplasia), cancer, and cervical warts caused by human papillomavirus.

Morbidity and mortality rates

Complications associated with colposcopy are extremely rare. There is a risk that the procedure will miss precancerous or cancerous tissues and thus prolong treatment until the cancer has become advanced. The American Cancer Society estimated that 11,150 new cases of cervical cancer were diagnosed in 2007 and 3,670 deaths could be attributed to the disease.

Alternatives

While the Pap test is an effective screening test for abnormal cell growth of the cervix, it is an inadequate diagnostic alternative to colposcopy because of the potential for false negative results (10–50%). In some instances, a repeat Pap test may be recommended before performing colposcopy (e.g., in the case of inflammation or no previous abnormal Pap test).

Resources

OTHER

"Colposcopy (Position Paper)." *American Academy of Family Physicians.* 2004 [cited February 12, 2008]. http://www.aafp.org/online/en/home/policy/policies/c/colposcopypositionpaper.html.

"Colposcopy." *MedlinePlus.* [cited February 12, 2008]. http://www.nlm.nih.gov/medlineplus/tutorials/colposcopy/htm/index.htm.

Garcia, Agustin A. "Cervical Cancer." *eMedicine.com.* December 12, 2007 [cited February 12, 2008]. http://www.emedicine.com/med/topic324.htm.

Pattan, Charles, Alissa Zuellig, Bophal Hong, Shironda Stewart, and Michael P. Grossman. "Colposcopy." *eMedicine.com.* July 22, 2005 [cited February 12, 2008]. http://www.emedicine.com/med/topic3298.htm.

ORGANIZATIONS

American College of Obstetricians and Gynecologists, 409 12th St., SW, P.O. Box 96920, Washington, DC, 20090-6920, (202) 638-5577, http://www.acog.org.

American Society for Colposcopy and Cervical Pathology, 152 West Washington Street, Hagerstown, MD, 21740, (301) 733-3640, (800) 787-7227, http://www.asccp.org.

Association of Women's Health, Obstetric, and Neonatal Nurses, 2000 L St., NW, Suite 740, Washington, DC, 20036, (202) 261-2400, (800) 673-8499, http://www.awhonn.org.

DES Action USA, 158 S. Stanwood Rd., Columbus, OH, 43209, (800) 337-9288, http://www.desaction.org.

Society of Gynecologic Oncologists, 230 West Monroe Street, Suite 710, Chicago, IL, 60606, (312) 235-4060, http://www.sgo.org.

Jennifer E. Sisk, M.A.
Stephanie Dionne Sherk
Tish Davidson, A.M.

Colpotomy

Definition

A colpotomy, also known as a vaginotomy, is a procedure by which an incision is made in the vagina.

Purpose

A colpotomy is performed either to visualize pelvic structures or to perform surgery on the fallopian tubes or ovaries.

Role of colpotomy in gynecologic surgery

Several gynecologic surgery protocols require a colpotomy as part of the overall surgical procedure. It is performed whenever the surgeon needs to access the vagina. Several of these surgeries include:

- Tubal sterilization. Sterilization is a procedure that can be performed using either abdominal or vaginal procedures. When a vaginal procedure is selected by the surgeon, he performs a colpotomy and may also insert a culdoscope to locate the tubes (culdoscopy), and close them off.

- Removal of myomas. Myomas are fibroid tumors of the muscle tissue of the uterus and they are sometimes removed vaginally by colpotomy.

- Removal of pelvic cysts and masses. In one treatment variant, patients may undergo a laparoscopy followed by a colpotomy for the vaginal extraction of the pelvic cyst or mass.

- Hysterectomy. One technique used to surgically remove the uterus combines three steps, an initial laparoscopic stage, followed by a vaginal stage, and a final laparoscopic stage. The colpotomy is performed during the second step to deliver the uterus into the vagina.

- Dysmenorrhea. Separation of the uterosacral ligaments via colpotomy is an approach that has been used for the relief of dysmenorrhea (painful menstruation).

- Complications in pregnancy and childbirth. Colpotomy may be used in the management of difficult pregnancies and childbirths.

Demographics

According to Professor V. Base-Smith at the University of Cincinnati College of Nursing, removal of the uterus is the second most commonly performed surgical procedure in the United States after cesarean delivery. Analysis of the demographics show that:

- 650,000 hysterectomies are performed annually, expected to reach approximately 834,000 by 2005.

- 6.1–8.6 per 1,000 women undergo hysterectomy per year.

- In the United States, the Northeast has the lowest hysterectomy rate, while the South has the highest rate.

- African-American women experience hysterectomy more frequently than European-American women.

The ratio of abdominal to vaginally performed hysterectomies is three to one, meaning that colpotomy is performed in one out of four **hysterectomy** procedures.

Female sterilization is a common contraception method. About 20,000 female sterilizations are carried out each year in Canada and nearly 10% of North

KEY TERMS

Anesthesia—A combination of drugs administered by a variety of techniques by trained professionals that provide sedation, amnesia, analgesia, and immobility adequate for the accomplishment of the surgical procedure with minimal discomfort, and without injury, to the patient.

Antiseptic—Substance preventing or stopping the growth of microorganisms.

Cul-de-sac—The closed end of a pouch.

Culdoscopy—Procedure by which a surgeon performs a colpotomy and inserts a culdoscope, an instrument with a light on the end, through the incision.

Culdocentesis—Removal of material from the pouch of Douglas, a deep peritoneal recess between the uterus and the upper vaginal wall, by means of puncture of the vaginal wall.

Cyst—A closed sac having a distinct membrane and developing abnormally in a body cavity or structure.

Dysmenorrhea—Painful menstruation.

Fallopian tubes—The pair of anatomical tubes that carry the egg from the ovary to the uterus.

Forceps—An instrument for grasping, holding firmly, or exerting traction upon objects especially for delicate operations.

Hysterectomy—Surgical removal of the uterus.

Laparoscopy—Visual examination of the inside of the abdomen by means of a laparoscope or surgery performed using a laparoscope.

Myoma—A tumor consisting of muscle tissue.

Ovary—One of the two essential female reproductive organs that produce eggs and sex hormones.

Pelvic—Located near the pelvis, the skeletal structure comprised of four bones that encloses the pelvic cavity.

Sterilization—To make sterile, meaning to deprive of the power of reproducing.

Uterus—The womb, an organ in females for containing and nourishing the young during development before to birth.

Vagina—A canal in the female body that leads from the cervix to the external orifice opening to the outside of the body.

Vulva—The external parts of the female genital organs that include the mons pubis, labia majora, labia minora, clitoris, vestibule of the vagina, bulb of the vestibule, and Bartholin's glands.

American women 30 years or older have been sterilized in a procedure that involved colpotomy.

Description

The patient is placed in a supine position on the operating table with her legs in stirrups and the incision site is prepared. An antiseptic solution, such as chlorhexidine, is applied to the skin using highly disinfected forceps and gauze swabs. The patient is covered with surgical drapes with the window positioned directly over the incision site. Throughout the procedure, the **vital signs** of the patient are monitored (blood pressure, pulse, respiratory rate) as well as her level of consciousness and blood loss. **Pain management** depends on the surgery that requires the colpotomy, and may involve local, regional, or **general anesthesia**. The incision is only made as large as necessary for the requirements of the overall surgery.

For example, when a decision has been made to remove a myoma by colpotomy, the procedure may proceed as follows:

- A small myoma screw is inserted into the myoma and a grasper with locking mechanism is placed on the lower edge of the wound.

- The myoma is directed toward the cul-de-sac using the myoma screw.

- A colpotomy is performed.

- The myoma is grasped and removed vaginally. During this part of the procedure, the surgeon examines whether the myoma extends into the uterine cavity.

- If it does, the uterus is guided to the colpotomy site. T-clamps are placed on the edges of the wounds and the fundus of the uterus is delivered, via the colpotomy incision, into the vagina.

- The uterus is sutured in three layers (endometrial, myometrial and serosal).

- The repaired uterus is returned to the abdominal cavity.

- The colpotomy incision is sutured.

Preparation

The procedure is explained to the patient within the broader context of the surgery that includes the colpotomy. Preoperative preparation includes whatever is required for the overall surgical procedure that will be performed.

Aftercare

Aftercare for colpotomy is associated with the overall surgery that required the colpotomy.

For example, if a colpotomy is performed for **tubal ligation** (female sterilization), the procedure takes only 15–30 minutes and women usually go home the same day. It may take a few days at home to recover. Sexual intercourse is usually postponed until the colpotomy incision is completely healed, and as advised by the doctor. The healing process usually requires several weeks and there are no visible scars. In the case of a colpotomy performed for myoma removal, aftercare is more elaborate with the patient's vital signs monitored in the **recovery room** until she regains consciousness.

Risks

Complications such as bleeding, infection, or reaction to the anesthetic, may occur as with any type of gynecological surgery.

Normal results

Colpotomy results are considered normal when the incision performed allows the surgeon to meet the goal of the overall surgical protocol.

Morbidity and mortality rates

Colpotomy morbidity rates are not reported. This is because the procedure represents one surgical process in an operation that involves other surgical peocedures. In the case of colpotomy performed in the context of tubal sterilization, morbidity with tubal ligation is 5%; mortality is less than four in 100,000 cases.

As for hysterectomies, a higher morbidity and mortality rate is associated with abdominal than with vaginal hysterectomy surgery, the latter procedure being the only one to involve colpotomy.

Alternatives

In the case of colpotomy used for tubal ligation procedures, **laparoscopy** or laparotomy procedures are currently the preferred technique, since fewer and fewer U.S. surgeons are trained to use colpotomy as an approach for sterilization.

Resources

BOOKS

Masterson, B. J. *Manual of Gynecologic Surgery (Comprehensive Manuals of Surgical Specialties).* New York: Springer Verlag, 1986.

Reiffenstahl, G., W. Platzer, and P.-G. Knapstein. *Vaginal Operations.* Philadelphia: Lippincott, Williams & Wilkins, 1996.

Stewart, E. G., and P. Spencer. *The V Book: A Doctor's Guide to Complete Vulvovaginal Health.* New York: Bantam Doubleday Dell Publishers, 2002.

PERIODICALS

Diakomanolis, E., A. Rodolakis, Z. Boulgaris, G. Blachos, and S. Michalas. "Treatment of Vaginal Intraepithelial Neoplasia With Laser Ablation and Upper Vaginectomy." *Gynecologic and Obstetric Investigation* 54 (2002): 17-20, 419-427.

Ghezzi, F., L. Raio, M. D. Mueller, T. Gyr, M. Buttarelli, and M. Franchi. "Vaginal Extraction of Pelvic Masses Following Operative Laparoscopy." *Surgical Endoscopy* 16 (December 2002): 1691-1696.

Goodlin, R. C. "In Defense of the Anterior Vaginotomy." *Journal of Reproductive Medicine* 47 (August 2002): 693-694.

Gortzak-Uzan, L., A. Walfisch, Y. Gortzak, M. Katz, M. Mazor, and M. Hallak. "Accidental Vaginal Incision During Cesarean Section. A Report of Four Cases."

Journal of Reproductive Medicine 46 (November 2001): 1017-1020.

Ou, C. S., A. Harper, Y. H. Liu, and R. Rowbotham. "Laparoscopic Myomectomy Technique. Use of Colpotomy and the Harmonic Scalpel." *Journal of Reproductive Medicine* 47 (October 2002): 849-853.

ORGANIZATIONS

American Association of Gynecological Laparoscopists. 13021 East Florence Avenue, Sante Fe Springs, CA 90670-4505. (800) 554-2245. www.aagl.com/.

American College of Obstetricians and Gynecologists. 409 12th Street, SW, Washington, DC 20024-2188. E-mail: resources@acog.org. www.acog.org/.

American Society for Colposcopy and Cervical Pathology. 20 West Washington Street, Suite 1, Hagerstown, MD 21740. (301) 733-3640. (800) 787-7227. www.asccp.org.

National Association for Women's Health. 300 W. Adams Street, Suite 328, Chicago, IL 60606-5101. (312) 786-1468. www.nawh.org/.

OTHER

"Culdocentesis and Colpotomy." *Managing Complications of Pregnancy and Childbirth: A Guide for Midwives and Doctors.* World Health Organization. [cited May 14, 2003]. http://www.who.int/reproductive-health/impac/Procedures/Culdocentesis_P69_P70.html.

National Women's Health Information Center. U.S. Department of Health and Human Services. [cited May 14, 2003]. http://www.4woman.org/.

Monique Laberge, Ph.D.

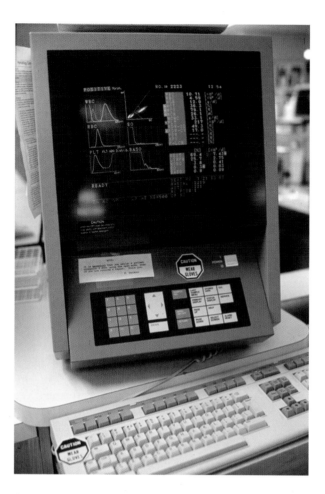

Computer monitor displaying a complete blood count with differential. *(Thomas Photography LLC / Alamy)*

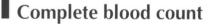

Complete blood count

Definition

A complete blood count (CBC) provides important information about the types and numbers of cells in the blood; in particular, information about red blood cells, white blood cells and platelets.

Purpose

The purpose of a CBC is to help physicians to diagnose conditions related to abnormalities in the blood such as infections and anemia.

Description

A complete blood count usually includes the following elements:

- Red blood cell count (also called RBC or erythrocyte count)

- Red blood cell indices - mean corpuscular volume (MCV, mean corpuscular hemoglobin (MCH) and mean corpuscular hemoglobin concentration (MCHC)

- Hemoglobin (also called Hgb)

- Hematocrit (also called HCT)

- White blood cell count (also called WBC or leukocyte count)

- Platelet count (also called thrombocyte count)

Red blood cells (erythrocytes) transport oxygen between the lungs and cells throughout the rest of the body. They also transport carbon dioxide back to the lungs so it can be exhaled. A low red cell count may be due to anemia and cells in the body may not be getting the oxygen that they need. A red blood cell count that is abnormally high may be due to an uncommon condition called polycythemia.

White blood cells (leukocytes) protect the body against infection. When an infection develops, white blood cells attack and destroy the pathogen (bacteria,

WHO PERFORMS THE PROCEDURE AND WHERE IS IT PERFORMED?

- A complete blood count is typically ordered by a family doctor, internist or surgeon but any physician may order one.
- A blood sample is usually obtained by a nurse, phlebotomist or medical technologist.
- The blood sample is tested or processed by a medical technologist.
- Results are usually reviewed, returned to the person being tested and interpreted by the physician initially ordering the complete blood count.

QUESTIONS TO ASK YOUR DOCTOR

- Why is a complete blood count needed?
- What do the results indicate for my health?
- What treatment options do I have?

virus, or other organism) causing it. White blood cells are larger than red blood cells but fewer in number. When a person has a bacterial infection, the number of white cells increases very quickly. The number of white blood cells is sometimes used to pinpoint an infection or to see how the body is reacting to cancer treatment.

Platelets (thrombocytes) are the smallest type of blood cell. They are essential to the process of blood clotting. When bleeding occurs, platelets swell, clump together, and form a sticky plug that helps to stop the bleeding. If the platelet count is too low, uncontrolled bleeding may occur. If the platelet count is too high, there is a chance of a blood clot forming in a blood vessel. Platelets may contribute to the process of hardening of the arteries (atherosclerosis).

There are three **red blood cell indices**: mean corpuscular volume (MCV), mean corpuscular hemoglobin (MCH), and mean corpuscular hemoglobin concentration (MCHC). They are measured by a laboratory instrument machine that calculates their values from other measurements in a complete blood count. The mean corpuscular volume reflects the average size of red blood cells. The mean corpuscular hemoglobin value reflects the quantity of hemoglobin in an average red blood cell. The mean corpuscular hemoglobin concentration reflects the concentration of hemoglobin in an average red blood cell. These numbers are used in diagnosing different types of anemia.

The hemoglobin value reflects the amount of hemoglobin in blood and is a good measure of the ability of a person's blood stream to carry oxygen throughout the body. A hemoglobin molecule comprises much of he volume of red blood cells. It carries oxygen and gives red blood cells their normal color.

The **hematocrit** value reflects the amount of space (volume) that red blood cells occupy in the blood. The value is given as a percentage of red blood cells in a volume of blood. For example, a hematocrit of 46 means that 46% of the blood's volume is comprised of red blood cells. Males and females have different normal hematocrit values.

Normal values for the elements of a complete blood count include the following:

- Red blood cell (erythrocyte) count: 4.2–5.9 million
- White blood cell (leukocyte) count: 4,300–10,800
- Platelet (thrombocyte) count: 150,000–400,000
- Mean corpuscular volume (MCV): 86–98
- Mean corpuscular hemoglobin (MCH): 27–32
- Mean corpuscular hemoglobin concentration (MCHC): 32–36%
- Hemoglobin (Hgb): 13–18 for men and 12–16 for women
- Hematocrit (HCT): 45–52% for men and 37–48% for women

A complete blood count can be ordered at any time.

Precautions

Precautions are generally not needed for a complete blood count.

At the time of drawing blood, the only precaution needed is to clean the venipuncture site with alcohol.

Side effects

The most common side effects of a complete blood count are minor bleeding (hematoma) or bruising at the site of venipuncture.

Interactions

There are no interactions for a complete blood count.

Resources

BOOKS

Fischbach, F. T. and M. B. Dunning. *A Manual of Laboratory and Diagnostic Tests.* 8th ed. Philadelphia: Lippincott Williams & Wilkins, 2008.

McGhee, M. *A Guide to Laboratory Investigations.* 5th ed. Oxford, UK: Radcliffe Publishing Ltd, 2008.

Price, C. P. *Evidence-Based Laboratory Medicine: Principles, Practice, and Outcomes.* 2nd ed. Washington, DC: AACC Press, 2007.

Scott, M.G., A. M. Gronowski, and C. S. Eby. *Tietz's Applied Laboratory Medicine.* 2nd ed. New York: Wiley-Liss, 2007.

Springhouse, A. M.. *Diagnostic Tests Made Incredibly Easy!* 2nd ed. Philadelphia: Lippincott Williams & Wilkins, 2008.

PERIODICALS

Amati, L., M. Chiloiro, E. Jirillo, and V. Covelli. "Early pathogenesis of atherosclerosis: the childhood obesity." *Current Pharmaceutical Design* 13, no. 36 (2007): 3696–3700.

James, T. R., H. L. Reid, and A. M. Mullings. "Are published standards for haematological indices in pregnancy applicable across populations: an evaluation in healthy pregnant Jamaican women." *BMC Pregnancy and Childbirth* 8, no. 1 (2008): 8–19.

Liao, S. C., M. F. Yang, and I. N. Lee. "Transforming laboratory data to improve medical care for patients with chronic kidney disease." *Journal of Nephrology* 21, no. 1 (2008): 74–80.

Lippi, G., A. Bassi, G. P. Solero, G. L. Salvagno, and G. C. Guidi. "Prevalence and type of preanalytical errors on inpatient samples referred for complete blood count." *Clinical Laboratory* 53, no. 9-12 (2007): 555–556.

ORGANIZATIONS

American Association for Clinical Chemistry. http://www.aacc.org/AACC/.

American Society for Clinical Laboratory Science. http://www.ascls.org/.

American Society of Clinical Pathologists. http://www.ascp.org/.

College of American Pathologists. http://www.cap.org/apps/cap.portal.

OTHER

American Clinical Laboratory Association. "Information about clinical chemistry." 2008 [cited February 24, 2008]. http://www.clinical-labs.org/.

Clinical Laboratory Management Association. "Information about clinical chemistry." 2008 [cited February 22, 2008]. http://www.clma.org/.

Lab Tests On Line. "Information about lab tests." 2008 [cited February 24, 2008]. http://www.labtestsonline.org/.

National Accreditation Agency for Clinical Laboratory Sciences. "Information about laboratory tests." 2008 [cited February 25, 2008]. http://www.naacls.org/.

L. Fleming Fallon, Jr, MD, DrPH

Computerized axial tomography *see* **CT scans**

Cone biopsy

Definition

A cone biopsy is a surgical procedure in which a cone-shaped tissue sample from the cervix is removed for examination. Also called cervical conization, a cone biopsy is done to diagnose cervical cancer or to remove cancerous or precancerous tissue.

Purpose

The cervix is the neck-shaped opening at the lower part of the uterus. The American Cancer Society estimated that in 2007, approximately 11,150 women would be diagnosed with cancer of the cervix, and 3,670 women would die of the disease. When cervical cancer is detected and treated in its early stages, however, the long-term rate of survival is almost 100%.

A cone biopsy is performed to diagnose cancer of the cervix or to detect precancerous changes. The procedure is often recommended if a Pap test indicates the presence of abnormal cells. In some cases, a cone biopsy may be used as a conservative treatment for cervical cancer for women who wish to avoid a **hysterectomy** (surgical removal of the uterus).

Demographics

The risk of developing cervical cancer increases with age through a woman's 20s and 30s; the risk

Cone biopsy

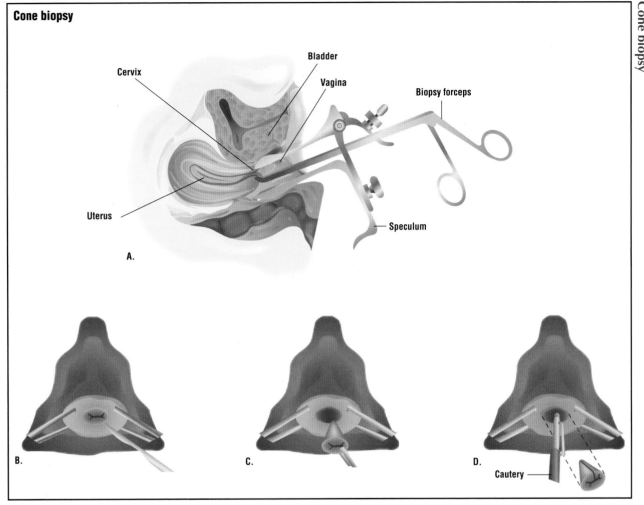

In a cone biopsy, the patient lies on her back, and a speculum is inserted into the vagina (A). The cervix is visualized, and a cone-shaped piece of the cervix is removed (B and C). A cauterizing tool is used to stop any bleeding (D). *(Illustration by GGS Information Services. Cengage Learning, Gale.)*

remains about the same for women over the age of 40. Minority women and women of low socioeconomic status have higher rates of cervical cancer and an increased mortality rate. According to the Centers for Disease Control and Prevention (CDC), African-American, Asian-American, and Hispanic women have a higher-than-average incidence of the disease, while African-American and Hispanic women have a higher rate of cervical cancer-related **death**.

Description

The procedure is performed with the patient lying on her back with her legs in stirrups. **General anesthesia** is commonly used, although regional (spinal or epidural) or **local anesthesia** may also be used. A speculum is inserted into the vagina to hold it open during surgery.

There are several different methods that may be used to perform a cone biopsy. Cold-knife conization is the removal of a cone-shaped wedge of tissue with a scalpel. The tissue may also be removed using a carbon dioxide laser, a procedure called laser conization. A loop electrosurgical excision procedure (LEEP) uses low-voltage, high-frequency radio waves to excise the tissue. Some surgeons choose to cover the open cervical tissue with flaps of tissue stitched into place.

The tissue sample will then be examined under a microscope for the presence of cancerous cells. If abnormal cells are found around the edge of the biopsy, then further surgery will be required to excise any remaining cancer. If there is evidence of invasive

WHO PERFORMS THE PROCEDURE AND WHERE IS IT PERFORMED?

A cone biopsy is usually performed by a gynecologist who specializes in the areas of women's general and reproductive health, pregnancy, labor and delivery, and prenatal testing. Tissue samples are analyzed by a pathologist who specializes in the diagnosis of diseases from microscopic analysis of cells and tissues. The procedure is generally done on an outpatient basis in a hospital or doctor's office.

cancer (i.e., the cancer has spread to surrounding tissues), then other treatments, such as more extensive surgery, chemotherapy, and/or radiation, may be recommended.

Diagnosis/Preparation

A number of tests may be performed prior to cone biopsy to determine if precancerous or cancerous cells exist. A Pap test involves scraping the cervix for a sample of cells and then staining and examining the cells for any abnormalities. **Colposcopy** is a procedure that allows a physician to examine a woman's cervix and vagina using a special microscope called a colposcope. A cervical biopsy involves the extraction of a smaller tissue sample and is less invasive than a cone biopsy. Based on the results of these tests, a cone biopsy may be indicated if moderate to severe cell abnormalities are found.

As cone biopsy is commonly performed under general anesthesia, the patient is usually instructed to refrain from eating and drinking after midnight on the day of surgery.

Aftercare

After the procedure, the patient may experience some cramping, discomfort, or mild to moderate bleeding. The biopsy site may take up to six weeks to completely heal. The patient will be instructed to avoid intercourse, tampons, and douches for at least three weeks following the procedure.

Risks

Bleeding during and after cone biopsy is the most common complication. Rarely, uncontrolled bleeding during the procedure may result in an emergency hysterectomy. Other potential complications include

reaction to the anesthesia, infection of the biopsy site, injury to the uterus or other tissues, cervical stenosis (when the cervical canal narrows or becomes closed), and failure to remove all cancerous tissue. If too much tissue is removed during a cone biopsy so that the internal opening of the cervix to the uterus (called the internal os) is affected, a woman may have difficulty carrying a pregnancy to term, increasing her risk of miscarriage or premature birth.

Normal results

Numerous studies have indicated that cone biopsy is successful in excising all cancerous tissue in 90% of patients with cervical cancer.

Morbidity and mortality rates

Between 2 and 8% of women who undergo a cone biopsy will experience bleeding for up to two weeks. One study found that cervical stenosis occurs at a rate of 3–8%, depending on the method of conization.

Alternatives

Cryotherapy (freezing and destroying of abnormal cells) or laser vaporization (using a laser to destroy abnormal cells) may be used to treat early-stage cancer. A hysterectomy may be necessary to remove more invasive cancer. In a subtotal hysterectomy, only the uterus is removed. In a radical hysterectomy, the uterus, cervix, ovaries, fallopian tubes, lymph nodes, and lymph channels are removed. The type of hysterectomy performed depends on how far the cancer has spread. In all cases, menstruation stops and a woman loses the ability to bear children.

Resources

BOOKS

Abeloff, M. D., et al. *Clinical Oncology.* 3rd ed. Philadelphia: Elsevier, 2004.

Gabbe, S. G., et al. *Obstetrics: Normal and Problem Pregnancies.* 5th ed. London: Churchill Livingstone, 2007.

Katz, V. L., et al. *Comprehensive Gynecology.* 5th ed. St. Louis: Mosby, 2007.

PERIODICALS

Brun, J. L., A. Youbi, and C. Hocke. "Complications, Sequellae and Outcome of Cervical Conizations: Evaluation of Three Surgical Techniques." *Journal of Gynecology and Obstetrics and Reproductive Biology* 31, no. 6 (January 10, 2002): 558–64.

ORGANIZATIONS

American Cancer Society. 1599 Clifton Road NE, Atlanta, GA 30329. (800) ACS-2345. http://www.cancer.org (accessed March 11, 2008).

American College of Obstetricians and Gynecologists. 409 12th St., S.W., PO Box 96920, Washington, D.C. 20090-6920. http://www.acog.org (accessed March 11, 2008).

OTHER

"All About Cervical Cancer: Overview." *American Cancer Society* 2003 [March 18, 2003]. http://www.cancer.org/docroot/CRI/CRI_2_1x.asp (accessed March 11, 2008).

National Cervical Cancer Coalition May 23, 2002 [cited March 18, 2003]. http://www.nccc-online.org/ (accessed March 11, 2008).

Nyirjesy, Istvan. "Conization of Cervix." *eMedicine* June 28, 2002 [cited March 18, 2003]. http://www.emedicine.com/med/topic3338.htm (accessed March 11, 2008).

Ries, L. A., et al., (eds). "SEER Cancer Statistics Review, 1973–1999." *National Cancer Institute* 2002 [cited March 18, 2003]. http://seer.cancer.gov/csr/1973_1999 (accessed March 11, 2008).

Stephanie Dionne Sherk
Rosalyn Carson-DeWitt, MD

Confidentiality *see* **Patient confidentiality**

Congenital glaucoma surgery *see* **Goniotomy**

Conization *see* **Cone biopsy**

Conscious sedation *see* **Sedation, conscious**

Continent ileostomy *see* **Ileoanal reservoir surgery**

Corneal keratoplasty *see* **Corneal transplantation**

Corneal transplantation

Definition

In corneal transplant, also known as keratoplasty, a patient's damaged cornea is replaced by the cornea from the eye of a human cadaver. This is the most common type of human **transplant surgery** and has the highest success rate. Eye banks acquire and store eyes from donors to supply the need for transplant corneas.

Purpose

Corneal transplant is used when vision is lost because the cornea has been damaged by disease or traumatic injury, and there are no other viable options. Some of the conditions that might require corneal transplant include the bulging outward of the cornea (keratoconus), a malfunction of the cornea's inner layer (Fuchs' dystrophy), and painful corneal swelling (pseudophakic bullous keratopathy). Other conditions that might make a corneal transplant necessary are tissue growth on the cornea (pterygium) and Stevens-Johnson syndrome, a skin disorder that can affect the eyes. Some of these conditions cause cloudiness of the cornea; others alter its natural curvature, which also can reduce vision quality.

Injury to the cornea can occur because of chemical burns, mechanical trauma, or infection by viruses, bacteria, fungi, or protozoa. The herpes virus produces one of the more common infections leading to corneal transplant.

Corneal transplants are used only when damage to the cornea is too severe to be treated with corrective lenses. Occasionally, corneal transplant is combined with other eye surgery, such as cataract surgery, to solve multiple eye problems with one procedure.

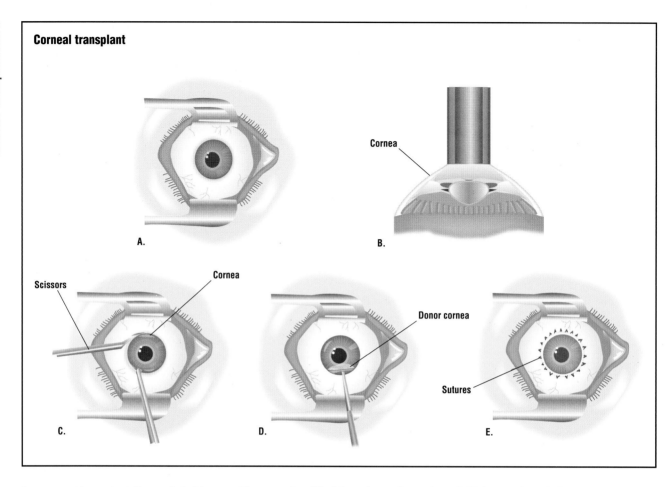

Corneal transplant

In a corneal transplant, the eye is held open with a speculum (A). A laser is used to make an initial cut in the existing cornea (B). The surgeon uses scissors to remove it (C), and a donor cornea is placed (D). It is stitched with very fine sutures (E). *(Illustration by GGS Information Services. Cengage Learning, Gale.)*

Demographics

The Eye Bank Association of America reported that corneal transplant recipients range in age from nine days to 103 years. In 2005, 31,952 corneal transplants were performed in the United States. The cost is usually covered in part by **Medicare** and health insurers, although the patient might be required to incur part of the cost for the procedure. All eye tissue is donated. It is illegal to buy or sell human tissue.

Description

The cornea is the transparent layer of tissue at the front of the eye. It is composed almost entirely of a special type of collagen. It normally contains no blood vessels, but because it contains nerve endings, cornea damage can be very painful.

In a corneal transplant, a disc of tissue is removed from the center of the eye and replaced by a corresponding disc from a donor eye. The circular incision is made using an instrument called a trephine, which resembles a cookie cutter. In one form of corneal transplant, penetrating keratoplasty (PK), the disc removed is the entire thickness of the cornea and so is the replacement disc.

The donor cornea is attached with extremely fine sutures. Surgery can be performed under **local anesthesia** that is confined to one area of the body, with the patient awake, or under **general anesthesia** that places the entire body of the patient in a state of unconsciousness. Corneal transplantation surgery takes about an hour to perform.

Over 90% of all corneal transplants in the United States are PK. In lamellar keratoplasty (LK), only the outer layer of the cornea is removed and replaced. LK has many advantages, including early suture removal and decreased infection risk. It is not as widely used as PK, however, because it is more time consuming and requires much greater technical ability by the surgeon.

KEY TERMS

Cadaver—The human body after death.

Cataract—A condition of cloudiness of the lens of the eye.

Cornea—The transparent layer of tissue at the very front of the eye.

Corticosteroids—Synthetic hormones widely used to fight inflammation.

Epikeratophakia—A procedure in which the donor cornea is attached directly onto the host cornea.

Epithelial cells—Cells that form a thin surface coating on the outside of a body structure.

Fibrous connective tissue—Dense tissue found in various parts of the body containing very few living cells.

Fuchs' dystrophy—A hereditary disease of the inner layer of the cornea.

Glaucoma—A vision defect caused when excessive fluid pressure within the eye damages the optic nerve.

Histocompatibility antigens—Proteins scattered throughout body tissues that are unique for almost every individual.

Keratoconus—An eye condition in which the cornea bulges outward, interfering with normal vision; usually both eyes are affected.

Pseudophakic bullous keratopathy (PBK)—Painful swelling of the cornea occasionally occurring after surgery to implant an artificial lens in place of a lens affected by cataract.

Retinal detachment—A serious vision disorder in which the light-detecting layer of cells inside the eye (retina) is separated from its normal support tissue and no longer functions properly.

Trephine—A small surgical instrument that is rotated to cut a circular incision.

A less common but related procedure called epikeratophakia involves suturing the donor cornea directly onto the surface of the existing host cornea. The only tissue removed from the host is the extremely thin epithelial cell layer on the outside of the host cornea. There is no permanent damage to the host cornea, and this procedure can be reversed. This procedure is mostly performed on children. In adults, the use of contact lenses can usually achieve the same goals.

Diagnosis/Preparation

Surgeons may discuss the need for corneal transplants after other viable options to remedy corneal trauma or disease have been discussed. No special preparation for corneal transplant is needed. Some ophthalmologists may request that the patient have a complete **physical examination** before surgery. Any active eye infection or eye inflammation usually needs to be brought under control before surgery. The patient may be asked to skip breakfast on the day of surgery.

Aftercare

Corneal transplant is often performed on an outpatient basis, although some patients need brief hospitalization after surgery. The patient will wear an eye patch at least overnight. An eye shield or glasses must be worn to protect the eye until the surgical wound has healed. The patient should avoid getting water in the eye while showering or bathing. Eye drops will be prescribed for the patient to use for several weeks after surgery. Some patients require medication for at least a year. These drops include **antibiotics** to prevent infection, as well as **corticosteroids** to reduce inflammation and prevent graft rejection.

For the first few days after surgery, the eye may feel scratchy and irritated. Vision will be somewhat blurry for as long as several months.

Sutures are often left in place for six months, and occasionally for as long as two years. Some surgeons may prescribe rigid contact lenses to reduce corneal astigmatism that follows corneal transplant.

Risks

Corneal transplants are highly successful, with over 90% of the operations in United States achieving restoration of sight. However, there is always some risk associated with any surgery. Complications that can occur include infection, glaucoma, retinal detachment, cataract formation, and rejection.

Graft rejection occurs in 5–30% of patients, a complication possible with any procedure involving tissue transplantation from another person (allograft). Allograft rejection results from a reaction of the patient's immune system to the donor tissue. Cell surface proteins called histocompatibility antigens trigger this reaction. These antigens are often associated with vascular tissue (blood vessels) within the graft tissue. Because the cornea normally contains no blood vessels, it experiences a very low rate of rejection. Generally, blood typing and tissue typing are not needed in

Corneal transplants are performed by an ophthalmologist, who is a corneal specialist and is expert at transplants and corneal diseases. Patients might be referred to a corneal specialist by their ophthalmologist or optometrist.

Surgery is performed in a hospital setting, usually on an outpatient basis. Some surgeons may also perform the procedure at an ambulatory surgery center designed for outpatient procedures. It is recommended that the patient have someone available to take him or her home, because patients are often groggy after the procedure.

corneal transplants, and no close match between donor and recipient is required. However, the Collaborative Corneal Transplantation Study found that patients at high risk for rejection could benefit from receiving corneas from a donor with a matching blood type.

Symptoms of rejection include persistent discomfort, sensitivity to light, redness, or a change in vision. If a rejection reaction does occur, it can usually be blocked by steroid treatment. Rejection reactions may become noticeable within weeks after surgery, but may not occur until 10 or even 20 years after the transplant. When full rejection does occur, the surgery will usually need to be repeated.

Although the cornea is not normally vascular, some corneal diseases cause vascularization (the growth of blood vessels) into the cornea. In patients with these conditions, careful testing of both donor and recipient is performed just as in transplantation of other organs and tissues such as hearts, kidneys, and bone marrow. In such patients, repeated surgery is sometimes necessary in order to achieve a successful transplant.

Normal results

Patients can expect restored vision after the healing process is complete. In some patients, this might take as long as a year. Patients with keratoconus, corneal scars, early bullous keratopathy, or corneal stromal dystrophies have the highest rate of transplant success. Corneal transplants for keratoconus patients have a success rate of more than 90%.

- Are there any alternatives that might restore my vision?
- What is the chance of rejection?
- How am I matched with the donor corneas?
- What is the screening process for donors?
- What physical restrictions will I have during the healing process?
- What are the chances of eye injury causing rejection?
- If the transplant is successful, how long will it be until vision is restored?
- Will I ever have to have another transplant?

Morbidity and mortality rates

While there is risk involved with any surgery, corneal transplants are relatively safe. In 2001, there was some concern about cornea donors transmitting Creutzfeldt-Jakob disease, a fatal neurological disease, after questions of infection arose in Europe. A study showed the risk of transmission in the United States was small, as was any infection risk from cornea donors. Currently, cornea donors are screened using medical standards of the Eye Bank Association of America. These guidelines restrict donors who died from unknown causes, or suffered from immune deficiency diseases, hepatitis, and other infectious diseases.

Transplant recipients may have to receive another transplant if the first is unsuccessful or if, after a number of years, the disease returns.

Alternatives

An increasingly popular alternative to corneal transplants is phototherapeutic keratectomy (PTK). This technique is now used to treat corneal scars and dystrophies, and some infections. Surgeons use an excimer laser and a computer to vaporize diseased tissue, leaving a smooth surface. New tissue begins growing immediately, and recovery takes only a few days. Patients must be carefully selected, however, and success is greatest if damage is restricted to the cornea's top layer.

Intrastromal corneal rings are implantable devices that could be used for some keratoconus patients. The rings are implanted and the procedure is reversible.

However, not much is known about long-term stability. Some companies also are developing synthetic corneas that are implanted using synthetic penetrating keratoplasty. This procedure may become more widely used for high-risk patients and those with severe chemical burns.

Resources

BOOKS

Boruchoff, S. Arthur, and Richard A. Thoft. "Keratoplasty: Lamellar and Penetrating." In *The Cornea*, edited by Gilbert Smolin and Richard A. Thoft. Boston: Little, Brown and Co., 1994.

Brightbill, Frederick S., ed. *Corneal Surgery*. St. Louis: Mosby, 1993.

Bruner, William E., Walter J. Stark, and A. Edward Maumenee. *Manual of Corneal Surgery*. New York: Churchill Livingstone, 1987.

Miller, Stephen J. H. *Parsons' Diseases of the Eye*, 18th ed. New York: Churchill Livingstone, 1990.

Vaughan, Daniel, ed. *General Ophthalmology*, 14th ed. Stamford: Appleton & Lange, 1995.

PERIODICALS

Kennedy, R. H., et al. "Eye Banking and Screening for Creutzfeldt-Jakob Disease." *Archives of Ophthalmology* 119 (May 2001): 721–6.

Watson, B. C., and G. L. White Jr. "Corneal Transplantation." *American Family Physician* 54 (Nov 1996): 1945–48.

ORGANIZATIONS

American Academy of Ophthalmology. 655 Beach Street, P.O. Box 7424, San Francisco, CA 94120-7424. http://www.aao.org (accessed March 11, 2008).

Eye Bank Association of America. 1015 Eighteenth Street NW, Suite 1010, Washington, D.C. 20036. (202) 775-4999. http://www.restoresight.org (accessed March 11, 2008).

OTHER

Asbell, Penny A., and Syed M. Ahmad. "New Techniques in Corneal Transplant." *Review of Ophthalmology*, May 15, 2002 [cited February 20, 2003]. http://www.revophth.com/index.asp?page = 1_94.htm (accessed March 11, 2008).

Cimberle, Michela. "New Type of Artificial Cornea Performs Better than Donor Grafts in High-Risk Cases." *Ocular Surgery News*, June 1, 2002 [cited February 23, 2003]. http://www.osnsupersite.com/view.asp?ID = 2346 (accessed March 11, 2008).

"Collaborative Corneal Transplantation Studies." *National Eye Institute*, October 21, 1999 [cited February 25, 2003]. http://www.nei.nih.gov/neitrials/static/study36.asp (accessed March 11, 2008).

"Corneal Transplantation." *Merck Manual of Diagnosis and Therapy*, [cited February 25, 2003]. http://www.merck.com/mmpe/index.html (accessed March 11, 2008).

"Facts About the Cornea and Corneal Disease." *National Eye Institute*, June 2001 [cited March 4, 2003]. http://www.nei.nih.gov/health/cornealdisease/ (accessed March 11, 2008).

"Cornea transplants: Restoring sight with donor tissue." *MayoClinic.com*. February 5, 2007. http://www.mayoclinic.com/health/cornea-transplant/EY00004 [accessed March 24, 2008].

Victor Leipzig, PhD
Mary Bekker
Fran Hodgkins

Coronary artery bypass graft surgery

Definition

Coronary artery bypass graft surgery (CABG) is a procedure in which one or more blocked coronary arteries are bypassed by a blood vessel graft to restore normal blood flow to the heart. These grafts usually come from the patient's own arteries and veins located in the leg, arm, or chest.

Purpose

Coronary artery bypass graft surgery, also called coronary artery bypass surgery and bypass operation, is performed to restore blood flow to the heart. This relieves chest pain and ischemia, improves the patient's quality of life, and, in some cases, prolongs the patient's life. The goals of the procedure are to relieve symptoms of coronary artery disease, enable the patient to resume a normal lifestyle, and lower the risk of a heart attack or other heart problems.

According to the American Heart Association, appropriate candidates for coronary artery bypass graft surgery include patients who:

- have blockages in at least two or three major coronary arteries, especially if the blockages are in arteries that feed the heart's left ventricle or are in the left anterior descending artery;

- have angina so severe that even mild exertion causes chest pain;

- have poor left ventricular function; and

- cannot tolerate percutaneous transluminal coronary angioplasty and do not respond well to drug therapy.

Angina—Also called angina pectoris, chest pain or discomfort that occurs when diseased blood vessels restrict blood flow to the heart.

Angiotensin-converting enzyme (ACE) inhibitor—A drug that lowers blood pressure by interfering with the breakdown of a protein-like substance involved in blood pressure regulation.

Aorta—The main artery that carries blood from the heart to the rest of the body. The aorta is the largest artery in the body.

Artery—A vessel that carries oxygen-rich blood to the body.

Atherectomy—A non-surgical technique for treating diseased arteries with a rotating device that cuts or shaves away obstructing material inside the artery.

Atrium (plural Atria)—The right or left upper chamber of the heart.

Beta blocker—An anti-hypertensive drug that limits the activity of epinephrine, a hormone that increases blood pressure.

Brachytherapy—The use of radiation during angioplasty to prevent the artery from narrowing again (a process called restenosis).

Calcium channel blocker—A drug that lowers blood pressure by regulating calcium-related electrical activity in the heart.

Cardiac rehabilitation—A structured program of education and activity offered by hospitals and other organizations.

Coronary artery disease—Also called atherosclerosis, it is a build-up of fatty matter and debris in the coronary artery wall that causes narrowing of the artery.

Echocardiogram—An imaging procedure used to create a picture of the heart's movement, valves, and chambers.

Graft—To implant living tissue surgically.

Homocysteine—An amino acid normally found in small amounts in the blood.

Ischemia—Decreased blood flow to an organ, usually caused by constriction or obstruction of an artery.

Lipoproteins—Substances that carry fat through the blood vessels for use or storage in other parts of the body.

Mammary artery—A chest wall artery that descends from the aorta and is commonly used for bypass grafts.

Radial artery—An artery located in the arm and used for bypass grafts.

Rotoblation—A non-surgical technique for treating diseased arteries.

Saphenous vein—A long vein in the thigh or calf commonly used for bypass grafts.

Stent—A device made of expandable, metal mesh that is placed (by using a balloon catheter) at the site of a narrowing artery; the stent stays in place to keep the artery open.

Sternum—Also called the breastbone, the sternum is the bone in the chest that is separated during open heart surgery.

Stress test—A test used to determine how the heart responds to stress.

Vein—A blood vessel that returns oxygen-depleted blood from various parts of the body to the heart.

Ventricle—A lower pumping chambers of the heart. There are two ventricles, right and left. The right ventricle pumps oxygen-poor blood to the lungs to be re-oxygenated. The left ventricle pumps oxygen-rich blood to the body.

Demographics

The American Heart Association estimated that in the United States in 2005, 469,000 coronary artery bypass procedures were performed on 261,000 individual patients. More than twice as many of these surgeries were performed on men than women. Fifteen thousand of these procedures were performed on people 15–44, 188,000 on people between ages 45 and 64, and the remainder on people age 65 and older.

Description

Coronary artery bypass graft surgery builds a detour around one or more blocked coronary arteries with a graft from a healthy vein or artery. The graft goes around the clogged artery (or arteries) to create new pathways for oxygen-rich blood to flow to the heart.

Procedure

After **general anesthesia** is administered, the surgeon removes the veins or prepares the arteries for grafting. The surgeon decides which grafts to use based on the location of the blockage, the amount of blockage, and the size of the patient's coronary arteries. If the saphenous vein is to be used for the graft, a series of incisions are made in the patient's thigh or calf. If the radial artery is to be used for the graft, incisions are made in the patient's forearm. More commonly, a segment of the internal mammary artery is used for the graft, and the incisions are made in the chest wall. The internal mammary arteries are often used because they have shown the best long-term results. The removal of veins or arteries for grafting does not deprive the area from which they are removed of adequate blood flow.

In traditional coronary artery bypass surgery, the surgeon makes an incision down the center of the patient's chest, cuts through the breastbone, and retracts the rib cage open to expose the heart. The patient is connected to a heart-lung bypass machine, also called a cardiopulmonary bypass pump, that takes over for the heart and lungs during the surgery. During this "on-pump" procedure, the heart-lung machine removes carbon dioxide from the blood and replaces it with oxygen. A tube is inserted into the aorta to carry the oxygenated blood from the bypass machine to the aorta for circulation to the body. The heart-lung machine allows heart contractions to be stopped, so the surgeon can operate on a still heart. Aortic clamps are used to restrict blood flow to the area of the heart where grafts will be placed so the heart is blood-free during the surgery. The clamps remain until the grafts are in place.

Some patients may be candidates for minimally invasive coronary artery bypass surgery or for off-pump bypass surgery. During minimally invasive surgery, smaller chest and graft removal incisions are used, promoting a quicker recovery and less risk of infection. Off-pump bypass surgery, also called beating heart surgery, is a surgical technique performed while the heart is still contracting (beating). The surgeon uses advanced equipment to stabilize portions of the heart and bypass the blocked artery while the rest of the heart keeps pumping and circulating blood through the body.

After the grafts are prepared, a small opening is made in the diseased coronary artery just below the blockage. Blood will be redirected through this opening once the graft is sewn in place. If a leg or arm vein is used, one end is connected to the coronary artery and the other to the aorta. If a mammary artery is used, one end is connected to the coronary artery while the other is already attached to the aorta and remains in place. The procedure is repeated on as many coronary

arteries as necessary. On average, three or four coronary arteries are bypassed during surgery. Blood flow is checked to assure the graft supplies adequate blood to the heart.

If the procedure was done "on-pump," electric shocks start the heart pumping again after the grafts have been completed. The heart-lung machine is turned off and the blood slowly returns to normal **body temperature**. After implanting pacing wires and inserting a chest tube to drain fluid, the surgeon closes the chest cavity. Sometimes a temporary pacemaker is attached to the pacing wires to regulate the heart rhythm until the patient's condition improves. After surgery, the patient is transferred to an **intensive care unit** (ICU) for close monitoring.

Diagnosis/Preparation

Diagnosis

The diagnosis of coronary artery disease is made after the patient's medical history is carefully reviewed, a physical exam is performed, and the patient's symptoms are evaluated. Tests used to diagnose coronary artery disease include:

- electrocardiogram;
- stress tests;
- cardiac catheterization;
- imaging tests such as a chest X-ray, echocardiography, or computed tomography (CT) scan; and
- blood tests to measure blood cholesterol, triglycerides, and other substances.

Preparation

The patient should quit smoking or using tobacco products before the surgery, and the patient needs to make the commitment to be a nonsmoker after the surgery. There are many **smoking cessation** programs available through hospital or community groups. A health care provider can provide more information about ways quit smoking.

Coronary artery bypass graft surgery should ideally be postponed for three months after a heart attack. Whenever possible, patients should be medically stable before the surgery. If the patient develops a cold, fever, or sore throat within a few days before the surgery, he or she should notify the surgeon's office.

During a preoperative appointment, usually scheduled one to two weeks before surgery, the patient will receive information about what to expect during the surgery and the recovery period. The patient will usually meet the cardiologist, anesthesiologist, nurse clinicians, and surgeon during this appointment or just before the procedure.

The evening before the surgery, the patient showers with antiseptic soap provided by the surgeon's office. After midnight, the patient should not eat or drink anything.

The patient is usually admitted to the hospital day the surgery is scheduled. The patient should bring a list of current medications, allergies, and appropriate medical records upon **admission to the hospital**.

Before the surgery, the patient is given a blood-thinning drug (usually heparin) that helps to prevent blood clots. A sedative is given the morning of surgery. The chest and the area from where the graft will be taken are shaved.

Coronary **angiography** will have been previously performed to show the surgeon where the arteries are blocked and where the grafts might best be positioned. Heart monitoring is initiated. The patient is given general anesthesia before the procedure.

The length of the procedure depends upon the number of arteries being bypassed, but it generally takes from three to five hours or sometimes longer.

Aftercare

Recovery in the hospital

The patient recovers in a surgical intensive care unit for one to two days after the surgery. The patient will be connected to chest and breathing tubes, a mechanical ventilator, a heart monitor, and other monitoring equipment. A urinary catheter will be in place to drain urine. The breathing tube and ventilator are usually removed about six hours after surgery, but the other tubes remain in place as long as the patient is in the intensive care unit.

Drugs are prescribed to control pain and infection and to prevent unwanted blood clotting. Daily doses of **aspirin** are started within 6–24 hours after the procedure.

The patient is closely monitored during the recovery period. **Vital signs** and other parameters such as heart sounds, oxygen, and carbon dioxide levels in arterial blood are checked frequently. The chest tube is checked to ensure that it is draining properly. The patient may be fed intravenously for the first day or two.

Chest physiotherapy is started after the ventilator and breathing tubes are removed. The therapy includes coughing, turning frequently, and taking deep breaths. Sometimes oxygen is delivered via a mask to help loosen and clear secretions from the lungs. Other exercises will be encouraged to improve the patient's circulation and prevent complications due to prolonged bed rest.

If there are no complications, the patient begins to resume a normal routine on the second day, including eating regular food, sitting up, and walking around a bit. Before being discharged from the hospital, the patient usually spends a few days under observation in a non-surgical unit. During this time, counseling is usually provided on eating right and starting a light **exercise** program to keep the heart healthy. The average hospital stay after coronary artery bypass graft surgery is five to seven days.

Recovery at home

INCISION AND SKIN CARE. The incision should be kept clean and dry. When the skin is healed, the incision should be washed with soapy water. The scar should not be bumped, scratched, or otherwise disturbed. Ointments, lotions, and **dressings** should not be applied to the incision unless specific instructions have been given to do so.

DISCOMFORT. While the incision scar heals, which takes one to two months, it may be sore. Itching, tightness, or numbness along the incision are common. Muscle or incision discomfort may occur in the chest during activity.

Swelling or aching may occur in the legs if the saphenous vein was used for the graft. Special support stockings may be needed to decrease leg swelling after surgery. While sitting, the patient should not cross the legs and the feet should be elevated. Walking daily, even if the legs are swollen, will help improve circulation and reduce swelling.

LIFESTYLE CHANGES. The patient needs to make several lifestyle changes after surgery, including:

- quitting smoking. Smoking causes damage to the bypass grafts and other blood vessels, increases the patient's blood pressure and heart rate, and decreases the amount of oxygen available in the blood.
- managing weight. Maintaining a healthy weight, by watching portion sizes and exercising, is important. Being overweight increases the work of the heart.
- participating in an exercise program. The exercise program is usually tailored for the patient, who will be encouraged to participate in a cardiac rehabilitation program supervised by exercise professionals.
- making dietary changes. Patients should eat a lot of fruits, vegetables, whole grains, and non-fat or low-fat dairy products, and reduce fat intake to less than 30% of all calories.

• taking medications as prescribed. Aspirin and other heart medications may be prescribed, and the patient may need to take these medications for life.

• following up with health care providers. The patient must schedule follow-up visits to determine how effective the surgery was, to confirm that progressive exercise is safe, and to monitor his or her recovery and control risk factors.

Risks

Coronary artery bypass graft surgery is major surgery and patients may experience any of the normal complications associated with major surgery and anesthesia, such as the risk of bleeding, pneumonia, or infection. Other possible complications include:

• graft closure or blockage;
• development of blockages in other arteries;
• damage to the aorta;
• long-term development of atherosclerotic disease of saphenous vein grafts;
• abnormal heart rhythms;
• high or low blood pressure;
• recurrence of angina;
• blood clots that can lead to a stroke or heart attack;
• kidney failure;
• depression or severe mood swings; and
• possible short-term memory loss, difficulty thinking clearly, and problems concentrating for long periods (these effects generally subside within six months after surgery).

There is a higher risk for complications in patients who:

• are heavy smokers;
• have a history of lung, kidney, or metabolic diseases;
• have diabetes;
• have had a recent heart attack; or
• have a history of angina, ventricular arrhythmias, congestive heart failure, cerebrovascular disease, or mitral regurgitation.

Normal results

Full recovery from coronary artery bypass graft surgery takes two to three months and is a gradual process. Upon release from the hospital, the patient will feel weak because of the extended bed rest in the hospital. Within a few weeks, the patient should begin to feel stronger.

Most patients are able to drive in three to eight weeks, after receiving approval from their physician.

Sexual activity can generally be resumed in three to four weeks, depending on the patient's rate of recovery.

It takes about six to eight weeks for the sternum to heal. During this time, the patient should not perform activities that cause pressure or weight on the breastbone or tension on the arms and chest. Pushing and pulling heavy objects (as in mowing the lawn) should be avoided and lifting objects more than 20 lbs (9 kg) is not permitted. The patient should not hold his or her arms above shoulder level for a long period, such as when doing household chores. The patient should try not to stand in one place for longer than 15 minutes. Stair climbing is permitted unless other instructions have been given. Within four to six weeks, people with sedentary office jobs can return to work. People with physical jobs, such as construction work or jobs requiring heavy lifting, must wait longer (up to 12 weeks) or may have to change careers.

About 90% of patients experience significant improvements after coronary artery bypass graft surgery. Patients experience full relief from chest pain and resume their normal activities in about 70% of the cases; the remaining 20% experience partial relief.

Coronary artery bypass surgery does not prevent coronary artery disease from recurring. For most people, the graft remains open for about 10–15 years. Therefore, lifestyle changes are strongly recommended and medications are prescribed to reduce the risk for the return of coronary artery disease. About 40% of patients have a new blockage within 10 years after surgery and require a second bypass, change in medication, or an interventional procedure.

Morbidity and mortality rates

The risk of **death** while in the hospital during and after coronary artery bypass graft surgery is 2–1%, although the rate varies among individual hospitals and surgeons. In 5–10% of coronary artery bypass graft surgeries, the bypass graft stops supplying blood to the bypassed artery within one year. Younger people who are healthy except for the heart disease achieve good results with bypass surgery. Patients who have poorer results from coronary artery bypass graft surgery include those over the age of 70, those who have poor left ventricular function, are undergoing a repeat surgery or other procedures concurrently, and those who continue smoking, do not treat high cholesterol or other coronary risk factors, or have another debilitating disease.

Over the long term, symptoms recur in only about 3–4% of patients per year. Five years after coronary artery bypass graft surgery, survival expectancy is

The surgery team for coronary artery bypass graft surgery includes the cardiovascular surgeon, assisting surgeons, a cardiovascular anesthesiologist, a perfusion technologist (who operates the heart-lung machine), and specially trained nurses. The surgery is performed in a hospital.

90%, at 10 years it is about 85%, at 15 years it is about 55%, and at 20 years it is about 40%.

Angina recurs in about 40% of patients after 10 years. In most cases, it is less severe than before the surgery and can be controlled with drug therapy. In patients who have had vein grafts, 40% of the grafts are severely obstructed 10 years after the procedure. Repeat coronary artery bypass graft surgery may be necessary, and is usually less successful than the first surgery.

Alternatives

All patients with coronary artery disease can help improve their condition by making lifestyle changes such as quitting smoking, losing weight if they are overweight, eating healthy foods, reducing blood cholesterol, exercising regularly, and controlling diabetes and high blood pressure.

All patients with coronary artery disease should be prescribed medications to treat their condition. Antiplatelet medications such as aspirin or clopidogrel (Plavix) are usually recommended. Other medications used to treat angina may include beta blockers, nitrates, and angiotensin-converting enzyme (ACE) inhibitors. Medications may also be prescribed to lower lipoprotein levels, since elevated lipoprotein levels have been associated with an increased risk of cardiovascular problems.

Treatment with vitamin E is not recommended because it does not lower the rate of cardiovascular events in people with coronary artery disease. Antioxidants such as vitamin C and beta-carotene show some signs of helping reduce coronary artery disease, but not enough rigorously documented information about their effects is available and they are not recommended for routine use. Treatment with folic acid and vitamins B_6 and B_{12} lowers homocysteine levels (reducing the risk for cardiovascular problems), but more studies are needed to determine if lowered homocysteine

QUESTIONS TO ASK THE DOCTOR

- Why is this surgery being performed?
- Am I a candidate for minimally invasive coronary artery bypass surgery?
- Which technique will be used during the surgery, the "on-pump" or "off-pump" technique?
- Who will be performing the surgery? How many years of experience does this surgeon have? How many other coronary artery bypass graft surgeries has this surgeon performed?
- Should I take my medications the day of the surgery?
- How long will I have to stay in the hospital after the surgery?
- After I go home from the hospital, how long will it take me to recover from surgery?
- What should I do if I experience chest discomfort or other symptoms similar to those I felt before surgery?
- What types of symptoms should I report to my doctor?
- How should I care for my incision?
- What types of medications will I have to take after surgery?
- When will I be able to resume my normal activities?
- If I have had the surgery once, can I have it again to correct future blockages?
- Are there any medications, foods, or activities I should avoid to prevent my symptoms from recurring?
- What lifestyle changes (including diet, weight management, exercise, and activity changes) are recommended after the procedure to improve my heart health?
- How often do I need to see my doctor for follow-up visits after the surgery?

levels correlate with a reduced rate of cardiovascular problems in treated patients.

Less invasive, nonsurgical interventional procedures, such as balloon **angioplasty**, stent placement, rotoblation, atherectomy, or brachytherapy, can be performed to open a blocked artery. These procedures may be the appropriate treatment for some patients before coronary artery bypass graft surgery is considered.

Enhanced external counterpulsation (EECP) may be a treatment option for patients who are not candidates for interventional procedures or coronary artery bypass graft surgery. During EECP, a set of cuffs is wrapped around the patient's calves, thighs, and buttocks. These cuffs gently but firmly compress the blood vessels in the lower limbs to increase blood flow to the heart. The inflation and deflation of the cuffs are electronically synchronized with the heartbeat and blood pressure using **electrocardiography** and blood pressure monitors. EECP may encourage blood vessels to open small channels to eventually bypass blocked vessels and improve blood flow to the heart. Not all patients are candidates for this procedure, and treatments, lasting one to two hours, must be repeated about five times a week for up to seven weeks.

Resources

BOOKS

Lichtenberg, Maggie. *The Open Heart Companion: Preparation and Guidance for Open-Heart Surgery Recovery.* Santa Fe, NM: Open Heart Publishing, 2006.

Sheridan, Brett C. *So You're Having Heart Bypass Surgery.* Hoboken, NJ: John Wiley, 2003.

OTHER

"Coronary Artery Bypass Surgery." *Medline Plus.* January 24, 2008 [cited January 29, 2008]. http://www.nlm.nih.gov/medlineplus/coronaryarterybypasssurgery.html.

MyHeartCentral.com. [cited March 16, 2008]. http://www.healthcentral.com/heart-disease/.

Your Total Health: Heart Health. http://yourtotalhealth.ivillage.com/heart-health.

ORGANIZATIONS

American College of Cardiology, Heart House2400 N Street, NW, Washington, DC, 20037, (800) 253-4636, http://www.acc.org.

American Heart Association, 7272 Greenville Ave., Dallas, TX, 75231, (800) 242-8721, http://www.americanheart.org.

The Cleveland Clinic Heart & Vascular Institute, 9500 Euclid Avenue, F25, Cleveland, OH, 44195, (866) 289-6911, http://www.clevelandclinic.org/heartcenter.

National Heart, Lung, and Blood Institute, P.O. Box 30105, Bethesda, MD, 20824-0105, (301) 592-8573, http://www.nhlbi.nih.gov.

Texas Heart Institute, Heart Information Service, P.O. Box 20345, Houston, TX, 77225-0345, (800) 292-2221, http://www.texasheartinstitute.org/.

Lori De Milto
Angela M. Costello
Tish Davidson, A.M.

Coronary stenting

Definition

A coronary stent is an artificial support device placed in the coronary artery to keep the vessel open after treatment for coronary artery disease. Also called atherosclerosis, coronary artery disease is a build-up of fatty matter and debris on the walls of the arteries. Over time, this buildup narrows the arteries and reduces blood supply to the heart.

The stent is usually a stainless steel mesh tube that is available in various sizes to match the size of the artery and hold it open after the blockage in the artery has been treated.

Purpose

The coronary stent is used to keep coronary arteries expanded, usually following a balloon **angioplasty** or other interventional procedure. Balloon angioplasty (also called percutaneous transluminal coronary angioplasty, or PTCA) and other interventional procedures are performed to open narrowed coronary arteries and improve blood flow to the heart. By forming a rigid support, the stent can prevent the vessel from reclosing (a process called restenosis) and reduce the need for coronary bypass surgery.

Demographics

According to the American Heart Association, 1,271,000 angioplasties were performed in the United States in 2005. There were 874,000 men and 397,000 women who had angioplasties in 2005. Stent placement is part of the majority of interventional procedures.

Description

Coronary stenting usually follows balloon angioplasty. After the patient receives a local anesthetic to numb the area, a **cardiac catheterization** procedure is performed in which a long, narrow tube (catheter) is passed through a sheath placed within a small incision in the femoral artery in the upper thigh. Sometimes, the catheter is placed in an artery in the arm.

A catheter with a small balloon at the tip is guided to the point of narrowing in the coronary artery. Contrast material is injected through the catheter so the physician can view the site where the artery is narrowed on a special monitor. When the balloon catheter is positioned at the location of the blockage in the coronary artery, it is slowly inflated to widen that

Coronary stenting

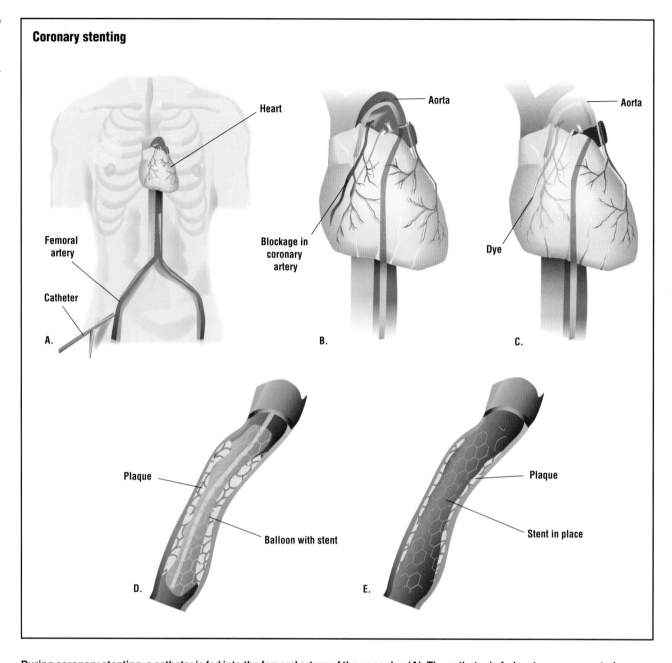

During coronary stenting, a catheter is fed into the femoral artery of the upper leg (A). The catheter is fed up to coronary arteries to an area of blockage (B). A dye is released, allowing visualization of the blockage (C). A stent is placed on the balloon-tipped catheter. The balloon is inflated, opening the artery (D). The stent holds the artery open after the catheter is removed (E). *(Illustration by GGS Information Services. Cengage Learning, Gale.)*

artery and compress the blockage or fatty area into the artery wall and stretch the artery open.

The stent is inserted into the artery with the balloon-tip catheter. The stent is flat when inserted so that it can travel through the artery. When the stent is correctly positioned in the coronary artery, the balloon is inflated, expanding the stent against the walls of the coronary artery. The balloon catheter is deflated and removed, leaving the stent permanently in place to hold the coronary artery open.

A cardiac **angiography** will follow to ensure that the stent is keeping the artery open.

In April 2003, the first drug-coated stent brand, the Cordis CYPHER, was approved for use by the U.S. Food and Drug Administration. Coated stents, also called drug-eluting stents, are stents that have

KEY TERMS

Angina—Also called angina pectoris, chest pain or discomfort that occurs when diseased blood vessels restrict blood flow to the heart.

Anticoagulant—A medication, also called a blood thinner, that prevents blood from clotting.

Atherectomy—A non-surgical technique for treating diseased arteries with a rotating device that cuts or shaves away obstructing material inside the artery.

Brachytherapy—The use of radiation during angioplasty to prevent the artery from narrowing again (a process called restenosis).

Cardiac angiography—A procedure used to visualize blood vessels of the heart.

Catheter—A long, thin flexible tube that can be inserted into the body; in this case, it is threaded to the heart.

Echocardiogram—An imaging procedure used to create a picture of the heart's movement, valves, and chambers.

Electrocardiogram (ECG, EKG)—A test that records the electrical activity of the heart.

Homocysteine—An amino acid normally found in small amounts in the blood.

Restenosis—The narrowing of a blood vessel after it has been opened, usually by balloon angioplasty.

Stress test—A test used to determine how the heart responds to stress.

Thrombosis—The development of a blood clot in the vessels, which may clog a blood vessel and stop the flow of blood.

- electrocardiogram;
- stress tests;
- cardiac catheterization;
- imaging tests such as a chest X-ray, echocardiography, or computed tomography (CT); and
- blood tests to measure blood cholesterol, triglycerides, and other substances.

Preparation

The patient should quit smoking or using tobacco products before the procedure, and should make the commitment to be a nonsmoker after the surgery. Most communities have a variety of free **smoking cessation** programs available. The patient can ask a health-care provider for more information about quitting smoking.

The patient is usually instructed to take **aspirin** or another blood-thinning medication for several days before the procedure. Aspirin can help decrease the possibility of blood clots forming at the stent.

It is advisable for the patient to arrange for transportation home because drowsiness may last several hours and driving is not permitted after the procedure.

After midnight the night before the procedure, the patient should not eat or drink anything.

The patient usually goes to the hospital the same day the procedure is scheduled, and should bring a list of current medications, allergies, and appropriate medical records upon **admission to the hospital**.

An intravenous needle will be inserted into a vein in the arm to deliver medications and fluids during the procedure. The catheter insertion site may be shaved. A sedative is given to make the patient drowsy and relaxed, but the patient will not be completely asleep during the procedure.

Aftercare

The procedure generally takes from 90 minutes to two hours to perform, but the preparation and recovery time add several hours to the overall procedure time. Although patients often go home the same day or the evening of the procedure, they should plan to stay at the hospital most of the day.

Recovery in the hospital

The patient is instructed to stay flat in bed without bending the legs so that the artery can heal from the insertion of the catheter. A stitch or collagen plug may be placed at the site of the catheter insertion to seal the wound and firm pressure may be applied to the area. A

been coated with drugs that help to ensure the blood vessel does not reclose. Some clinical studies have found that these drug coated stents can reduce the rate of blood vessel reclosing from about one third down to as low as 3%.

Diagnosis/Preparation

Diagnosis

The diagnosis of coronary artery disease is made after the patient's medical history is carefully reviewed, a physical exam is performed and the patient's symptoms are evaluated. Tests used to diagnose coronary artery disease include:

flat position is required for two to six hours after the procedure. A health-care provider will help the patient get out of bed for the first time when the doctor approves it. The patient will be allowed to eat after he or she is able to get out of bed.

The patient is closely monitored during the recovery period. **Vital signs** and other parameters such as the heart's rhythm and electrical activity as well as oxygen and carbon dioxide levels in arterial blood are checked frequently. A catheter may be placed to drain urine during the recovery period.

A blood thinner may be given to the patient intravenously for the first few hours after the procedure to prevent clotting.

Recovery at home

Medications are prescribed to control pain. Minor chest discomfort is common after the procedure; however, the patient should notify the health-care provider if severe chest, arm, or back discomfort is experienced. Some bleeding and bruising near the catheter insertion site are also common after the procedure. Severe bleeding should be reported to a health-care provider immediately. If bleeding occurs, the patient should dial 911 and lay down immediately. The dressing covering the area should be removed and firm pressure should be applied to the area until help arrives.

Ointments, lotions, and **dressings** should not be applied to the catheter insertion site unless specific instructions have been given.

Medications are prescribed to prevent unwanted blood clotting. Daily doses of aspirin or other anticoagulant medications are started after the procedure and are continued after the patient goes home.

The patient should not have any **magnetic resonance imaging** (MRI) tests for six months after the procedure, because the magnetic field may move the stent.

LIFESTYLE CHANGES. The patient needs to make several lifestyle changes after surgery, including:

- Quitting smoking. Smoking causes damage to blood vessels, increases the patient's blood pressure and heart rate, and decreases the amount of oxygen available in the blood.
- Managing weight. Maintaining a healthy weight by watching portion sizes and exercising is important. Being overweight increases the work of the heart.
- Participating in an exercise program. The exercise program is usually tailored for the patient, who will be encouraged to participate in a cardiac rehabilitation program supervised by exercise professionals.

- Making dietary changes. Patients should eat a lot of fruits, vegetables, grains, and non-fat or low-fat dairy products, and reduce fats to less than 30% of all calories. A diet low in cholesterol and vitamin K (to prevent interference with the anticoagulant medication) may be recommended.
- Taking medications as prescribed. Aspirin and other heart medications may be prescribed, and the patient may need to take these medications for life.
- Managing other health conditions such as diabetes or high blood pressure. Taking medications as prescribed and following the doctor's guidelines are very important ways for the patient to manage his or her health.
- Following up with health-care providers. The patient needs to regularly see the physician to monitor his or her recovery and control risk factors. Routine stress testing is a part of the follow-up treatment to detect restenosis that may occur without symptoms.

Risks

Although coronary stents greatly reduce the risk of restenosis following balloon angioplasty, there is still some risk that the stented artery may close.

Serious complications are uncommon, but may include infection, damage to the heart or blood vessels, and blood clots. Anticlotting medication is given after stent placement to prevent the risk of blood clots. Less serious complications include bleeding, swelling, or bruising where the catheter was placed.

Normal results

The patient usually goes home the day or evening of the procedure, but sometimes an overnight stay in the hospital is necessary so monitoring can be continued. Patients should have someone to take them home after the procedure; driving is not recommended for at least 24 hours after the procedure.

Fatigue and weakness are common after the procedure. The patient should limit activities for the first two days after the procedure and can gradually resume normal activities by the end of the week.

For the first week after the procedure, pushing and pulling heavy objects (as in mowing the lawn) should be avoided, and lifting objects more than 20 lbs (9 kg) is not permitted. Stair climbing is permitted unless other instructions have been given.

Balloon angioplasty and the placement of a stent does not prevent coronary artery disease from recurring; therefore, lifestyle changes are strongly recommended and medications are prescribed to further reduce this risk.

WHO PERFORMS THE PROCEDURE AND WHERE IS IT PERFORMED?

A team of specialized heart doctors (cardiologists), nurses, and technicians trained in stent placement perform this procedure. Stent placement usually takes place in the hospital setting in a special lab called the catheterization laboratory. It may also be performed in an intensive care unit, emergency room (such as for treatment of a heart attack), or other special procedure room.

Morbidity and mortality rates

Death is extremely rare as a result of the stent placement procedure. There is some risk of embolism, a blockage in an artery in the brain caused by a clot or loosened debris. Embolism can cause stroke.

Sometimes a blockage returns to the treated coronary artery (restenosis). If restenosis occurs, it usually happens within the first six months after the procedure. If the patient has previously experienced restenosis, there is an increased risk that it will recur. Repeat blockages can be treated with other interventional procedures; **coronary artery bypass graft surgery** may be needed.

Alternatives

All patients with coronary artery disease can help improve their condition by making lifestyle changes such as quitting smoking, losing weight if they are overweight, eating healthy foods, reducing blood cholesterol, exercising regularly, and controlling diabetes and high blood pressure.

All patients with coronary artery disease should be prescribed medications to treat their condition. Antiplatelet medications such as aspirin or clopidogrel (Plavix) are usually recommended. Medications may also be prescribed to lower lipoprotein levels, since elevated lipoprotein levels have been associated with an increased risk of cardiovascular problems.

Treatment with vitamin E is not recommended because it does not lower the rate of cardiovascular events in people with coronary artery disease. Although antioxidants such as vitamin C, beta-carotene, and probucol show promising results, they are not recommended for routine use. Treatment with folic acid and vitamins B_6 and B_{12} lowers homocysteine levels (reducing the risk for cardiovascular problems), but more

QUESTIONS TO ASK THE DOCTOR

- Why is this procedure being performed?
- Should I take my medications the day of the procedure?
- Can I eat or drink the day of the procedure? If not, how long before the procedure should I stop eating or drinking?
- When can I drive after the procedure?
- What should I wear the day of the procedure?
- Will I be awake during the procedure?
- Will I have to stay in the hospital after the procedure?
- When can I resume my normal activities?
- When will I find out the results?
- What if the procedure was not successful?
- If I have had the procedure once, can I have it again to treat coronary artery disease?
- Will I have any pain or discomfort after the procedure? If so, how can I relieve this pain or discomfort?
- Are there any medications, foods, or activities I should avoid to prevent my symptoms from recurring?

studies are needed to determine if lowered homocysteine levels correlate with a reduced rate of cardiovascular problems in treated patients.

Other interventional procedures used to open a blocked artery include rotoblation, brachytherapy, and atherectomy.

Coronary artery bypass graft surgery is a treatment option that is considered when medications and interventional therapies do not adequately treat coronary artery disease. During coronary artery bypass graft surgery, a blood vessel graft to restore normal blood flow to the heart is used to bypass one or more blocked coronary arteries. These grafts usually come from the patient's own arteries and veins located in the leg, arm, or chest.

Enhanced external counterpulsation (EECP) may be a treatment option for patients who are not candidates for interventional procedures or coronary artery bypass graft surgery. During EECP, a set of cuffs is wrapped around the patient's calves, thighs, and buttocks. These cuffs gently but firmly compress the blood vessels in the lower limbs to increase blood flow to the heart. The inflation and deflation of the cuffs are electronically synchronized with the heartbeat and blood pressure using **electrocardiography** and blood pressure monitors. EECP may encourage blood vessels to open small channels to eventually bypass blocked vessels and improve blood flow to the heart. Not all patients are candidates for this procedure, and treatments, lasting one to two hours, must be repeated about five times a week for up to seven weeks.

Resources

BOOKS

Ellis, Stephen G., and David R. Holmes, Jr., eds. *Strategic Approaches in Coronary Intervention,* 3rd ed. Philadelphia: Lippincott Williams & Wilkins, 2006.

King, Spencer B., and Alan C. Yeung. *Interventional Cardiology* New York: McGraw-Hill Professional, 2006.

Timmins, Fiona. *Contemporary Issues in Coronary Care Nursing,* 4th ed. New York: Routledge, 2005.

PERIODICALS

Jenkins, R. "No Need to Rush Stents in Stable CAD." *Australian Doctor* (April 6, 2007): 3.

Pfisterer, M., O. Bertel, P. O. Bonetti, H. P. Brunner-La Rocca, et al. "Drug-Eluting or Bare-Metal Stents for Large Coronary Vessel Stenting? The BASKET-PROVE (Prospective Validation Examination) Trial: Study Protocol and Design." *American Heart Journal* 155, no. 4 (April 2008): 609–614.

ORGANIZATIONS

American College of Cardiology, Heart House2400 N. Street NW, Washington, DC, 20037, (800) 253-4636, http://www.acc.org.

American Heart Association, 7272 Greenville Avenue, Dallas, TX, 75231, (800) 242-8721, http://www.americanheart.org.

Cleveland Clinic Heart Center, 9500 Euclid Avenue, Cleveland, OH, 44195, (800) 223-2273, http://www.clevelandclinic.org/heartcenter.

National Heart, Lung and Blood Institute, National Institutes of Health, P.O. Box 30105, Bethesda, MD, 20824-0105, NHLBIinfo@nhlbi.nih.gov, http://www.nhlbi.nih.gov.

Cindy L. A. Jones, Ph.D.
Angela M. Costello
Robert Bockstiegel

Corpus callosotomy

Definition

Corpus callosotomy is a treatment for epilepsy, in which a group of fibers connecting the two sides of the brain, called the corpus callosum, is cut.

Purpose

Corpus callosotomy is used to treat epilepsy that is unresponsive to drug treatments. A person with epilepsy may be considered a good candidate for one type of epilepsy surgery or another if he or she has seizures that are not adequately controlled by drug therapy, and has tried at least two (perhaps more, depending on the treatment center's guidelines) different anti-epileptic drugs.

The seizures of epilepsy are due to unregulated spreading of electrical activity from one part of the brain to other parts. In many people with epilepsy, this activity begins from a well-defined focal point, which can be identified by electrical testing. Surgical treatment of focal-origin seizures involves removal of the brain region containing the focal point, usually in a procedure called temporal lobectomy. In other people, no focal point is found, or there may be too many to remove individually. These patients are most likely to receive corpus callosotomy.

The purpose of a corpus callosotomy is to prevent spreading of seizure activity from one half of the brain to the other. The brain is divided into two halves, or hemispheres, that are connected by a thick bundle of nerve fibers, the corpus callosum. When these fibers are cut, a seizure that begins in one hemisphere is less likely to spread to the other. This can reduce the frequency of seizures significantly.

The initial surgery may cut the forward two-thirds of the corpus callosum, leaving the rest intact. If this does not provide sufficient seizure control, the remaining portion may be cut.

Demographics

Corpus callosotomy is most often performed for children with "drop attacks," or atonic seizures, in which a sudden loss of muscle tone causes the child to fall to the floor. It is also performed in people with uncontrolled generalized tonic-clonic, or grand mal, seizures, or with massive jerking movements. Of the 20,000 to 70,000 people in the United States considered candidates for any type of epilepsy surgery, approximately 5,000 receive surgery per year. Between 1985 and 1990, more than 800 corpus callosotomies were performed, and the number has increased since then. Corpus callosotomy is performed by a special neurosurgical team, at a regional epilepsy treatment center.

Description

During corpus callosotomy, the patient is under **general anesthesia**, lying on the back. The head is fixed in place with blunt pins attached to a rigid

WHO PERFORMS THE PROCEDURE AND WHERE IS IT PERFORMED?

Corpus callosotomy is performed by a neurosurgeon in a hospital operating room.

QUESTIONS TO ASK THE DOCTOR

- Are there any drugs that we haven't tried that may be effective?
- How long until I can return to school or work?
- Am I a candidate for any other epilepsy surgery?

structure. The head is shaved either before or during the procedure.

Incisions are made in the top of the skull to remove a flap of bone, exposing the brain. The outer covering is cut, and the two hemispheres are pulled slightly apart to expose the corpus callosum. The fibers of the corpus callosum are cut, taking care to avoid nearby arteries and ventricles (fluid-filled cavities in the brain).

Once the cut is made and any bleeding is controlled, the brain covering, bone, and scalp are closed and stitched.

Diagnosis/Preparation

The candidate for any type of epilepsy surgery will have had a wide range of tests prior to surgery. These include **electroencephalography** (EEG), in which electrodes are placed on the scalp, on the brain surface, or within the brain to record electrical activity. EEG is used to attempt to locate the focal point(s) of the seizure activity.

Several neuroimaging procedures are used to obtain images of the brain. These may reveal structural abnormalities that the neurosurgeon must be aware of. These procedures may include **magnetic resonance imaging** (MRI), x rays, computed tomography (CT) scans, or **positron emission tomography (PET)** imaging.

Neuropsychological tests may be done to provide a baseline against which the results of the surgery are measured. A Wada test may also be performed. In this test, a drug is injected into the artery leading to one half of the brain, putting it to sleep, allowing the neurologist to determine where language and other functions in the brain are localized, which may be useful for predicting the result of the surgery.

Aftercare

The patient remains in the hospital for about a week, possibly more depending on any complications that have occurred during surgery and on the health of the patient. There may be some discomfort afterwards. Tylenol with codeine may be prescribed for pain. Bending over should

be avoided if possible, as it may lead to headache in the week or so after the procedure. Ice packs may be useful for pain and itchiness of the sutures on the head. Another several weeks of convalescence at home are required before the patient can resume normal activities. Heavy lifting or straining may continue to cause headaches or nausea, and should be avoided until the doctor approves. A diet rich in fiber can help avoid constipation, which may occur following surgery. Patients remain on anti-seizure medication at least for the short term, and may continue to require medication.

Risks

There is a slight risk of infection or hemorrhage from the surgery, usually less than 1%. Disconnection of the two hemispheres of the brain can cause some neuropsychological impairments such as decreased spontaneity of speech (it may be difficult to bring the right words into one's mind) and decreased use of the non-dominant hand. These problems usually improve over time. Complete cutting of the corpus callosotomy produces more long-lasting, but very subtle deficits in connecting words with images. These are usually not significant, or even noticed, by the patient.

Normal results

Patients typically experience a marked reduction in number and severity of seizures, with a small percentage of people becoming seizure free. Drop attacks may be eliminated completely in approximately 70% of patients. Other types of seizure are also reduced by 50% or more from corpus callosotomy surgery.

Morbidity and mortality rates

Serious morbidity or mortality occurs in 1% or less of patients. Combined major and minor complication rates are approximately 20%.

Alternatives

Newer anti-seizure medications have partially replaced corpus callosotomy. Focal epilepsy is treated with focal surgery such as temporal lobectomy or **hemispherectomy**. Vagus nerve stimulation is an alternative for some patients.

Resources

BOOKS

Devinsky, O. *A Guide to Understanding and Living with Epilepsy.* Philadelphia: EA Davis, 1994.

ORGANIZATIONS

Epilepsy Foundation. www.epilepsyfoundation.org.

Richard Robinson

Corticosteroids

Definition

Corticosteroids are a group of natural and synthetic analogs (chemical cousins) of the hormones secreted by the pituitary gland, also known as the hypothalamic-anterior pituitary-adrenocortical (HPA) axis. These analogs include glucocorticoids, which are anti-inflammatory agents with a large number of other functions; mineralocorticoids, which control salt and water balance primarily through action on the kidneys; and corticotropins, which control secretion of hormones by the pituitary gland. First introduced in 1949 for the treatment of rheumatoid arthritis, corticosteroids are widely used in the twenty-first century to treat conditions as varied as asthma, lung infections in AIDS patients, bacterial meningitis, and cancer-related pain.

Purpose

Glucocorticoids have multiple effects, and are used for a large number of conditions. They affect glucose (sugar) utilization and fat metabolism, bone development, and are potent anti-inflammatory agents. They may be used for replacement of natural hormones in patients with pituitary deficiency (Addison's disease), as well as for a wide number of other conditions including arthritis, asthma, anemia, various cancers, eye disease (uveitis), inflammatory bowel disease, and skin inflammations. Additional uses include inhibition of nausea and vomiting after chemotherapy, treatment of septic shock, treatment of spinal cord injuries, and treatment of hirsutism (excessive hair growth). The choice of drug will vary with the condition.

Cortisone and hydrocortisone, which have both glucocorticoid and mineralocorticoid effects, are the drugs of choice for replacement therapy of natural hormone deficiency. Synthetic compounds, which have greater anti-inflammatory effects and less effect on salt and water balance, are usually preferred for other purposes. These compounds include dexamethasone, which is almost exclusively glucocorticoid in its actions, as well as prednisone, prednisolone, betamethasone, triamcinolone, and others. Glucocorticoids are formulated in oral dosage forms, topical creams and ointments, oral and nasal inhalations, rectal foams, and ear and eye drops.

Mineralocorticoids control the retention of sodium in the kidneys. In mineralocorticoid deficiency, there is excessive loss of sodium through the kidneys, with resulting water loss. Fludrocortisone (Florinef) is the only drug available for treatment of mineralocorticoid deficiency, and is available only in an oral form.

Corticotropin (ACTH, adrenocorticotropic hormone) stimulates the pituitary gland to release cortisone. A deficiency of corticotropic hormone will have the same effects as a deficiency of cortisone. The hormone, which is available under the brand names Acthar and Actrel, is used for diagnostic testing to determine the cause of a glucocorticoid deficiency. It is rarely used for replacement therapy, however, since direct administration of glucocorticoids may be easier and offers better control over dosages.

Recommended dosage

Dosage of glucocorticoids varies with the specific drug, the route of administration, the condition being treated, and the patient's individual metabolism.

Fludrocortisone, for use in replacement therapy, is normally dosed at 0.1 mg/day. Some patients require higher doses. It should normally be taken in conjunction with cortisone or hydrocortisone.

ACTH, when used for diagnostic purposes, is given as 10–25 units by intravenous solution over eight hours. A long-acting form, which may be used for replacement therapy, is given by subcutaneous (SC) or intramuscular (IM) injection at a dose of 40–80 units every 24–72 hours.

Precautions

The most significant risk associated with administration of glucocorticoids is suppression of natural corticosteroid secretion. When the artificial hormones are administered, they suppress the secretion of ACTH, which in turn reduces the secretion of the natural hormones. The extent of suppression varies with dose, drug potency, duration of treatment, and individual patient response. While suppression is seen primarily with drugs

KEY TERMS

Addison's disease—A rare endocrine disorder in which the adrenal gland does not produce enough steroid hormones.

Addisonian crisis—A medical emergency resulting from severe adrenal insufficiency. It can be caused by sudden withdrawal from oral glucocorticoid medications, as well as from damage to the adrenal gland itself. Untreated Addisonian crisis can be fatal.

Cortisol—A corticosteroid hormone produced by the adrenal gland.

Cushing's syndrome—A condition resulting from excess cortisol in the body, characterized by high blood pressure, a round "moon" face, excessive sweating, thinning of the skin and easy bruising, and the growth of fat pads around the shoulders and back of the neck. It was first described in 1932 by Harvey Cushing, an eminent American surgeon.

Hallucination—A false or distorted perception of objects, sounds, or events that seems real. Hallucinations usually result from drugs or mental disorders.

Hirsutism—Excessive or increased growth of facial or body hair in women resembling the male pattern of hair distribution.

Hormone—A substance that is produced in one part of the body, then travels through the bloodstream to another part of the body where it has its effect.

Hypertension—High blood pressure.

Hypotension—Low blood pressure.

Inflammation—Pain, redness, swelling, and heat that usually develop in response to injury or illness.

Ointment—A thick spreadable substance that contains medicine and is meant to be used on the outside of the body.

Pregnancy category—A system of classifying drugs according to their established risks for use during pregnancy. The classifications are categories A, B, C, D, and X.

Chronic overdose of glucocorticoids leads to Cushingoid syndrome, which is clinically identical to Cushing's syndrome. The only difference is that in Cushingoid, the excessive steroids are from drug therapy rather than excessive glandular secretion of cortisol. Symptoms vary, but most people have upper body obesity, a rounded "moon" face, increased fat around the neck, and thinning arms and legs. In its later stages, this condition leads to weakening of bones and muscles with rib and spinal column fractures.

The short-term adverse effects of corticosteroids are generally mild, and include indigestion, increased appetite, insomnia, and nervousness. There are also a very large number of infrequent adverse reactions, the most significant of which is drug-induced paranoia. Delirium, depression, menstrual irregularity, and increased hair growth are also possible.

Long-term use of topical glucocorticoids can result in thinning of the skin or permanent damage to the retina of the eye. Oral steroid inhalations may cause fungal overgrowth in the oral cavity. Patients must be instructed to rinse their mouths carefully after each dose.

Corticosteroids are included in pregnancy category C. The pregnancy category system classifies drugs according to their established risks for use during pregnancy. Corticosteroids have caused congenital malformations in animal studies, including cleft palate. Breastfeeding while taking these medications should be avoided.

Because fludrocortisone has glucocorticoid activity as well as mineralocorticoid action, the same hazards and precautions apply to fludrocortisone as to the glucocorticoids. Overdose of fludrocortisone may also cause edema (swelling), hypertension, and congestive heart failure.

Corticotropin has all the same risks as the glucocorticoids. Prolonged use may cause reduced response to the stimulatory effects of corticotropin.

Warnings

Patients with the following conditions should use corticosteroids with caution:

- osteoporosis or any other bone disease
- current or past tuberculosis
- glaucoma or cataracts
- infections of any type (virus, bacteria, fungus, ameba)
- sores in the nose or recent nose surgery (if using nasal spray forms of corticosteroids)
- an underactive or overactive thyroid gland

administered systemically, it can also occur with topical drugs such as creams and ointments, or drugs administered by inhalation. Abrupt cessation of corticosteroids may result in acute adrenal crisis (Addisonian crisis) which is marked by dehydration with severe vomiting and diarrhea, sudden sharp pain in the abdomen, lower back, or legs, hypotension, convulsions, mental confusion, and loss of consciousness. Acute adrenal crisis is potentially fatal.

- liver disease
- stomach or intestine problems
- diabetes
- heart disease
- high blood pressure
- high cholesterol
- kidney disease or kidney stones
- myasthenia gravis
- systemic lupus erythematosus (SLE)
- emotional problems
- skin conditions that cause the skin to be thinner and bruise more easily

Interactions

Corticosteroids interact with many other drugs a patient might take; they reduce the effectiveness of vaccination in some patients. Patients taking **barbiturates** as sleep medications may need higher doses of corticosteroids. Smoking reduces the effectiveness of inhaled corticosteroids. Patients should inform their doctor about all other medications (both prescription and over-the-counter) they take, and discuss possible interactions.

Resources

BOOKS

Abrams, Anne C., Carol B. Lammon, and Sandra S. Pennington. *Clinical Drug Therapy: Rationales for Nursing Practice*, 8th ed. Philadelphia: Lippincott Williams and Wilkins, 2007.

Griffith, H. W., and S. Moore. *2001 Complete Guide to Prescription and Nonprescription Drugs.* New York: Berkely Publishing Group, 2001.

Neal, Michael J. *Medical Pharmacology at a Glance*, 5th ed. Malden, MA: Blackwell Publishing, 2005.

PERIODICALS

Bacharier, L. B., H. H. Raissy, L. Wilson, et al. "Long-term Effect of Budesonide on Hypothalamic-Pituitary-Adrenal Axis Function in Children with Mild to Moderate Asthma." *Pediatrics* 113 (June 2004): 1693–1699.

Greenwood, B. M. "Corticosteroids for Acute Bacterial Meningitis." *New England Journal of Medicine* 357 (December 13, 2007): 2507–2509.

Hubbard, R., et al. "Use of Inhaled Corticosteroids and the Risk of Fracture." *Chest* 130 (October 2006): 1082–1088.

Kroon, L. A. "Drug Interactions with Smoking." *American Journal of Health-System Pharmacy* 64 (September 15, 2007): 1917–1921.

Rodrigo, G. J. "Rapid Effects of Inhaled Corticosteroids in Acute Asthma: An Evidence-based Evaluation." *Chest* 130 (November 2006): 1301–1311.

Zoorob, Roger J., and Dawn Cender. "A Different Look at Corticosteroids." *American Family Physician* 58 (August 1998): 443–450.

ORGANIZATIONS

American Academy of Allergy, Asthma and Immunology. 611 East Wells Street, Milwaukee, WI 53202. Telephone: (414) 272–6071. Web site: http://www.aaaai.org (accessed March 11, 2008).

Arthritis Foundation. 1330 West Peachtree Street, Suite 100, Atlanta, GA 30309. (800) 283-7800 or (404) 872-7100. http://www.arthritis.org/index.php (accessed March 11, 2008).

Asthma and Allergy Foundation of America. 1125 15th Street NW, Suite 502, Washington, DC 20005. Telephone: (800) 727–8462. Web site: http://www.aafa.org (accessed March 11, 2008).

National Heart, Lung and Blood Institute. National Institutes of Health, P.O. Box 30105, Bethesda, MD 20824-0105. Telephone: (301) 592-8573. http://www.nhlbi.nih.gov/ (accessed March 11, 2008).

U.S. Food and Drug Administration (FDA). 5600 Fishers Lane, Rockville, MD 20857-0001. (888) INFO-FDA (1-888-463-6332). http://www.fda.gov/ (accessed March 11, 2008).

Samuel Uretsky, PharmD
Rebecca Frey, PhD

Cosmetic surgery *see* **Plastic, reconstructive, and cosmetic surgery**

Cotrel-Dubousset spinal instrumentation *see* **Spinal instrumentation**

CPR *see* **Cardiopulmonary resuscitation**

Craniofacial reconstruction

Definition

Craniofacial reconstruction refers to a group of procedures used to repair or reshape the face and skull of a living person, or to create a replica of the head and face of a dead or missing person. The word "craniofacial" is a combination of "cranium," which is the medical word for the upper portion of the skull, and facial. Craniofacial reconstruction is sometimes called orbital-craniofacial surgery; "orbital" refers to the name of the bony cavity in the face that surrounds the eyeball.

Purpose

Craniofacial reconstruction has several different purposes depending on the group of patients or

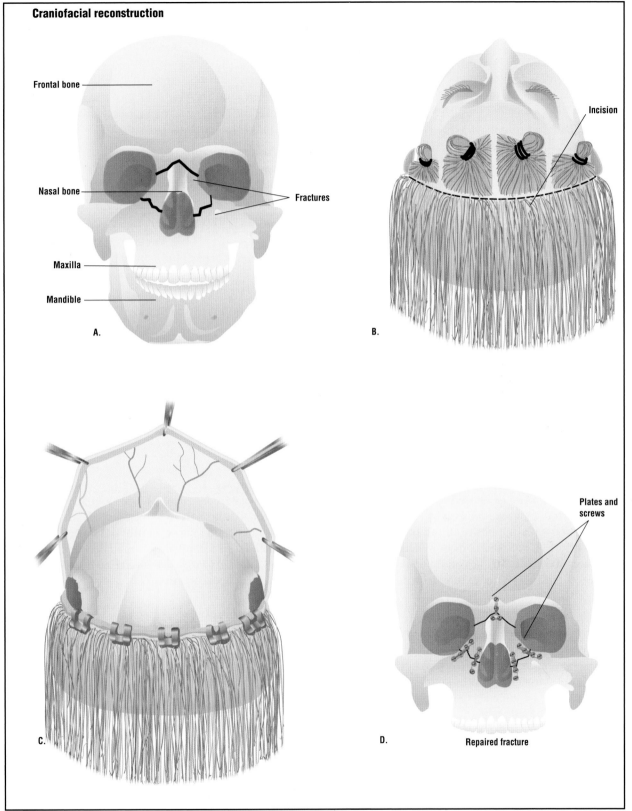

Craniofacial reconstruction

Frontal bone

Nasal bone

Maxilla

Mandible

Fractures

A.

Incision

B.

Plates and screws

Repaired fracture

C.

D.

To repair severe fractures around the nasal bone (A), an incision is made into the patient's skin at the top of the head (B). The skin is pulled off the face to expose the fracture (C), which then can be repaired with plates and screws (D). *(Illustration by GGS Information Services. Cengage Learning, Gale.)*

Cleft palate—A birth defect in which the roof of the mouth is open because the two sides of the palate failed to join together during fetal development.

Congenital—Present at the time of birth.

Craniosynostosis—Premature closing of the sutures joining the skull bones.

Cranium—The large, rounded upper part of the skull that encloses the brain.

Down syndrome—A congenital disorder caused by a mutation of human chromosome 21 in which there are three chromosomes (trisomy) instead of the usual pair.

Flap—A piece of tissue used for grafting that has kept its own blood supply.

Forensic—Referring to legal or courtroom proceedings.

Frontal bone—The part of the skull that lies behind the forehead.

Le Fort fracture—A term that refers to a system for classifying fractures of the facial bones into three groups according to the region affected.

Mandible—The horseshoe-shaped bone that forms the lower jaw.

Maxilla—The facial bone that forms the upper jaw and holds the upper teeth.

Microsurgery—Surgery performed under a microscope on nerves and other very small structures with the help of special instruments.

Orbit—The bony cavity in the face that surrounds and protects the eyeball.

Suture—A type of body joint that is found only in the skull; the surfaces of the bones in the skull are held together by a thin layer of fibrous connective tissue.

Treacher Collins syndrome—A disorder that affects facial development and hearing, thought to be caused by a gene mutation on human chromosome 5; sometimes called mandibulofacial dysotosis.

Zygoma—The cheek bone in the front of the face below the eye socket, it is connected to the frontal bone of the forehead and the maxilla (upper jaw); sometimes called the os zygomaticum or zygomatic bone.

persons in question. In children, craniofacial reconstruction is done to repair abnormalities in the shape of the child's skull and facial features resulting from birth defects or genetic disorders. It is also done to repair traumatic injuries resulting from accidents or child abuse. Craniofacial reconstruction in children requires special techniques and planning because the surgeon must allow for future growth of the child's facial bones and skull.

In adults, craniofacial reconstruction is most commonly done following head or facial trauma, but it is also performed on cancer patients who have lost part of the bony structures or soft tissue of the face following tumor surgery. In both adults and children, the reconstruction is intended to restore the functioning of the patient's mouth, jaw, and sensory organs as well as improve his or her appearance. Craniofacial reconstruction is a complicated procedure because the surgeon is operating on a part of the body that contains the brain and upper part of the spinal cord, the eyes, and other sensory organs, and the opening of the patient's airway—all within a small space.

The third major application of craniofacial reconstruction is in forensic medicine and anthropology. Forensic is a term that refers to legal matters. Physicians who specialize in forensic science study the remains of people who have died to establish not only the cause of **death** but in some cases, the identity of the dead person. Craniofacial reconstruction is one approach to this identification. Anthropologists, the scientists who study the origins and cultural development of humans, make use of craniofacial reconstruction to understand what prehistoric people looked like and to compare them with present-day humans.

Demographics

Birth defects and genetic disorders

About 7%, or 227,500, of the children born each year in the United States are affected by birth defects of the head and face. According to the American Society of Plastic Surgeons, 37,732 procedures were performed to repair birth defects in 2001, an increase of 2% over the number of surgeries in 2000.

The demographics of specific birth defects affecting the head and face vary; some are considered rare disorders. Figures for some of the disorders most likely to be treated surgically include:

• Cleft palate. Cleft lip or palate is the fourth most common birth defect affecting American children, one in every 700 newborns. The male-female ratio is two to one in children of all races. Asian-American children have a higher than average incidence of cleft palate, while African-American children have a lower than average incidence.

- Down syndrome. Down syndrome is the most common congenital disorder caused by a chromosomal abnormality; it occurs in one in every 900 infants. Children with Down syndrome have facial characteristics that typically include slanted eyes, a flattened nasal bridge, small rounded ears, and a large protruding tongue. There are about 350,000 people in the United States with Down syndrome.

- Treacher Collins syndrome. This congenital disorder is caused by a mutation on human chromosome 5 that can arise spontaneously or be inherited from the parents. The craniofacial abnormalities in Treacher Collins include an abnormally small jaw and airway that can cause breathing problems; the ears may also be malformed or missing. Treacher Collins syndrome affects one in every 10,000 infants.

- Apert and Crouzon syndromes. These two disorders are sometimes grouped together because they are both characterized by craniosynostosis, which is the medical term for premature closing of the sutures (seams) in the bones at the top of the skull. Children with these syndromes have misshapen heads and a sunken-in appearance to the face. They also have breathing problems and malpositioning of the teeth caused by deformed facial bones. Apert syndrome is very rare, affecting only one child in every 150,000. Crouzon syndrome occurs in one out of every 25,000 infants.

Traumatic injuries

Traumatic injuries to the face and head can include blunt trauma, lacerations (tears), and burns. Heat, chemicals, or electricity may cause burns. According to the American Burn Institute, there are 1.1 million burn injuries each year in the United States that are serious enough to require medical treatment. In 2001, 16,879 adults needed **plastic surgery** to repair burn injuries, while 24,298 required maxillofacial surgery for injuries to the face and jaw.

Prior to the early 1980s, when more rigorous seat belt laws were passed, most severe facial injuries in the United States resulted from automobile accidents. As of 2003, however, 70% of facial injuries treated in urban hospitals are caused by assaults; at least 10% of fractured facial bones in women are the result of domestic violence. Falls cause a significant number of facial injuries in small children and the elderly. Another common source of facial trauma in children is animal bites.

Cancer patients

Cancers of the head and neck affect about 55,000 Americans each year; about 13,000 of these patients die. These cancers include cancers of the skin of the face, the esophagus, the larynx (voice box), the mouth, and the nasal passages. Most of these cancers are preventable because they result from prolonged exposure to either sunlight (facial skin) or tobacco (mouth, throat, nose, and larynx). Men are two to four times as likely to develop cancers of the mouth and throat as women.

Description

General background

Craniofacial reconstruction dates back to the late nineteenth century, when doctors in Germany and France first used it to produce more accurate images of the faces of certain famous people who had died before the invention of photography. Early craniofacial reconstructions included those of Bach, Dante, Kant, and Raphael. The technique was then applied to reconstructing the appearance of prehistoric humans for museums and research institutions. An important contribution to the field was the publication in 1901 of three major papers on the classification of facial fractures by René Le Fort, a French surgeon. Le Fort identified the lines of weakness in the facial bones where fractures are most likely to occur. Traumatic injuries of the facial bones are still classified as Le Fort I, II, and III fractures. A Le Fort I fracture runs across the maxilla, or upper jaw; a Le Fort II fracture is pyramidal in shape, breaking the cheekbone below the orbit (eye socket) and running across the bridge of the nose; a Le Fort III fracture separates the frontal bone behind the forehead from the zygoma (cheekbone) as well as breaking the nasal bridge. A Le Fort III fracture is sometimes called a craniofacial separation.

In the 1920s, British physicians pioneered the application of facial reconstruction to unsolved criminal cases and to treating World War I veterans who had been disfigured in combat. Prior to the invention of the computer, craniofacial reconstruction was done either by applying soft clay to the skull (or a cast of the skull) to recreate the person's features, or by making a two-dimensional drawing over a photograph or x-ray picture of the skull. It was difficult for surgeons operating on mutilated patients to predict the outcome of the operation from these two-dimensional sketches.

The first attempts at craniofacial reconstruction in children with congenital abnormalities were made in the late 1940s by Sir Harold Gillies, a British plastic surgeon who had treated disfigured World War II veterans. More recent advances in craniofacial reconstruction include improved understanding of the soft tissues of the face and better surgical techniques for repairing injuries to these tissues; the invention of surgical plastics that can be used instead of bone grafts to fill in missing pieces of bone; new techniques for fixing the facial bones in place during the healing process; and computerized imaging programs that help the surgeon analyze the patient's facial abnormality or injury. Some of these programs allow doctors to download data directly from x rays, computed tomography (CT) scans, or other diagnostic imaging programs in order to plan the operation and have a clearer picture of the results. In the case of children, computer imaging can be used to estimate the future growth lines of a child's skull and facial bones as well as his or her present condition. Orthodontists and other dental specialists have developed additional imaging programs that provide more details about the mouth and jaw area than can be obtained from **CT scans** and x-ray studies.

Craniofacial reconstruction of birth defects and genetic abnormalities

Craniofacial reconstruction in children with congenital abnormalities of the head and face is preceded by a consultation between the surgeon, other specialists, and the child's parents. It is important to determine the exact cause of the child's deformities, since some abnormalities may be found in as many as 150 different genetic disorders. Following the diagnosis, a comprehensive treatment plan is made that includes long-term psychosocial as well as surgical follow-up. Craniofacial reconstruction in children is complex because the surgeon must allow for changes in the proportions of the child's face and skull as he or she matures as well as attempt to make the facial features look as normal as possible. It is difficult to provide a general description of craniofacial surgery in children because there are many variables among children diagnosed with the same disorder as well as a large number of different disorders requiring craniofacial reconstruction. Reconstructions in children, however, are always done under **general anesthesia** and usually take between three and six hours to complete.

Craniofacial reconstruction following trauma or surgery

Craniofacial reconstruction following trauma is a highly individualized process, depending on the nature and location of the patient's injuries. Emergency workers are trained to evaluate and clear the patient's airway before treating facial injuries as such; severe injuries to the midface and lower face frequently result in airway blockage caused by blood, loose teeth or bone fragments, or the tongue falling backward toward the windpipe. The trauma team may have to intubate the patient or perform an emergency **cricothyroidotomy** in order to help the patient breathe. The second priority in treating traumatic facial injuries is controlling severe bleeding.

Imaging studies of craniofacial injuries may need to be postponed for 24–72 hours in order to treat injuries to other organ systems. Over 60% of patients with severe facial trauma have other serious injuries in the head, chest, or abdomen; this high rate reflects the tremendous forces needed to fracture the human frontal bone, zygoma, and maxilla. In particular, a doctor who is examining a patient with severe facial trauma will be particularly concerned about damage to the brain, the spinal column in the neck region, and the eyes. All Le Fort II and III fractures have the potential for permanent damage to the eyes. There are specific maneuvers that the doctor can perform to assess the location and severity of bone fractures, possible dislocation of the jaw, and injury to the eyes and nose before taking an x ray or CT scan.

When the patient is out of immediate danger, x-ray studies and computed tomography (CT) scans are taken of the craniofacial injuries. Three-dimensional scans assist the surgeon in analyzing the fractures and the condition of the other structures in the face and head. Imaging studies can be used to generate computer images for plastic or metal implants to be matched to the patient's injuries for filling in sections of missing bone.

Surgery following facial trauma may take as long as four to 14 hours, as the goal is to repair as much as possible in one operation. The surgeon may use bone grafts, taking bone from other parts of the body to repair the facial bones, or fill in smaller areas of missing bone with hydroxyapatite cement or polymer implants. Broken facial bones are held in place with titanium miniplates and surgical screws. This technique is called rigid fixation; it often does away with the need to wire the jaws in place, and it speeds the patient's recovery. Lacerations (tears) in the skin are usually simply closed with **stitches**, although the surgeon will be careful to minimize scarring. If large areas of skin are missing, the surgeon will cut a flap, which is a section of living tissue carrying its own blood supply, from another area of the patient's body and transplant it to the face. Some facial injuries may require the assistance of a neurosurgeon, oral surgeon, or ophthalmologist.

Cancers on the skin of the face are usually removed and closed with a few stitches, although skin flaps may be required if the area of the face that is affected is large. Cancers of the head or neck may require bone grafts as well as skin flaps after the tumor has been removed. **Reconstructive surgery** after cancer treatment may involve the use of a microscope and special instruments to rejoin the facial blood vessels and nerve fibers. This technique, which is known as **microsurgery**, is done to preserve the function of the muscles in the face as well as restoring the patient's appearance as much as possible.

Diagnosis/Preparation

Diagnosis of the need for craniofacial reconstruction depends on the cause of the abnormality, injury, or disfigurement. The obstetrician or the child's pediatrician will often make the diagnosis of craniofacial abnormalities in children at the time of delivery. Some genetic disorders that are associated with congenital facial abnormalities, including Down syndrome and Treacher Collins syndrome, can be detected before birth by chromosomal analysis. In adults, the diagnosis is usually made by trauma surgeons in the emergency room or by physicians who have treated the patient for cancer.

Imaging studies, including x-ray photographs, CT scans, and **magnetic resonance imaging** (MRI), are used to analyze the patient's abnormalities or injuries before the operation in order to plan the surgery. The surgeon may also consult a neurosurgeon or ophthalmologist if the abnormality or injury involves the functioning of the patient's brain, spinal cord, or eyes.

Aftercare

Medical and surgical

Children who have had reconstructive surgery for congenital abnormalities are usually taken to a pediatric **intensive care unit** for a day or two, and remain in the hospital for a total of four to five days. Adults who have had reconstructive surgery following trauma may be monitored in an intensive care unit for one to two days after the operation, particularly if they required special treatment for airway problems. The total length of the hospital stay varies according to the severity of the patient's other injuries; some burn victims may be hospitalized for several months.

Short-term aftercare includes medications for pain, changes of surgical **dressings**, breathing exercises, and **antibiotics** to reduce the possibility of infection. Patients with injuries to the jaw or mouth may be given special semi-liquid or soft diets. Children are restricted from swimming for two months after reconstructive surgery and from more active sports for six months.

Long-term follow-up may include revision surgery six to 12 months after facial trauma. In the case of children, the patient will be followed until his or her growth is complete; most will need periodic consultations with an orthodontist as well as with the plastic surgeon. A dentist or an oral surgeon should check on patients who have had craniofacial surgery following trauma during their recovery to make sure that the teeth and jawbones are in proper alignment. All Le Fort fractures (I, II, and III) involve damage to the patient's normal occlusion (bite pattern).

Some patients may choose to have **cosmetic surgery** to remove or minimize facial scars after healing is complete, usually about six months after the reconstructive operation.

Psychological

The psychological aftereffects of a disfiguring congenital abnormality or post-traumatic injury are often problematic. Craniofacial reconstruction in children with congenital syndromes typically includes ongoing psychological assessment and counseling to help the parents as well as the child cope with feelings of guilt as well as deal with teasing or ridicule from others. Many parents blame themselves for their child's condition if it is associated with a genetic disorder. Children who have had a disfiguring injury often develop post-traumatic stress disorder (PTSD), depression, or anxiety. One study found that 98% of children between the ages of three and 12 who had been disfigured by accidents or dog bites had symptoms of PTSD within five days of the traumatic event. A year later, 44% of the children still had symptoms, and 21% met the full diagnostic criteria for PTSD. Psychiatric symptoms in children are often intensified as the youngsters reach adolescence and become even more preoccupied with their appearance.

Adult patients also have high rates of depression, PTSD, or anxiety disorders following craniofacial reconstruction. Support groups as well as individual psychotherapy appear to be effective in helping people learn to live with disfiguring injuries or the aftermath of cancer surgery. Specific concerns include coping with awkward social situations as well as internal feelings of guilt or anger. Some researchers have reported that men find it harder to adjust to facial disfigurement than women, possibly because males in Western societies are not encouraged to discuss concerns about their appearance.

Risks

Some of the risks of craniofacial reconstruction are common to all surgical procedures done under

WHO PERFORMS THE PROCEDURE AND WHERE IS IT PERFORMED?

Craniofacial reconstruction of congenital abnormalities requires a team of medical specialists, including plastic surgeons, maxillofacial surgeons, neurosurgeons, dentists, ophthalmologists, and psychiatrists. These procedures can be done in a department of plastic surgery in a teaching hospital; increasingly, however, they are being performed in separate clinics or institutes that specialize in craniofacial reconstruction in children.

Craniofacial reconstruction following trauma is started as soon as possible once the patient's general condition is stable. Although at one time surgeons delayed the treatment of disfiguring injuries for several weeks, recent studies have found that early treatment gives better results as well as minimizing the need for revision plastic surgery. These procedures can be started in a hospital emergency room or done in a specialized trauma center. Facial injuries resulting from burns or electrical trauma may be treated at special burn centers.

Craniofacial reconstruction following cancer treatment is done in specialized departments of plastic and reconstructive surgery within larger hospitals. Many of these are teaching hospitals associated with major medical schools.

Forensic craniofacial reconstruction is done in specialized facilities in university departments of anthropology or in laboratories related to the criminal justice system.

general anesthesia. These include bleeding, breathing problems, bruises underneath the skin, reactions to the anesthesia, and infection.

Risks that are specific to craniofacial reconstruction include damage to the nerves in the face and head; visible scarring; bone graft failure; and the need for further surgery.

Risk factors that can affect the results of craniofacial reconstruction include:

- poor nutrition
- HIV infection
- a weakened immune system
- damage to the skin from radiation therapy

QUESTIONS TO ASK THE DOCTOR

- Am I likely to need further surgery after recovery from craniofacial reconstruction?
- How normal can I expect to look at the end of the process?
- What are the risks of permanent damage to my eyesight or hearing?
- Does the hospital or clinic have a support group for people who have undergone craniofacial reconstruction?

- a connective tissue disease, such as lupus or scleroderma
- smoking
- time elapsed between a traumatic injury and surgical treatment
- poor blood circulation in the affected area

Normal results

Normal results of craniofacial reconstruction vary, depending on the type of injury or defect. Good results include improvement or restoration of the general shape of the patient's head or face; improving or maintaining the functioning of the eyes, ears, nose, mouth, and teeth; and a more nearly normal appearance to the face.

Morbidity and mortality rates

Morbidity and mortality rates vary widely, depending on the patient's age, general health, and the cause of the injury or abnormality.

Alternatives

There are no mainstream alternatives to craniofacial reconstruction in the treatment of birth defects, traumatic injuries, or disfigurement resulting from cancer surgery.

DNA analysis can be used together with craniofacial reconstruction to help identify badly disfigured or damaged human remains.

Resources

BOOKS

"Chromosomal Abnormalities." In Section 19, Chapter 261 in *The Merck Manual of Diagnosis and Therapy*, edited by Mark H. Beers, and Robert Berkow. Whitehouse Station, NJ: Merck Research Laboratories, 1999.

Colucciello, Stephen A., MD. "Maxillofacial Trauma." In Chapter 138 in *The Emergency Medicine Reports Textbook of Adult and Pediatric Emergency Medicine,* edited by Gideon Bosker. Atlanta, GA: American Health Consultants, 2000.

"Musculoskeletal Abnormalities." In Section 19, Chapter 261 in *The Merck Manual of Diagnosis and Therapy,* edited by Mark H. Beers, and Robert Berkow. Whitehouse Station, NJ: Merck Research Laboratories, 1999.

Nafte, Myriam. *Flesh and Bone: An Introduction to Forensic Anthropology,* Chapter 7, "Reconstructing Identity." Durham, NC: Carolina Academic Press, 2000.

Sargent, Larry. *The Craniofacial Surgery Book.* Chattanooga, TN: Erlanger Health System, 2000.

PERIODICALS

Cordeiro, P. G., and J. J. Disa. "Challenges in Midface Reconstruction." *Seminars in Surgical Oncology,* 19 (October–November 2000): 218–225.

Eppley, B. L. "Craniofacial Reconstruction with Computer-Generated HTR Patient-matched Implants: Use in Primary Bony Tumor Excision." *Journal of Craniofacial Surgery,* 13 (September 2002): 650–657.

Eufinger, H., and M. Wehmoller. "Microsurgical Tissue Transfer and Individual Computer-aided Designed and Manufactured Prefabricated Titanium Implants for Complex Craniofacial Reconstruction." *Scandinavian Journal of Plastic and Reconstructive Surgery and Hand Surgery,* 36 (2002): 326–331.

Girotto, J. A., et al. "Long-term Physical Impairment and Functional Outcomes After Complex Facial Fractures." *Plastic and Reconstructive Surgery,* 108 (August 2001): 312–327.

Hunt, J. A., and P. C. Hobar. "Common Craniofacial Anomalies: The Facial Dysostoses." *Plastic and Reconstructive Surgery,* 110 (December 2002): 1714–1725.

Kos, M., et al. "Midfacial Fractures in Children." *European Journal of Pediatric Surgery,* 12 (August 2002): 218–225.

Leong, K., C. L. Nastala, and P. T. Wang. "Cosmetic Aspects of Cranial Reconstruction." *Neurosurgery Clinics of North America,* 13 (October 2002): 491–503.

Lorenz, R. R., et al. "Hydroxyapatite Cement Reconstruction in the Growing Craniofacial Skeleton: An Experimental Model." *Journal of Craniofacial Surgery,* 13 (November 2002): 802–808.

Moreira-Gonzalez, A., et al. "Clinical Outcome in Cranioplasty: Critical Review in Long-term Follow-up." *Journal of Craniofacial Surgery,* 14 (March 2003): 144–153.

Papadoupoulos, M. A., et al. "Three-dimensional Craniofacial Reconstruction Imaging." *Oral Surgery, Oral Medicine, Oral Pathology, Oral Radiology, and Endodontics,* 93 (April 2002): 382–393.

Parsa, Tatiana, Arthur Adamo, and Yvette Calderon. "Initial Evaluation and Management of Maxillofacial Injuries." *eMedicine,* August 28, 2002 [March 8, 2003].

Rusch, M. D., et al. "Psychological Adjustment in Children After Traumatic Disfiguring Injuries: A 12-month Follow-up." *Plastic and Reconstructive Surgery,* 106 (December 2000): 1451–1458.

Sarwer, D. B., and C. E. Crerand. "Psychological Issues in Patient Outcomes." *Facial Plastic Surgery: FPS,* 18 (May 2002): 125–133.

Strumas, N., O. Antonyshyn, C. B. Caldwell, and J. Mainprize. "Multimodality Imaging for Precise Localization of Craniofacial Osteomyelitis." *Journal of Craniofacial Surgery,* 14 (March 2003): 215–219.

Thompson, A., and G. Kent. "Adjusting to Disfigurement: Processes Involved in Dealing with Being Visibly Different." *Clinical Psychology Review,* 21 (July 2001): 663–682.

Vanezis, M., and P. Vanezis. "Cranio-Facial Reconstruction in Forensic Identification—Historical Development and a Review of Current Practice." *Medicine, Science, and the Law,* 40 (July 2000): 197–205.

Yucel, A., et al. "Malignant Tumors Requiring Maxillectomy." *Journal of Craniofacial Surgery,* 11 (September 2000): 418–429.

ORGANIZATIONS

American Burn Association. 625 North Michigan Avenue, Suite 1530, Chicago, IL 60611. (312) 642-9260. www.ameriburn.org.

American Cleft Palate-Craniofacial Association. 104 South Estes Drive, Suite 204, Chapel Hill, NC 27514. (919) 933-9044. www.cleftline.org.

American Society of Plastic Surgeons (ASPS). 444 East Algonquin Road, Arlington Heights, IL 60005. (847) 228-9900. www.plasticsurgery.org.

FACES: The National Craniofacial Association. P. O. Box 11082, Chattanooga, TN 37401. (800) 332-2373. www.faces-cranio.org.

Federal Bureau of Investigation (FBI), Laboratory Division. J. Edgar Hoover Building, 935 Pennsylvania Avenue, NW, Washington, DC 20535-0001. www.fbi.gov/hq/lab/labhome.htm.

National Down Syndrome Society (NDSS). 666 Broadway, New York, NY 10012. (212) 460-9330 or (800) 221-4602. www.ndss.org.

National Organization for Rare Disorders (NORD). 55 Kenosia Avenue, P. O. Box 1968, Danbury, CT 06813-1968. (203) 744-0100. www.rarediseases.org.

University of Maryland Medical Center, R. Adams Cowley Shock Trauma Center. 22 South Greene Street, Baltimore, MD 21201. (410) 328-2757 or (800) 373-4111. www.umm.edu/shocktrauma.

OTHER

Tuncay, Orhan C., M. Nuveen, C. X. Nguyen, and J. Slattery. "The Development of a System for Three-Dimensional Imaging and Animation of the Craniofacial Complex." *Greater Philadelphia Society of Orthodontists Newsletter,* June 2000 [March 24, 2003]. www.gpso. org/newsletter/3d_imaging.html.

Rebecca Frey, PhD

Craniotomy

Definition

A craniotomy is a procedure to remove a lesion in the brain through an opening in the skull (cranium).

Purpose

A craniotomy is a type of brain surgery. It is the most commonly performed surgery for brain **tumor removal**. It also may be done to remove a blood clot (hematoma), to control hemorrhage from a weak, leaking blood vessel (cerebral aneurysm), to repair arteriovenous malformations (abnormal connections of blood vessels), to drain a brain abscess, to relieve pressure inside the skull, to perform a biopsy, or to inspect the brain.

Demographics

Because craniotomy is a procedure that is utilized for several conditions and diseases, statistical information for the procedure itself is not available. However, because craniotomy is most commonly performed to remove a brain tumor, statistics concerning this condition are given. Approximately 90% of primary brain cancers occur in adults, more commonly in males between 55 and 65 years of age. Tumors in children peak between the ages of three and 12. Brain tumors are presently the most common cancer in children (four out of 100,000).

Description

There are two methods commonly utilized by surgeons to open the skull. Either an incision is made at the nape of the neck around the bone at the back (occipital bone) or a curving incision is made in front of the ear that arches above the eye. The incision penetrates as far as the thin membrane covering the skull bone. During skin incision the surgeon must seal off many small blood vessels because the scalp has a rich blood supply.

The scalp tissue is then folded back to expose the bone. Using a high-speed drill, the surgeon drills a

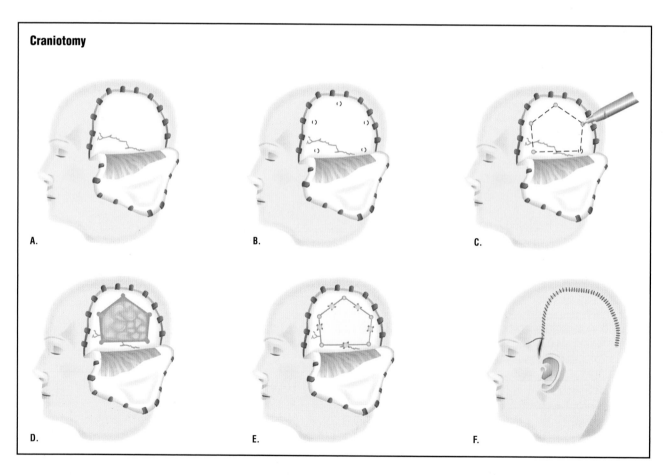

Craniotomy

In a craniotomy, the skin over a part of the skull is cut and pulled back (A). Small holes are drilled into the skull (B), and a special saw is used to cut the bone between the holes (C). The bone is removed, and a tumor or other defect is visualized and repaired (D). The bone is replaced (E), and the skin closed (F). *(Illustration by GGS Information Services. Cengage Learning, Gale.)*

KEY TERMS

Abscess—A localized collection of pus or infection that is walled off from the rest of the body.

Arteriogram—An x-ray study of an artery that has been injected with a contrast dye.

Arteriovenous malformation—Abnormal, direct connection between the arteries and veins. Arteriovenous malformations can range from very small to large.

Cerebral aneurysm—An abnormal, localized bulge in a blood vessel that is usually caused by a congenital weakness in the wall of the vessel.

Cranium—Skull; the bony framework that holds the brain.

Computed tomography (CT)—An imaging technique that produces three-dimensional pictures of organs and structures inside the body using a 360° x-ray beam.

Edema—An accumulation of watery fluid that causes swelling of the affected tissue.

Hematoma—An accumulation of blood, often clotted, in a body tissue or organ, usually caused by a break or tear in a blood vessel.

Hemorrhage—Very severe, massive bleeding that is difficult to control.

Magnetic resonance imaging (MRI)—An imaging technique that uses magnetic fields and radio waves to create detailed images of internal body organs and structures, including the brain.

WHO PERFORMS THE PROCEDURE AND WHERE IS IT PERFORMED?

The procedure is performed in a hospital with a neurosurgery department and an intensive care unit. The procedure is performed by a board certified neurosurgeon, who has completed two years of general surgery training and five years of neurosurgical training.

- CT (computed tomography, uses x-rays and injection of an intravenous dye to visualize the lesion)
- MRI (magnetic resonance imaging, uses magnetic fields and radio waves to visualize a lesion)
- arteriogram (an x-ray of blood vessels injected with a dye to visualize a tumor or cerebral aneurysm)

Before surgery the patient may be given medication to ease anxiety and to decrease the risk of seizures, swelling, and infection after surgery. Blood thinners (Coumadin, heparin, **aspirin**) and **nonsteroidal anti-inflammatory drugs** (ibuprofen, Motrin, Advil, aspirin, Naprosyn, Daypro) have been correlated with an increase in blood clot formation after surgery. These medications must be discontinued at least seven days before the surgery to reverse any blood thinning effects. Additionally, the surgeon will order routine or special laboratory tests as needed. The patient should not eat or drink after midnight the day of the surgery. The patient's scalp is shaved in the **operating room** just before the surgery begins.

Aftercare

Craniotomy is a major surgical procedure performed under **general anesthesia**. Immediately after surgery, the patient's pupil reactions are tested, mental status is assessed after anesthesia, and movement of the limbs (arms/legs) is evaluated. Shortly after surgery, breathing exercises are started to clear the lungs. Typically, after surgery patients are given medications to control pain, swelling, and seizures. Codeine may be prescribed to relive headache. Special leg stockings are used to prevent blood clot formation after surgery. Patients can usually get out of bed in about a day after surgery and usually are hospitalized for five to 14 days after surgery. The **bandages** on the skull are removed and replaced regularly. The sutures closing the scalp are removed by the surgeon, but the soft wires used to reattach the portion of the skull that was removed are permanent and require no further

pattern of holes through the cranium (skull) and uses a fine wire saw to connect the holes until a segment of bone (bone flap) can be removed. This gives the surgeon access to the inside of the skill and allows him to proceed with surgery inside the brain. After removal of the internal brain lesion or other procedure is completed, the bone is replaced and secured into position with soft wire. Membranes, muscle, and skin are sutured into position. If the lesion is an aneurysm, the affected artery is sealed at the leak. If there is a tumor, as much of it as possible is resected (removed). For arteriovenous malformations, the abnormality is clipped and the repair redirects the blood flow to normal vessels.

Diagnosis/Preparation

Since the lesion is in the brain, the surgeon uses imaging studies to definitively identify it. Neuroimaging is usually accomplished by the following:

attention. Patients should keep the scalp dry until the sutures are removed. If required (depending on area of brain involved), occupational therapists and physical therapist assess, the patient's status postoperatively and help the patient improve strength, daily living skills and capabilities, and speech. Full recovery may take up to two months, since it is common for patients to feel fatigued for up to eight weeks after surgery.

Risks

The surgeon will discuss potential risks associated with the procedure. Neurosurgical procedures may result in bleeding, blood clots, retention of fluid causing swelling (edema), or unintended injury to normal nerve tissues. Some patients may develop infections. Damage to normal brain tissue may cause damage to an area and subsequent loss of brain function. Loss of function in specific areas can cause memory impairment. Some other examples of potential damage that may result from this procedure include deafness, double vision, numbness, paralysis, blindness, or loss of the sense of smell.

Normal results

Normal results depend on the cause for surgery and the patient's overall health status and age. If the operation was successful and uncomplicated recovery is quick, since there is a rich blood supply to the area. Recovery could take up to eight weeks, but patients are usually fully functioning in less time.

Morbidity and mortality rates

There is no information about the rates of diseases and **death** specifically related to craniotomy. The operation is performed as a neurosurgical intervention for several different diseases and conditions.

Alternatives

There are no alternative treatments if a neurosurgeon deems this procedure as necessary.

Resources

BOOKS

Connolly, E. Sanders, ed. *Fundamentals of Operative Techniques in Neurosurgery.* New York: Thieme Medical Publishers, 2002.

Greenberg, Mark S. *Handbook of Neurosurgery.* 5th ed. New York: Thieme Medical Publishers, 2000.

Miller, R. *Anesthesia.* 5th ed. Philadelphia, PA: Churchill Livingstone, 2000.

PERIODICALS

Gebel, J. M., and W. J. Powers. "Emergency Craniotomy for Intracerebral Hemorrhage: When Doesn't It Help and Does It Ever Help?" *Neurology* 58 (May 14, 2002): 1325-1326.

Mamminen, P., and T. K. Tan. "Postoperative Nausea and Vomiting After Craniotomy for Tumor Surgery: A Comparison Between Awake Craniotomy and General Anesthesia." *Journal of Clinical Anesthesia* 14 (June 2002): 279-283.

Osguthorpe, J. D., and S. Patel, eds. "Skull Base Tumor Surgery." *Otolaryngologic Clinics of North America* 34 (December 2001).

Rabinstein, A. A., J. L. Atkinson, and E. F. M. Wijdicks. "Emergency Craniotomy in Patients Worsening Due to Expanded Cerebral Hematoma: To What Purpose?" *Neurology* 58 (May 14, 2002): 1367-1372.

ORGANIZATIONS

American Association of Neurological Surgeons. 5550 Meadowbrook Drive, Rolling Meadows, IL 60008. (888) 566-AANS (2267). Fax: (847) 378-0600. E-mail: info@aans.org. http://www.neurosurgery.org/aans/index.asp.

Laith Farid Gulli, M.D., M.S.
Nicole Mallory, M.S., PA-C
Robert Ramirez, B.S.

Creatine kinase test *see* **Cardiac marker tests**

Creatine phosphokinase (CPK)

Definition

Creatine phosphokinase or CPK is an enzyme found in cells that is used to turn creatine into phosphate. This phosphate is a quick source of cellular energy. Muscle cells are the primary source of CPK in the body. The CPK test measures the amount of CPK present in the bloodstream.

Purpose

Because damaged muscle tissue releases CPK into the blood, the detected levels are an indication of the extent and time of the damage. There are different forms of CPK (CPK isoenzymes) that can help determine what tissue has been damaged.

Precautions

There are many variables that contribute to the amount of enzymes present in the bloodstream, including a person's activity level and even if a person is taking a certain type of medication or drug. In a healthy adult, the normal range of total CPK falls between 22 to 198 (units per liter). CPK levels higher than this indicate that muscle damage has occurred. If the CPK test result is elevated, further tests are performed to determine where the muscle damage occurred. There are many causes for elevated levels of CPK. For this reason, the general total CPK test is only approximately 70% accurate. The CPK isoenzyme testing is more specific and therefore approximately 90% accurate.

Drugs that may increase CPK levels:

- Ampicillen
- Anticoagulants
- Alcohol
- Cocaine
- Aspirin
- Morphine
- Furosemide
- Dexamethasone
- Clofibrate
- Amphotericin B
- Isotretinoin (acne treatment)
- Some anesthetics

Description of CPK Isoenzyme Testing

CPK is composed of three different isoenzymes:

- CPK-1 (CPK-BB) is concentrated in the brain and lungs
- CPK-2 (CPK-MB)is found mostly in heart tissue
- CPK-3 (CPK-MM)is found mostly in skeletal muscle

If the level of CPK-1 is elevated that would indicate that the damage occurred to the brain or lung tissue. For the brain, this could mean, a stroke, brain cancer, brain injury, or a seizure. For the lungs, elevated levels could indicate a pulmonary embolism. If the level of CPK-2 is elevated, that would indicate that the damage has occurred in the heart tissue. For the heart, this could mean a heart attack has occurred.

CPK-2 levels rise 3-6 hours after a heart attack, peak at 12-24 hours and will return to normal 12-48 hours after tissue damage occurs. Elevated CPK-2 levels could also indicate other heart trauma, myocarditis, or electrical injuries. CPK-3 levels that are elevated usually indicate an injury or stress to skeletal muscle. For skeletal muscle this could indicate strenuous exercise, seizures, injury or trauma to muscle tissue, multiple intramuscular injections, myositis or muscular dystrophy. Individuals who are affected with certain types of muscular dystrophy may have levels of CPK as high as 15,000 to 35,000 (units per liter).

Preparation

CPK levels are obtained by a routine blood draw. There is no preparation for the blood draw, except that individuals should avoid vigorous or prolonged exercise prior to the test. The test may be repeated several times over a period of time to look for significant rising or falling of the CPK levels.

Aftercare

Aftercare following a routine blood test consists of care of the area around the puncture site. Pressure is applied for a few seconds prior to covering the wound with a bandage.

Risks

The risks associated with routine blood draw include bruising, swelling or excessive bleeding from the puncture site and dizziness or fainting may occur during or shortly after the blood draw.

Normal Results

As stated above, in a healthy adult, the normal range of total CPK falls between 22 to 198 (units per liter).

Resources

BOOKS

Segen, J.C. and J. Wade. *Patient's Guide to Medical Tests: Everything You Need to Know About the Tests Your Doctor Orders.* New York, Checkmark Books, 2002.

PERIODICALS

Kymak, Y. "Creatine Phosphokinase Values During Isotretinoin Treatment For Acne." *International Journal of
Dermatology* 47 (April 2008): 398–401.

OTHER

GeneTests, 9725 Third Avenue NE, Suite 602, Seattle, WA
98115. Funded by the National Institutes of Health.
http://www.genetests.org.

Medline Plus, A service of the U.S. National Library of
Medicine and the NIH, 8600 Rockville Pike, Bethesda,
MD 20894. http://www.nlm.nih.gov/medlineplus/ency/
article/003503.htm.

Renee Laux, M.S.

Creatinine test *see* **Kidney function tests**

Cricothyroidotomy

Definition

Cricothyroidotomy is usually regarded as an
emergency surgical procedure in which a surgeon or
other trained person cuts a hole through a membrane
in the patient's neck into the windpipe in order to
allow air into the lungs. Cricothyroidotomy is a sub-
type of surgical procedure known as a **tracheotomy**; in
some situations, it is considered an elective alternative
to other types of tracheotomy.

Purpose

The primary purpose of a cricothyroidotomy is to
provide an emergency breathing passage for a patient
whose airway is closed by traumatic injury to the neck;
by burn inhalation injuries; by closing of the airway
due to an allergic reaction to bee or wasp stings; or by
unconsciousness. It may also be performed in some
seriously ill patients with structural abnormalities in
the neck. Some surgeons consider a cricothyroidotomy to be preferable to a standard tracheotomy in
treating patients in an **intensive care unit**.

Demographics

The demographics of cricothyroidotomies are difficult to establish because the procedure is relatively
uncommon in the general population, even in emergency situations. In the emergency room, the incidence
varied between 1.7% and 2.7%. A study found that
nine of a group of 1,560 patients admitted for blunt or
penetrating injuries of the neck required emergency
cricothyroidotomies, or about 0.5%.

Another study found that the most important
single cause of injuries requiring emergency cricothyroidotomy was traffic accidents (51%), followed by
gunshot and knife wounds (29%); falls (5%); and
criminal assault (5%).

Most cricothyroidotomies are performed on adolescent and young adult males, because this group accounts
for the majority of cases of neck trauma in the United
States. It is estimated that injuries to the neck account
for 5–10% of all serious traumatic injuries.

Description

There are two basic types of cricothyroidotomy: needle cricothyroidotomy and surgical cricothyroidotomy.

Needle cricothyroidotomy

In a needle cricothyroidotomy, a syringe with a
needle attached is used to make a puncture hole
through the cricothyroid membrane that overlies the
trachea. After the needle has reached the trachea, a
catheter is passed over the needle into the windpipe
and attached to a bag-valve device.

Surgical cricothyroidotomy

In a surgical cricothyroidotomy, the doctor or
other emergency worker makes an incision through
the cricothyroid membrane into the trachea in order
to insert a piece of tubing for ventilating the patient.

Diagnosis/Preparation

The primary concerns in emergency medical treatment are sometimes known as the ABCs: airway patency
(openness), breathing, and circulation. Keeping the airway patent is critical to an injured person's survival. The
signs of a blocked airway in people are obvious, including a bluish complexion (cyanosis); noisy breathing,
unusual breath sounds, or choking; emotional agitation
or panic; and often loss of consciousness.

In an emergency situation, the following are considered reasons for performing a cricothyroidotomy
first, rather than attempting to open or clear the
patient's airway by other methods:

• Major injuries to the face or jaw, such as multiple
  fractures of the jawbone or severe fractures of the
  patient's midface. In many cases of facial injury, the
  airway is blocked by broken teeth or fragments of
  bone from the jaw and cheekbones.

• Burns in or around the mouth.

• A neurological disorder or damage that has caused
  the patient's teeth to clamp shut.

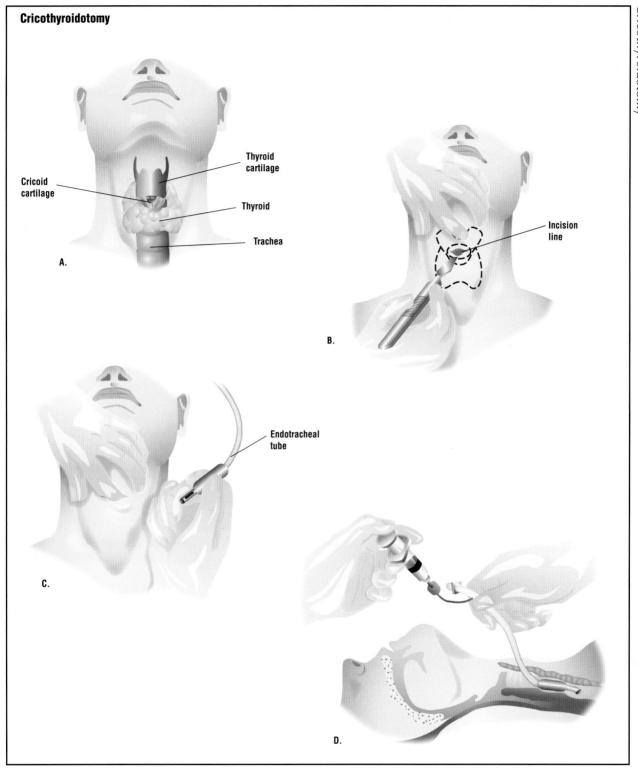

Cricothyroidotomy

A.

Cricoid
cartilage

Thyroid
cartilage

Thyroid

Trachea

B.

Incision
line

C.

Endotracheal
tube

D.

To perform a cricothyroidotomy, the surgeon into the cricoid cartilage of the throat (B). The incision is held open while an endotracheal tube is inserted (C). The tube is secured in the trachea to maintain an airway for the patient (D). *(Illustration by GGS Information Services. Cengage Learning, Gale.)*

KEY TERMS

Airway—The passageway through the mouth, nose, and throat that allows air to enter and leave the lungs; the term can also refer to a tube or other artificial device used to create an air passageway into and out of the lungs when the patient is under general anesthesia or unable to breathe properly.

Cricoid cartilage—A ring-shaped piece of cartilage that forms the lower and rear parts of the voice box or larynx; it is sometimes called the annular cartilage because of its shape.

Cricothyroid membrane—The piece of connective tissue that lies between the thyroid and cricoid cartilages.

Cyanosis—A bluish discoloration of the skin, caused by a loss of oxygen content in the blood.

Endotracheal intubation—A procedure in which a tube is inserted into the trachea in order to administer anesthesia or ventilate the patient.

Hypercarbia—An excess of carbon dioxide in the blood.

Patency—Being wide open, as in a patient's airway.

Pneumothorax—A condition in which air or gas has accumulated in the space in the chest around the lungs.

Subglottic stenosis—An abnormal narrowing of the trachea below the level of the vocal cords.

Thyroid cartilage—The largest cartilage in the human larynx, or voice box. It is sometimes called the Adam's apple.

Trachea—The windpipe.

Tracheotomy—The surgical creation of an opening into the windpipe through the neck; it is also called a tracheostomy.

Transtracheal jet ventilation (TTJV)—A technique for ventilating a patient that involves passing oxygen under pressure through a catheter that has been passed through the patient's cricothyroid membrane.

Ventilate—To assist a patient's breathing by use of a mechanical device or surgical procedure.

- Fractured larynx. Fractures of the larynx most commonly result from automobile or motorcycle accidents, but also occur in cases of strangulation or attempted suicide by hanging.

- Larynx swollen shut by allergic reaction to bee or wasp venom.

Preparation

The first steps in preparation are the same for needle and surgical cricothyroidotomies. The patient is positioned lying on the back with a towel under the shoulders and the neck stretched backward (hyperextended). If the patient is conscious, he or she is given a local anesthetic. The doctor then palpates, or feels, the patient's throat for the thyroid cartilage, or Adam's apple. This piece of cartilage is an anatomical landmark for this procedure, which means that it is a structure that is relatively easy to identify and serves as a reference point for other structures. In men, the Adam's apple is easy to find by running the finger down the center of the neck. In women, however, the thyroid cartilage is less prominent. Below the thyroid cartilage is a softer area about the width of a finger; this is the cricothyroid membrane, which is a piece of tissue lying between the thyroid cartilage above it and the cricoid cartilage below it.

When the doctor has located the cricothyroid membrane, he or she will scrub the skin over it with a povidone-iodine solution to prevent infection.

Needle cricothyroidotomy

In a needle cricothyroidotomy, the doctor uses a 12- or 14-gauge catheter and needle assembly. The needle is advanced through the cricothyroid cartilage at a 45-degree angle until the trachea is reached. When the doctor is able to withdraw air through the syringe, he or she knows that the catheter is in the correct spot. The catheter is then pushed forward over the needle, which is then removed. An endotracheal tube connector is then fitted onto the end of the catheter and connected to a bag-valve unit with an oxygen reservoir.

A needle cricothyroidotomy will supply the patient with enough oxygen for about 40–45 minutes; it is a time-limited technique because it does not allow the efficient escape of carbon dioxide from the bloodstream. It will, however, help to ventilate the patient until he or she can be taken to a hospital or trauma center.

Needle cricothyroidotomy is the only form of this procedure that can be done in children under 12 years of age. The reason for this restriction is that the upper part of the trachea is not fully developed in children, and a surgical incision through the cricothyroid membrane increases the risk of the child's developing subglottic stenosis, which is a condition in which the trachea is abnormally narrow below the level of the vocal cords due to an overgrowth of soft tissue. It is often seen in children who were intubated as infants.

Surgical cricothyroidotomy

In a surgical cricothyroidotomy, the doctor steadies the patient's thyroid cartilage with one hand and makes a horizontal (transverse) incision across the cricothyroid membrane. The incision is deepened until the airway is reached. The doctor then rotates the edge of the scalpel 90° in order to open the incision to receive an endotracheal or tracheotomy tube. A hemostat or surgical clamp may be used to hold the incision open while the doctor prepares to insert the tube through the opening into the trachea. After checking the tube to make certain that it is in the proper location, the doctor tapes it in place. If necessary, the doctor may use suction to clear the patient's airway.

In some emergency situations, the doctor or other medical professional may not have an antiseptic available to cleanse the skin over the patient's throat, and may have to use any sharp-edged implement that is handy to make the incision. Emergency cricothyroidotomies have been performed with scissors, hunting or pocketknives, razor blades, broken glass, and the jagged edges of a lid from a tin can. The airway has been held open with such objects as paper clips, nail clippers, the plastic barrel from a ballpoint pen, and a piece of plastic straw from a sports water bottle.

Aftercare

Needle cricothyroidotomy

A needle cricothyroidotomy must be replaced by a formal surgical tracheotomy or other means of ventilating the patient within 45 minutes.

Surgical cricothyroidotomy

A surgical cricothyroidotomy can be left in place for about 24 hours, but should be replaced within that time period by a formal tracheotomy performed in a hospital **operating room**.

Other aspects of aftercare depend on the cause of the airway blockage and the nature of the patient's injuries. The head and neck contain major blood vessels, a large portion of the central nervous system, the organs of sight, smell, hearing, and taste, and the central airway—all within a relatively small area. Injuries to the face and neck often require treatment by specialists in neurology,

trauma surgery, otolaryngology, ophthalmology, and **plastic surgery** as well as by specialists in emergency medicine.

Risks

Needle cricothyroidotomy

The risks of a needle cricothyroidotomy include:

- external scar from needle puncture
- bleeding
- accidental perforation of the esophagus
- hypercarbia (overly high levels of carbon dioxide in the blood)

Surgical cricothyroidotomy

The risks of surgical cricothyroidotomy include:

- large visible external scar from the incision
- subglottic stenosis
- bleeding
- accidental perforation of the esophagus
- fracture of the larynx
- pneumothorax, a condition in which air has entered the space around the lungs
- damage to the vocal cords resulting in hoarseness or a changed voice

Normal results

Needle cricothyroidotomy

Normal results for a needle cricothyroidotomy would be adequate ventilation of a patient with a blocked airway for a brief period of time of about 45 minutes.

Surgical cricothyroidotomy

Normal results of a surgical cricothyroidotomy would be adequate ventilation in emergency circumstances of a patient with a blocked airway for a period of about 24 hours.

Morbidity and mortality rates

In general, cricothyroiditomy has a very low mortality rate, even when performed outside a hospital. By contrast, the mortality rate for patients who lose airway patency is 33%. Overall, emergency cricothyroidotomy is considered an effective way to create an emergency surgical airway with low overall morbidity.

WHO PERFORMS THE PROCEDURE AND WHERE IS IT PERFORMED?

Under ideal circumstances, a cricothyroidotomy would be performed in a hospital emergency room, ICU, or trauma center by a general surgeon, otolaryngologist, or anesthesiologist. Because it is an emergency procedure, however, a medical student, physician's assistant, paramedic, or nurse may also perform cricothyroidotomies. Many trauma centers require paramedics and nurses specializing in emergency medicine to practice performing cricothyroidotomies at least twice a year in a clinical laboratory in order to keep their skill level high. Since the procedure is risky but uncommon, it is important for emergency personnel to feel comfortable with the equipment and techniques required.

Military personnel are trained to perform emergency cricothyroidotomies in combat situations. There are also cases reported of cricothyroidotomies being done in emergencies by civilian bystanders with some medical training.

Alternatives

Cricothyroidotomy is generally considered a procedure of last resort, to be performed when other ways of opening the patient's airway have failed or are unavailable. It is frequently done if **endotracheal intubation** has been attempted and failed, or if intubation cannot be performed due to the nature of the patient's injuries. Endotracheal intubation is a procedure in which a breathing tube is introduced directly into the trachea through the patient's mouth or nose with the help of a laryngoscope. It is most commonly done during **general anesthesia**, but can also be performed to help the patient breathe.

One alternative to cricothyroidotomy is a technique known as transtracheal jet ventilation (TTJV). In TTJV, a syringe is used to introduce a catheter through the patient's cricothyroid membrane. The catheter is connected to a high-pressure oxygen supply. In hospital settings, TTJV has about the same rate of complications as a surgical cricothyroidotomy. Its disadvantages are that it cannot be used outside a hospital setting and it takes longer to perform. A surgical cricothyroidotomy can be performed in 30 seconds to two minutes; TTJV takes twice to three times as long to perform.

QUESTIONS TO ASK THE DOCTOR

- Am I likely to have lasting side effects from this emergency procedure?

Resources

BOOKS

Gomella, Leonard G., and Alan T. Lefor. *Surgery On Call*, 3rd ed. New York: McGraw-Hill/Appleton & Lange, 2001.

PERIODICALS

Adams, B. D., and W. L. Whitlock. "Bystander Cricothyroidotomy Performed with an Improvised Airway." *Military Medicine* 167 (January 2002): 76–78.

Bennett, John D. C. "Securing the Airway in Burns." *Journal of Burns* 1 (2002): 1 [cited March 8, 2003]. www.journalofburns.com.

Flynn, Sean. "How to Save a Soldier." *New York Times Magazine* March 16, 2003. www.nytimes.com/2003/03/16/magazine/16BATTLE.html.

Francois, B., et al. "Complications of Tracheostomy Performed in the ICU: Subthyroid Tracheostomy vs Surgical Cricothyroidotomy." *Chest* 123 (January 2003): 151–158.

Gillespie, M. B., and D. W. Eisele. "Outcomes of Emergency Surgical Airway Procedures in a Hospital-wide Setting." *Laryngoscope* 109 (November 1999): 1766–1769.

Hayden, S. R., and E. A. Panacek. "Procedural Competency in Emergency Medicine: The Current Range of Resident Experience." *Academic Emergency Medicine* 6 (July 1999): 728–735.

Janson, Paul, and Richard Iseke. "Hymenoptera Stings." *eMedicine* July 26, 2002 [cited March 9, 2003]. www.emedicine.com/med/topic1058.htm.

Levy, David, and Robert Buckman. "Neck Trauma." *eMedicine* June 21, 2001 [cited March 8, 2003]. www.emedicine.com/emerg/topic331.htm.

Parsa, Tatiana, Arthur Adamo, and Yvette Calderon. "Initial Evaluation and Management of Maxillofacial Injuries." *eMedicine* August 28, 2002 [cited March 8, 2003]. www.emedicine.com/med/topic3222.htm.

Rehm, C. G., et al. "Cricothyroidotomy for Elective Airway Management in Critically Ill Trauma Patients with Technically Challenging Neck Anatomy." *Critical Care* 6 (December 2002): 531–535.

Torres, Manuel. "Case Study: Airway and Facial Trauma." *Stat Page: Newsletter of the Center for Emergency Medicine*, 8 (February 1997): 6–7.

Vassiliu, P., et al. "Aerodigestive Injuries of the Neck." *American Surgeon* 67 (January 2001): 75–79.

ORGANIZATIONS

Center for Emergency Medicine. 230 McKee Place, Suite 500, Pittsburgh, PA 15213. (412) 647-5300. www.centerem.com.

National Association of Emergency Medical Technicians (NAEMT). P. O. Box 1400, Clinton, MS 39060-1400. (800) 34-NAEMT. www.naemt.org.

University of Maryland Medical Center, R. Adams Cowley Shock Trauma Center. 22 South Greene Street, Baltimore, MD 21201. (410) 328-2757 or (800) 373-4111. www.umm.edu/shocktrauma.

OTHER

Jaberi, Mahmood, Kimberley Mitchell, and Colin Mackenzie. *Cricothyroidotomy: Good, Bad, or Ugly?* Third Place Scientific Award, 14th Trauma Anesthesia and Critical Care Symposium, San Diego, CA, May 17, 2001.

Rebecca Frey, PhD

Cryosurgery *see* **Cryotherapy**

Cryosurgery for retinal detachment *see* **Retinal cryopexy**

Cryotherapy

Definition

Cryotherapy is a technique that uses an extremely cold liquid or instrument to freeze and destroy abnormal cells that require removal. The technique has been in use since the turn of the century, but modern techniques have made it widely available to dermatologists and primary care doctors. The technique is also known as cryocautery or cryosurgery.

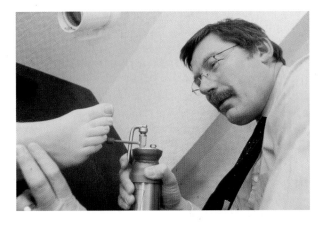

A doctor using cryotherapy to remove warts from patient's foot. (*Pulse Picture Library, Inc./Phototake. Reproduced by permission.*)

Purpose

Cryotherapy is used to destroy a variety of benign skin growths, such as warts, precancerous lesions (actinic keratoses), and malignant lesions (basal cell and squamous cell cancers). It has been used at several medical centers for tumors of the prostate, liver, lung, breast, and brain as well as for cataracts, gynecological problems, and other diseases. The goal of cryotherapy is to freeze and destroy targeted skin growths while preserving the surrounding skin from injury.

Description

In dermatology applications, there are three main techniques used in cryotherapy. In the simplest technique, usually reserved for warts and other benign skin growths, the physician dips a cotton swab or other applicator into a cup containing a "cryogen" such as liquid nitrogen and applies it directly to the skin growth to freeze it. At a temperature of $-320°F$ ($-196°C$), liquid nitrogen is the coldest cryogen available. The goal is to freeze the skin growth as quickly as possible, and then let it thaw slowly to cause maximum destruction of the skin cells. A second application may be necessary depending on the size of the growth. In another approach, a device is used to direct a small spray of liquid nitrogen or other cryogen directly onto the skin growth. Freezing may last from five to 20 seconds, depending on the size of the lesion. A second freeze-thaw cycle may be required. Sometimes, the physician inserts a small needle connected to a **thermometer** into the lesion to make certain the lesion is cooled to a temperature low enough to guarantee maximum destruction. In a third option, liquid nitrogen or another cryogen is circulated through a probe to cool it to low temperatures. The probe is then brought into direct contact with the skin lesion to freeze it. The freeze time can take two to three times longer than with the spray technique.

When used for cancer treatment, cryotherapy is usually performed as follows: for external tumors, liquid nitrogen is applied directly to the cancer cells with a cotton swab or spraying device; for internal tumors, liquid nitrogen is circulated through an instrument called a cryoprobe that is placed in contact with the tumor. To guide the cryoprobe and to monitor the freezing of the cells, the treating physician uses **ultrasound** to guide his work and spare nearby healthy tissue.

Preparation

No extensive preparation is required prior to cryotherapy. The area to be treated should be clean and

Actinic keratosis—A crusty, scaly precancerous skin lesion caused by damage from the sun; frequently treated with cryotherapy.

Basal cell cancer—The most common form of skin cancer that usually appears as one or several nodules having a central depression; it rarely spreads (metastasizes), but is locally invasive.

Cervical cryotherapy—Surgery performed after a biopsy has confirmed abnormal cervical cells (dysplasia).

Cryogen—A substance with a very low boiling point, such as liquid nitrogen, used in cryotherapy treatment.

Melanoma—The most dangerous form of skin cancer.

Squamous cell cancer—A form of skin cancer that usually originates in sun-damaged areas or pre-existing lesions; at first local and superficial, it may later spread to other areas of the body.

Ultrasound—Imaging technique by which computerized moving pictures of the body are generated by high-frequency sound waves.

dry, but sterile preparation is not necessary. Patients should know that they will experience some pain at the time of the freezing, but **local anesthesia** is usually not required. In dermatology applications, the physician may want to reduce the size of certain growths such as warts prior to the cryotherapy procedure, and may have patients apply salicylic acid preparations to the growth over several weeks. Sometimes, the physician will pare away some of the tissue using a device called a curette or a scalpel. In the case of **cervical cryotherapy**, the procedure is not performed during, or from two to three days before, the menstrual period.

Aftercare

In dermatology applications, redness, swelling, and the formation of a blister at the site of cryotherapy are all expected results of the treatment. A gauze dressing is applied, and patients should wash the site three or four times daily while fluid continues to ooze from the wound, usually for five to 14 days. A dry crust will form that falls off by itself. Wounds on the head and neck may take four to six weeks to heal, but those on the body, arms, and legs can take longer. Some patients experience pain at the site following the treatment. This can usually be eased with **acetaminophen** (Tylenol),

Cryotherapy is performed by the treating physician, who may be a gynecologist (cervical cryotherapy) or a dermatologist (wart removal) or an oncologist (tumor removal). The procedure is usually carried out on an outpatient basis, but may require a hospital setting depending on the condition requiring the cryotherapy.

though in some cases a stronger pain reliever may be required.

Risks

In dermatology applications, cryotherapy poses little risk and can be well tolerated by elderly and other patients who are not good candidates for other surgical procedures. As with other surgical procedures, there is some risk of scarring, infection, and damage to underlying skin and tissue. These risks are generally minimal in the hands of experienced physicians.

Care should be taken, however, in subjecting people with diabetes or certain circulation problems to cryotherapy for growths located on their lower legs, ankles, and feet. In these patients, healing can be poor and the risk of infection can be higher than for other patients.

Although cryotherapy is a relatively low-risk procedure, some side effects may occur as a result of the treatment. They include:

- Infection—though uncommon, infection is more likely on the lower legs where healing can take several months.
- Pigmentary changes—both hypopigmentation (lightening of the skin) and hyperpigmentation (darkening of the skin) are possible after cryotherapy. Both generally last a few months, but can be longer lasting.
- Nerve damage—though rare, damage to nerves is possible, particularly in areas where they lie closer to the surface of the skin, such as the fingers, the wrist, and the area behind the ear. Reports suggest this will disappear within several months.

In cancer treatment, cryosurgery does have side effects, although they may be less severe than those associated with conventional surgery or radiation therapy. Cryosurgery of the liver may cause damage to the bile ducts or major blood vessels, which can lead to heavy bleeding or infection. Cryosurgery for prostate cancer may affect the urinary system. It also may cause incontinence (lack of control over urine flow) and impotence (loss of sexual function), although these side effects are often temporary. Cryosurgery for cervical tumors has not been shown to affect fertility, but this possibility is under study. More studies must be conducted to determine the long-term effects of cryosurgery as a cancer treatment approach.

Normal results

Some redness, swelling, blistering, and oozing of fluid are all common results of cryotherapy. Healing time can vary depending on the site treated and the cryotherapy technique used. When cryogen is applied directly to the growth, healing may occur in three weeks. Growths treated on the head and neck with the spray technique may take four to six weeks to heal, while growths treated on other areas of the body may take considerably longer. Cryotherapy boasts high success rates in permanently removing skin growths; even for malignant lesions such as squamous cell and basal cell cancers, studies have shown a cure rate of up to 98%. For certain types of growths, such as some forms of warts, repeat treatments over several weeks are necessary to prevent the growth's return.

Alternatives

Alternatives to cryotherapy depend on the specific medical condition being treated. A general alternative is the use of conventional surgical procedures.

Resources

BOOKS

Chan, Paul D., David M. Thomas, and Elizabeth K. Stanford. *Outpatient and Primary Care Medicine.* Mission Viejo, CA: Current Clinical Strategies, 2008.

Jackson, Arthur D., Graham Colver, and Rodney Dawber. *Cutaneous Cryosurgery: Principles and Clinical Practice,* 3rd ed. UK: Informa Healthcare, 2005.

Korpan, N. N. *Basics of Cryosurgery.* New York: Springer Verlag, 2002.

PERIODICALS

Housman, T. S., and J. L. Jorizzo. "Anecdotal Reports of Three Cases Illustrating a Spectrum of Resistant Common Warts Treated with Cryotherapy Followed by Topical Imiquimod and Salicylic Acid." *Journal of the American Academy of Dermatology* 47 (October 2002): 217–220.

Otte, J. W., M. A. Merrick, C. D. Ingersoll, and M. L. Cordova. "Subcutaneous Adipose Tissue Thickness Alters Cooling Time during Cryotherapy." *Archives of Physical and Medical Rehabilitation* 83 (November 2002): 1501–1505.

Uchio, Y., M. Ochi, A. Fujihara, N. Adachi, J. Iwasa, and Y. Sakai. "Cryotherapy Influences Joint Laxity and Position Sense of the Healthy Knee Joint." *Archives of Physical and Medical Rehabilitation* 84 (January 2003): 131–135.

Wozniacka, A., A. Omulecki, and J. D. Torzecka. "Cryotherapy in the Treatment of Angiolymphoid Hyperplasia with Eosinophilia." *Medical Science Monitor* 9 (January 2003): CS1–CS4.

OTHER

Scott Moses. "Cryotherapy." *Family Practice Notebook.* March 10, 2008. http://www.fpnotebook.com/DER/Procedure/Crythrpy.htm [Accessed April 11, 2008].

ORGANIZATIONS

American Academy of Dermatology, 930 N. Meacham Road, P.O. Box 4014, Schaumburg, IL, 60168-4014, (847) 330-0230, (847) 240-1859, http://www.aad.org.

American Society for Dermatologic Surgery, 555 Meadowbrook Drive, Suite 120, Rolling Meadows, IL, 60008, (847) 956-0900, http://www.asds.net.

Richard H. Camer
Monique Laberge, Ph.D.
Laura Jean Cataldo, R.N., Ed.D.

Cryotherapy for cataracts

Definition

Cryosurgery, or **cryotherapy**, is a technique that destroys abnormal tissue by freezing the cells. Cryotherapy can be used in the treatment of cataracts.

Purpose

The procedure is used to treat cataracts. A cataract is a form of clouding that develops in the lens of the eye. The crystalline lens consists mainly of protein matter and water. Normally, the protein is packed so as to allow light to pass through the lens. A cataract forms when protein molecules start aggregating and clump together, eventually clouding the lens and blocking light. If left untreated, cataracts may eventually cause blindness. Cryotherapy is performed to remove the clouding protein matter from the lens.

Demographics

According to the National Institutes of Health, more than 50% of people over the age of 80 in the United States have a cataract or have had cataract surgery. Some estimates put this figure at 70% or more. Women are affected by cataracts more often than men. African Americans suffer impaired vision from both cataracts and glaucoma at twice the rate of Caucasian Americans, primarily due to lack of treatment.

Description

Cryotherapy involves the application of a very cold probe to the outside of the eye, which, because of the thin nature of the eye wall (sclera), transmits the freezing temperature to the retina. The intense cold stimulation to the retina can seal abnormal leaky retinal blood vessels. This technique is indicated for the treatment of cataracts that obscure the passage of light into the eye, thus limiting the effectiveness of techniques such as laser therapy.

Cryotherapy uses a cryogenic substance, such as liquid nitrogen, to freeze the cataract. At a temperature of -320°F (-196°C), liquid nitrogen is the coldest cryogenic substance available. The ophthalmologist uses a device to direct a small spray of liquid nitrogen directly onto the cataract. Freezing may last from 5 to 20 seconds, depending on the size of the cataract. A second freeze-thaw cycle may be required. Sometimes, the ophthalmologist will insert a small needle connected to a **thermometer** to make certain the cataract is cooled to a low enough temperature to guarantee destruction. In another option, liquid nitrogen or another cryogen is circulated through a probe to cool it to low temperatures. The probe is then brought into direct contact with the cataract to freeze it. The freeze time can take two to three times longer than with the spray technique.

Diagnosis/Preparation

In order to see the back of the eye properly, the examining ophthalmologist uses two powerful microscopes, the slit lamp and ophthalmoscope. Eye drops are also often used to make the pupil bigger, so that

---

---

the back of the eye can be seen more clearly. The effect of these drops wears off after a few hours. Once a cataract has been diagnosed and has progressed to the point that it is interfering with daily activities and normal lifestyle, an appointment is made to treat the cataract.

For cryotherapy, the patient may be asked to skip breakfast, depending on the time of surgery. Upon arrival for cryotherapy, he or she is given eye drops, and perhaps medications to help relax. A local or topical anesthetic is used to make the procedure painless. The patient may see light and movement, but will not be able to see the cryotherapy when it is performed. The skin around the eye is thoroughly cleansed, and sterile coverings are placed around the patient's head.

Aftercare

After cryotherapy, a patch is placed over the operated eye and the patient is asked to rest for a while. The attending physician checks to see if there are any problems, such as bleeding. Most people who have cataract cryotherapy go home the same day. Arrangements for transportation home should be made because individuals cannot drive after cataract surgery. After the procedure, the doctor schedules exams to check the progress of the vision. Eyedrops or pills may be given to help healing and to control pressure inside the eye. The patient is also asked to wear an eye shield or eyeglasses to help protect the eye, and he or she is told to avoid rubbing or pressing on the eye, and to not lift heavy objects because bending increases pressure in the

---

WHO PERFORMS THE PROCEDURE AND WHERE IS IT PERFORMED?

Cryotherapy can be done in the treating doctor's office. The doctor is usually an ophthalmologist, specialized in the treatment of cataracts. An ophthalmologist is a physician who specializes in the medical and surgical care of the eyes and visual system and in the prevention of eye disease and injury. He has completed four or more years of college premedical education, four or more years of medical school, one year of internship, and three or more years of specialized medical, surgical, and refractive training and experience in eye care.

QUESTIONS TO ASK THE DOCTOR

- Will my vision improve?
- What are the risks of cryotherapy?
- What is the likely hood of pain during or after surgery?
- How long will it take to recover from the surgery?
- What are the likely side-effects of cryotherapy?
- How much cryotherapy do you perform each year for cataracts?

eye. Walking, climbing stairs, and light household chores can be performed.

Risks

Narcotic analgesia may be required after the procedure to relieve pain. Cryotherapy also causes significant swelling of the eye and eyelid, which makes postoperative assessment difficult. Problems after cryotherapy are rare, but can occur and may include infection, bleeding, inflammation (pain, redness, swelling), loss of vision, or light flashes. With careful medical attention, these problems usually can be treated successfully.

Normal results

Surgical treatment for cataracts usually results in excellent vision; however, if other problems are present besides the cataract, as, for example, degeneration of the retina or optic nerve, results will not be as favorable.

Alternatives

The alternative treatment for cataracts is surgical cataract removal, which is one of the most common surgical procedures performed in the United States. Approximately 90% of patients who undergo this surgery experience improved vision. Two procedures are commonly used to surgically remove a cataract: phacoemulsification and extracapsular surgery. During phacoemulsification a small cut is made in the cornea, and a probe that emits ultrasonic waves is inserted into the eye. The ultrasonic waves break up the lens, which is then suctioned out of the eye. During extracapsular the doctor makes a larger cut in the eye and removes the majority of the lens in one piece.

There are no medications, dietary supplements, exercises, or optical devices that have been shown to prevent or cure cataracts.

Resources

BOOKS

Chang, David F., and Howard Gimbel. *Cataracts: A Patient's Guide to Treatment.* Omaha, NE: Addicus Books, 2004.

Hockwin, O., M. Kojima, N. Takahashi, and D. H. Sliney, eds. *Progress in Lens and Cataract Research.* New York: Karger, 2002.

Malhotra, Raman. *Cataract.* New York: Butterworth Heinemann, 2008.

PERIODICALS

Medow, Norman B. "Cryotherapy: A Fall from Grace, But Not a Crash." *Ophthalmology Times* 30, no. 20 (October 15, 2005): 66.

OTHER

Cataract Brochure. American Academy of Ophthalmology. 2002.

ORGANIZATIONS

American Academy of Ophthalmology, P.O. Box 7424, San Francisco, CA, 94120-7424, (415) 561-8500, http://www.aao.org.

New England Ophthalmological Society, P.O. Box 9165, Boston, MA, 02114, (617) 227-6484, http://www.neos-eyes.org.

Monique Laberge, Ph.D.
Robert Bockstiegel

Cryotherapy for the cervix *see* **Cervical cryotherapy**

CSF analysis *see* **Cerebrospinal fluid (CSF) analysis**

CT-myelogram *see* **Myelography**

CT scans

Definition

Computed tomography (CT) scans are completed with the use of a 360-degree X-ray beam and computer production of images. These scans allow for cross-sectional views of body organs and tissues. Computed tomography is also known as computerized axial tomography or CAT scan.

Purpose

CT scans are used to image a wide variety of body structures and internal organs. Since the 1990s, CT equipment has become more affordable and available. In some diagnoses, CT scans have become the first imaging exam of choice. Because the computerized image is so sharp, focused, and three-dimensional, many tissues can be better differentiated than on standard X-rays. Common CT indications include:

- Sinus studies—the CT scan can show details of sinusitis and bone fractures. Physicians may order a CT scan of the sinuses to provide an accurate map for surgery.

- Brain studies—brain scans can detect tumors, strokes, and hematomas (collections of blood that have escaped from the vessels). The introduction of CT scanning, especially spiral CT, has helped reduce the need for more invasive procedures such as cerebral angiography.

- Body scans—CT scans of the body will often be used to observe abdominal organs, such as the liver, kidneys, adrenal glands, spleen, pancreas, biliary tree and lymph nodes, and extremities.

- Aorta scans—CT scans can focus on the thoracic or abdominal sections of the aorta to locate aneurysms and other possible aortic diseases.

- Chest scans—CT scans of the chest are useful in distinguishing tumors and in detailing accumulation of fluid in chest infections.

Description

Computed tomography is a combination of focused x-ray beams, a detector array, and computerized production of an image. Introduced in the early 1970s, this radiologic procedure has advanced rapidly and is now widely used, sometimes in the place of standard X-rays.

KEY TERMS

Aneurysm—The bulging of the blood vessel wall. Aortic aneurysms are the most dangerous. Aneurysms can break and cause bleeding.

Contrast (agent, medium)—A substance injected into the body that delineates certain structures that would otherwise be hard or impossible to see on the radiograph (film).

Gantry—A name for the portion of a CT scanner which houses the X-ray tube and detector array used to capture image information and send it to the computer.

Hematoma—A collection of blood that has escaped from the vessels. It may clot and harden, causing pain to the patient.

Hydrocephalus—Abnormal dilatation of fluid-containing ventricles in the brain.

Metastasis—Secondary cancer, or cancer that has spread from one body organ or tissue to another.

Radiologist—A medical doctor specially trained in radiology (X-ray) interpretation and its use in the diagnosis of disease and injury.

Spiral CT—Also referred to as helical CT, this method allows for continuous 360-degree X-ray image capture.

Thoracic—Refers to the chest area. The thorax runs between the abdomen and neck and is encased in the ribs.

CT equipment

A CT scan may be performed in a hospital or outpatient imaging center. Although the equipment looks large and intimidating, it is very sophisticated and fairly comfortable. The patient is asked to lie on a narrow table that slides into the center of the scanner, called the gantry. The scanner looks like a square doughnut with a round opening in the middle, which allows the X-ray beam to rotate around the patient. The scanner's gantry section may also be tilted slightly to allow for certain cross-sectional angles.

CT procedure

The patient will feel the table move very slightly as the precise adjustments for each sectional image are made. A technologist watches the procedure from a window and views the images on a monitor.

It is essential that the patient lie very still during the procedure to prevent motion blurring. In some studies, such as chest CT scans, the patient will be asked to hold his or her breath during image capture.

Following the procedure, films of the images are usually printed for the radiologist and referring physician to review. A radiologist can also interpret CT exams on a special viewing console. The procedure time will vary in length depending on the area being imaged. Average study times are from 30 to 60 minutes. Some patients may be concerned about claustrophobia, but the width of the gantry portion of the scanner is wide enough to preclude problems with claustrophobia, in most instances.

The CT image

Traditional X-rays image organs in two dimensions, with the possibility that organs in the front of the body are superimposed over those in the back. CT scans allow for a more three-dimensional effect. Some have compared CT images to slices in a loaf of bread. Precise sections of the body can be located and imaged as cross-sectional views. The technologist's console displays a computerized image of each section captured by the X-ray beam and detector array. Thus, various densities of tissue can be easily distinguished.

Contrast agents

Contrast agents are often used in CT exams and in other radiology procedures to demonstrate certain anatomic details that otherwise may not be seen easily. Some contrast agents are natural, such as air or water. Other times, a water-based contrast agent is administered for specific diagnostic purposes. Barium sulfate is commonly used in gastrointestinal procedures. The patient may drink this contrast medium, or receive it in an enema. Oral and rectal contrasts are usually given when examining the abdomen or gastrointestinal tract, and not used when scanning the brain or chest. Iodine-based contrast media are the most widely used intravenous contrast agents and are usually administered through an antecubital (in front of the elbow) vein.

If contrast agents are used in the CT exam, these will be administered several minutes before the study begins. Abdominal CT patients may be asked to drink a contrast medium. Some patients may experience a salty taste, flushing of the face, warmth, slight nausea, or hives from an intravenous contrast injection. Technologists and radiologists have equipment and training to help patients through these minor reactions and to handle more severe reactions. Severe reactions to contrast agents are rare, but do occur.

Spiral CT

Spiral CT, also called helical CT, is a newer version of CT scanning that is continuous in motion and allows for three-dimensional re-creation of images. For example, traditional CT allows the technologist to take slices at very small and precise intervals one after the other. Spiral CT allows for a continuous flow of images, without stopping the scanner to move to the next image slice. A major advantage of spiral CT is higher resolution and the ability to reconstruct images anywhere along the length of the study area. The procedure also speeds up the imaging process, meaning less time for the patient to lie still. The ability to image the contrast medium more rapidly after it is injected and when it is at its highest level, is another advantage of the spiral CT scans high speed.

Some facilities have both spiral and conventional CT available. Although spiral is more advantageous for many applications, conventional CT is still a superior and precise method for imaging many tissues and structures. The physician will evaluate which type of CT works best for the specific exam purpose.

Preparation

If a contrast medium must be administered, the patient may be asked to fast from about four to six hours prior to the procedure. This is so if a patient experiences nausea, vomiting will not occur. Patients will usually be given a hospital gown to wear during the procedure. All metal and jewelry must be removed to avoid artifacts on the film. Pregnant women or those who could possibly be pregnant should not have a CT scan unless the diagnostic benefits outweigh the risks. Contrast agents are often used in CT exams and the use of these agents should be discussed with the medical professional prior to the procedure. Patients may be asked to sign a consent form concerning the administration of contrast media. One common ingredient in contrast agents, iodine, can cause allergic reactions. Patients who are known to be allergic to iodine (or shellfish) should inform the physician prior to the CT scan.

Aftercare

No aftercare is generally required following a CT scan. Immediately following the exam, the technologist will continue to watch the patient for possible adverse contrast reactions. Patients are instructed to advise the technologist of any symptoms, particularly respiratory difficulty. The site of contrast injection will be bandaged and may feel tender following the exam. Hives may develop later and usually do not require treatment.

Risks

Radiation exposure from a CT scan is similar to, though higher than, that of a conventional X-ray. Although this is a risk to pregnant women, the exposure to other adults is minimal and should produce no effects. Severe contrast reactions are rare, but they are a risk of many CT procedures. There is also a small risk of renal failure in high-risk patients.

Normal results

Normal findings on a CT exam show bone, the most dense tissue, as white areas. Tissues and fluid will appear as various shades of gray, and fat will be dark gray or black. Air will also look black and darker than fat tissue. Intravenous, oral, and rectal contrast appear as white areas. The radiologist can determine if tissues and organs appear normal by the different gradations of the gray scale. In CT, the images that can cut through a section of tissue or organ provide three-dimensional viewing for the radiologist and referring physician.

Abnormal results may show different characteristics of tissues within organs. Accumulations of blood or other fluids where they do not belong may be detected. Radiologists can differentiate among types of tumors throughout the body by viewing details of their makeup.

Sinus studies

The increasing availability and lowered cost of CT scanning has led to its increased use in sinus studies, either as a replacement for a sinus X-ray or as a follow-up to an abnormal sinus radiograph. The sensitivity of CT allows for location of areas of sinus infection, particularly chronic infection, and is useful for planning prior to functional **endoscopic sinus surgery**. CT scans can show the extent and location of tiny fractures of the sinus and nasal bones. Foreign bodies in the sinus and nasal area are also easily detected by CT. CT imaging of the sinuses is important in evaluating trauma or disease of the sphenoid bone (the wedge-shaped bone at the base of the skull). Sinus tumors will show as shades of gray indicating the difference in their density from that of normal tissues in the area.

Brain studies

The precise differences in density allowed by CT scanning can clearly show tumors, strokes, or other lesions in the brain area as altered densities. These lighter or darker areas on the image may indicate a tumor or hemorrhage within the brain. Different types of tumors can be identified by the presence of edema, by the tissue's density, or by abnormal contrast enhancement. Congenital abnormalities in children, such as hydrocephalus, may also be confirmed with CT. Hydrocephalus is suggested by enlargement of the fluid structures, called ventricles, of the brain.

Body scans

The body scan can identify abnormal body structures and organs. Throughout the body, a CT scan may indicate tumors or cysts; enlarged lymph nodes; abnormal collections of fluid, blood, or fat; and metastasis of cancer. Fractures or damage to soft tissues can be more easily seen on the sensitive images produced by CT scanning. Liver conditions, such as cirrhosis, abscess, and fatty liver, may be observed with a CT body scan.

The aorta

CT provides the ability to visualize and measure the thickness of the aorta, which is very helpful in diagnosing aortic aneurysms. The use of contrast will help define details within the aorta. In addition, increased areas of density can identify calcification, which helps differentiate between acute and chronic problems. An abnormal CT scan may indicate signs of aortic clots. Aortic rupture is suggested by signs, such as a hematoma around the aorta or the escape of blood or contrast from its cavity.

Chest scans

In addition to those findings which may indicate aortic aneurysms, chest CT studies can show other problems in the heart and lungs. The computer will not only show differences between air, water, tissues, and bone, but will also assign numerical values to the various densities. Mass lesions in the lungs may be indicative of tuberculosis or tumors. CT will help distinguish between the two. Enlarged lymph nodes in the chest area may indicate lymphoma. Spiral CT is particularly effective at identifying pulmonary emboli (clots in the lung's blood vessels).

Resources

BOOKS
Karthikevan, D., and Deepa Chegu. *Step by Step CT Scan.* Kent, UK: Anshan Ltd., 2006

Springhouse Corporation. *Illustrated Guide to Diagnostic Tests.* Springhouse, PA: Springhouse Corporation, 1998.

PERIODICALS

Beauchamp, N., et al. "Imaging of Acute Cerebral Ischemia." *Radiology* 212 (August 1999): 307–324.

OTHER

RadiologyInfo. http://www.radiologyinfo.org.

ORGANIZATIONS

American College of Radiology, 1891 Preston White Drive, Reston, VA, 20191, (800) 227-5463, http://www.acr.org.

Stephen John Hage, A.A.A.S., R.T(R), F.A.H.R.A.
Lee Alan Shratter, M.D.
Laura Jean Cataldo, R.N., Ed.D.

Curettage and electrosurgery

Definition

Curettage is the surgical removal of growths or tissue from the wall of a body cavity or other surface, using a spoon-like instrument with a sharp edge called a curette. Electrosurgery is a procedure that cuts, destroys, or cauterizes tissue using a high-frequency electric current applied locally with a pencil-shaped metal instrument or needle. When the two procedures are combined, the surgery is referred to as curettage and electrosurgery.

Purpose

The general purpose of curettage is to scrape an area free of undesirable tissue. The purposes of electrosurgery are to destroy benign and malignant lesions, control bleeding, and cut or excise tissue.

Specifically, a curettage and electrosurgery procedure is used to treat the following conditions:

- benign skin lesions, such as angiomas, nevis, and warts
- actinic keratoses (AKs), which are premalignant skin lesions
- skin cancers, chiefly basal cell carcinoma (BCC) and cutaneous squamous cell carcinoma (SCC)
- genital warts that result from human papillomavirus (HPV) infection

Demographics

Curettage—with or without electrosurgery—is the second most commonly used treatment in the United

KEY TERMS

Anesthesia—A combination of drugs administered by a variety of techniques by trained professionals that provide sedation, amnesia, analgesia, and immobility adequate for the accomplishment of the surgical procedure with minimal discomfort, and without injury, to the patient.

Anesthetics—Drugs or methodologies used to make a body area free of sensation or pain.

Basal cell carcinoma—Basal cell carcinoma is the most common malignant tumor, affecting more than 800,000 people annually in the United States.

Curettage—Procedure performed with a curette, a spoon-shaped instrument used to scrape tissue.

Cutaneous squamous cell carcinoma—Malignant skin tumor of the epidermis or its appendages.

States. (Cryosurgery is the most commonly used treatment in the United States.)

Approximately 15% of actinic keratoses develop into squamous cell carcinoma. Based on current demographics in the United States, the incidence of actinic keratoses is expected to increase. Older individuals are more likely than younger ones to have actinic keratoses, because cumulative sun exposure increases with age. A survey of older Americans found keratoses in more than half of all men and more than a third of women between the ages of 65 and 74 who had a high degree of lifetime sun exposure. Some medical experts believe that the majority of people who live to the age of 80 have AKs.

Basal cell carcinoma is the most common form of skin cancer and the most common of all types of cancer. It affects about 800,000 individuals in the United States each year. BCC is primarily caused by chronic exposure to sunlight and until recently those most often affected were older, especially older men who worked outdoors. In the last several decades, the incidence of BCC among younger people has increased. So has the number of cases in women. However, many more men are still affected by BCC than women.

Squamous cell carcinoma is the second most common form of skin cancer, affecting more than 200,000 Americans each year. It too is most often caused by chronic exposure to sunlight.

Genital human papillomavirus infection is the most common sexually transmitted disease in the United States with about 55 million new cases reported each year. Genital warts are the most easily recognized sign of HPV infection, but many people with HPV infection never develop genital warts. Both drugs and surgery are used to treat genital warts, but the warts often come back after treatment because the treatment only removes the warts and does not cure the underlying infection.

Description

In the case of AK, the procedure is carried out under **local anesthesia** to reduce discomfort during curettage. First, the surgeon uses a curette to scrape off the undesirable AK cells down to the level of uninvolved tissue. This is followed by electrosurgery to widen the area of AK cell destruction and removal, and to cauterize the wound to limit bleeding.

In the treatment of skin cancers, curettage is used to scrape away the tumor cells and then an extra margin of surrounding tissue is destroyed by electrosurgery. These steps may be repeated several times in the same treatment session. Curettage and electrosurgery are considered suitable for small primary lesions on sun-exposed skin. It is less effective in the case of recurrent lesions that have attendant scar tissue. Tumors that have spread into subcutaneous tissues or subcutaneous fat are less likely to be cured when treated with this procedure.

The major techniques that may be involved in the electrosurgery step include electrodesiccation (removal of water), fulguration (production of a spark to destroy tissue), electrocoagulation (forming blood clots to stop bleeding), and electrosection (cutting). Electrosurgery can be used to incise, to shave, and to remove lesions. The correct output power is determined by starting at low power and increasing the power level until the desired result is achieved (destruction, coagulation, or cutting).

Diagnosis/Preparation

Skin biopsies and histologic examination confirm diagnoses for AKs and skin cancers such as basal cell carcinoma. A recommendation for curettage and electrosurgery is made following patient evaluation.

Injectable lidocaine is administered before most curetttage and electrosurgical procedures. Lidocaine is often used together with epinephrine to further reduce blood loss. Anesthesia may not be necessary when small lesions are being treated. Another alternative is to use a mixture of local anesthetics, containing 2.5% lidocaine and 2.5% prilocaine, in a cream base. The cream is applied to the skin at least one hour before the procedure to achieve topical anesthesia.

> ## WHO PERFORMS THE PROCEDURE AND WHERE IS IT PERFORMED?
>
> Curettage and electrosurgery is done in a hospital or clinic, although most physicians have small electrosurgical units in their offices to treat benign lesions. The procedure is usually performed by a dermatologist or dermatologic surgeon. The American Academy of Family Physicians and several private organizations offer basic training sessions in electrosurgery.

Aftercare

After the procedure, the patient is advised to keep the wound clean and dry. The healing process takes at least several weeks or longer, depending on the size of the wound and other factors. Electrosurgery produces two types of skin wounds—partial- and full-thickness wounds. Partial-thickness wounds result from the electrodesiccation of skin lesions and the curettage and desiccation of basal cell carcinomas. These wounds may be cleansed daily and then covered with an antibiotic ointment that provides a moist environment for new tissue growth. The wound may then be covered with common adhesive **bandages**. Full-thickness wounds require closure with sutures.

Risks

As with every type of surgical procedure, there is a risk of infection. **Antibiotics** are not routinely given, but some physicians believe they may minimize the risk. Other potential risks include:

- Subcutaneous bleeding. If it occurs, subcutaneous bleeding may create a hematoma and require the wound to be reopened and drained.

- Temporary or permanent nerve damage. This may result from excision in an area with extensive nerves.

- Wounds that reopen. If this occurs, the risk of infection and scarring increases.

- Scarring.

Normal results

Curettage and electrosurgery results in the removal of the targeted skin lesion, AK, skin cancer, or genital wart and in the formation of a minor wound that heals rapidly after the procedure.

Alternatives

Alternative treatment for AKs include:

- cryosurgery, the most common method of treating AKs in the United States
- dermabrasion, a procedure performed with an instrument that removes skin with a rapidly rotating brush
- laser removal, a treatment that uses the infrared beam of a carbon dioxide laser to destroy AK cells
- surgical excision, an uncommon treatment for AKs, used only if the lesions are very thick or difficult to remove by other means

Alternative treatment for skin cancers include:

- cryosurgery, a treatment that uses subfreezing temperature to destroy the tumor
- surgical excision, a procedure useful for both primary and recurrent tumors
- Mohs micrographic surgery, a treatment used to deal with some recurrent lesions
- laser surgery, a procedure that uses a laser to excise or destroy the tumor
- radiation therapy, a treatment that is useful for definitive treatment of primary tumors and some recurrent cancers
- interferon therapy, a drug therapy that prevents the growth of cancerous cells
- photodynamic therapy, a treatment in which the patient is given a photoactive compound followed by photoirradiation

Resources

BOOKS

Duffy, S., and G. V. Cobb. *Practical Electrosurgery*. Philadelphia: Lippincott, Williams and Wilkins, 1994.

PERIODICALS

Gonzalez, D. I., C. M. Zahn, M. G. Retzloff, W. F. Moore, E. R. Kost, and R. R. Snyder. "Recurrence of Dysplasia After Loop Electrosurgical Excision Procedures With Long-term Follow-up." *American Journal of Obstetrics and Gynecology* 184 (February 2001): 315–321.

Moniak, C. W., S. Kutzner, E. Adam, J. Harden, and R. H. Kaufman. "Endocervical Curettage in Evaluating Abnormal Cervical Cytology." *Journal of Reproductive Medicine* 45 (April 2000): 285–292.

Sheridan, A. T., and R. P. Dawber. "Curettage, Electrosurgery and Skin Cancer." *Australasian Journal of Dermatology* 41 (February 2000): 19–30.

Werlinger, K. D., G. Upton, and A. Y. Moore. "Recurrence Rates of Primary Nonmelanoma Skin Cancers Treated by Surgical Excision Compared to Electrodesiccation-curettage in a Private Dermatological Practice." *Dermatology and Surgery* 28 (December 2002): 1138–1142.

Williams, D. L., C. Dietrich, and J. McBroom. "Endocervical Curettage when Colposcopic Examination is Satisfactory and Normal." *Obstetrics and Gynecology* 95 (June 2000): 801–803.

ORGANIZATIONS

American Academy of Dermatology Association. 1350 I Street NW, Suite 880, Washington, DC 20005. (202) 842-3555. http://www.aadassociation.org/.

American College of Obstetricians and Gynecologists. 409 12th St., S.W., PO Box 96920 Washington, D.C. 20090-6920. (312) 786-1468. http://www.acog.com/.

American Society for Dermatologic Surgery (ASDS). 5550 Meadowbrook Dr., Suite 120, Rolling Meadows, IL 60008. (847) 956-0900. http://www.asds-net.org.

National Association for Women's Health. 300 W. Adams Street, Suite 328, Chicago, IL 60606-5101. (312) 786-1468. http://www.nawh.org/.

OTHER

CANCERLIT: NIH Cancer Information Center. [cited May 14, 2003]. http://www.cancer.gov/CancerInformation/cancerliterature.

National Women's Health Information Center. [cited May 14, 2003]. http://www.4woman,org/.

The Skin Cancer Foundation. [cited May 14, 2003]. http://www.skincancer.org/.

Monique Laberge, Ph.D.

Cyclocryotherapy

Definition

Cyclocryotherapy (CCT) is a procedure that employs temperatures as low as -112°F (-80°C) to destroy the ciliary body, an organ in the anterior chamber of the eye behind the iris, which produces aqueous fluid. A certain

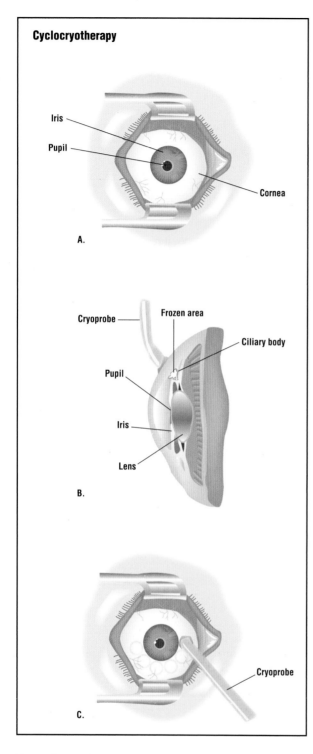

Cyclocryotherapy

Iris

Pupil

Cornea

A.

Cryoprobe

Frozen area

Ciliary body

Pupil

Iris

Lens

B.

Cryoprobe

C.

For cyclocryotherapy, the patient's eyelids are first retracted (A). A cryoprobe is applied to the outside of the eyeball in the area surrounding the iris (B). The probe freezes ciliary bodies in 50-60 seconds. The probe is applied to adjoining sites in a semicircle around the iris during one treatment (C). *(Illustration by GGS Information Services. Cengage Learning, Gale.)*

amount of fluid is required to maintain the integrity of the eye, but an increase in intraocular fluid leads to an elevation in intraocular pressure (IOP); elevated IOP is a major cause of glaucoma. Ablation, or destruction, of part of the ciliary body lowers the IOP by decreasing the fluid or aqueous humor within the eye and thus helping to control glaucoma. The main purpose of CCT is to treat uncontrolled or refractory glaucoma. It is also used to reduce ocular pain in some patients with end-stage glaucoma.

Glaucoma is a general term used to describe a group of potentially blinding diseases, the main sign of which is a relatively high intraocular pressure. This increase in IOP causes damage to the optic nerve and the surrounding retinal tissue. In end-stage glaucoma, a patient's visual field is severely restricted. The increased intraocular pressure usually is caused by increased aqueous fluid in the eye. Treatment of glaucoma involves medical or surgical strategies to either increase the outflow of fluid from the eye, or to decrease the production of fluid in the eye, in an attempt to lower the IOP. The objective of glaucoma treatment is to attain an intraocular fluid level low enough such that damage to the optic nerve does not occur, yet is high enough such that the integrity of the eye is not sacrificed.

CCT is a last-resort treatment for patients in whom conventional medical and surgical techniques to control glaucoma have failed. Medical treatment involves the use of eyedrops that may be administered from one to four times a day. Surgical techniques are used to treat glaucoma when the number of eyedrops becomes cumbersome to the patient, or if patient compliance with medical therapy is difficult, or if medical therapy is not effective in lowering the IOP. One non-cyclodestructive surgical technique is filtration surgery, a procedure in which an outlet for the aqueous fluid is made through the sclera, the white fibrous covering of the anterior part of the eye. Another such procedure is argon laser trabeculoplasty, in which laser burns are made on the trabecular meshwork, the major drainage system to increase the number of drainage ports from the eye. Both these procedures promote outward flow of the intraocular fluid, decreasing the IOP.

In congenital glaucoma, other procedures that open up the fluid flow within the eye such as **goniotomy** or trabeculotomy are performed. Many patients with congenital glaucoma, due to a defect in the interior structure of the eye, have a limited ability to drain the aqueous fluid sufficiently. For pediatric patients, trabeculoplasty is not successful because the maturing eye will attempt to close the outlet. CCT may be performed on patients for which cyclophotocoagulation, another method of cyclodestruction, is not an option or not available. Many patients on whom this technique is employed have neovascular glaucoma, a type of glaucoma that is a result of uncontrolled diabetes or hypertension.

Purpose

The main purpose of CCT is to treat uncontrolled or refractory glaucoma. It is also used to reduce pain in some patients with end-stage glaucoma. This procedure lowers the intraocular pressure by destroying the source of intraocular fluid, the ciliary body, and subsequently lowering the intraocular pressure, as well as decreasing the pain of patients with some glaucomas, the most notable of which is neovascular glaucoma.

Demographics

Patients who undergo CCT are patients for whom certain techniques such as filtration surgery are contraindicated or for which other medical and surgical procedures have not been successful. Patients with neovascular glaucoma and congenital glaucoma make up a large percentage of the patients who undergo CCT. Because of the risks involved, cyclocryotherapy should not be performed on patients who have the potential for good vision, or on individuals who have had cataract surgery with intraocular lens implantation. CCT is a last-resort technique employed on patients for whom all other strategies have failed.

Description

Cyclocryotherapy is usually performed while the patient is awake and supine (laying down on the back). Prior to doing CCT, the doctor will inject an anesthetic into the posterior part of the eye; however, CCT may be performed under **general anesthesia** for anxious adults and for children. In performing the procedure, the surgeon locates the ciliary body with a lighted instrument and then applies a cryoprobe with a temperature of -112°F (-80°C) to the sclera of the eye. This probe is applied to the eye several times in a clockwise manner, using moderate pressure, carefully avoiding the area of the eye where the extraocular muscles, which control movement of the eye, attach to the eye. Each application by the probe lasts 50–60 seconds and usually only half of the eye is treated during the initial attempt; for less severe glaucoma and in older patients who respond better to this treatment, only a quarter of the eye will be treated. The surgeon leaves at least one quadrant of the eye untreated.

Immediately after surgery, a steroid is injected into the eye to reduce inflammation, and an eyedrop or ointment such as atropine is applied to the eye to maintain dilation of the eye. Some surgeons may inject into the eye an anesthetic that numbs the entire eye, including the muscles. This injection has many risks associated with it, such as a droopy eyelid and an increased risk of corneal ulcers.

Diagnosis/Preparation

Cyclocryotherapy is a procedure of last resort in glaucoma patients. When all other therapies available to the patient have failed, CCT is considered, especially if the patient's vision is poor, i.e., less than 20/200, since there is a high risk of vision loss associated with this procedure. Patients and/or legal guardians of the patient are informed of the inherent risks and benefits, and CCT is performed only after **informed consent**. In preparation for CCT, the patient continues with all glaucoma medications up to the day of the procedure.

Aftercare

It is important that the patient continue with most topical glaucoma medications after surgery because a significant spike in IOP is expected after cyclocryotherapy. Glaucoma medications that should not be continued include miotics, which constrict the pupil and thus act in opposition to atropine, and drops derived from prostaglandins, which have very limited effect in some forms of glaucoma, especially neovascular glaucoma. Steroids are administered to the eye to reduce the risk of inflammation. Atropine, which dilates or enlarges the pupil and decreases post-operative discomfort, may be used a few times a day. Atropine and steroids are continued for a month after surgery.

As the retrobulbar anesthesia wears off, usually within 12 hours, **acetaminophen** (Tylenol) may be required for pain. In patients for whom the potential for good vision is unlikely and in whom the CCT is done to eliminate pain, the doctor may inject alcohol into the eye for continued pain relief.

Patients are seen for follow-up visits at a minimum of one day, one week, and one month after surgery. Sometimes the procedure needs to be repeated and, if this is the case, it should be done no sooner than one month after the first attempt. The area that was treated initially is treated again and may be expanded to include a third quadrant.

Risks

The risks of this procedure are greater than for other types of glaucoma treatment. The most common side effect is pain after the procedure. A common risk of CCT is hypotony, which is a low level of fluid in the eye that can lead to phthisis bulbi, a condition in which the fluid level in the eye reaches a dangerously low level, such that the integrity of the eye is compromised. Other risks to consider are retinal detachment, inflammation of the iris, cataract formation, macular edema, and swelling of the cornea. The risk of inflammation within the eye is greater for diabetics. Loss of visual acuity, including total vision loss, is an associated risk of any of the previously mentioned risks and occurs in up to 67% of patients.

Patients with darker irises will have more side effects from this procedure, and pediatric patients with aniridia, or no iris, also have an increased rate of complications. Individuals who are aphakic, meaning they have had cataract extraction without a subsequent intraocular lens implantation, have fewer complications than patients with an intact lens.

Normal results

Normal results of cyclocryotherapy would be a reduction in the IOP and decreased intraocular pain. The overall success rate of CCT to reduce IOP in glaucoma patients is reported to be from 34% to 92%. Approximately 70% of patients with neovascular glaucoma have an IOP reduction of at least 50%. A determination of whether or not the surgery has been effective may not be clear until a month after CCT is performed; retreatment is required in up to one-third of adult patients. Repeated procedures increase the success of

---

WHO PERFORMS THE PROCEDURE AND WHERE IS IT PERFORMED?

This procedure is performed by an ophthalmologist in an office setting. Many ophthalmologists who perform glaucoma surgery have had an additional year of subspecialty training specific to the treatment of glaucoma.

---

the surgery. CCT is successful in 90% of patients after a second surgery and in 95% after the third treatment. Among pediatric patients who undergo CCT, the success rate is only 30–44%, as the ciliary body of the child is more resistant to damage by **cryotherapy**, and thus repeat applications are more common.

Morbidity and mortality rates

Within four years of treatment, hypotony will occur in up to 12% of all patients who undergo CCT, but is seen in up to 40% of patients with neovascular glaucoma. Up to two-thirds of patients will lose some visual acuity after CCT; many of them will have vision worse than 20/400. About 20% of patients who have had cyclocryotherapy will develop cataracts.

Alternatives

An alternative to cyclocryotherapy is cyclophotocoagulation. This is another cyclodestructive procedure that employs the thermal energy of a laser instead of the freezing temperature of cryotherapy to ablate, or destroy, a part of the ciliary body. Cyclophotocoagulation is performed with the patient seated at the slit lamp biomicroscope. The eye is anesthesized prior to performing the procedure. In one type of cyclophotocoagulation, a fiberoptic laser endoscope is passed into the eye to help the surgeon visualize the interior of the eye. The energy of a laser passes through the endoscope and destroys the ciliary body directly. In another type of cyclodestruction, the energy of a diode laser is applied to the ciliary body through the sclera without the use of an endoscope.

Cyclophotocoagulation is as effective as CCT without as many of the complications inherent in CCT. The risks of transient elevation of intraocular inflammation and intraocular inflammation itself are decreased with this procedure over CCT for adult patients, but the risks associated with this procedure for pediatric patients are comparable to CCT. The

---

cyclophotocoagulation procedure is not as painful as CCT.

Surgical removal of the part of the ciliary body is another alternative that is not often used. It is effective in lowering IOP, but the rate of complications such as hemorrhages in the vitreous, hypotony, and retinal detachment is high.

Therapeutic **ultrasound** can also be used to reduce the IOP in glaucoma patients, though the mechanism in which the IOP is lowered in this procedure is not clear.

In end-stage neovascular glaucoma patients who have no useful vision, medical treatment of pain control may sometimes be attained with the use of atropine and topical steroids alone. Retrobulbar injection of alcohol is sometimes necessary and, as a last resort in painful eyes without useful vision, enucleation, or removal, of the eye is required.

Resources

BOOKS

Albert, Daniel M. *Principles and Practice of Ophthalmology,* 2nd ed. Philadelphia, PA: W.B. Saunders Company, 2000.

Azuara-Blanco, Augusto. *Handbook of Glaucoma.* London: Martin Dunitz Ltd., 2002.

Epstein, Daniel, et al. *Glaucoma.* Baltimore, MD: Williams and Wilkins, 1997.

Jaffe, Norman S. *Atlas of Ophthalmic Surgery.* London: Mosby-Wolfe, 1996.

Kanski, Jack. *Glaucoma: A Colour Manual of Diagnosis and Treatment,* 2nd ed. Oxford: Butterworth Heinemann, 1996.

Ritch, Robert, et al. *The Glaucomas* Vol. 2 Clinical Sciences. St. Louis, MO: Mosby Yearbook, 1996.

Ritch, Robert, et al. *The Glaucomas.* Vol. 3 Glaucoma Therapies. St. Louis, MO: Mosby Yearbook, 1996.

PERIODICALS

Deepak, Gupta. "Surgical Update, Part III The Fallback Options When IOP Won't Drop." *Review of Optometry* (February 15, 2003): 79–86.

Sivak-Calcott, M. D., et al. "Evidence-based Recommendations for the Diagnosis and Treatment of Neovascular Glaucoma." *Ophthalmology* 108 (October 2001): 1767–1778.

Wagle, Nikhil. "Long-term Outcome of Cyclocryotherapy for Refractory Pediatric Glaucoma." *Ophthalmology* 105 (October 1998): 1921–7.

OTHER

Cyclotherapy for Endstage Glaucoma. <http.wills-glaucoma. org/cyclo.htm>.

Pediatric Glaucoma. http://www.childrens.org/MSO/dept/ lnav/view.asp?nav + 554.

Martha Reilly, OD

Cyclosporine *see* **Immunosuppressant drugs**

Cyst removal *see* **Ganglion cyst removal**

Cystectomy

Definition

Cystectomy is a surgical procedure that removes all or part of the urinary bladder, the muscular organ that collects urine from the kidneys for excretion at a later time. Partial or segmental cystectomy removes part of the bladder; simple cystectomy removes the entire bladder; and radical cystectomy removes the bladder as well as other pelvic organs or structures.

Purpose

Cystectomy is most commonly performed to treat cancer of the bladder. Once a patient has been diagnosed with bladder cancer, a staging system is used to indicate how far the cancer has spread and determine appropriate treatments. Superficial tumors isolated to the inner lining of the bladder (stage 0 or I) may be treated with non-surgical therapies such as chemotherapy or radiation, or with partial or simple cystectomy. Radical cystectomy is the standard treatment for cancer that has invaded the bladder muscle (Stage II, III, or IV). Muscle-invasive cancer accounts for 90% of all bladder cancers.

Other conditions that may require cystectomy include interstitial cystitis (chronic inflammation of the bladder), endometriosis that has spread to the bladder, severe urinary dysfunction, damage to the bladder from radiation or other treatments, or excessive bleeding from the bladder.

Demographics

Approximately 56,500 cases of urinary bladder cancer are diagnosed in the United States annually, with approximately 12,600 men and women **dying** of the disease each year. Men are more often diagnosed with bladder cancer (2.6 men for each woman diagnosed), and they also have a higher mortality rate (two men for each woman that dies). The average age that the disease is diagnosed is 65 years.

More cases of bladder cancer are found among white men and women. The Centers for Disease Control and Prevention (CDC) reported that from 1992–1999, whites were diagnosed with bladder cancer at a rate of 21.9 per 100,000 persons, while African Americans had a rate of only 12.4 per 100,000. The mortality rate, however, is similar among white and African-American patients (4.5 and 4.1 per 100,000 persons), respectively.

Description

Partial cystectomy

During partial or segmental cystectomy, only the area of the bladder where the cancer is found is removed. This allows for most of the bladder to be preserved. Because the cancer must not have spread to the bladder muscle and must be isolated to one area, partial cystectomy is only used infrequently for the patients who meet these select criteria.

The patient is first placed under **general anesthesia**. After an incision is made into the lower abdomen, the bladder is identified and isolated. The surgeon may choose to perform the operation with the bladder remaining inside the abdominal cavity (transperitoneal approach) or with the bladder lifted outside of the abdominal cavity (extraperitoneal approach). The

cancerous area is excised (cut out) with a 0.8 in (2 cm) margin to ensure that all abnormal cells are removed. The bladder is then closed with **stitches**. The pelvic lymph nodes may also be removed during the procedure. After the cancerous tissue is removed, it is examined by a pathologist to determine if the margins of the tissue are clear of abnormal cells.

Simple or radical cystectomy

While partial cystectomy is considered a bladder-conserving surgery, simple and radical cystectomy involves the removal of the entire bladder. In the case of radical cystectomy, other pelvic organs and structures are also removed because of the tendency of bladder cancer to spread to nearby tissues. After the patient is placed under general anesthesia, an incision is made into the lower abdomen. Blood vessels leading to and from the bladder are ligated (tied off), and the bladder is divided from the urethra, ureters, and other tissues holding it in place. The bladder may then be removed.

The surgical procedure for radical cystectomy differs between male and female patients. In men, the prostate, seminal vesicles, and pelvic lymph nodes are removed with the bladder. In women, the uterus, fallopian tubes, ovaries, anterior (front) part of the vagina, and pelvic lymph nodes are removed with the bladder. If the surgery is being performed as a treatment for cancer, the removed tissues may be examined for the presence of abnormal cells.

Urinary diversion

Once the bladder is removed, a new method for excreting urine must be created. One commonly used approach is the ileal conduit. A piece of the small intestine is removed, cleaned, and tied at one end to form a tube. The other end is used to form a stoma, an opening through the abdominal wall to the outside. The ureters are then connected to the tube. Urine produced by the kidneys flows down the ureters, into the tube, and through the stoma. The patient wears a bag to collect the urine.

For continent cutaneous diversion, a pouch is constructed out of portions of the small and large intestine; the ureters are connected to the pouch and a stoma is created through the abdominal wall. Urine is removed by inserting a thin tube (catheter) into the stoma when the pouch is full. Alternatively, a similar pouch called a neobladder may be created, attached to both the ureters and the urethra, in an attempt to preserve as close to normal bladder function as possible.

Diagnosis/Preparation

The medical team will discuss the procedure and tell the patient where the stoma will appear and what it will look like. The patient will receive instruction on caring for a stoma and bag. A period of fasting and an enema may be required.

Aftercare

After the operation, the patient is given fluid-based nutrition until the intestines begin to function normally again. **Antibiotics** are given to prevent infection. The nature of cystectomy means that there will be major lifestyle changes for the person undergoing the operation. Men may become impotent if nerves controlling penile erection are cut during removal of the bladder. Infertility is a consequence for women undergoing radical cystectomy because the ovaries and uterus are removed. Most women who undergo cystectomy, however, are postmenopausal and past their childbearing years.

Patients are fitted with an external bag that connects to the stoma and collects the urine. The bag is generally worn around the waist under the clothing. It takes a period of adjustment to get used to wearing the bag. Because there is no bladder, urine is excreted as it is produced. The stoma must be treated properly to ensure that it does not become infected or blocked. Patients must be trained to care for their stoma. Often, there is a period of psychological adjustment to the major change in lifestyle created by the stoma and bag. Patients should be prepared for this by their physician.

Risks

As with any major surgery, there is a risk of infection; in this case, infection of the intestine is especially dangerous as it can lead to peritonitis (inflammation of the membrane lining the abdomen). In the case of partial cystectomy, there is a risk of urine leakage from the bladder incision site. Other risks include injury to nearby organs, complications associated with general

anesthesia (such as respiratory distress), excessive blood loss, sexual dysfunction, or urinary incontinence (inadvertent leakage of urine).

Normal results

During a successful partial cystectomy, the cancerous or damaged area of the bladder is removed and the patient retains urinary control. A successful simple or radical cystectomy results in the removal of the bladder and the creation of a urinary diversion, with little or no effect on sexual function. Intestinal function returns to normal and the patient learns proper care of the stoma and bag. He or she adjusts to lifestyle changes and returns to a normal routine of work and recreation.

Morbidity and mortality rates

The overall rate of complications associated with radical cystectomy may be as high as 25–35%; major complications occur at a rate of 5%. The rate of radical cystectomy-related deaths is 1–3%. Partial cystectomy has a complication rate of 11–29%. Some studies have placed the rate of cancer reoccurrence after partial cystectomy at 40–80%.

Alternatives

Transurethral resection (TUR) is one method that may be used to treat superficial bladder tumors. A cystoscope (a thin, tubular instrument used to visualize the interior of the bladder) is inserted into the bladder through the urethra and used to remove any cancerous tissue. Non-surgical options include chemotherapy and radiation.

Resources

BOOKS

Walsh, Patrick C., et al., eds. *Campbell's Urology*, 8th ed. Philadelphia: Elsevier Science, 2002.

PERIODICALS

"Bladder Cancer, Part III: Treatment Approaches in Current Practice and in Evaluation." *Future Oncology* 6, no. 5 (April 30, 2001): 1322–40.

Carrion, Rafael, and John Seigne. "Surgical Management of Bladder Carcinoma." *Cancer Control: Journal of the Moffitt Cancer Center* 9, no. 4 (October 31, 2002): 284–92.

ORGANIZATIONS

American Cancer Society. 1599 Clifton Road NE, Atlanta, GA 30329. (800) ACS-2345. http://www.cancer.org.

Cancer Information Service, National Cancer Institute. Building 31, Room 10A19, 9000 Rockville Pike, Bethesda, MD 20892. (800) 4-CANCER. http://www.nci.nih.gov/cancerinfo/index.html.

OTHER

"All About Bladder Cancer." *American Cancer Society,* 2003 [cited April 4, 2003]. http://www.cancer.org/docroot/CRI/CRI_2x.asp.

"Cancer Facts and Figures, 2002." *American Cancer Society,* 2002 [cited April 4, 2003]. http://www.cancer.org/downloads/STT/CancerFacts&Figures2002TM.pdf.

Eggner, Scott, and Steven Campbell. "Cystectomy, Radical." *eMedicine,* August 1, 2001 [cited April 4, 2003]. http://www.emedicine.com/med/topic3061.htm.

Feng, Adrian H. "Cystectomy, Partial." *eMedicine,* February 8, 2002 [cited April 4, 2003]. http://www.emedicine.com/med/topic3043.htm.

Ries, L. A. G., et al., eds. "SEER Cancer Statistics Review." *National Cancer Institute,* 2002 [cited April 4, 2003]. <http://seer.cancer.gov/csr/1973_1999>.

John T. Lohr, PhD
Stephanie Dionne Sherk

Cystocele repair

Definition

A cystocele is the protrusion or prolapse of the bladder into the vagina. A number of surgical interventions are available to treat cystoceles.

Purpose

A prolapse occurs when an organ falls out of its normal anatomical position. The pelvic organs normally have tissue (muscle, ligaments, etc.) holding them in place. Certain factors, however, may cause those tissues to weaken, leading to prolapse of the organs. A cystocele may be the result of a central or lateral (side) defect. A central defect occurs when the bladder protrudes into the center of the anterior (front) wall of the vagina due to a defect in the pubocervical fascia (fibrous tissue that separates the bladder and vagina). The pubocervical fascia is also attached on each side to tough connective tissue called the arcus tendineus; if a defect occurs close to this attachment, it is called a lateral or paravaginal defect. A central and lateral defect may be present simultaneously. The location of the defect determines what surgical procedure is performed.

Factors that are linked to cystocele development include age, repeated childbirth, hormone deficiency, menopause, constipation, ongoing physical activity, heavy lifting, and prior **hysterectomy**. Symptoms of bladder prolapse include stress incontinence (inadvertent leakage of urine with physical activity), urinary frequency, difficult urination, a vaginal bulge, vaginal pressure or pain, painful sexual intercourse, and lower back pain. Urinary incontinence is the most common symptom of a cystocele.

Surgery is generally not performed unless the symptoms of the prolapse have begun to interfere with daily life. A staging system is used to grade the severity of a cystocele. A stage I, II, or III prolapse descends to progressively lower areas of the vagina. A stage IV prolapse descends to or protrudes through the vaginal opening. Surgery is generally reserved for stage III and IV cystoceles.

Demographics

Approximately 22.7 out of every 10,000 women will undergo pelvic prolapse surgery. The rate is highest among women between 60 and 69 years of age (42 per 10,000); the mean age of patients is 54.6. White women undergo pelvic prolapse surgery at a rate of 19.6 per 10,000 and a mean age of 54.3, while 6.4 per 10,000 African American women have surgery at a mean age of 49.3.

A 2002 study indicated cystocele repair accounts for 8% of all prolapse repair surgeries; in 1997, approximately 18,500 cystocele repairs were performed. Cystocele repair was combined with **rectal prolapse repair** in 10% of prolapse surgeries, with hysterectomy (surgical removal of the uterus) in 6%, and with both procedures in 16%.

Description

The goals of cystocele repair are to relieve a patient's symptoms, to improve or maintain urinary and sexual function, to return pelvic structures to their original position, and to prevent the formation of new defects. The anatomical structures involved in a cystocele may be approached vaginally, abdominally, or laparoscopically.

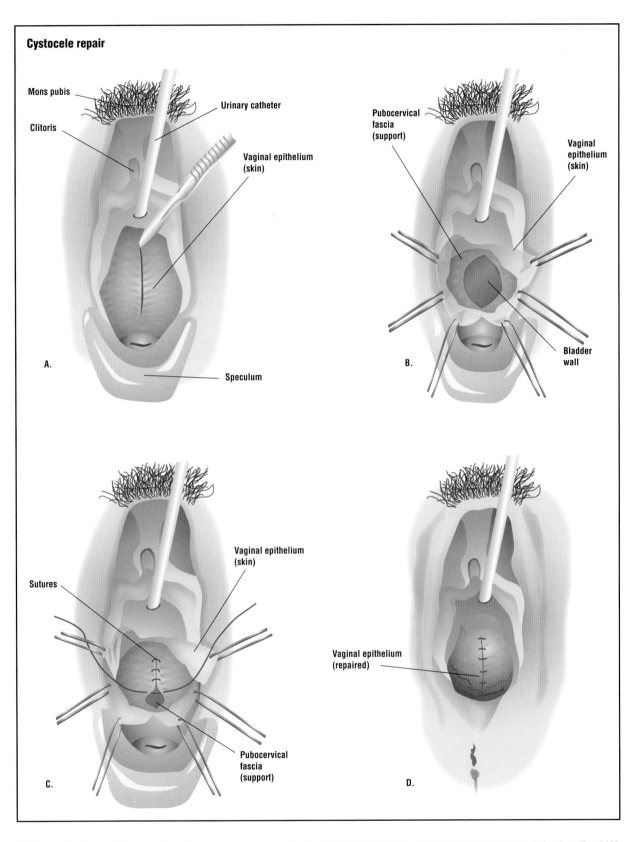

Cystocele repair

A.

Mons pubis

Clitoris

Urinary catheter

Vaginal epithelium (skin)

Speculum

B.

Pubocervical fascia (support)

Vaginal epithelium (skin)

Bladder wall

C.

Sutures

Vaginal epithelium (skin)

Pubocervical fascia (support)

D.

Vaginal epithelium (repaired)

In this cystocele repair by anterior colporrhaphy, a speculum is used to hold open the vagina, and the cystocele is visualized (A). The wall of the vagina is cut open to reveal an opening in the supporting structures, or fascia (B). The defect is closed (C), and the vaginal skin is repaired (D). *(Illustration by GGS Information Services. Cengage Learning, Gale.)*

KEY TERMS

Burch procedure—A surgical procedure, also called retropubic colposuspension, in which the neck of the bladder is suspended from nearby ligaments with sutures. It is performed to treat urinary incontinence.

Colporrhapy—A surgical procedure in which the vagina is sutured.

Ligaments—Tough fibrous connective tissue.

Magnetic resonance imaging—A specialized imaging technique used to visualize internal structures; it is considered superior to the standard x ray.

Pubocervical fascia—Fibrous tissue that separates the vagina and the bladder.

Ultrasound—A procedure that uses high-frequency sound waves to visualize structures in the human body.

Speculum—A retractor used to separate the walls of the vagina and aid in visual examination.

Vaginal repair

Anterior **colporrhaphy** is the most common procedure to repair a central defect. The patient is first given general or regional anesthesia. A speculum is inserted into the vagina to hold it open during the procedure. An incision is made into the vaginal skin and the defect in the underlying fascia is identified. The vaginal skin is separated from the fascia and the defect is folded over and sutured (stitched). Any excess vaginal skin is removed and the incision is closed with **stitches**.

Lateral defects may be repaired vaginally or abdominally. During a vaginal paravaginal repair, the approach and initial incision are similar to anterior colporrhaphy. The defect to the fascia is located and reattached to the arcus tendineus using sutures. The incision may then be stitched closed.

Abdominal and laparoscopic repair

A cystocele caused by a lateral defect may be treated through an abdominal incision made transversely (from side to side) just above the pubic hairline. The space between the pubic bone and bladder is identified and opened and the pubocervical fascia reattached to the arcus tendineus using methods similar to the vaginal paravaginal repair. In some cases, a retropubic colposuspension is performed during the same surgery. Also called a Burch procedure, colposuspension treats urinary incontinence by suspending the bladder neck to nearby ligaments with sutures. Other surgical treatments for incontinence may be combined with paravaginal repair.

A lateral defect may also be repaired by **laparoscopy**, a surgical procedure in which a laparoscope (a thin, lighted tube) and various instruments are inserted into the abdomen through small incisions. A patient's recovery time following laparoscopic surgery is shorter and less painful than following a traditional laparotomy (a larger surgical incision into the abdominal cavity).

Diagnosis/Preparation

Physical examination is most often used to diagnose a cystocele. A speculum is inserted into the vagina and the patient is asked to strain or sit in an upright position; this increase in intra-abdominal pressure maximizes the degree of prolapse and aids in diagnosis. The physician then inspects the walls of the vagina for prolapse or bulging.

In some cases, a physical examination cannot sufficiently diagnose pelvic prolapse. For example, cystography may be used to determine the extent of a cystocele; the bladder is filled by urinary catheter with contrast medium and then x rayed. **Ultrasound** or **magnetic resonance imaging** may also be used to visualize the pelvic structures.

Women who have gone through menopause may be given six weeks of estrogen therapy prior to surgery; this is thought to improve circulation to the vaginal walls and thus improve recovery time. **Antibiotics** may be administered to decrease the risk of postsurgical infection. An intravenous (IV) line is placed and a Foley catheter is inserted into the bladder directly preceding surgery.

Aftercare

A Foley catheter may remain for one to two days after surgery. The patient is given a liquid diet until normal bowel function returns. The patient also is instructed to avoid activities for several weeks that cause strain on the surgical site; these include lifting, coughing, long periods of standing, sneezing, straining with bowel movements, and sexual intercourse.

Risks

Risks of cystocele repair include potential complications associated with anesthesia, infection, bleeding, injury to other pelvic structures, dyspareunia (painful intercourse), recurrent prolapse, and failure to correct the defect.

WHO PERFORMS THE PROCEDURE AND WHERE IS IT PERFORMED?

Cystocele repair is usually performed in a hospital operating room by a gynecologist, urologist, or urogynecologist. A gynecologist is a medical doctor who specializes in the areas of women's general and reproductive health, pregnancy, and labor and childbirth. A urologist is a medical doctor who specializes in the diagnosis and treatment of diseases of the urinary tract and genital organs. A urogynecologist studies aspects of both fields.

QUESTIONS TO ASK THE DOCTOR

- What defect is causing the cystocele?
- What surgical procedure is recommended for treatment?
- Will other procedures be performed to treat urinary incontinence (e.g. Burch procedure)?
- What nonsurgical alternatives are available?
- How soon after surgery may normal activities be resumed?

Normal results

A woman usually is able to resume normal activities, including sexual intercourse, in about four weeks after the procedure. After successful cystocele repair, symptoms recede, although a separate procedure may be needed to treat stress incontinence.

Morbidity and mortality rates

The risk of cystocele recurrence following surgical repair depends on the procedure used to treat it. Anterior colporrhaphy is associated with a 0–20% rate of recurrence; this rate is higher when colporrhaphy is combined with other surgical procedures. Abdominal paravaginal repair results in a 5% chance of recurrence, while vaginal paravaginal repair has the highest recurrence rate (7–22%).

Alternatives

Surgery is generally reserved for more severe cystoceles. Milder cases may be treated by a number of medical interventions. The physician may recommend that the patient do Kegel exercises, a series of contractions and relaxations of the muscles in the perineal area. These exercises are thought to strengthen the pelvic floor and may help prevent urinary incontinence.

A pessary, a device that is inserted into the vagina to help support the pelvic organs, may be recommeded. Pessaries come in different shapes and sizes and must be fitted to the patient by a physician. Hormone replacement therapy may also be prescribed if the woman has gone through menopause; hormones may improve the quality of the supporting tissues in the pelvis.

Resources

BOOKS

Ryan, Kenneth J., et al. *Kistner's Gynecology and Women's Health,* 7th ed. St. Louis, MO: Mosby, Inc., 1999.

Walsh, Patrick C., et al. *Campbell's Urology,* 8th ed. Philadelphia: Elsevier Science, 2002.

PERIODICALS

Brown, Jeanette S., L. Elaine Waetjen, Leslee L. Subak, David H. Thom, Stephen Van Den Eeden, and Eric Vittinghoff. "Pelvic Organ Prolapse Surgery in the United States, 1997." *American Journal of Obstetrics and Gynecology* 186 (April 2002): 712–6.

Cespedes, R. Duane, Cindy A. Cross, and Edward J. McGuire. "Pelvic Prolapse: Diagnosing and Treating Cystoceles, Rectoceles, and Enteroceles." *Medscape Women's Health eJournal* 3 (1998).

Viera, Anthony, and Margaret Larkins-Pettigrew. "Practice Use of the Pessary." *American Family Physician* 61 (May 1, 2000): 2719–2726.

ORGANIZATIONS

American Board of Obstetrics and Gynecology. 2915 Vine Street, Dallas, TX 75204. (214) 871-1619. http://www.abog.org.

American Urological Association. 1120 North Charles Street, Baltimore, MD 21201. (410) 727-1100. http://www.auanet.org.

OTHER

"Cystocele (Fallen Bladder)." *National Kidney and Urologic Diseases Information Clearinghouse.* March 2002 [cited April 11, 2003]. http://www.niddk.nih.gov/health/urolog/summary/cystocel.

Miklos, John. "Vaginal Prolapse Relaxation." *OBGYN.net.* 2002 [cited April 11, 2003]. http://www.obgyn.net/urogyn/urogyn.asp?page=/urogyn/articles/miklos-vagprolapse.

Stephanie Dionne Sherk

Cystoscopy

Definition

Cystoscopy (cystourethroscopy) is a diagnostic procedure that uses a cystoscope, which is an endoscope especially designed for urological use to examine the bladder, lower urinary tract, and prostate gland. It can also be used to collect urine samples, perform biopsies, and remove small stones.

Purpose

Cystoscopy is performed by urologists to examine the entire bladder lining and take biopsies of any questionable areas. Cystoscopy may be prescribed for patients who display the following conditions:

- blood in the urine (hematuria)
- inability to control urination (incontinence)
- urinary tract infection (UTI)
- signs of congenital abnormalities in the urinary tract
- suspected tumors in the bladder
- bladder or kidney stones
- signs or symptoms of an enlarged prostate
- pain or difficulty urinating (dysuria)
- disorders of or injuries to the urinary tract
- symptoms of interstitial cystitis

Blood and urine studies, in addition to x rays of the kidneys, ureters, and bladder, may be performed before a cystoscopy to obtain as much diagnostic information as possible. During the cystoscopy, a retrograde pyelogram may also be performed to examine the kidneys and ureters.

Description

There are two types of cystoscopes used to carry out the procedure, a rigid type and a flexible type. Both types are used for the same purposes and differ only in their method of insertion. The rigid type requires that the patient adopt the lithotomy position, meaning that the patient lies on his or her back with knees up and apart. The flexible cystoscope does not require the lithotomy position.

A cystoscopy typically lasts from 10–40 minutes. The patient is asked to urinate before surgery and advised that relaxing pelvic muscles will help make this part of the procedure easier. A well-lubricated flexible or rigid cystoscope (urethroscope) is passed through the urethra into the bladder where a urine sample is taken. There may be some discomfort as the instrument is inserted. Fluid is then injected to inflate the bladder and allow the urologist to examine the entire bladder wall. The cystoscope uses a lighted tip for guidance and enables biopsies to be taken or small stones to be removed through a hollow channel in the cystoscope.

During a cystoscopy, the urologist may remove bladder stones or kidney stones, gather tissue samples, and perform x-ray studies. To remove stones, an instrument that looks like a tiny basket or grasper is inserted through the cystoscope so that small stones can be extracted through the scope's channel. For a biopsy, special forceps are inserted through the cystoscope to pinch off a tissue sample. Alternatively, a small brush-like instrument may be inserted to scrape off some tissue. To perform x-ray studies such as a retrograde pyelogram, a dye is injected into the ureter by way of a catheter passed through the cystoscope. After completion of all required tests, the cystoscope is removed.

Preparation

Before cytoscopy, patients may be asked to give a urine sample to check for infection and to avoid urinating for an hour before the procedure. A sedative may be given about one hour prior to the operation to help the patient relax. The region of the urethra is cleansed and a local anesthetic is applied. Spinal or **general anesthesia** may also be used for the procedure. Distension of the bladder with fluid is particularly painful, and if it needs to be done, as in the case of evaluating interstitial cystitis, general anesthesia is required. A signed consent form is necessary for this procedure.

Aftercare

After removal of the cystoscope, the urethra is usually sore, and patients should expect to feel a burning sensation while urinating for one or two days following the procedure. To alleviate discomfort or pain, patients may be prescribed pain medication, and **antibiotics** may also be required to prevent infection. Minor pain may also be treated with over-the-counter, nonprescription drugs such as **acetaminophen**. To relieve discomfort, patients may be advised to drink two 8-oz glasses of water each hour for two hours and to take a warm bath to relieve the burning feeling. If not able to bathe, they may be advised to hold a warm, damp washcloth over the urethral opening.

Patients who have undergone a cystoscopy are instructed to:

- take warm baths to relieve pain.
- rest and refrain from driving for several days, especially if general anesthesia was used.

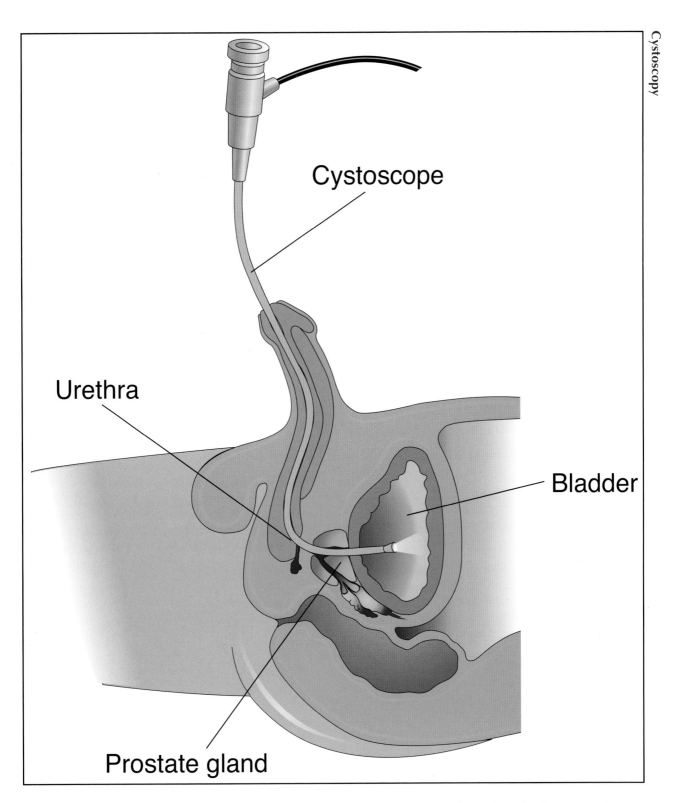

Cystoscope

Urethra

Bladder

Prostate gland

Cystoscopy is a diagnostic procedure which is used to view the bladder, collect urine samples, and examine the prostate gland. This procedure also enables biopsies to be taken. The primary instrument used in cystoscopy is the cystoscope, a tube which is inserted through the penis into the urethra, and ultimately into the bladder. *(Illustration by Electronic Illustrators Group. Cengage Learning, Gale.)*

KEY TERMS

Anesthetic—A drug that causes loss of sensation. It is used to lessen the pain of surgery and other medical procedures.

Bladder—The bladder is located in the lower part of the abdomen; it is a structure like a small balloon that collects urine for temporary storage and is emptied from time to time by urinating.

Catheter—A tubular, flexible surgical instrument for withdrawing fluids from (or introducing fluids into) a body cavity, especially one for introduction into the bladder through the urethra for the withdrawal of urine.

Cystoscope—Endoscope especially designed for urological use to examine the bladder, lower urinary tract, and prostate gland.

Diverticula—A pouch or sac occurring normally or from a herniation or defect in a membrane.

Endoscope—A highly flexible, thin viewing instrument used to see inside body cavities.

Endoscopy—A minimally invasive procedure that involves examination of body organs or cavities using an endoscope.

Interstitial cystitis—A chronic inflammatory condition of the bladder involving symptoms of bladder pain, frequent urination, and burning during urination.

Retrograde pyelogram—A pyelography or x-ray technique in which a dye is injected into the kidneys through the ureters.

Ureter—The tube that carries urine from each kidney to the bladder.

Urethra—The tube that carries urine from the bladder to outside the body. In females, the urethral opening is between the vagina and clitoris; in males, the urethra travels through the penis, opening at the tip.

Urogynecologist—A physician that specializes in female medical conditions concerning the urinary and reproductive systems.

Uroradiologist—A radiologist that specializes in diagnostic imaging of the urinary tract and kidneys.

- expect any blood in the urine to clear up in one to two days.
- avoid strenuous exercise during recovery.
- postpone sexual relations until the urologist determines that healing is complete.

Risks

As with any surgical procedure, there are some risks involved with a cystoscopy. Complications may include profuse bleeding, a damaged urethra, a perforated bladder, a urinary tract infection, or an injured penis.

Patients should contact their physician if they experience any of the following symptoms after the procedure, including pain, redness, swelling, drainage, or bleeding from the surgical site; signs of generalized infection, which may include headache, muscle aches, dizziness, or an overall ill feeling and fever; nausea or vomiting; or difficult or painful urination.

Cystoscopy is a commonly performed procedure, but it is an invasive technique that involves small yet significant risk. If anesthesia is required, there is additional risk, particularly for people who are obese, smoke, or are in poor health. Those undergoing anesthesia must inform the doctor of any medications they are taking.

Normal results

A successful cystoscopy includes a thorough examination of the bladder and collection of urine samples for cultures. If no abnormalities are seen, the results are indicated as normal. In this case, the bladder wall appears smooth and the bladder is seen to be of normal size, shape, and position, without obstructions, growths, or stones.

The treating physician can tell the patient what was seen inside the bladder right after the procedure. If a biopsy sample was taken, this will take several days to be examined and tested.

Cystoscopy allows the urologist to detect inflammation of the bladder lining, prostatic enlargement, or tumors. If these are seen, further evaluation or biopsies may be needed. Cystoscopy with bladder distention can also evaluate interstitial cystitis. Bladder stones, urethral strictures, diverticula, or congenital abnormalities can also be detected.

Alternatives

There are procedures that can provide some information about the lining of the bladder, for example, x rays; however, none of these provide as much information to the doctor as a cystoscopy.

WHO PERFORMS THE PROCEDURE AND WHERE IS IT PERFORMED?

Cystoscopy is typically performed on an outpatient basis, but up to three days of recovery in the hospital is sometimes required. The procedure can be performed in a hospital, doctor's office, cystoscopy suite, or urology office, depending on the condition of the patient and the anesthesia required. If general anesthesia is required, an anesthesiologist is present to administer the anesthesia and monitor the patient. The cystoscopy procedure is performed by a urologist, urologic surgeon, or urogynecologist, with assistance from nurses experienced in urologic procedures. If x rays are taken during the procedure, a uroradiologist or radiologic technologist is required to operate the x-ray equipment. Biopsy tissue samples are sent to the clinical laboratory for examination by a pathologist.

QUESTIONS TO ASK THE DOCTOR

- What will happen during the procedure?
- How do I prepare for cytoscopy?
- Will cystoscopy hurt?
- How long will the test last?
- How many cytoscopies do you perform each year?
- Are there any risks associated with the procedure?

Resources

BOOKS

Khatri, V. P., and J. A. Asensio. *Operative Surgery Manual* 1st ed. Philadelphia: Saunders, 2003.

Townsend, C. M., et al. *Sabiston Textbook of Surgery* 17th ed. Philadelphia: Saunders, 2004.

Wein, A. J., et al. *Campbell-Walsh Urology* 9th ed. Philadelphia: Saunders, 2007.

PERIODICALS

Fraczyk, L., H. Godfrey, and R. Feneley. "Flexible Cystoscopy: Outpatients or Domiciliary?" *British Journal of Community Nursing* 7 (February 2002): 69–74.

Jabs, C. F., and H. P. Drutz. "The Role of Intraoperative Cystoscopy in Prolapse and Incontinence Surgery." *American Journal of Obstetrics and Gynecology* 185 (December 2001): 1368–1371.

Kwon, C. H., R. Goldberg, S. Koduri, and P. K. Sand. "The Use of Intraoperative Cystoscopy in Major Vaginal and Urogynecologic Surgeries." *American Journal of Obstetrics and Gynecology* 187 (December 2002): 1471–1472.

Payne, D. A., and R. C. Kockelbergh. "Improving the View at Flexible Cystoscopy." *Annals of The Royal College of Surgeons of England* 85 (March 2003): 132–138.

Sant, Grannum R., and Philip M. Hanno. "Interstitial Cystitis: Current Issues and Controversies in Diagnosis." *Urology* 57, Supplement 6A (June 2001): 82–88.

Satoh, E., N. Miyao, H. Tachiki, and Y. Fujisawa. "Prediction of Muscle Invasion of Bladder Cancer by Cystoscopy." *European Urology* 41 (February 2002): 178–181.

ORGANIZATIONS

American Urologic Association Foundation. P. O. Box 79183, Baltimore, MD 21279-0183. (800) 242-2383. http://www.auafoundation.org (accessed March 11, 2008).

American Urological Association. 1120 North Charles Street, Baltimore, MD 21201. (410) 727-1100. http://www.auanet.org (accessed March 11, 2008).

Interstitial Cystitis Association. 51 Monroe Street, Suite 1402, Rockville, MD 20850. (301) 610-5300. http://www.ichelp.org (accessed March 11, 2008).

Society of Urologic Nurses and Associates. East Holly Avenue, Box 56, Pitman, NJ 08071-0056. (609) 256-2335. http://suna.inurse.com/ (accessed March 11, 2008).

OTHER

"Cystoscopy." *Harvard Medical School.* http://www.health.harvard.edu/fhg/diagnostics/cysto/cystoWhat.shtml (accessed March 11, 2008).

"Cystoscopy." *Medline Plus.* http://www.nlm.nih.gov/medlineplus/ency/article/003903.htm (accessed March 11, 2008).

"What Is IC? Interstitial Cystitis Fact Sheet." *Interstitial Cystitis Association.* http://www.ichelp.org/whatisic/ICFActSheet.html (accessed March 11, 2008).

Jennifer E. Sisk
Monique Laberge, PhD
Rosalyn Carson-DeWitt, MD